Hearing Impairment: An Evidence-Based Approach

Hearing Impairment: An Evidence-Based Approach

Editor: Sophie Silva

AMERICAN
MEDICAL PUBLISHERS
www.americanmedicalpublishers.com

AMERICAN
MEDICAL PUBLISHERS
www.americanmedicalpublishers.com

Cataloging-in-Publication Data

Hearing impairment : an evidence-based approach / edited by Sophie Silva.
p. cm.
Includes bibliographical references and index.
ISBN 978-1-63927-408-6
1. Hearing disorders. 2. Hearing impaired. 3. Ear--Diseases. 4. Otolaryngology. I. Silva, Sophie.
RF290 .H43 2022
617.8--dc23

American Medical Publishers,
41 Flatbush Avenue,
1st Floor, New York,
NY 11217, USA

ISBN 978-1-63927-408-6 (Hardback)

Contents

Preface

Hearing impairment is the partial or total loss of hearing. Chronic ear infections are considered to be the chief cause of hearing impairment. Syphilis, rubella and cytomegalovirus infections can also result in hearing loss in children. The diagnosis of hearing loss is established on the basis of hearing tests. If a person is insensitive to sound around 25 decibels even in one ear, it is classified as hearing impairment. Hearing loss is of three types - sensorineural hearing loss, conductive hearing loss and mixed hearing loss. 50% of all cases of hearing loss occurring globally are largely preventable through public health actions. All newborns should be tested for hearing loss. By providing proper care during pregnancy, immunization, avoiding certain medications and loud noise, hearing loss may be prevented. For those with hearing impairment, sign language, cochlear implants, lip reading, hearing aids and subtitle use must be promoted. There exists no treatment for the sensorineural hearing loss arising due to genetic defects, age or noise. Certain surgical interventions such as correction of superior semicircular canal dehiscence, surgical excision or vestibular schwannoma or acoustic neuroma, stapedotomy and stapedectomy, etc. may be used for the remedy of the condition. This book is compiled in such a manner, that it will provide an in-depth evidence-based approach to the understanding of hearing impairment. From theories to research to practical applications, case studies related to all contemporary topics of relevance to this condition have been included in this book. With state-of-the-art inputs by acclaimed experts of audiology, this book targets students and professionals.

The researches compiled throughout the book are authentic and of high quality, combining several disciplines and from very diverse regions from around the world. Drawing on the contributions of many researchers from diverse countries, the book's objective is to provide the readers with the latest achievements in the area of research. This book will surely be a source of knowledge to all interested and researching the field.

In the end, I would like to express my deep sense of gratitude to all the authors for meeting the set deadlines in completing and submitting their research chapters. I would also like to thank the publisher for the support offered to us throughout the course of the book. Finally, I extend my sincere thanks to my family for being a constant source of inspiration and encouragement.

Editor

1

Hydrogen-Saturated Saline Protects Intensive Narrow Band Noise-Induced Hearing Loss in Guinea Pigs through an Antioxidant Effect

Liwei Chen[1], Ning Yu[1]*, Yan Lu[1], Longjun Wu[2], Daishi Chen[1], Weiwei Guo[1], Lidong Zhao[1], Mingbo Liu[1], Shiming Yang[1], Xuejun Sun[3], Suoqiang Zhai[1]*

1 Department of Otolaryngology Head and Neck Surgery, Chinese PLA General Hospital, Beijing, China, **2** Department of Otolaryngology Head and Neck Surgery, Wenzhou Medical College, Wenzhou, Zhejiang Province, China, **3** Department of Diving Medicine, Faculty of Naval Medicine, Second Military Medical University, Shanghai, China

Abstract

The purpose of the current study was to evaluate hydrogen-saturated saline protecting intensive narrow band noise-induced hearing loss. Guinea pigs were divided into three groups: hydrogen-saturated saline; normal saline; and control. For saline administration, the guinea pigs were given daily abdominal injections (1 ml/100 g) 3 days before and 1 h before narrow band noise exposure (2.5–3.5 kHz 130 dB SPL, 1 h). The guinea pigs in the control group received no treatment. The hearing function was assessed by the auditory brainstem response (ABR) and distortion product otoacoustic emission (DPOAE) recording. The changes of free radicals in the cochlea before noise exposure, and immediately and 7 days after noise exposure were also examined. By Scanning electron microscopy and succinate dehydrogenase staining, we found that pre-treatment with hydrogen-saturated saline significantly reduced noise-induced hair cell damage and hearing loss. We also found that the malondialdehyde, lipid peroxidation, and hydroxyl levels were significantly lower in the hydrogen-saturated saline group after noise trauma, indicating that hydrogen-saturated saline can decrease the amount of harmful free radicals caused by noise trauma. Our findings suggest that hydrogen-saturated saline is effective in preventing intensive narrow band noise-induced hearing loss through the antioxidant effect.

Editor: Bruce Riley, Texas A&M University, United States of America

Funding: This project was supported by the National Natural Science Fundation of China (No. 81241034, No. 81271081, No.30971199, http://www.nsfc.gov.cn). The funders had no role in study design, data collection and analysis, decision to publish, or preparation of the manuscript.

Competing Interests: The authors have declared that no competing interests exist.

* E-mail: yuning12@sina.com (NY); zhaisq@plagh.com.cn (SQZ)

Introduction

With the development of modern industry, environmental noise can cause permanent hearing loss in human. Noise-induced hearing loss (NIHL) is a sensorineural hearing deficit that is mainly caused by a strong noise stimulus. It is well known that oxidative stress within the cochlea produces large amounts of free radicals and is a major molecular mechanism underlying noise-induced deafness [1]. Moreover, the oxidative stress is also associated with age-related hearing loss and aminoglycoside-induced hearing loss [2,3,4].

Previous studies demonstrated that hydrogen can selectively reduce hydroxyl, peroxynitrite, and especially hydroxyl radicals, the most toxic reactive oxygen species, to inhibit oxidative stress, thus acting as an antioxidant reagent [5]. Recently, it has been found that hydrogen-saturated medium could significantly reduce antimycin A induced ROS and lipid peroxidation in hair cells, to promote hair cell survival *in vitro* [6]. Oral or intraperitoneal induction of hydrogen-rich saline can also reduce NIHL and hair cell damage *in vivo* [7,8]. An intensive 2.5–3.5 kHz sound is one type of narrow band noise that is usually used as a warning sound and may induce a strong uncomfortable feeling which can cause severe hair cell injury and hearing loss. In this study, the effect of hydrogen-saturated saline on narrow band noise-induced hearing loss was investigated. Our results showed that hydrogen-saturated saline can act as an antioxidant reagent to protect against intensive narrow band noise-induced hearing loss.

Materials and Methods

1. Animals

Healthy adult albino guinea pigs (250–300 g) of either sex were used for the experiments. Albino guinea pigs were randomly assigned to 1 of 3 experimental groups: (1) hydrogen-saturated saline (1 ml/100 g) was administered intraperitoneally 3 days (once a day) and 1 h before noise exposure (hydrogen-saturated saline group, n = 20); (2) normal saline (0.9%) was administered to the same number of guinea pigs by the same method as the control (normal saline group, n = 20); and (3) guinea pigs that did not receive any noise exposure or treatment were used as the normal control (control group, n = 15). All of the animals were bought from Vital River Laboratory Animal Technology Co. Ltd. (Beijing, China). Care and use of the animals in this study was approved by the Institutional Animal Care and Use Committee of the Chinese PLA General Hospital.

2. Preparation of Hydrogen-saturated Saline

Hydrogen-saturated saline was prepared as described previously [9]. Briefly, hydrogen was dissolved in normal saline for 2 h under high pressure (0.4 MPa) to supersaturation using a self-designed hydrogen-saturated water-producing apparatus. The saturated hydrogen saline was stored under atmospheric pressure at 4°C in an aluminum bag without dead volume. Hydrogen-saturated saline was freshly prepared each week to ensure a constant concentration >0.6 mM.

3. Noise Exposure and Procedures

The animals were exposed to a warning sound, which is a narrow band noise centered at 2.5–3.5 kHz (Sound Spotlight System 2000; China ASX Technology Co., Ltd., Beijing). The animals were exposed to the noise at a level of 130 dB SPL for 1 h. Alert, non-anesthetized animals were placed in a special restraint cage and the distance from the noise generator to both ears was set at 1 m to ensure that each ear received noise exposure of equal intensity. The noise levels were calibrated with a sound level meter (B&K type 2209) and a condenser microphone (B&K type 4136).

4. Auditory Brainstem Response (ABR) Measurements

Electrophysiologic measurements were made in a double-walled soundproof room. The ABR threshold value was examined in each group before noise exposure, and immediately and 1, 3, 7, and 14 days after noise exposure. Hearing was evaluated with Tucker-Davis Technologies hardware and software (TDT System III, Alachua, FL, USA). Briefly, non-anesthetized animals were placed in a special restraint cage, and ABRs were subcutaneously recorded with sterile electrode needles. The reference electrode was inserted beneath the pinna of the ear, the ground beneath the opposite ear, and the active electrode beneath the skin at the vertex. ABRs were evoked with clicks. Band-pass was filtered between 100 and 3000 Hz. Stimulus levels varied in descending steps of 5 dB. At each level, 1024 responses were averaged. The hearing threshold was confirmed until the wave III disappeared.

5. Measurement of the Distortion Product Otoacoustic Emission (DPOAE)

The DPOAE was examined before noise exposure, and 7 and 14 days after noise exposure. Briefly, the DPOAE was recorded using a Madsen Capella Distortion Product Otoacoustic Emission System (Madsen Capella, Taastrup, Denmark). Briefly, non-anesthetized animals were placed in a special restraint cage and the earpiece was inserted into the ear canal for DPOAE testing. Two frequency transducers were used to deliver the primary tones, f_1 and f_2, to the ear canal through flexible tubes connected to the earpiece. The f_2/f_1 ratio was set at 1.2. The DPOAE input/output functions were measured at f_2 frequencies of 500, 750, 1000, 1500, 2000, 3000, 4000, 6000, and 8000 Hz with the same intensity of L2/L1 = 55/65 dB.

6. Scanning Electron Microscopy (SEM)

On the 14th day after noise trauma, the animals were sacrificed by decapitation and the cochleae were removed. Round and oval windows of the cochleae were perforated with a sharp pick. The peri-lymphatic space was perfused with 2.5% glutaraldehyde in 0.1 M PBS, and each specimen was placed in glutaraldehyde solution overnight. The cochleae were washed three times with PBS. The specimens were fixed with 1% OsO_4 for 15 min. The samples were then washed in PBS three times. The tissues were serially dehydrated in 50%, 70%, 90%, and 100% ethanol. After critical point drying with CO_2 and sputter-coating with gold, the tissues were examined using a Hitachi S-4800 scanning electron microscope.

7. Histologic Analysis of the Cochlea

On the 7th day after noise trauma, the animals were sacrificed and the cochleae were removed. The round window membrane was opened, and succinate dehydrogenase (SDH) staining solution (1:1:2 0.2 M sodium succinate, 0.2 M PBS [pH 7.6], and 0.1% tetranitro-blue tetrazolium) was gently perfused through the round and oval windows. Subsequently, the cochleae were immersed in SDH solution for 60 min at 37°C. The specimens were later fixed with 4% formalin for 24 h. The sensory epithelium was removed from the cochlea in 0.01 M PBS and mounted in glycerin on glass slides as surface preparations. The sensory epithelium was viewed with a light microscope (Olympus BX51, Tokyo, Japan) and photographed with a highly sensitive camera (Olympus DP-72) at 400× magnification using DP2-BSW software.

8. Detection of Lipid Peroxidation (LPO), Malondialdehyde (MDA), and Hydroxyl (·OH) Levels in the Cochlea

The frozen cochlear tissues were harvested and homogenized immediately 5 times at 5000 rotations per min for 30 sec by a high-speed homogenizer in an ice bath in 10 volumes of physiologic saline. The homogenates were centrifuged at 6000 G for 10 min at 4°C. The levels of LPO, MDA, and ·OH in the supernatant were detected using the corresponding assay kits according to the manufacturer's recommendations. Each sample consisted of 10 cochleae from 5 guinea pigs.

9. Statistical Analysis

All data are expressed as the mean ± standard deviation (SD). Data were analyzed using an unpaired t-test (Student's t-test) for two groups and a one-way ANOVA with Bonferroni *post hoc* tests for multiple comparisons, as noted in the figure legends (SPSS 13.0 software). $P<0.05$ were deemed statistically significant.

Results

1. ABR

Before noise exposure, ABR tests confirmed that guinea pigs had normal hearing function. Immediately after intensive narrow band noise exposure (130 dB SPL for 1 h), the guinea pigs in the hydrogen-saturated saline group had an average ABR threshold shift of 54 dB SPL. The guinea pigs in the normal saline group had an average ABR threshold shift of 62 dB SPL. The ABR was subsequently tested 1, 3, 7, and 14 days after noise exposure. The results showed that guinea pigs in the hydrogen-saturated saline group had less of an ABR threshold shift compared to the guinea pigs in the normal saline group (Fig. 1).

2. DPOAE

The DPOAE amplitudes were tested to assess the noise damage to the outer hair cells (Fig. 2). After noise exposure, the amplitude of DPOAE at 1–8 kHz significantly decreased in the groups. Seven days after noise damage, the guinea pigs in the hydrogen saline group had less of a decrease in DPOAE amplitudes at frequencies of 0.5–4 kHz compared to the guinea pigs in the control group. Fourteen days after noise exposure, the DPOAE amplitude at frequencies of 0.5, 0.75, 1, 2, 3, and 4 kHz for the guinea pigs in the hydrogen-saturated saline group were significantly higher than the normal saline group.

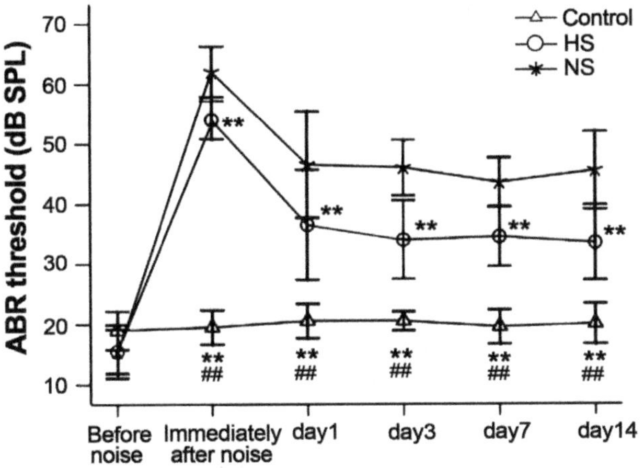

Figure 1. Noise-induced ABR threshold shifts. Immediately after noise exposure (130 dB SPL for 1 h), the ABR threshold of the hydrogen-saturated saline and normal saline groups was 54 dB and 62 dB, respectively. The ABR was subsequently tested 14 days after noise exposure. The hydrogen-saturated saline group had less of an ABR threshold shift compared to the normal saline group, 3, 7, and 14 days after noise exposure. HS: hydrogen-saturated saline group; NS: normal saline group. **P<0.01: vs. NS; ##P<0.01: control vs. HS.

3. Scanning Electron Microscopy

Scanning electron microscopy showed that the morphology of hair cells was minimally damaged in the guinea pigs treated with hydrogen-saturated saline. In contrast, the inner hair cell stereocilia were missing in some regions in the normal saline group, and the outer hair cell stereocilia were severely damaged by noise trauma with a large number prostrate or missing. The damage was more evident in the 3rd row of outer hair cells in the basal turns of the cochlea (Fig. 3). Thus, the scanning electron microscopy results are also consistent with the ABR and DPOAE results.

4. Succinate Dehydrogenase (SDH) Staining

Seven days after noise exposure, guinea pigs were sacrificed for immunohistochemical examination. The cochleae were stained with SDH. The hair cells of the hydrogen-saturated saline group were minimally damaged, and the staining of the SDH was also stronger than the normal saline group. Instead, the hair cells of the normal saline group had a large percentage of damage. Interestingly, the damaged hair cells of the normal saline group were mostly dropsical, with a minimal percentage of missing cells (Fig. 4).

5. Free Radical Detection

The free radical levels were measured in the cochleae before noise exposure, and immediately and 7 days after noise exposure (Fig. 5). Immediately and 7 days after noise exposure, the levels of expression of LPO and MDA were significantly lower in the cochleae of the hydrogen-saturated saline group as compared to the normal saline group. Immediately after noise exposure, the levels of OH in the guinea pigs pre-treated with hydrogen-saturated saline were significantly lower than the guinea pigs pre-treated with normal saline. Interestingly, the difference was abolished 7 days after noise exposure.

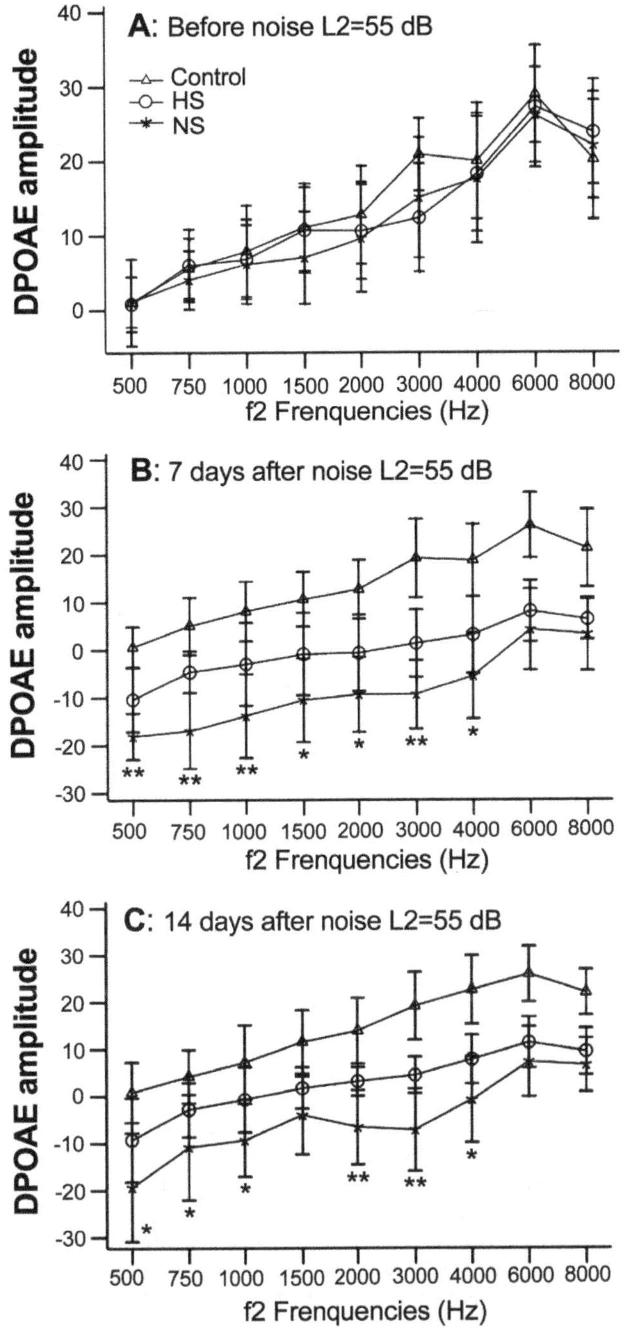

Figure 2. DPOAE amplitudes were detected before and after noise exposure. (A) The average DPOAE amplitudes were normal in the three groups before noise exposure. (B) The average DPOAE amplitudes were markedly decreased 7 days after noise exposure. There were significant differences in the mean DPOAE amplitudes between the hydrogen-saturated and normal saline groups at frequencies of 0.5–4 kHz. (C) 14 days after noise exposure, the DPOAE amplitudes of the hydrogen-saturated saline group were significantly better than the normal saline group, especially at frequencies of 0.5, 0.75, 1, 2, 3, and 4 kHz. HS: hydrogen-saturated saline group; NS: normal saline group; *P<0.05, **P<0.01: hydrogen-saturated saline group vs. normal saline group.

Discussion

Direct mechanical damage and indirect metabolic damage are recognized as major causes of noise-induced deafness. The

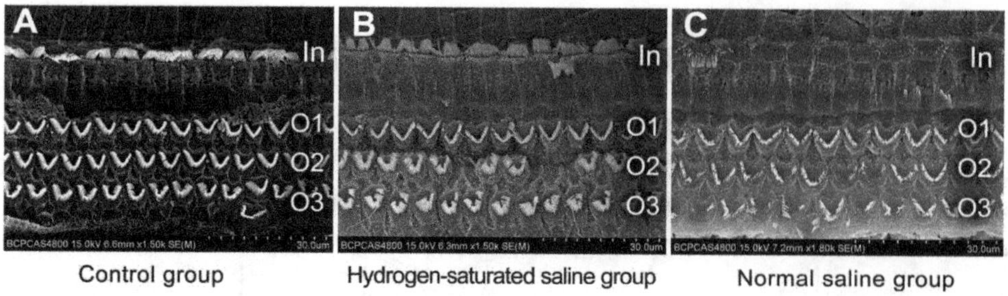

Figure 3. SEM findings after noise exposure. Fourteen days after noise trauma, scanning electron microscopy was performed. After pre-treatment with hydrogen-saturated saline, damage to the stereocilia of hair cells decreased significantly compared with the normal saline group. (A) Control group. (B) Hydrogen-saturated saline group. (C) Normal saline group. In: inner hair cell layer. O1–3: outer hair cell layers.

excessive expression of ROS after noise trauma in the cochlea is recognized as the most important factor causing cochlear damage [10]. Lim and Melnick [11] first proposed that noise causes metabolic changes in the cochlea, damages the inner ear structure, and results in deafness. Yamane et al. [12] first discovered that free radicals are generated in inner ear tissues after noise exposure. Subsequent studies have confirmed that excessive production of free radicals is a major cause of cochlear hearing loss [13,14,15]. It has also been reported that free radicals are widely generated in various cochlear tissues, including vascular vessels, outer hair cells, spiral ganglion cells, and supporting tissues, and the expression of free radicals after noise exposure can persist for 2 weeks [16,17,18]. Thus, preventing the generation of free radicals and the application of antioxidant drugs are critical in reducing NIHL. A series of studies have shown that antioxidants, such as R-phenylisopropyladenosine (R-PIA), glutathione monoethylester, salicylate, acetyl-L-carnitine (ALCAR), and N-L-acetylcysteine (NAC), as well as free radical scavengers (vitamins A, C and E), can prevent hair cell damage and hearing loss induced by noise trauma [19,20,21,22,23]; however, these drugs have limited protective effects as they do not cross the lipid membrane barriers, thus inefficiently scavenging free radicals [1].

In recent years hydrogen has been used as a new reagent of antioxidants to protect tissues in various organs [24]. Studies have shown that there are several benefits to using hydrogen as a potential antioxidant; specifically, hydrogen can effectively neutralize ·OH in living cells, easily diffuse into the cytosol, mitochondria, or nucleus through biomembranes, and quickly spread to the target area to achieve the goal of highly efficient anti-free radical effects [5]. These characteristics of hydrogen suggest that hydrogen may cross the blood-labyrinth barrier to reach the cochlear hair cells, thus making hydrogen an ideal cochlear antioxidant.

It has been shown that hydrogen-saturated medium can significantly reduce antimycin A-induced ROS, and subsequent LPO in hair cells *in vitro* and increased hair cell survival [6], providing a theoretic basis for research on the prevention and treatment of NIHL with hydrogen. In the present study, we found that pre-treatment with hydrogen-saturated saline not only reduced temporary hearing threshold shifts, but also prevented permanent hearing threshold shifts. Fourteen days after noise exposure, the hydrogen-saturated saline group showed better ABR and DPOAE results. After hearing testing, electron microscopy showed that the stereocilia of hair cell were scattered, lying prostrate, and even missing in the normal saline group, whereas the stereocilia were minimally damaged in the hydrogen-saturated saline group. The results of SDH staining were also superior in the hydrogen-saturated saline group to the normal saline group, suggesting that hydrogen protected the function of mitochondria and maintained a normal tricarboxylic acid cycle, thus protecting noised-induced hair cell damage in the cochlea. These morphologic results are consistent with the results of audiologic testing.

It has been reported that a nearly 4-fold increase in ·OH radicals in outer hair cells within 1–2 h of noise exposure [14]. MDA and LPO levels increase after noise trauma is detected [25,26]. To verify if the protective effect of hydrogen-saturated saline against noise-induced hearing loss is due to its antioxidant effects, we examined the free radicals before noise exposure, and immediately and 7 days after noise exposure. We found that immediately and 7 days after noise exposure, cochlear LPO and MDA content in the normal saline group were higher than the hydrogen-saturated saline group. Immediately after noise exposure, the cochlear ·OH content in the normal saline group was also significantly higher than the hydrogen-saturated saline group. Seven days after noise exposure, however, the difference was not statistically significant. We speculate that hydrogen can decrease the amount of harmful free radicals caused by noise trauma. We cannot provide direct experimental evidence demonstrating how hydrogen removes these harmful free radicals; however, it is clear that hydrogen is an antioxidant. Our experiments show that hydrogen has a significant protective effect against intensive

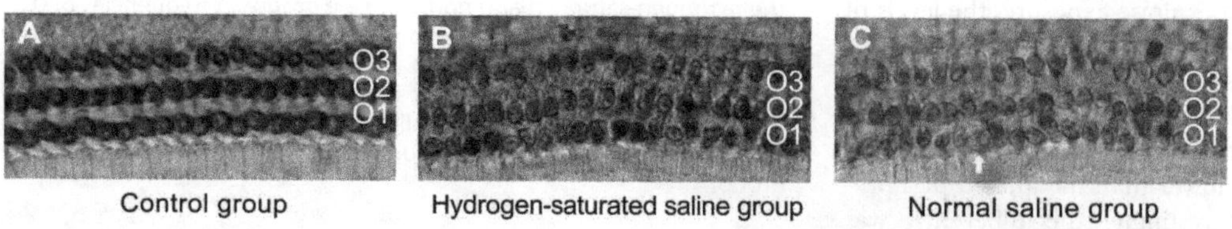

Figure 4. Surface preparation of the organ of Corti in the basal turn stained with SDH. Seven days after noise exposure, the cochleae were stained with SDH. The staining and the morphology of the hair cells in the hydrogen-saturated saline group were superior to the normal saline group. (A) Control group. (B) Hydrogen-saturated saline group. (C) Normal saline group. O1–3: outer hair cell layers. " ↑ ": dropsical hair cells.

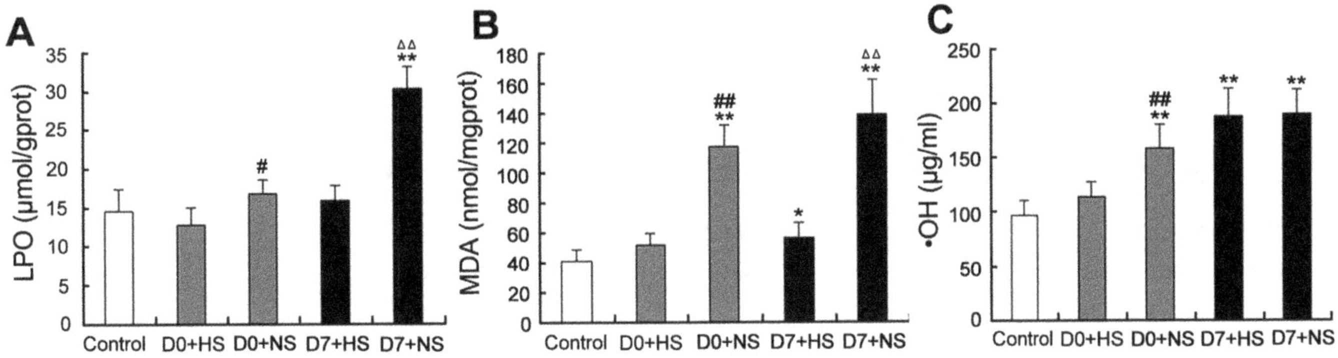

Figure 5. Free radicals in the cochleae were detected after noise exposure. (A, B) After noise exposure, the LPO and MDA levels of the normal saline group were significantly higher than the hydrogen-saturated saline group. (C) Immediately after noise exposure, the content of ·OH in the cochleae of the normal saline group was significantly higher than the hydrogen-saturated saline group. The difference was abolished by the 7th day after noise exposure. D0/D7+HS: immediately/7days after noise exposure of hydrogen-saturated saline group. D0/D7+NS: immediately/7days after noise exposure of normal saline group. *P<0.05, **P<0.01: vs. control. #P<0.05, ##P<0.01: D0+NS vs. D0+HS. ΔP<0.05, ΔΔP<0.01: D7+NS vs. D7+HS.

narrow band noise-induced hair cell damage, and the protective effect of hydrogen is via an antioxidant mechanism.

Currently, there are only two studies involving hydrogen protection on NIHL [7,8]. In those studies, the intensity of noise used was 115 dB SPL, which was markedly less than the 130 dB SPL used in present study. The administration time of hydrogen was significantly longer (6 and 14 days), as compared to 3 days and 1 h before noise exposure in the current study. Our experiments showed that a small amount of hydrogen and a short period of administration is sufficient to protect intensive narrow band noise-induced hearing loss in guinea pigs. Future studies are needed to optimize the time points and the amount of administration, even the signal pathway to deepen our understandings of the antioxidant effect of hydrogen in the cochlea.

Author Contributions

Conceived and designed the experiments: SQZ NY. Performed the experiments: LWC YL LJW DSC WWG LDZ MBL XJS SMY. Analyzed the data: LWC NY DSC. Wrote the paper: LWC NY.

References

1. Le Prell CG, Yamashita D, Minami SB, Yamasoba T, Miller JM (2007) Mechanisms of noise-induced hearing loss indicate multiple methods of prevention. Hear Res 226: 22–43.
2. Poirrier AL, Pincemail J, Van Den Ackerveken P, Lefebvre PP, Malgrange B (2010) Oxidative stress in the cochlea: an update. Curr Med Chem 17: 3591–3604.
3. Warchol ME (2010) Cellular mechanisms of aminoglycoside ototoxicity. Curr Opin Otolaryngol Head Neck Surg 18: 454–458.
4. Fetoni AR, Picciotti PM, Paludetti G, Troiani D (2011) Pathogenesis of presbycusis in animal models: a review. Exp Gerontol 46: 413–425.
5. Ohsawa I, Ishikawa M, Takahashi K, Watanabe M, Nishimaki K, et al. (2007) Hydrogen acts as a therapeutic antioxidant by selectively reducing cytotoxic oxygen radicals. Nat Med 13: 688–694.
6. Kikkawa YS, Nakagawa T, Horie RT, Ito J (2009) Hydrogen protects auditory hair cells from free radicals. Neuroreport 20: 689–694.
7. Lin Y, Kashio A, Sakamoto T, Suzukawa K, Kakigi A, et al. (2011) Hydrogen in drinking water attenuates noise-induced hearing loss in guinea pigs. Neurosci Lett 487: 12–16.
8. Zhou Y, Zheng H, Ruan F, Chen X, Zheng G, et al. (2012) Hydrogen-rich saline alleviates experimental noise-induced hearing loss in guinea pigs. Neuroscience 209: 47–53.
9. Sun Q, Cai J, Liu S, Liu Y, Xu W, et al. (2011) Hydrogen-rich saline provides protection against hyperoxic lung injury. J Surg Res 165: e43–49.
10. Hu BH, Henderson D, Nicotera TM (2002) Involvement of apoptosis in progression of cochlear lesion following exposure to intense noise. Hear Res 166: 62–71.
11. Lim DJ, Melnick W (1971) Acoustic damage of the cochlea. A scanning and transmission electron microscopic observation. Arch Otolaryngol 94: 294–305.
12. Yamane H, Nakai Y, Takayama M, Iguchi H, Nakagawa T, et al. (1995) Appearance of free radicals in the guinea pig inner ear after noise-induced acoustic trauma. Eur Arch Otorhinolaryngol 252: 504–508.
13. Ohlemiller KK, McFadden SL, Ding DL, Flood DG, Reaume AG, et al. (1999) Targeted deletion of the cytosolic Cu/Zn-superoxide dismutase gene (Sod1) increases susceptibility to noise-induced hearing loss. Audiol Neurootol 4: 237–246.
14. Ohlemiller KK, Wright JS, Dugan LL (1999) Early elevation of cochlear reactive oxygen species following noise exposure. Audiol Neurootol 4: 229–236.
15. Ohlemiller KK, McFadden SL, Ding DL, Lear PM, Ho YS (2000) Targeted mutation of the gene for cellular glutathione peroxidase (Gpx1) increases noise-induced hearing loss in mice. J Assoc Res Otolaryngol 1: 243–254.
16. Henderson D, Bielefeld EC, Harris KC, Hu BH (2006) The role of oxidative stress in noise-induced hearing loss. Ear Hear 27: 1–19.
17. Mattson MP (2000) Apoptosis in neurodegenerative disorders. Nat Rev Mol Cell Biol 1: 120–129.
18. Yamashita D, Jiang HY, Schacht J, Miller JM (2004) Delayed production of free radicals following noise exposure. Brain Res 1019: 201–209.
19. Hu BH, Zheng XY, McFadden SL, Kopke RD, Henderson D (1997) R-phenylisopropyladenosine attenuates noise-induced hearing loss in the chinchilla. Hear Res 113: 198–206.
20. Hight NG, McFadden SL, Henderson D, Burkard RF, Nicotera T (2003) Noise-induced hearing loss in chinchillas pre-treated with glutathione monoethylester and R-PIA. Hear Res 179: 21–32.
21. Yamashita D, Jiang HY, Le Prell CG, Schacht J, Miller JM (2005) Post-exposure treatment attenuates noise-induced hearing loss. Neuroscience 134: 633–642.
22. Kopke R, Bielefeld E, Liu J, Zheng J, Jackson R, et al. (2005) Prevention of impulse noise-induced hearing loss with antioxidants. Acta Otolaryngol 125: 235–243.
23. Le Prell CG, Hughes LF, Miller JM (2007) Free radical scavengers vitamins A, C, and E plus magnesium reduce noise trauma. Free Radic Biol Med 42: 1454–1463.
24. Zhang JY, Liu C, Zhou L, Qu K, Wang R, et al. (2012) A review of hydrogen as a new medical therapy. Hepatogastroenterology 59: 1026–1032.
25. Kaygusuz I, Ozturk A, Ustundag B, Yalcin S (2001) Role of free oxygen radicals in noise-related hearing impairment. Hear Res 162: 43–47.
26. Ohinata Y, Miller JM, Altschuler RA, Schacht J (2000) Intense noise induces formation of vasoactive lipid peroxidation products in the cochlea. Brain Res 878: 163–173.

2

Reversible Induction of Phantom Auditory Sensations through Simulated Unilateral Hearing Loss

Roland Schaette[1]*, Charlotte Turtle[2], Kevin J. Munro[2]

1 Ear Institute, University College London, London, United Kingdom, 2 School of Psychological Sciences, University of Manchester, Manchester, United Kingdom

Abstract

Tinnitus, a phantom auditory sensation, is associated with hearing loss in most cases, but it is unclear if hearing loss causes tinnitus. Phantom auditory sensations can be induced in normal hearing listeners when they experience severe auditory deprivation such as confinement in an anechoic chamber, which can be regarded as somewhat analogous to a profound bilateral hearing loss. As this condition is relatively uncommon among tinnitus patients, induction of phantom sounds by a lesser degree of auditory deprivation could advance our understanding of the mechanisms of tinnitus. In this study, we therefore investigated the reporting of phantom sounds after continuous use of an earplug. 18 healthy volunteers with normal hearing wore a silicone earplug continuously in one ear for 7 days. The attenuation provided by the earplugs simulated a mild high-frequency hearing loss, mean attenuation increased from <10 dB at 0.25 kHz to >30 dB at 3 and 4 kHz. 14 out of 18 participants reported phantom sounds during earplug use. 11 participants presented with stable phantom sounds on day 7 and underwent tinnitus spectrum characterization with the earplug still in place. The spectra showed that the phantom sounds were perceived predominantly as high-pitched, corresponding to the frequency range most affected by the earplug. In all cases, the auditory phantom disappeared when the earplug was removed, indicating a causal relation between auditory deprivation and phantom sounds. This relation matches the predictions of our computational model of tinnitus development, which proposes a possible mechanism by which a stabilization of neuronal activity through homeostatic plasticity in the central auditory system could lead to the development of a neuronal correlate of tinnitus when auditory nerve activity is reduced due to the earplug.

Editor: Eleni Vasilaki, University of Sheffield, United Kingdom

Funding: This study was supported by the British Tinnitus Association (www.tinnitus.org.uk). The funders had no role in study design, data collection and analysis, decision to publish, or preparation of the manuscript.

Competing Interests: The authors have declared that no competing interests exist.

* E-mail: r.schaette@ucl.ac.uk

Introduction

Tinnitus is a phantom auditory sensation, the perception of a sound in the absence of a corresponding sound source. In most cases, tinnitus is associated with hearing loss [1,2], but whether hearing loss actually causes tinnitus has not been clarified yet. Animal models have demonstrated that cochlear damage can lead to behavioural evidence for tinnitus [3,4] and to the development of increased spontaneous activity of neurons in the central auditory system (see [5] for a review), which has been interpreted as a putative neuronal correlate for the phantom auditory sensation [6]. However, which mechanisms in the brain trigger the development of tinnitus has remained largely unclear.

Computational modelling studies have recently illustrated how cochlear damage might lead to the development of increased spontaneous neuronal activity as observed in animal models of tinnitus [7,8]. In the models, the development of neural correlates of tinnitus constitutes a side-effect of a stabilization of the mean activity in central auditory neurons through homeostatic plasticity: hearing loss reduces AN activity with a concomitant reduction in excitatory drive to the central auditory system. When homeostatic mechanisms restore average neuronal activity to normal levels by increasing excitation and reducing inhibition, the resulting increase in response gain in the central auditory system causes an amplification of spontaneous neural activity, leading to spontaneous neuronal hyperactivity and the generation of a tinnitus percept. The model's prediction of tinnitus frequencies closely match subjects' perceived tinnitus pitch [9]. It follows from the model that reduction of auditory nerve activity, and not cochlear damage as such, might be the determining factor for the development of tinnitus.

It has been long known that complete auditory deprivation can induce tinnitus-like phantom sounds in healthy, normal-hearing volunteers [10,11]. After several minutes of complete silence in an anechoic chamber or sound-proof booth, participants reported auditory sensations, and the descriptions of the sounds were very similar to those given by tinnitus patients. After leaving the anechoic chamber, the phantom sounds disappeared. This suggests that normal mechanisms of adaptation and plasticity in the brain could also be involved in the development of tinnitus. However, complete auditory deprivation presents a rather drastic scenario, corresponding to profound deafness. It has not been explored yet whether partial deprivation similar to a mild-to-moderate hearing loss typically associated with natural ageing or noise damage, also leads to the perception of phantom sounds. In our previous studies on the effects of unilateral auditory deprivation through an earplug on acoustic reflex thresholds, participants often complained about ringing in their ears after wearing the earplug continuously for several days. We thus studied the occurrence of phantom sounds in 18 healthy volunteers without hearing loss who wore an earplug in one ear for 7 days.

Methods

This study was approved by the ethics committee of the University of Manchester, and all participants gave written informed consent. The investigation of phantom sounds after earplug usage was embedded in a study on changes in acoustic reflex thresholds and perceived loudness through earplugs (which were assessed on day 1, 7, 8 and 14). 18 volunteers (age range 20–28 years, mean age 23.5±0.44 years; 11 female) were recruited into the study. Participants were required to have normal hearing, i.e. thresholds of <20 dB HL from 0.25 kHz to 8 kHz, and no asymmetry >10 dB between ears at any frequency. A short health questionnaire was used to screen for other conditions, and persons reporting tinnitus were excluded from the study. Pure tone audiometry was performed with an Aurical clinical audiometer and TDH-39 supra-aural headphones. Hearing thresholds were tested at 0.25, 0.5, 1, 2, 4 and 8 kHz. Normal middle ear function was ensured through tympanometry using a GSI TympStar middle ear analyser; participants were required to have middle ear pressure between +50 and −50 daPa and middle ear compliance of 0.3 to 1.6 cm^3. All equipment was calibrated to accepted standards.

Participants wore a silicone putty ear plug in one ear for 7 days. Each participant was randomly assigned to plug either the left or the right ear, and the participants were instructed to wear the earplug continuously. Sound attenuation of the earplug i.e., the difference in ear canal sound level with and without the earplug in situ, was measured using a clinical probe tube microphone system and a broadband signal of 75 dB SPL. This method was also used to confirm that participants fitted the earplug with a maximum attenuation difference of 3 dB at 1 kHz and 2 kHz when fitting it themselves. At the end of the session, participants were given an "earplug logbook" to record earplug usage (expected to be continuous except for removal for cleaning). They were also told that there might be a possibility of experiencing phantom sounds during earplugs usage, and they were asked to take a note about their occurrence in the logbook. We deliberately did not mention tinnitus in all explanations about phantom sounds to avoid this strongly suggestive term.

All participants who perceived a phantom sound on day 7 underwent a characterisation of the phantom sound using a modified version of the tinnitus spectrum approach [12]. Comparison sounds (pure tones of 0.5, 1, 2, 4, 8, 12, and 16 kHz) were generated using custom-made MATLAB software and were presented to the control ear via Sennheiser HD650 headphones. The comparison tones where first matched to the loudness of the phantom sound using a single-interval adaptive procedure [13]. During loudness matching, sound intensity was limited to levels ≤100 dB SPL. After loudness matching, each sound was presented three times, in random order, and participants were asked to rate the similarity between the pitch of the comparison sound and their phantom sound on a scale of 0–10, with 0 for "completely different" and 10 for "extremely similar". For comparison tones of 16 kHz, we could not achieve a loudness match for all participants, and thus the results for this frequency were excluded from further analysis.

Computational Model

To model the development of phantom sounds after earplug-induced auditory deprivation, we employed a computational model of tinnitus development comprising the first stages of auditory processing [7,8,9]. The model was organised in frequency channels, with 10 channels per octave. In each channel, we modelled the probability distribution of sound intensities (in units of decibels) by a Gaussian distribution with a mean intensity of 40 dB HL and a standard deviation of 25 dB. The average population response of the auditory nerve fibres in each frequency channel was then modelled by a population rate-intensity function $f(I)$ that was assumed to be tuned to the sound intensity distribution (see [7,8,9] for more details).

The effects of sound attenuation through an earplug providing ΔI_{ep} dB attenuation were emulated by shifting the normal AN fibre population response $f(I)$ to higher sound intensities:

$$f_{ep}(I) = f(I - \Delta I_{ep})$$

The resulting rate-intensity functions with and without earplugs are shown in Fig. 2b. Using the probability distribution of sound intensities, the effect of sound attenuation on the mean activity of the auditory nerve fibre population was calculated numerically.

The central auditory system stage of the model is based on the circuit that has been proposed for the dorsal cochlear nucleus [14], where projection neurons (PNs) receive inhibition from narrow- (NBI) and wide-band inhibitor (WBI) neurons (Fig. 2a, see [8,9] for more details). The strengths of these two inhibitory projections, which are controlled by the gain factors g_n and g_w, was adjusted such that the projection neurons displayed type III response properties, as we had shown previously that model neurons with these response properties develop tinnitus-related hyperactivity after hearing loss [8]. The mean firing rates of the model neurons in the central auditory system stage of the model, and how they were changed by the earplug, were determined numerically.

Homeostatic plasticity was implemented in the model by simultaneously scaling the strength of the excitatory and inhibitory synapses onto principal neurons in opposite directions [15,16]. In the model, homeostatic plasticity was assumed to act in PNs in the cochlear nucleus (see [7,8,9] for more details on how homeostasis was implemented in the model). Homeostatic plasticity was assumed to stabilize a certain target level of the mean activity, which we defined as the mean activity of a PN receiving input from an unplugged ear and an undamaged cochlea. The change in excitation and inhibition required to restore the mean activity to its target level during earplug-induced auditory deprivation was determined numerically.

Data analysis and model simulations were performed using MATLAB (The MathWorks Inc., Natick, Massachusetts). All error bars are given as ± s.e.m.

Results

18 participants with normal hearing (mean hearing thresholds are shown in Fig. 1a) wore an earplug in one ear for 7 days. The earplugs provided attenuation similar to a mild high-frequency hearing loss, mean attenuation increased from <10 dB at 0.25 kHz to >30 dB at 3 and 4 kHz (Fig. 1b). Fourteen participants reported phantom sounds during the 7 days of earplug usage. The descriptions of the phantom sounds can be found in Table 1. Eleven participants reported phantom sounds while still wearing the earplug on day 7. In these participants, detailed characterisations of the phantom sounds were obtained using the tinnitus spectrum method [12]. The mean tinnitus spectra showed that phantom sounds were generally high-pitched; the highest similarity ratings were obtained for comparison tones at 8 and 12 kHz (Fig. 1c). After the earplug was taken out, the phantom sounds disappeared in all participants. At the end day 7,

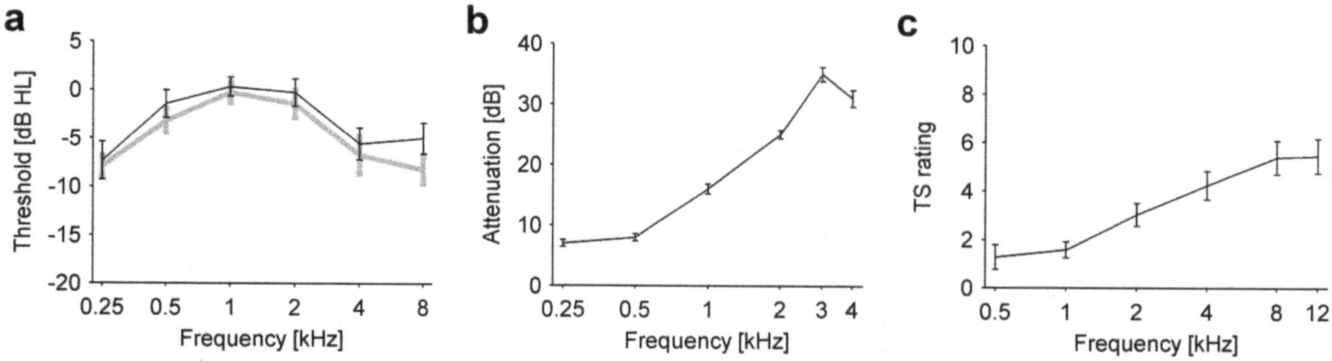

Figure 1. Audiograms, earplug attenuation characteristics, and characterization results for the phantom auditory sensations. a) Mean pure tone hearing thresholds (in dB hearing level) for left (grey line) and right ears (black line) of all participants (n = 18). All error bars denote ± s.e.m. **b)** Mean attenuation provided by the earplugs (n = 18). **c)** Mean tinnitus spectrum (TS) rating of the participants who perceived a stable phantom sound on day 7 (n = 11).

four participants reported still being aware of a sound in the previously-plugged ear. Only one participant reported hearing phantom sounds on day 8, and no participant reported phantom sounds on day 14.

In order to understand how attenuation through an ear-plug could lead to the occurrence of phantom sounds, we employed a computational model of the first stages of auditory processing (Fig. 2a) that we had originally developed to model tinnitus-related changes in the auditory brainstem after cochlear damage [7,8]. Here, only one additional parameter was introduced to the model in order to capture the effects of sound attenuation through the earplug by shifting the auditory nerve rate-vs.-intensity functions to higher sound intensities (Fig. 2b, see also Methods). All parameters of the model relating to the central auditory pathways remained unchanged to previous versions of the model [7,8]. In a first run of simulations, we only considered "model earplugs" with a flat attenuation profile, i.e. the degree of attenuation was identical for all frequency channels, varying attenuation from 0 to 50 dB. We found that attenuation reduced the mean activity in both the AN (Fig. 2c) and the central auditory system stage of the model (Fig. 2d, grey line), and the degree of activity reduction was proportional to the attenuation provided by the earplug.

In the model, we assumed that the mean activity levels of principal neurons (PNs) in the central auditory system were stabilized by homeostatic plasticity. After the model's ear had been plugged, homeostatic plasticity thus tried to compensate for the decrease in PN activity by increasing excitation and decreasing inhibition. When homeostasis restored the mean activity of the PNs in the model cochlear nucleus to the healthy target level (Fig. 2d, black line), the resulting increase in neuronal response gain also caused an over-amplification of spontaneous input from the auditory nerve, leading to increased spontaneous firing rates in

Table 1. Occurrence and description of phantom auditory sensations (PAS).

Subject number	Occurrence of PAS during the week	Description of PAS	PAS present on day 7 for tinnitus spectrum
1	Yes	Fluctuating tone	Yes
2	Yes	Ringing	Yes
3	Yes	Ringing/tones	Yes
4	Yes	Low-pitched buzz	No
5	Yes	Humming & low ringing	Yes
6	Yes	Ringing	Yes
7	Yes	Ringing	Yes
8	Yes	Trains and whistles first, then ringing	No
9	Yes	Humming	No
10	No	/	/
11	No	/	/
12	Yes	Ringing and a high-pitched beep	Yes
13	No	/	/
14	Yes	Humming, cracking, ringing	No
15	No	/	/
16	Yes	High-pitched	Yes
17	Yes	Ringing	Yes
18	Yes	High-pitched buzz	Yes

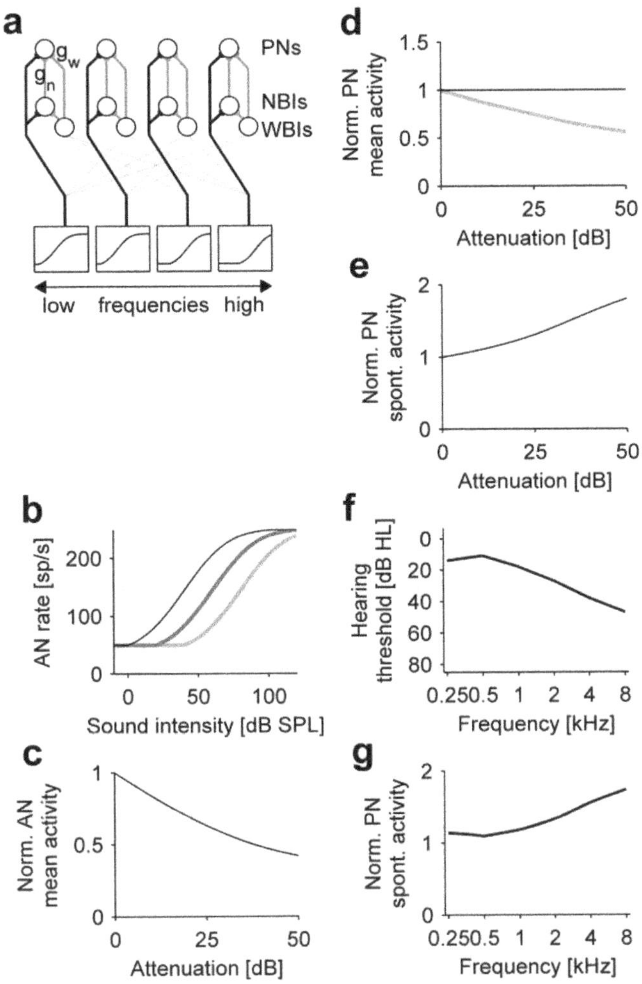

Figure 2. A computational model illustrates how attenuation through an earplug could lead to the development of a neural correlate of phantom sounds. a) Architecture of the model covering auditory nerve (bottom) and cochlear nucleus (middle) with projection neurons (PNs), narrow- (NBIs) and wide band inhibitor neurons (WBIs), 4 frequency channels are shown. Circles denote neurons, black lines excitatory and grey lines inhibitory connections. The strength of inhibition from WBIs and NBIs onto the PNs is determined by the gain factors g_w and g_n. **b**) Attenuation through an earplug is modelled by shifting AN rate-vs.-intensity functions to higher intensities, two different degrees of attenuation are shown (black line – normal, dark grey line –20 dB attenuation, light grey line –40 dB attenuation). **c**) The mean AN activity is reduced in proportion to the degree of attenuation. **d**) Attenuation reduces the mean activity of the principal neurons in the CN stage of the model (grey line). By increasing excitation and decreasing inhibition, homeostatic plasticity is able to restore the mean activity to its healthy target level (black line). **e**) As a side-effect of activity stabilization through homeostatic plasticity, spontaneous firing rates in the model PNs are increased in dependence upon the degree of attenuation. **f**) Average hearing thresholds of our participants with the earplug in place. **g**) After homeostatic plasticity has compensated for the earplug-induced decrease in mean activity, the PNs in the CN stage of the model display a pattern of increased spontaneous activity in the high frequency range.

the cochlear nucleus PNs (Fig. 2e). Such hyperactivity could be a neural substrate for the perception of phantom sounds. The degree of elevation of the spontaneous activity was proportional to the amount of attenuation provided by the earplug (Fig. 2e). To directly relate the model to our experimental results, we evaluated its prediction for the mean hearing threshold curve of our participants with the ear plug in place (Fig. 2f). This curve was estimated by adding the mean attenuation values of the earplugs (Fig. 1b) to the mean hearing threshold curve (Fig. 1a). As the attenuation value for 8 kHz could not be measured due to technical limitations, we estimated it based on data from a previous study [17]. For auditory deprivation as induced by the earplugs, the model predicted a hyperactivity profile that peaked at high frequencies (Fig. 2g), thus showing a pattern similar to the 'tinnitus spectra' obtained for the phantom sounds experienced by our participants (Fig. 1c). Finally, also in the model the development of phantom sounds was fully reversible, spontaneous firing rates decreased back to the healthy normal level when the "model earplug" was taken out.

Discussion

Our results demonstrate that unilateral auditory deprivation similar to a mild high-frequency hearing loss is sufficient to induce phantom auditory sensations in healthy normal hearing subjects without tinnitus. This suggests that auditory deprivation (not necessarily involving cochlear damage), and the concomitant reduction of auditory nerve activity, could be the dominant factor for the development of phantom sounds. The characteristics of the phantom auditory sensations perceived by our participants were very similar to tinnitus: Firstly, the descriptions of the phantom sounds resembled those of tinnitus sounds given by tinnitus patients [2]. Secondly, the mean tinnitus spectrum reached its highest values at 8 and 12 kHz, which is similar to tinnitus spectra of tinnitus patients with mild hearing loss [18]. Using a computational model, we have illustrated how plasticity mechanisms that stabilize neuronal activity levels in the central auditory system could lead to the development of a neural correlate of tinnitus during auditory deprivation.

The participants in our study wore earplugs in one ear only. Bilateral earplugs were not tested due to ethical considerations, as plugging both ears could increase the probability of dangerous situations, e.g. in traffic. Thus, the phantom auditory sensations perceived by our participant could have developed in reaction to decreased input from the ipsilateral ear, the imbalance between the ears, or both. Given that binaural deprivation in a sound-proof booth also gives rise to phantom sounds [10,11], we would expect to obtain similar results when both ears are plugged.

In the recruitment information sheet for the study, our participants were informed that they might experience phantom sounds while their ear was plugged, and this suggestion itself might have increased the incidence of phantom sounds, e.g. by focussing attention. One way of addressing this problem would be to use a control group wearing non-attenuating earplugs. However, a non-attenuating earplug can be easily recognized by the wearer. Alternatively, a future study could employ earplugs with different degrees of attenuation to study whether the occurrence of phantom sounds depends on the degree of attenuation, which was beyond the means of our current study. Moreover, it also remains to be shown if a similar relation between phantom sound characteristics and attenuation profile can also be obtained when only low frequencies are attenuated, which would support a true frequency-specific adaptation effect. However, we believe that the fact that the phantom sounds were stable enough to run a full tinnitus spectrum characterisation in 11/18 participants, that their pitch generally matched the attenuation characteristics of the earplugs, and that the phantom sounds disappeared in all participants after removing the earplug, already support a causal relation between plugging the ear and the occurrence of phantom sounds.

Several mechanisms might contribute to the occurrence of phantom sounds while the ear is plugged: Firstly, an intrinsic tinnitus could have been unmasked through the reduction of AN input caused by the earplug. However, as the earplug does not change the spontaneous activity of the auditory nerve, and thus not the neural activity coding for silence, changes in the central auditory system would still be required to give rise to a conscious tinnitus percept. Secondly, the neuronal response gain in the central auditory system could have been increased in response to the auditory deprivation. The resulting over-amplification of spontaneous activity in this scenario could account for the occurrence of phantom sounds. It has been shown recently that earplug-induced unilateral auditory deprivation lowers the acoustic reflex threshold in the ipsilateral ear, a physiological change indicative of increased gain in the auditory brainstem [17]. A putative mechanism for increased gain has been demonstrated in animal experiments: plugging one ear for 24 hours lead to an increase in excitation and a decrease in inhibition in the cochlear nucleus, both of which were completely reversible [19]. These plastic changes would be consistent with the activation of homeostatic plasticity, a mechanism that is believed to stabilize the mean neuronal activity on time scales of hours to days by scaling the strength of excitatory and inhibitory synapses and regulating intrinsic neuronal excitability [16,20,21].

Homeostatic plasticity is also a key factor in our computational model for the development of tinnitus [7,9]. Homeostatic plasticity and similar gain adaptation mechanisms have also been explored in other models of tinnitus generation [22,23], which could therefore be expected to give similar predictions for the effects of earplugs. It follows from our model that earplugs could also induce phantom sounds (Fig. 2), as verified experimentally in this study. However, not all participants perceived phantom sounds while their ears were plugged, even though our model would always predict an increase in spontaneous activity in the auditory brainstem. This discrepancy can be understood in the light of a recent theory of tinnitus, which postulates that pathological changes in spontaneous neuronal activity in the auditory brainstem are only a pre-requisite for tinnitus, whereas conscious perception of tinnitus requires additional changes at the cortical level and a failure of thalamic gating mechanisms [24]. As not all of our participants perceived 'tinnitus' during earplug usage, the putative mechanisms involved in the gating of a 'brainstem tinnitus' could be studied using the earplug paradigm.

When auditory nerve activity was 'renormalized' by removing the earplug, the phantom auditory sensations disappeared in all participants. This is consistent with the mechanism of activity stabilization in our model. Thus, one might conclude that tinnitus (occurring in association with hearing loss) could be decreased by renormalizing or simply increasing AN activity through increased acoustic stimulation, delivered for example through a hearing aid. However, there are technical and biological limitations for the renormalization of auditory nerve activity after cochlear damage. Firstly, the limited frequency range of current ear-level devices restricts the frequency range where AN activity can be increased through amplification, and we have shown recently that this factor influences the effectiveness of tinnitus management through hearing aids and noise generators [25]. Secondly, severe damage to the cochlear transducing cells or/and associated neurones, i.e. cochlear dead regions [26], will often preclude a complete renormalization of auditory nerve activity by means of acoustic stimulation. In these cases, electrical stimulation of the remaining auditory nerve fibres might be a more promising option. We hope that our demonstration that the perception of phantom sounds can be triggered by a reduction of auditory nerve activity independent of cochlear damage will open up new perspectives for the understanding of phantom auditory sensations and inspire new approaches for the treatment of tinnitus.

Author Contributions

Conceived and designed the experiments: RS KJM. Performed the experiments: CT RS. Analyzed the data: RS CT. Wrote the paper: RS KJM.

References

1. Axelsson A, Ringdahl A (1989) Tinnitus - a study of its prevalence and characteristics. Br J Audiol 23: 53–62.
2. Nicolas-Puel C, Faulconbridge RL, Guitton M, Puel JL, Mondain M, et al. (2002) Characteristics of tinnitus and etiology of associated hearing loss: a study of 123 patients. The international tinnitus journal 8: 37–44.
3. Kaltenbach JA, Zacharek MA, Zhang J, Frederick S (2004) Activity in the dorsal cochlear nucleus of hamsters previously tested for tinnitus following intense tone exposure. Neurosci Lett 355: 121–125.
4. Brozoski TJ, Bauer CA, Caspary DM (2002) Elevated fusiform cell activity in the dorsal cochlear nucleus of chinchillas with psychophysical evidence of tinnitus. J Neurosci 22: 2383–2390.
5. Kaltenbach JA (2011) Tinnitus: Models and mechanisms. Hear Res 276: 52–60.
6. Roberts LE, Eggermont JJ, Caspary DM, Shore SE, Melcher JR, et al. (2010) Ringing ears: the neuroscience of tinnitus. J Neurosci 30: 14972–14979.
7. Schaette R, Kempter R (2006) Development of tinnitus-related neuronal hyperactivity through homeostatic plasticity after hearing loss: a computational model. Eur J Neurosci 23: 3124–3138.
8. Schaette R, Kempter R (2008) Development of hyperactivity after hearing loss in a computational model of the dorsal cochlear nucleus depends on neuron response type. Hear Res 240: 57–72.
9. Schaette R, Kempter R (2009) Predicting tinnitus pitch from patients' audiograms with a computational model for the development of neuronal hyperactivity. J Neurophysiol 101: 3042–3052.
10. Heller MF, Bergman M (1953) Tinnitus aurium in normally hearing persons. Ann Otol Rhinol Laryngol 62: 73–83.
11. Del Bo L, Forti S, Ambrosetti U, Costanzo S, Mauro D, et al. (2008) Tinnitus aurium in persons with normal hearing: 55 years later. Otolaryngol Head Neck Surg 139: 391–394.
12. Norena A, Micheyl C, Chery-Croze S, Collet L (2002) Psychoacoustic characterization of the tinnitus spectrum: implications for the underlying mechanisms of tinnitus. Audiol Neurootol 7: 358–369.
13. Lecluyse W, Meddis R (2009) A simple single-interval adaptive procedure for estimating thresholds in normal and impaired listeners. J Acoust Soc Am 126: 2570–2579.
14. Young ED, Davis KA (2002) Circuitry and function of the dorsal cochlear nucleus. In: Oertel D, Fay RR, Popper AN, eds. Integrative functions in the mammalian auditory pathway. New York: Springer. pp 121–157.
15. Turrigiano GG, Leslie KR, Desai NS, Rutherford LC, Nelson SB (1998) Activity-dependent scaling of quantal amplitude in neocortical neurons. Nature 391: 892–896.
16. Kilman V, van Rossum MC, Turrigiano GG (2002) Activity deprivation reduces miniature IPSC amplitude by decreasing the number of postsynaptic GABA(A) receptors clustered at neocortical synapses. J Neurosci 22: 1328–1337.
17. Munro KJ, Blount J (2009) Adaptive plasticity in brainstem of adult listeners following earplug-induced deprivation. J Acoust Soc Am 126: 568–571.
18. Roberts LE, Moffat G, Baumann M, Ward LM, Bosnyak DJ (2008) Residual inhibition functions overlap tinnitus spectra and the region of auditory threshold shift. J Assoc Res Otolaryngol 9: 417–435.
19. Whiting B, Moiseff A, Rubio ME (2009) Cochlear nucleus neurons redistribute synaptic AMPA and glycine receptors in response to monaural conductive hearing loss. Neuroscience 163: 1264–1276.
20. Turrigiano GG (1999) Homeostatic plasticity in neuronal networks: the more things change, the more they stay the same. Trends Neurosci 22: 221–227.
21. Desai NS, Rutherford LC, Turrigiano GG (1999) Plasticity in the intrinsic excitability of cortical pyramidal neurons. Nat Neurosci 2: 515–520.
22. Chrostowski M, Yang L, Wilson HR, Bruce IC, Becker S (2011) Can homeostatic plasticity in deafferented primary auditory cortex lead to travelling waves of excitation? J Comput Neurosci 30: 279–299.
23. Parra LC, Pearlmutter BA (2007) Illusory percepts from auditory adaptation. J Acoust Soc Am 121: 1632–1641.
24. Rauschecker JP, Leaver AM, Muhlau M (2010) Tuning out the noise: limbic-auditory interactions in tinnitus. Neuron 66: 819–826.

3

Newborn Genetic Screening for Hearing Impairment: A Preliminary Study at a Tertiary Center

Chen-Chi Wu[1,2], Chia-Cheng Hung[2,5], Shin-Yu Lin[2], Wu-Shiun Hsieh[3], Po-Nien Tsao[3], Chien-Nan Lee[4], Yi-Ning Su[2,5]*, Chuan-Jen Hsu[1]

1 Department of Otolaryngology, National Taiwan University Hospital, Taipei, Taiwan, **2** Department of Medical Genetics, National Taiwan University Hospital, Taipei, Taiwan, **3** Department of Pediatrics, National Taiwan University Hospital, Taipei, Taiwan, **4** Department of Obstetrics and Gynecology, National Taiwan University Hospital, Taipei, Taiwan, **5** Graduate Institute of Clinical Genomics, National Taiwan University College of Medicine, Taipei, Taiwan

Abstract

Universal newborn hearing screening (UNHS) is of paramount importance for early identification and management of hearing impairment in children. However, infants with slight/mild, progressive, or late-onset hearing impairment might be missed in conventional UNHS. To investigate whether genetic screening for common deafness-associated mutations could assist in identifying these infants, 1017 consecutive newborns in a tertiary hospital were subjected to both newborn hearing screening using a two-step distortion-product otoacoustic emissions (DPOAE) screening and newborn genetic screening (NGS) for deafness. The NGS targeted 4 deafness-associated mutations commonly found in the Taiwanese population, including p.V37I (c.109G>A) and c.235delC of the *GJB2* gene, c.919-2A>G of the *SLC26A4* gene, and mitochondrial m.1555A>G of the 12S rRNA gene. The results of the NGS were then correlated to the results of the NHS. Of the 1017 newborns, 16 (1.6%) had unilateral DPOAE screening failure, and 22 (2.2%) had bilateral DPOAE screening failure. A total of 199 (19.6%) babies were found to have at least 1 mutated allele on the NGS for deafness, 11 (1.1%) of whom were homozygous for *GJB2* p.V37I, 6 (0.6%) compound heterozygous for *GJB2* p.V37I and c.235delC, and 1 (0.1%) homoplasmic for m.1555A>G, who may potentially have hearing loss. Among them, 3 babies, 5 babies, and 1 baby, respectively, passed the NHS at birth. Comprehensive audiological assessments in the 9 babies at 3 months identified 1 with slight hearing loss and 2 with mild hearing loss. NGS for common deafness-associated mutations may identify infants with slight/mild or potentially progressive hearing impairment, thus compensating for the inherent limitations of the conventional UNHS.

Editor: Markus Schuelke, Charité Universitätsmedizin Berlin, NeuroCure Clinical Research Center, Germany

Funding: This study was supported by a research grant from the National Science Council of the Executive Yuan of the Republic of China (NSC-97-2314-B-002-092-MY3; NSC-99-2314-B-002-063-MY3; 99-2622-B-002-002-CC2; 100-2622-B-002-003-CC2). The funders had no role in study design, data collection and analysis, decision to publish, or preparation of the manuscript.

Competing Interests: The authors have declared that no competing interests exist.

* E-mail: ynsu@ntu.edu.tw

Introduction

Hearing loss is one of the most common congenital disorders, with approximately 1 in 1000 newborns affected by bilateral moderate, severe or profound (i.e. >40dBHL) permanent congenital hearing loss (PCHL) [1,2]. If the criterion of hearing loss is lowered to 15 dBHL, 0.88% of the school-aged population have slight or mild bilateral sensorineural hearing impairment (SNHI) [3]. There is solid evidence that moderate (or more severe) hearing impairment exerts a negative impact on speech, language, and cognitive development [2], and early identification and management may be of great benefit to these children, through improved language, communication, mental health, and employment prospects [4]. Although several risk factors (such as prolonged NICU admission and congenital infections) are associated with PCHL, about 50% of infants with PCHL do not have any known risk factors [5,6], mandating the implementation of universal newborn hearing screening (UNHS) for both newborns with and without risk factors. The feasibility, cost-efficiency, and benefits of UNHS were supported by several studies [1,7,8,9]. However, UNHS may suffer from 3 inherent limitations. First, since the target condition for the majority of UNHS programs is permanent hearing loss >35 dBHL, children with slight or mild hearing loss will be missed [10]. Second, children with late-onset or progressive hearing loss may not be identified by UNHS, because their hearing is normal or near-normal at birth. Third, even in countries where UNHS has been implemented, it is difficult to approach and screen specific subgroups of infants, such as those born outside of hospitals [11].

With recent advancement in the molecular genetics of hearing impairment, it has been demonstrated that more than 50% of children with SNHI have attributable genetic factors [12], making genetic testing a powerful tool for addressing hearing-impaired children. Among a plethora of deafness genes discovered in the past decade (The Hereditary Hearing Loss Homepage, http://hereditaryhearingloss.org/), mutations in certain genes, such as *GJB2* (or *Cx26*) (MIM *121011), *SLC26A4* (or *PDS*) (MIM *605646), and the mitochondrial 12S rRNA gene (or *MTRNR1*) (MIM *561000) have been shown to be much more prevalent than other genes [13]. Some common *GJB2* mutations, such as p.M34T, p.V37I, and p.L90P are associated with mild-to-moderate SNHI [14]. *SLC26A4* mutations contribute to Pendred syndrome (PS, MIM #274600) or non-syndromic hearing loss (DFNB4, MIM #600791), and some affected patients have progressive or fluctuating hearing loss [15,16,17]. Patients with the most common mitochondrial 12S rRNA mutation, m.1555A>G, also demonstrate great variation in the severity of hearing loss progression with age [18]. In other words, some common deafness-associated mutations are associated with mild and/or progressive hearing loss. Accordingly, in this study, we hypothesize that the application of newborn genetic screening for common deafness-associated mutations may compensate for the inherent limitations of UNHS.

Methods

Recruitment and study design

From 2009 to 2010, 1017 consecutive newborns in the National Taiwan University Hospital were enrolled in the study. All newborns were subjected to both newborn hearing screening (NHS) and newborn genetic screening (NGS) for deafness. The results of the NGS were then correlated to the results of the NHS. Written informed consent for participation in the project was obtained from the parents of all infants, and all procedures were approved by the Research Ethics Committee of the National Taiwan University Hospital.

Newborn hearing screening

The babies received a two-step hearing screening using distortion-product otoacoustic emissions (DPOAEs) recorded with a GSI 60 DPOAE system (Grason-Stadler Inc., Milford, NH, USA). The first step of the screening was performed at 48 hours after birth to prevent debris and vernix in the external ear canal from interfering with the DPOAE measurement [19]. Babies who failed to pass the initial screening, either for one or for both ears, were given a second chance to repeat the DPOAE screening before they were discharged from the hospital. Those failing to pass the second step of the hearing screening, either for one or for both ears, were referred to the outpatient clinic for further assessment. The referral rate of the NHS was determined by the proportion of infants who failed both steps of the DPOAE screening.

Newborn genetic screening for deafness

A bloodspot was obtained within 1 hour after birth. Sample of blood from the heel stick from each infant was spotted onto QIAcard FTA One Spot (Qiagen). For newborn screening, three 3-mm-diameter bloodspots from each blood spot on FTA paper were punched out and used. All DNA samples were extracted using the Chemagic DNA Blood Kit (Chemagen), according to the manufacturer's instructions.

Using our previously generated epidemiologic database [20], the four most common deafness-associated mutations in the Taiwanese population, p.V37I (c.109G>A) and c.235delC of *GJB2*, c.919-2A>G of *SLC26A4*, and mitochondrial m.1555A>G, were included in the NGS panel. In terms of the allele frequency in the hearing-impaired population, these 4 mutations amount to >80% of the known deafness-associated mutations in Taiwanese individuals [20,21].

The four mutations were screened using the real-time polymerase chain reaction (PCR) assay with fluorescence resonance energy transfer (FRET) hybridization probes in a LightCycler 480 instrument (Roche) (Fig. 1). The real-time PCR was performed using two primers and two adjacent fluorescent hybridization probes. One probe was labeled with fluorescein at the 3′-end as the donor, and the other probe (acceptor) was labeled with LightCycler (LC) Red fluorophore at the 5′-end, which was phosphorylated at the 3′-end. Real-time PCR was performed in a total volume of 10 μL containing 1 μL of DNA, 3 mM of $MgCl_2$, 0.25 μM of each primer, 0.25 of μM fluorescein probe, 0.25 μM of LC Red fluorophore probe, and 1× LightCycler FastStart DNA Master Hybridization Probes Mix (Roche), as provided by the manufacturer. The cycling conditions for real-time PCR in LiC480 were as follows: 95°C for 10 min followed by 50 cycles of denaturation at 95°C for 10 s with a temperature transition rate of 4.4°C/s, annealing at 56°C for 10 s with a temperature transition rate of 2.2°C/s, and extension at 72°C for 10 s, with a temperature transition rate of 4.4°C/s.

Audiological assessments after discharge

For infants who failed the NHS, another DPOAE test was performed within 1 month after discharge, and those failing to pass the test again were referred to a pediatric otologist for comprehensive audiological assessments at 3 months. The comprehensive audiological assessments included a behavioral observation audiometry (BOA) in a sound field using warble tones, narrow band noise, and live voice; DPOAE testing; and a diagnostic auditory brainstem response (ABR, Nicolet, Bravo, Madison, WI, USA) under sedation to determine the hearing thresholds at 0.5, 1, 2, and 4 kHz [22]. The hearing level of the better ear calculated by four-tone average (0.5, 1, 2, and 4 kHz) was labeled as slight (16~25 dBHL), mild (26~40 dBHL), moderate (41~70 dBHL), severe (71~95 dBHL), or profound (>95 dBHL) (GENDEAF: http://audiology.unife.it/www.gendeaf.org/index.html) [3].

For infants who passed the NHS but segregated for 2 mutated *GJB2* alleles (i.e., with the p.V37I/p.V37I, p.V37I/c.235delC, and c.235delC/c.235delC genotypes), 2 mutated *SLC26A4* alleles (i.e., with the c.919-2A>G/c.919-2A>G genotype), or the m.1555A>G mutation (i.e., homoplasmic or heteroplasmic), comprehensive audiological assessments including BOA, DPOAE, and ABR were also performed at 3 months to confirm their audiological phenotypes.

Genetic examination in hearing impaired infants and heterozygous infants

For hearing-impaired infants who revealed an inconclusive genotype in NGS (i.e., segregating 0 or only 1 mutated *GJB2* or *SLC26A4* allele), mutation screening of both exons of *GJB2*, all of the 21 exons of *SLC26A4*, and the whole mitochondrial 12S rRNA gene was completed by direct sequencing [20]. For infants who passed the NHS but carried heterozygous *GJB2* mutations, direct sequencing of the coding region of *GJB2* was also performed.

Results

Results of newborn hearing screening

Results of the two-step NHS in the 1017 subjects are summarized in Table 1. Among the 1017 babies, 979 (96.3%) were screened as normal when they bilaterally passed both steps of the DPOAE testing. Of the remaining 38 babies, 16 (1.6%) had unilateral DPOAE screening failure, and 22 (2.2%) had bilateral DPOAE screening failure. The referral rate of the two-step NHS was 3.7%.

Results of newborn genetic screening for deafness

Of the 1017 subjects, a total of 199 (19.6%) were screened as having at least 1 mutated allele according to the NGS for deafness. Table 2 summarizes their genotypes. As for the *GJB2* mutations, 17 subjects (1.7%) had two mutated alleles, 11 (1.1%) of whom were homozygous for p.V37I and 6 (0.6%) compound heterozygous for p.V37I and c.235delC. None (0%) were homozygous for c.235delC. Nineteen subjects (1.9%) were shown to have 1 c.235delC allele, and 156 subjects (15.3%) were heterozygous for

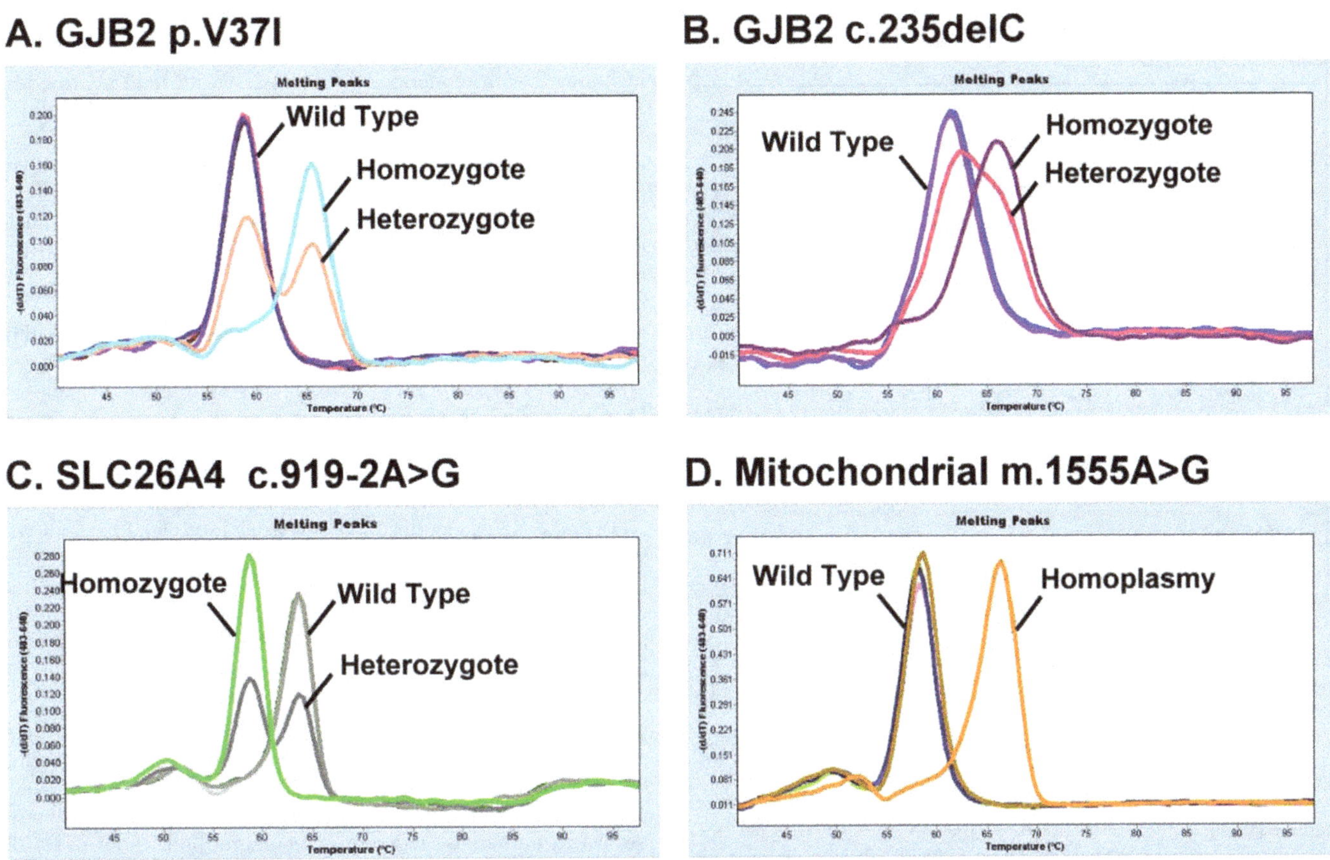

Figure 1. Melting curve analysis of real-time hybridization with FRET probes for the four most common deafness-associated mutations in the Taiwanese population. A, p.V37I of the *GJB2* gene; B, c.235delC of the *GJB2* gene; C, c.919-2A>G of the *SLC26A4* gene; and D, mitochondrial m.1555A>G.

p.V37I. The high carrier rate of *GJB2* p.V37I in this newborn cohort was compatible to that observed in a normal control population in our previous report [23]. In relation to the *SLC26A4* c.919-2A>G mutation, 6 subjects (0.6%) were heterozygous for c.919-2A>G and none (0%) were homozygotes. One subject (0.1%) was found to have the m.1555A>G mutation, with the mutation load detected as "homoplasmy" in hybridization probe testing, which was later confirmed using a restriction enzyme digestion method [24]. None of the 1017 babies segregated for mutations in 2 different genes for deafness, according to NGS.

Analysis of NHS results according to genotypes in NGS

The results of NHS in subjects with different genotypes in NGS are shown in Table 3. Among the 11 babies homozygous for the *GJB2* p.V37I mutation and the 6 babies compound heterozygous for *GJB2* p.V37I and c.235delC, 8 (73%) and 1 (17%), respectively, failed to pass the NHS. In other words, 3 babies homozygous for p.V37I and 5 babies compound heterozygous for p.V37I and c.235delC, with potential hearing problems, were

Table 1. Newborn hearing screening in the 1017 subjects.

OAE results	No. of subjects (%)
Bilateral pass	979 (96.3)
Unilateral failure	16 (1.6)
Bilateral failure	22 (2.2)
Total	1017 (100)
Referral rate	38 (3.7)

Table 2. Newborn genetic screening in the 1017 subjects.

Genotype	No. of subjects (%)
GJB2	
p.V37I/p.V37I	11 (1.1)
p.V37I/c.235delC	6 (0.6)
c.235delC/c.235delC	0 (0)
p.V37I/wt	156 (15.3)
c.235delC/wt	19 (1.9)
SLC26A4	
c.919-2A>G/c.919-2A>G	0 (0)
c.919-2A>G/wt	6 (0.6)
Mitochondrial 12S rRNA	
m.1555A>G	1 (0.1)
No mutation identified	818 (80.4)

wt, wild type.

Table 3. Newborn hearing screening results in subjects with different genotypes.

Genotype	Total (n)	No. of subjects NHS pass (n)	NHS failure (n)	Failure rate (%)
GJB2				
p.V37I/p.V37I	11	3	8	73
p.V37I/c.235delC	6	5	1	17
p.V37I/wt	156	148	8	5
c.235delC/wt	19	18	1	5
SLC26A4				
c.919-2A>G/wt	6	6	0	0
Mitochondrial 12S rRNA				
m.1555A>G	1	1	0	0

NHS, newborn hearing screening; wt, wild type.

not detected by NHS, indicating that NGS could identify an additional subgroup of affected newborns outside the target area of NHS.

The failure rates of NHS in the 156 *GJB2* p.V37I heterozygotes and 19 c.235delC heterozygotes were 5% (n = 8) and 5% (n = 1), respectively. Both exons of *GJB2* were then sequenced in the 9 heterozygous babies who failed to pass NHS, yet we did not identify any mutation in the second *GJB2* allele. Likewise, a second *GJB2* mutation was not detected in the other 166 heterozygous babies who passed NHS, indicating that they were probably coincidental carriers of the mutations.

None (0%) of the 6 babies heterozygous for *SLC26A4* c.919-2A>G failed to pass NHS. Probably these babies were only carriers. However, the possibility of Pendred syndrome or non-syndromic DFNB4 could not be completely excluded, because PS or DFNB4 patients might be born with normal hearing or minimal hearing loss, with their hearing deteriorating later during childhood or adolescence [25]. The only subject who was homoplasmic for the mitochondrial m.1555A>G mutation passed the NHS, implying that the hearing of this baby at birth might still be normal or near normal and could not be detected by NHS.

Audiological assessments after discharge

Among the 38 infants who failed the NHS, 9 (24%) segregated for 2 mutated *GJB2* alleles (including 8 p.V37I homozygotes and 1 p.V37I/c.235delC compound heterozygote), 9 (24%) segregated for 1 mutated *GJB2* allele (including 8 p.V37I heterozygotes and 1 c.235delC heterozygote), and 20 (53%) segregated for none of the 4 deafness-associated mutations (Table 4). Six of the 9 babies with 2 mutated *GJB2* alleles revealed bilateral hearing loss at 3 months, including 2 with moderate hearing loss, 3 with mild hearing loss and 1 with slight hearing loss. The other 3 babies with 2 mutated *GJB2* alleles revealed normal hearing at 3 months. Nevertheless, a close observation of hearing is still warranted in these 3 babies because progressive hearing loss is a common feature in patients with p.V37I [26]. One of the 9 babies with 1 mutated *GJB2* allele demonstrated bilateral moderate hearing loss at 3 months, and 1 of the 20 babies with no mutation detected by NGS showed unilateral profound hearing loss.

Comprehensive audiological assessments were also completed in the 9 infants who passed the NHS but segregated for 2 mutated *GJB2* alleles or homoplasmic m.1555A>G mutation (Table 5). One baby (NGS0071) showed slight hearing loss at 3 months, whereas 2 babies (NGS0032 and NGS0379) showed mild hearing loss at 3 months.

The clinical utility of NGS was summarized in the flow from NHS and NGS to identification of hearing loss (Fig. 2). Among the 979 newborns who passed NHS, 9 were identified to have potential hearing deficits by NGS. Of these 9, 3 were identified with slight/mild hearing loss at 3 months with diagnostic ABR. In other words, NGS might be useful for identifying slight/mild hearing loss that was not detected by conventional NHS.

Genetic examination in hearing impaired infants

As shown in Table 4, 1 baby with bilateral moderate hearing loss harbored only a mutated *GJB2* allele, and 1 baby with unilateral profound hearing loss had none of the 4 deafness-associated mutations. Mutation screening of both exons of *GJB2*, all 21 exons of *SLC26A4*, and the whole mitochondrial 12S rRNA gene, was performed in the 2 babies, yet no mutation was identified.

Discussion

In the present study, we developed a high throughput genetic screening tool to screen 4 common deafness-associated mutations in the Taiwanese population, and applied it to a prospective cohort of 1017 newborns. Our preliminary results revealed that NGS for deafness might compensate for the inherent limitations of conventional UNHS, including failure to identify infants with slight or mild hearing loss, as well as failure to identify infants who may potentially have late-onset or progressive hearing loss during childhood or adolescence.

There have been disputes with regard to whether the goal of UNHS should be to find out infants with slight or mild hearing loss [10,27]. Several studies demonstrated that slight/mild bilateral SNHI might also have a negative impact on academic performance [28], attention capacity [29], and language skills [30] of children. In a study arguing that slight/mild bilateral SNHI might

Table 4. Audiological results (at 3 m) in infants failing NHS.

Genotype	Total (n)	Loss F/U (n)	Normal hearing (n)	Unilateral (n)	Bilateral (n)
2 mutated *GJB2* alleles	9	0	3	0	6[a]
1 mutated *GJB2* allele	9	1	7	0	1[b]
No mutation detected	20	3	16	1[c]	0

[a]Including 2 babies with moderate hearing loss, 3 with mild hearing loss and 1 with slight hearing loss.
[b]The baby revealed bilateral moderate hearing loss.
[c]The baby revealed unilateral profound hearing loss.

Table 5. Audiological results (at 3 m) in infants passing NHS but segregating for an abnormal genotype.

					ABR threshold (dBHL)					
Subject no.	**Sex**	**Genotype**	**Laterality**	**DPOAE results**	**0.5 k Hz**	**1 k Hz**	**2 k Hz**	**4 k Hz**	**average**	**Audiometry shape**
NGS0032	M	*GJB2* p.V37I/c.235delC	bil. symmetric	bil. pass	25	30	30	30	28.8	flat
NGS0071	F	*GJB2* p.V37I/c.235delC	bil. symmetric	bil. pass	15	15	15	20	16.3	flat
NGS0072	F	*GJB2* p.V37I/p.V37I	bil. symmetric	bil. pass	15	10	15	15	13.8	flat
NGS0379	F	*GJB2* p.V37I/c.235delC	bil. symmetric	bil. pass	30	35	35	35	33.8	flat
NGS0586	F	m.1555A>G	bil. symmetric	bil. pass	15	10	10	15	12.5	flat
NGS0598	F	*GJB2* p.V37I/c.235delC	bil. symmetric	bil. pass	10	10	10	15	11.3	flat
NGS0736	M	*GJB2* p.V37I/p.V37I	bil. symmetric	bil. pass	10	5	5	10	7.5	flat
NGS0830	F	*GJB2* p.V37I/c.235delC	bil. symmetric	bil. pass	10	10	10	10	10	flat
NGS0961	M	*GJB2* p.V37I/p.V37I	bil. symmetric	bil. pass	10	10	5	10	8.75	flat

not affect language, reading, behavior, or health-related quality of life, phonological short-term memory and phonological discrimination were reported to be poorer in children with slight/mild bilateral SNHI [3]. However, including slight/mild losses within the target population of UNHS indicates that the screening program should be altered to achieve higher sensitivity, which inevitably will reduce the specificity of UNHS and greatly increase referral and false-positive rates [27]. To circumvent this difficulty, efforts have been made to ascertain the risk factors for slight/mild SNHI, disclosing that conventional risk factors for neonatal hearing loss, such as craniofacial anomaly, family history of childhood hearing loss and perinatal illness, were not strongly predictive of slight/mild SNHI [31]. On the other hand, the present study provides evidence that NGS, by detecting subjects with genetic mutations associated with mild-to-moderate SNHI, might help in identifying slight/mild SNHI not targeted by conventional UNHS. Although there is still no unanimous consensus concerning the standard management of infants with

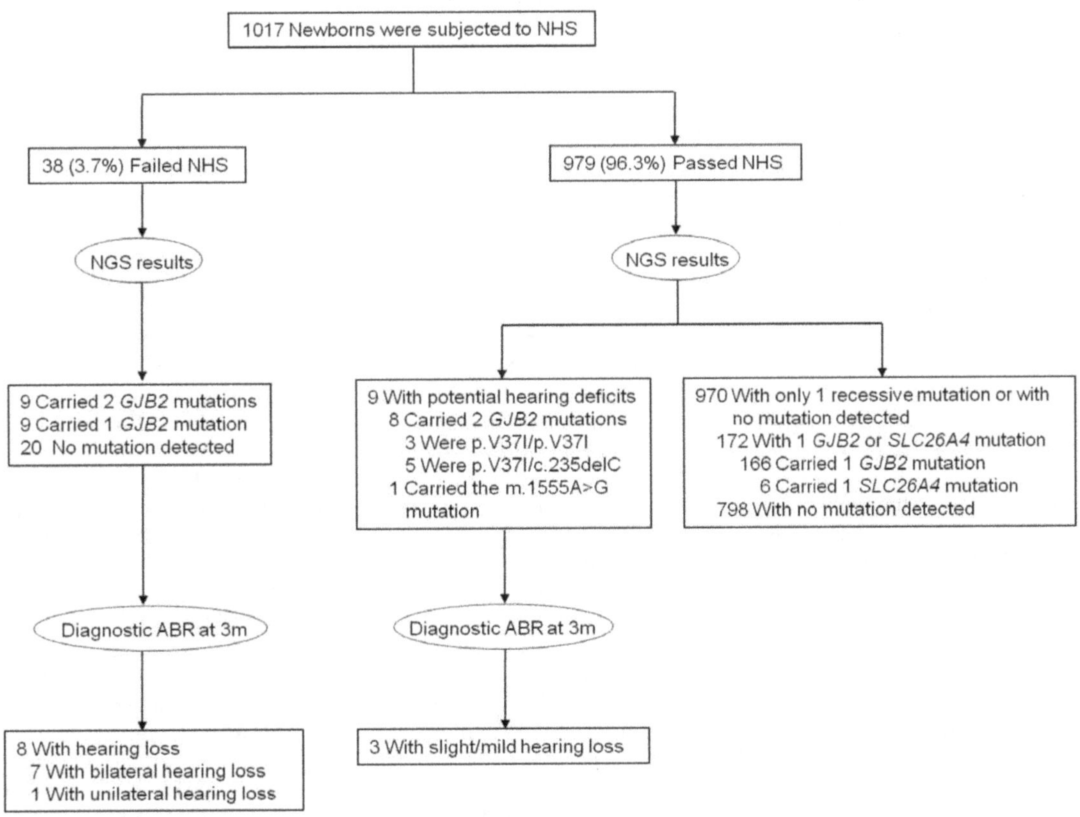

Figure 2. From newborn hearing screening (NHS) and newborn genetic screening (NGS) to identification of hearing loss. Among the 979 newborns who passed NHS, 9 were identified to have potential hearing deficits by NGS. Of these 9, 3 were identified with slight/mild hearing loss at 3 months with diagnostic ABR. ABR, auditory brainstem response.

slight/mild SNHI, referral to early intervention, speech and language monitoring, and provision of resources to parents are recommended [32,33]. Infants diagnosed as having slight/mild SNHI in the present cohort were referred to rehabilitation facilities for further consultation with an audiologist and a speech pathologist. Even if parents chose not to have their baby fit with a hearing aid immediately, they were provided with information about how to optimize the listening environment for their baby.

To identify infants and children with late-onset or progressive hearing loss at the earliest possible time is also considered important and has been included in the national Early Hearing Detection and Intervention (EHDI) goals (http://www.cdc.gov/ncbddd/ehdi/nationalgoals.htm). However, there is still no efficient way to achieve this goal [11]. In a recent report, progressive hearing impairment was noted in 7 (39%) of the 18 patients who were either homozygous for p.V37I mutation or segregated for a p.V37I allele in compound heterozygosity with a truncating allele, indicating that progression is a common feature for p.V37I [26]. In a Japanese cohort, it was also reported that p.V37I was found mainly in patients diagnosed at a higher age [34]. Progressive hearing loss has also been reported among patients with other *GJB2* mutations, such as p.M34T [35,36]. These lines of evidence highlight the clinical utility of NGS for certain *GJB2* mutations in identifying infants who are likely to have late-onset or progressive hearing loss, necessitating a close observation of hearing in these affected individuals. The potential benefits of identifying subjects with *SLC26A4* mutations or the mitochondrial m.1555A>G mutation might even be greater. For subjects with *SLC26A4*-mutation-associated Pendred syndrome or non-syndromic DFNB4, attacks of acute sensorineural hearing loss could be prevented by avoiding head trauma or abrupt barometric pressure changes [25], thus halting the progression or fluctuation of hearing impairment. The severity of hearing loss due to m.1555A>G mutation is modulated by several factors [24]. Especially, the use of aminoglycosides should be avoided in individuals with the mutation, because m.1555A>G is well established as a predisposing factor for aminoglycoside ototoxicity [37].

Interestingly, a recent study reported 32 of 108 cochlear implant (CI) recipients (29.6%) born in Illinois during or after 2003 passed UNHS, demonstrating the limitation of the current UNHS in early identification of delayed-onset SNHI [38]. The authors also pointed out that this problem could not be solved by recent JCIH guidelines, which suggest reevaluation by 24 to 30 months of age in children with known risk factors who pass UNHS [38]. Repeated hearing screening in all children provides a solution, but it might be rather costly as well as unfeasible once the babies are discharged from hospitals or clinics. On the other hand, NGS might be helpful in identifying a group of children with increased risk in developing SNHI for whom a close audiological assessment should be implemented. In the Illinois series, a substantial proportion of CI recipients would have been identified by NGS, since among the 32 CI recipients who passed UNHS, 6 were diagnosed as having connexin mutations, and 7 were found to have cochlear malformations, which might be associated with *SLC26A4* mutations.

With regard to the difficulty in approaching and screening specific subgroups of infants such as those born outside of hospitals, NGS might also serve as an alternative solution. Obtaining a few drops of blood from a heel stick within the first 2 or 3 days of life is a minimally invasive procedure, and can be conducted by a nurse or a midwife with basic training. In addition, the new generation of DNA cards, such as filter blotters, Guthrie cards, and FTA cards, are easy to collect, transport, and store.

Offering parents reproductive choices (prenatal diagnosis) has been considered a benefit of expanded newborn screening programs [39]. Although this might be true for certain rare diseases, its clinical implications in deafness should be scrutinized with caution. Some deaf advocates argue that deafness is not a disability, and are against screening for hearing defects [40]. Even for hearing parents of deaf children, it has been documented that few of them would use genetic information to terminate an affected pregnancy, although most recorded a positive attitude toward prenatal genetic testing for deafness [41,42].

New ethical questions might emerge with the institution of NGS for deafness, including risks of discrimination or stigmatization, respect for autonomy of persons to make their own decisions, and parental anxiety resulting from a false positive test or the carrier status of a recessive mutation, as other newborn screening panels [39]. For hereditary hearing impairment, of which the majority of cases are inherited in an autosomal recessive manner, identification of healthy carriers could be of special concern because it might lead to unjustified parental anxiety about the health of their baby [43]. In the present study, 175 babies were found to carry 1 *GJB2* mutation, and 6 babies were found to carry 1 *SLC26A4* mutation; among them, 9 babies and no baby failed the NHS at birth, respectively. These 9 babies were managed as other newborns who failed the NHS according to the national guidelines, i.e., another DPOAE test within 1 month after discharge, followed by comprehensive audiological assessments at 3 months if indicated. Seven of the 9 babies had normal hearing at 3 months (Table 4), and were regarded as coincidental carriers, given the high frequency of the *GJB2* p.V37I allele in the Taiwanese population and the absence of a second *GJB2* mutation in these babies. One baby revealed bilateral moderate hearing loss at 3 months, and genetic counseling was performed as hearing-impaired patients with only 1 *GJB2* mutated allele detected [44]. By contrast, for carriers who passed the NHS, no further audiological studies were performed. The great majority of these babies were p.V37I heterozygotes, and were regarded as coincidental carriers given the high frequency of the *GJB2* p.V37I allele in the Taiwanese population. The parents were assured that their babies were not at an increased risk of developing hearing impairment, and access to genetic counseling was provided whenever necessary to minimize potential stress for families.

Of special note, deafness-associated mutations should be adjusted if NGS for deafness is to be implemented in other populations because different ethnic groups show different mutation spectra for each deafness gene. Although mutations of the connexin 26-encoding *GJB2* gene are the most common cause of hereditary hearing loss in most world populations, they occur at different frequencies across populations. To screen *GJB2* mutations in Caucasians, c.35delG, p.M34T, and p.L90P should be included in the screening panel instead of p.V37I and c.235delC, since these mutations are more common in Caucasians [14]. Likewise, to screen *GJB2* mutations in Ashkenazi Jews, c.167delT should be included [45]. Leading to Pendred syndrome, the most common form of syndromic deafness [46], as well as to DFNB4, a common form of non-syndromic deafness with enlarged vestibular aqueduct (EVA), mutations of *SLC26A4* might be the second most frequent cause of hereditary hearing loss worldwide. Common *SLC26A4* mutations also differ across populations. To screen *SLC26A4* mutations, p.T416P and c.1001+1G>A should be covered in populations of northern European ethnicity [47,48,49,50], whereas p.H723R should be included if screening is to be performed in Japanese [51] or Koreans [52]. The m.1555A>G mutation appears to be a common cause of hearing impairment worldwide, and has been reported in 2–5% of sensorineural hearing-impaired Caucasians [53,54], Japanese [55], and Southeast Asians [56]. In a European birth cohort unselected for hearing loss, the prevalence of m.1555A>G was as high as 1 in 520 [57], attesting to the necessity for conducting national genetic screening prior to aminoglycoside administration. For Spanish subjects, the p.Q829X mutation of the *OTOF* gene (MIM *603861) should be added due to its high prevalence in patients with prelingual SNHI [58].

Some limitations of the present study deserve discussion. First, only common, known deafness-associated mutations are included in the current screening panel. This might lead to a false assurance in individuals with rare or novel mutations because of normal NGS results. This limitation, however, might be overcome with the advent of the next-generation sequencing technology, as massively parallel sequencing has recently been proven as an effective tool for addressing hereditary hearing loss [59]. Second, as a preliminary report, the present study documented the audiological results in 9 infants passing NHS, but segregating for an abnormal genotype, until 3 months. Although 3 of them were confirmed as having slight/mild SNHI, the follow-up period of 3 months is apparently too short to elucidate the frequency of late-onset hearing loss. Long-term follow-up of the present cohort is thus necessary to delineate correlations between NHS and NGS findings. Third, genetic heterogeneity of hereditary hearing loss might preclude a precise interpretation of NGS results. For instance, genetic diagnosis is complicated by the fact that 10%–50% of affected subjects with *GJB2* mutations carry only 1 mutant allele. Although the del(*GJB6-D13S1830*) mutation, through eliminating a *cis*-regulatory element of *GJB2*, provided an explanation for the deafness in as many as 30%–70% of affected *GJB2* heterozygotes in some populations [60,61], the etiology remained unclear for the others. These affected heterozygotes pose a diagnostic dilemma: their hearing loss might be attributed to an unrecognized *GJB2* mutation, or they might be merely coincidental carriers with hearing loss unrelated to *GJB2*. Similarly, it is also difficult to interpret the genetic results in babies who passed NHS and segregated only 1 mutated *GJB2* allele on NGS, although it can be inferred that a greater proportion of these babies are coincidental carriers as compared to "affected" heterozygotes. Nonetheless, NGS for deafness is still useful in identifying babies with 2 mutated *GJB2* alleles, for whom the genetic diagnosis is more straightforward. These babies require a close audiological observation or intervention because their genotypes are associated with mild-to-moderate, progressive, or late-onset hearing impairment.

In a retrospective report, it was demonstrated that some patients with 2 *GJB2* mutations could not be identified with UNHS [62]. By contrast, the present study might be the first prospective study to have conducted hearing screening in conjunction with genetic screening in all newborns and longitudinal follow-up of these infants. For babies with a definite genetic diagnosis on NGS (i.e., with 2 mutated *GJB2* alleles, 2 mutated *SLC264* alleles, homoplasmic or heteroplasmic m.1555A>G mutation) who reveal normal hearing at 3 months, comprehensive audiological evaluation will be repeated at 1 year, whereas for normal hearing babies with 1 mutated *GJB2* or *SLC264* allele, adequate genetic counseling will be implemented, and additional genetic study (such as sequencing of the whole gene) will be provided whenever necessary. Once hearing impairment develops in these babies, the management protocol will be switched to the conventional management protocol for pediatric SNHI regardless of their genotypes. Long-term follow-up of this cohort might provide insight into how and to what extent genetic mutations exert their influence on the development of pediatric hearing impairment, as well as provide important audiological information about the natural history of specific genetic mutations, such as the *GJB2* p.V37I mutation.

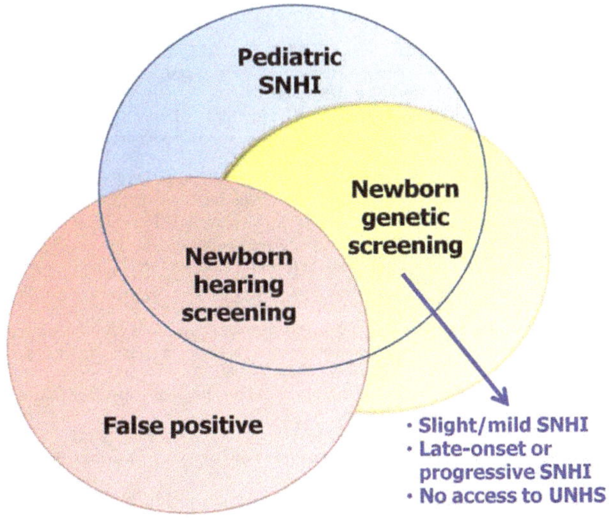

Figure 3. Clinical utility of newborn genetic screening (NGS) for deafness. NGS for common deafness-associated mutations, by detecting subjects with mutations associated with mild-to-moderate, progressive, or late-onset hearing impairment, may compensate for the inherent limitations of conventional universal newborn hearing screening (UNHS), including failure to identify infants with slight or mild hearing loss, as well as failure to identify infants who potentially have late-onset or progressive hearing loss during their childhood or adolescence. For infants born outside of hospitals and who do not have an access to UNHS at birth, NGS may also serve as an alternative. SNHI, sensorineural hearing impairment.

In conclusion, the present study revealed that NGS for common deafness-associated mutations, by detecting subjects with mutations associated with mild-to-moderate, progressive, or late-onset hearing impairment, might compensate for the inherent limitations of conventional UNHS (Fig. 3). For infants born outside of hospitals and who do not have access to UNHS at birth, NGS might also serve as an alternative. The benefits of NGS for deafness would be maximized with the construction of a well-designed infrastructure to support testing, counseling, education, treatment, and follow-up. Despite its clinical utility, the authors would like to emphasize that the role of NGS for deafness is to augment the armamentarium of UNHS instead of replacing UNHS, given that a genetic cause could not be identified in many hearing-impaired children. To our knowledge, this pilot report might be among the first to demonstrate the clinical utility of NGS for deafness. A nation-wide screening is currently underway to confirm the long-term benefits of NGS for the detection of deafness.

Acknowledgments

We wish to thank all subjects and their parents for participating in the study.

Author Contributions

Conceived and designed the experiments: C-CW W-SH C-NL Y-NS. Performed the experiments: C-CW C-CH C-JH. Analyzed the data: ?C-CW Y-NS. Contributed reagents/materials/analysis tools: S-YL P-NT. Wrote the paper: C-CW C-CH.

References

1. Kennedy CR, McCann DC, Campbell MJ, Law CM, Mullee M, et al. (2006) Language ability after early detection of permanent childhood hearing impairment. N Engl J Med 354: 2131–2141.
2. Thompson DC, McPhillips H, Davis RL, Lieu TL, Homer CJ, et al. (2001) Universal newborn hearing screening: summary of evidence. JAMA 286: 2000–2010.
3. Wake M, Tobin S, Cone-Wesson B, Dahl HH, Gillam L, et al. (2006) Slight/mild sensorineural hearing loss in children. Pediatrics 118: 1842–1851.
4. Yoshinaga-Itano C, Sedey AL, Coulter DK, Mehl AL (1998) Language of early- and later-identified children with hearing loss. Pediatrics 102: 1161–1171.
5. Wessex Universal Neonatal Hearing Screening Trial Group (1998) Controlled trial of universal neonatal screening for early identification of permanent childhood hearing impairment. Lancet 352: 1957–1964.
6. Kennedy C, McCann D, Campbell MJ, Kimm L, Thornton R (2005) Universal newborn screening for permanent childhood hearing impairment: an 8-year follow-up of a controlled trial. Lancet 366: 660–662.
7. Barsky-Firkser L, Sun S (1997) Universal newborn hearing screenings: a three-year experience. Pediatrics 99: E4.
8. Vohr BR, Carty LM, Moore PE, Letourneau K (1998) The Rhode Island Hearing Assessment Program: experience with statewide hearing screening (1993–1996). J Pediatr 133: 353–357.
9. Mason JA, Herrmann KR (1998) Universal infant hearing screening by automated auditory brainstem response measurement. Pediatrics 101: 221–228.
10. Johnson JL, White KR, Widen JE, Gravel JS, James M, et al. (2005) A multicenter evaluation of how many infants with permanent hearing loss pass a two-stage otoacoustic emissions/automated auditory brainstem response newborn hearing screening protocol. Pediatrics 116: 663–672.
11. White KR, Forsman I, Eichwald J, Munoz K (2010) The evolution of early hearing detection and intervention programs in the United States. Semin Perinatol 34: 170–179.
12. Smith RJ, Bale JF, Jr., White KR (2005) Sensorineural hearing loss in children. Lancet 365: 879–890.
13. Hilgert N, Smith RJ, Van Camp G (2009) Forty-six genes causing nonsyndromic hearing impairment: which ones should be analyzed in DNA diagnostics? Mutat Res 681: 189–196.
14. Snoeckx RL, Huygen PL, Feldmann D, Marlin S, Denoyelle F, et al. (2005) GJB2 mutations and degree of hearing loss: a multicenter study. Am J Hum Genet 77: 945–957.
15. Everett LA, Glaser B, Beck JC, Idol JR, Buchs A, et al. (1997) Pendred syndrome is caused by mutations in a putative sulphate transporter gene (PDS). Nat Genet 17: 411–422.
16. Li XC, Everett LA, Lalwani AK, Desmukh D, Friedman TB, et al. (1998) A mutation in PDS causes non-syndromic recessive deafness. Nat Genet 18: 215–217.
17. Mori T, Westerberg BD, Atashband S, Kozak FK (2008) Natural history of hearing loss in children with enlarged vestibular aqueduct syndrome. J Otolaryngol Head Neck Surg 37: 112–118.
18. Kokotas H, Petersen MB, Willems PJ (2007) Mitochondrial deafness. Clin Genet 71: 379–391.
19. Chang KW, Vohr BR, Norton SJ, Lekas MD (1993) External and middle ear status related to evoked otoacoustic emission in neonates. Arch Otolaryngol Head Neck Surg 119: 276–282.
20. Wu CC, Chen PJ, Chiu YH, Lu YC, Wu MC, et al. (2008) Prospective mutation screening of three common deafness genes in a large Taiwanese Cohort with idiopathic bilateral sensorineural hearing impairment reveals a difference in the results between families from hospitals and those from rehabilitation facilities. Audiol Neurootol 13: 172–181.
21. Wu CC, Lu YC, Chen PJ, Liu AY, Hwu WL, et al. (2009) Application of SNaPshot multiplex assays for simultaneous multigene mutation screening in patients with idiopathic sensorineural hearing impairment. Laryngoscope 119: 2411–2416.
22. Wu CC, Lee YC, Chen PJ, Hsu CJ (2008) Predominance of genetic diagnosis and imaging results as predictors in determining the speech perception performance outcome after cochlear implantation in children. Arch Pediatr Adolesc Med 162: 269–276.
23. Hwa HL, Ko TM, Hsu CJ, Huang CH, Chiang YL, et al. (2003) Mutation spectrum of the connexin 26 (GJB2) gene in Taiwanese patients with prelingual deafness. Genet Med 5: 161–165.
24. Wu CC, Chiu YH, Chen PJ, Hsu CJ (2007) Prevalence and clinical features of the mitochondrial m.1555A>G mutation in Taiwanese patients with idiopathic sensorineural hearing loss and association of haplogroup F with low penetrance in three families. Ear Hear 28: 332–342.
25. Jackler RK, De La Cruz A (1989) The large vestibular aqueduct syndrome. Laryngoscope 99: 1238–1242; discussion 1242–1233.
26. Chan DK, Schrijver I, Chang KW (2010) Connexin-26-associated deafness: Phenotypic variability and progression of hearing loss. Genet Med 12: 174–181.
27. Kennedy C, Kimm L, Thornton R, Davis A (2000) False positives in universal neonatal screening for permanent childhood hearing impairment. Lancet 356: 1903–1904.
28. Bess FH, Dodd-Murphy J, Parker RA (1998) Children with minimal sensorineural hearing loss: prevalence, educational performance, and functional status. Ear Hear 19: 339–354.
29. Hick CB, Tharpe AM (2002) Listening effort and fatigue in school-age children with and without hearing loss. J Speech Lang Hear Res 45: 573–584.
30. Davis JM, Elfenbein J, Schum R, Bentler RA (1986) Effects of mild and moderate hearing impairments on language, educational, and psychosocial behavior of children. J Speech Hear Disord 51: 53–62.
31. Cone BK, Wake M, Tobin S, Poulakis Z, Rickards FW (2010) Slight-mild sensorineural hearing loss in children: audiometric, clinical, and risk factor profiles. Ear Hear 31: 202–212.
32. McKay S, Gravel JS, Tharpe AM (2008) Amplification considerations for children with minimal or mild bilateral hearing loss and unilateral hearing loss. Trends Amplif 12: 43–54.
33. Joint Committee on Infant Hearing (2007) Year 2007 position statement: Principles and guidelines for early hearing detection and intervention programs. Pediatrics 120: 898–921.
34. Tsukada K, Nishio S, Usami S (2010) A large cohort study of GJB2 mutations in Japanese hearing loss patients. Clin Genet 78: 464–470.
35. Pollak A, Skorka A, Mueller-Malesinska M, Kostrzewa G, Kisiel B, et al. (2007) M34T and V37I mutations in GJB2 associated hearing impairment: evidence for pathogenicity and reduced penetrance. Am J Med Genet A 143A: 2534–2543.
36. Marlin S, Feldmann D, Blons H, Loundon N, Rouillon I, et al. (2005) GJB2 and GJB6 mutations: genotypic and phenotypic correlations in a large cohort of hearing-impaired patients. Arch Otolaryngol Head Neck Surg 131: 481–487.
37. Hutchin T, Haworth I, Higashi K, Fischel-Ghodsian N, Stoneking M, et al. (1993) A molecular basis for human hypersensitivity to aminoglycoside antibiotics. Nucleic Acids Res 21: 4174–4179.
38. Young NM, Reilly BK, Burke L (2011) Limitations of universal newborn hearing screening in early identification of pediatric cochlear implant candidates. Arch Otolaryngol Head Neck Surg 137: 230–234.
39. Dhondt JL (2010) Expanded newborn screening: social and ethical issues. J Inherit Metab Dis 33: S211–217.
40. Levy N (2002) Deafness, culture, and choice. J Med Ethics 28: 284–285.
41. Brunger JW, Murray GS, O'Riordan M, Matthews AL, Smith RJ, et al. (2000) Parental attitudes toward genetic testing for pediatric deafness. Am J Hum Genet 67: 1621–1625.
42. Withrow KA, Burton S, Arnos KS, Kalfoglou A, Pandya A (2008) Consumer motivations for pursuing genetic testing and their preferences for the provision of genetic services for hearing loss. J Genet Couns 17: 252–260.
43. Lewis S, Curnow L, Ross M, Massie J (2006) Parental attitudes to the identification of their infants as carriers of cystic fibrosis by newborn screening. J Paediatr Child Health 42: 533–537.
44. Lipan M, Ouyang X, Yan D, Angeli S, Du LL, et al. (2011) Clinical comparison of hearing-impaired patients with DFNB1 against heterozygote carriers of connexin 26 mutations. Laryngoscope 121: 811–814.
45. Morell RJ, Kim HJ, Hood LJ, Goforth L, Friderici K, et al. (1998) Mutations in the connexin 26 gene (GJB2) among Ashkenazi Jews with nonsyndromic recessive deafness. N Engl J Med 339: 1500–1505.
46. Batsakis JG, Nishiyama RH (1962) Deafness with sporadic goiter. Pendred's syndrome. Arch Otolaryngol 76: 401–406.
47. Coyle B, Reardon W, Herbrick JA, Tsui LC, Gausden E, et al. (1998) Molecular analysis of the PDS gene in Pendred syndrome. Hum Mol Genet 7: 1105–1112.
48. Campbell C, Cucci RA, Prasad S, Green GE, Edeal JB, et al. (2001) Pendred syndrome, DFNB4, and PDS/SLC26A4 identification of eight novel mutations and possible genotype-phenotype correlations. Hum Mutat 17: 403–411.
49. Pryor SP, Madeo AC, Reynolds JC, Sarlis NJ, Arnos KS, et al. (2005) SLC26A4/PDS genotype-phenotype correlation in hearing loss with enlargement of the vestibular aqueduct (EVA): evidence that Pendred syndrome and non-syndromic EVA are distinct clinical and genetic entities. J Med Genet 42: 159–165.
50. Choi BY, Stewart AK, Madeo AC, Pryor SP, Lenhard S, et al. (2009) Hypo-functional SLC26A4 variants associated with nonsyndromic hearing loss and enlargement of the vestibular aqueduct: genotype-phenotype correlation or coincidental polymorphisms? Hum Mutat 30: 599–608.
51. Tsukamoto K, Suzuki H, Harada D, Namba A, Abe S, et al. (2003) Distribution and frequencies of PDS (SLC26A4) mutations in Pendred syndrome and nonsyndromic hearing loss associated with enlarged vestibular aqueduct: a unique spectrum of mutations in Japanese. Eur J Hum Genet 11: 916–922.
52. Park HJ, Shaukat S, Liu XZ, Hahn SH, Naz S, et al. (2003) Origins and frequencies of SLC26A4 (PDS) mutations in east and south Asians: global implications for the epidemiology of deafness. J Med Genet 40: 242–248.
53. Hutchin TP, Thompson KR, Parker M, Newton V, Bitner-Glindzicz M, et al. (2001) Prevalence of mitochondrial DNA mutations in childhood/congenital onset non-syndromal sensorineural hearing impairment. J Med Genet 38: 229–231.
54. Kupka S, Toth T, Wrobel M, Zeissler U, Szyfter W, et al. (2002) Mutation A1555G in the 12S rRNA gene and its epidemiological importance in German, Hungarian, and Polish patients. Hum Mutat 19: 308–309.
55. Usami S, Abe S, Akita J, Namba A, Shinkawa H, et al. (2000) Prevalence of mitochondrial gene mutations among hearing impaired patients. J Med Genet 37: 38–40.
56. Malik SG, Pieter N, Sudoyo H, Kadir A, Marzuki S (2003) Prevalence of the mitochondrial DNA A1555G mutation in sensorineural deafness patients in island Southeast Asia. J Hum Genet 48: 480–483.

57. Bitner-Glindzicz M, Pembrey M, Duncan A, Heron J, Ring SM, et al. (2009) Prevalence of mitochondrial 1555A→G mutation in European children. N Engl J Med 360: 640–642.
58. Migliosi V, Modamio-Hoybjor S, Moreno-Pelayo MA, Rodriguez-Ballesteros M, Villamar M, et al. (2002) Q829X, a novel mutation in the gene encoding otoferlin (OTOF), is frequently found in Spanish patients with prelingual non-syndromic hearing loss. J Med Genet 39: 502–506.
59. Shearer AE, DeLuca AP, Hildebrand MS, Taylor KR, Gurrola J, 2nd, et al. (2010) Comprehensive genetic testing for hereditary hearing loss using massively parallel sequencing. Proc Natl Acad Sci U S A 107: 21104–21109.
60. Del Castillo I, Moreno-Pelayo MA, Del Castillo FJ, Brownstein Z, Marlin S, et al. (2003) Prevalence and evolutionary origins of the del(GJB6-D13S1830) mutation in the DFNB1 locus in hearing-impaired subjects: a multicenter study. Am J Hum Genet 73: 1452–1458.
61. Rodriguez-Paris J, Schrijver I (2009) The digenic hypothesis unraveled: the GJB6 del(GJB6-D13S1830) mutation causes allele-specific loss of GJB2 expression in cis. Biochem Biophys Res Commun 389: 354–359.
62. Norris VW, Arnos KS, Hanks WD, Xia X, Nance WE, et al. (2006) Does universal newborn hearing screening identify all children with GJB2 (Connexin 26) deafness? Penetrance of GJB2 deafness. Ear Hear 27: 732–741.

4

A *MITF* Mutation Associated with a Dominant White Phenotype and Bilateral Deafness in German Fleckvieh Cattle

Ute Philipp[1], Bettina Lupp[1], Stefanie Mömke[1], Veronika Stein[2], Andrea Tipold[2], Johanna Corinna Eule[3], Jürgen Rehage[4], Ottmar Distl[1]*

1 Institute for Animal Breeding and Genetics, University of Veterinary Medicine Hannover, Hannover, Germany, **2** Clinic for Small Animals, University of Veterinary Medicine Hannover, Hannover, Germany, **3** Small Animal Clinic, Freie Universität Berlin, Berlin, Germany, **4** Clinic for Cattle, University of Veterinary Medicine Hannover, Hannover, Germany

Abstract

A dominantly inherited syndrome associated with hypopigmentation, heterochromia irides, colobomatous eyes and bilateral hearing loss has been ascertained in Fleckvieh cattle (German White Fleckvieh syndrome). This syndrome has been mapped to bovine chromosome (BTA) 22 using a genome-wide association study with the bovine high density single nucleotide polymorphism array. An R210I missense mutation has been identified within *microphthalmia-associated transcription factor* (*MITF*) as responsible for this syndrome. The mutation is located in the highly conserved basic region of the protein and causes a negative-dominant effect. *SOX10* and *PAX3* promoter binding site mutations in *MITF* could be ruled out as causative for the German White Fleckvieh syndrome. Molecular characterization of this newly detected bovine syndrome means a large animal model is now available for the Tietz syndrome in humans.

Editor: Xiuhcun (Cindy) Tian, University of Connecticut, USA, United States of America

Funding: The authors have no support or funding to report.

Competing Interests: The authors have declared that no competing interests exist.

* E-mail: ottmar.distl@tiho-hannover.de

Introduction

A German Fleckvieh cattle family has been ascertained segregating for a white coat phenotype. Examination of these animals revealed a phenotype similar to incomplete albinism. Incomplete albinism in cattle is characterized by white coat color, pigmentless skin, heterochromia irides and white-yellowish hooves and horns [1,2]. Incomplete albino cattle have previously been noted in Herefords and Hereford crossbreds. This condition has been considered as an autosomal dominant trait [3]. The German Fleckvieh investigated here distinguishes from Herefords and their crossbreds with incomplete albinism in that the German White Fleckvieh exhibited profound bilateral deafness. The German White Fleckvieh represents the first reported dominant white cattle with heterochromia irides and bilateral hearing loss. In dogs, white coat color and heterochromia irides are often associated with congenital sensorineural deafness [4]. Phenotypes similar to these dominant white cattle are known in humans as Waardenburg Syndrome Type 2A (WS2A) [5] and Tietz syndrome (TS) [6–8]. WS2A and TS are auditory-pigmentary syndromes caused by dominantly acting mutations in the *MITF* gene [9]. Patients with WS2A are experiencing sensorineural hearing loss of varying degrees and show heterochromia irides, early greying and a white forelock and in some cases vestibular dysfunction [5,9]. Tietz syndrome differs in its phenotype from WS2A in some respects. Deafness is always congenital, profound and bilateral, depigmentation is generalized rather than patchy, but irides are not heterochromatic. Fundus hypopigmentation and vestibular dysfunction are similar in both syndromes, WS2A and TS [6–9]. The objectives of this study were to characterize the phenotypes of German White Fleckvieh and to identify the mutation responsible for this newly detected phenotype in cattle using genome-wide association analyses and re-sequencing of *MITF*, the most likely candidate gene.

Results

Phenotypic characterization of the animals

The German White Fleckvieh cattle family exhibited pure white coat color, pink skin without any darker spots or ghost patterns, yellow-white hooves, white horns, pigmentless muzzle, anus, eyelids, eye lashes, cilia, nictitating membranes and conjunctivae (Figure 1). The irides were pale blue in the central part and white towards the periphery (Figure 2). Pupils exhibited typical albinotic light reflection and the ocular fundus was completely or nearly completely albinotic using direct ophthalmoscopy (Figure 3). Optic disks were enlarged and irregular. The white animals were bilaterally deaf. We could not observe behavioural reactions or Preyer's reflex on different sounds. Sensorineural hearing loss could be confirmed using brainstem auditory evoked response (BAER) tests in two young bulls. The mode of inheritance appeared autosomal dominant with full penetrance and all white cattle could be traced to the same white founder dam (Figure 4).

Mapping the associated genomic region

A genome-wide association study (GWAS) using the *bovine* high density Illumina bead chip with 774,660 single nucleo-

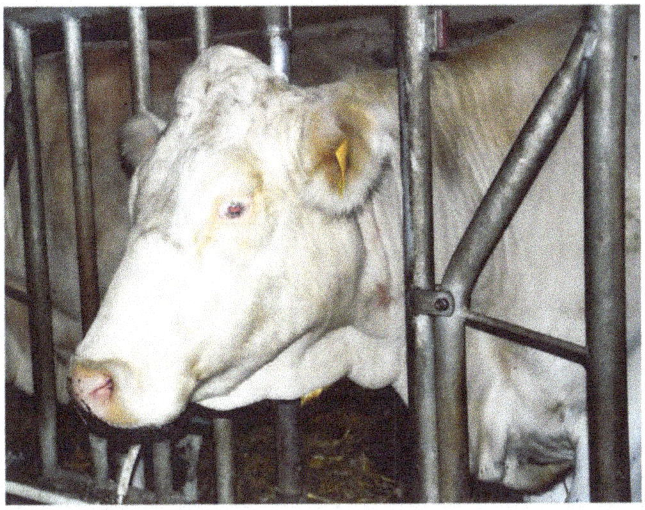

Figure 1. German White Fleckvieh cow exhibiting a colour mutation similar to incomplete albinism with irises being pale blue in the central part and white towards the periphery as well as pigmentless muzzle, eyelashes and eyelids.

tide polymorphisms (SNPs) and TASSEL [10,11] revealed the genome-wide most significantly ($-\log_{10}P_{raw} = 254.4$; $-\log_{10}P_{Bonferroni\text{-}adjusted} = 248.6$) associated region on bovine chromosome (BTA) 22 at 33.422, 36.052 and 36.060 Mb (Figure S1). Haplotypes were estimated using these three SNPs and the procedure HAPLOTYPE of SAS/Genetics, version 9.2. The haplotypes of dominant white animals were consistent with inheritance of the mutation from the common founder dam and one joint haplotype for the alleles associated with the dominant white mutation could be confirmed (Table S1). The alleles of the associated haplotype were uncommon in German Fleckvieh and not present in the spotted animals related with German White Fleckvieh.

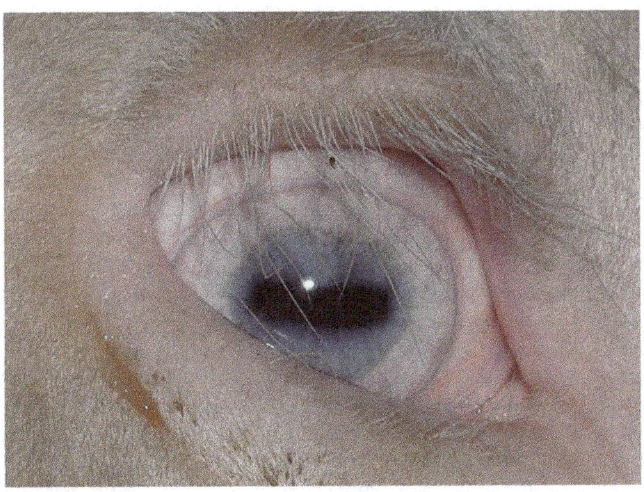

Figure 2. Heterochromia irides with the central iris appearing blue and white towards the periphery in the right eye of a German White Fleckvieh bull. Cilia, eyelashes, eyelids, nictitating membrane and conjunctiva are white.

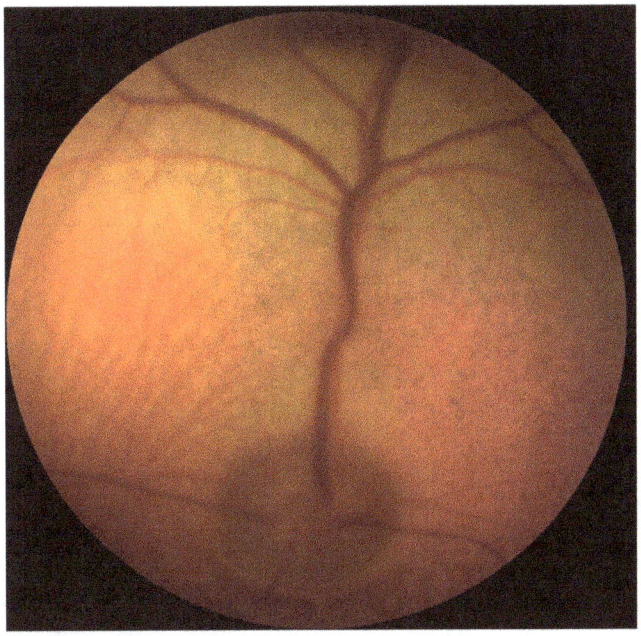

Figure 3. Ocular fundus of the left eye of a German White Fleckvieh bull showing a subalbinotic fundus with large areas of choriodal hypopigmentation. Choriodal vessels and white sclera are visible due to the transparent choriodal layer.

Identification of the associated mutation

Among 13 genes contained in the associated interval on BTA22 of Btau 4.0/5.2 (Ensemble, http://www.ensembl.org/index.html), we considered the *microphthalmia-associated transcription factor* (*MITF*) gene at 32,353,746–32,387,234 bp as the most plausible candidate. MITF is essential for the development and post-natal survival of melanocytes. All *MITF* mutations reported in humans and mice affect melanocytes to a varying degree, retinal pigment epithelial cells and a few osteoclasts. The resulting phenotypic changes are characterized by pigmentary defects of skin, coat and eyes, deafness and in some instances osteopetrosis or hyperosteosis [9]. We could not see genome-wide significant signals in the GWAS at BTA2, 5, 6, 12, 15, and 29 where possible candidate genes other than *MITF* are located on the bovine genome assembly. Thus, possible candidates for white coat colour (*KIT* on BTA6, *KITLG* on BTA5, *PMEL* on BTA5, *TYR* on BTA29) and other Waardenburg syndromes (WS) including *PAX3* (WS1, WS3; on BTA2), *EDNRB* (WS4a; on BTA12), *EDN3* (WS4b; on BTA13) and *SOX10* (WS2e, WS4c; on BTA5) could be clearly excluded. MITF is a transcription factor of the basic helix-loop-helix zipper (bHLH-Zip) family of proteins controlling differentiating and development of melanocytes, osteoclasts and mast cells [12]. We sequenced all exons of all *in silico* identified bovine *MITF* isoforms (Table S2, Figure S2). A missense mutation (c.629G>T, p.210R>I) was identified within exon 7 of the bovine *MITF* M-Form (NM_001001150) for which all German White Fleckvieh animals were heterozygous (Figure 5). Furthermore, this mutation was not detected in 383 non-completely white controls from ten different breeds (Table S3). *In silico* analysis using Polyphen predicted a probably damaging effect on the protein with a PSIC score difference of 3.065. The c.629G>T mutation is localized within the region encoding the basic region of the MITF protein involved in DNA binding. The basic domain is highly conserved between all species including vertebrates and invertebrates (Table 1) [9]. In

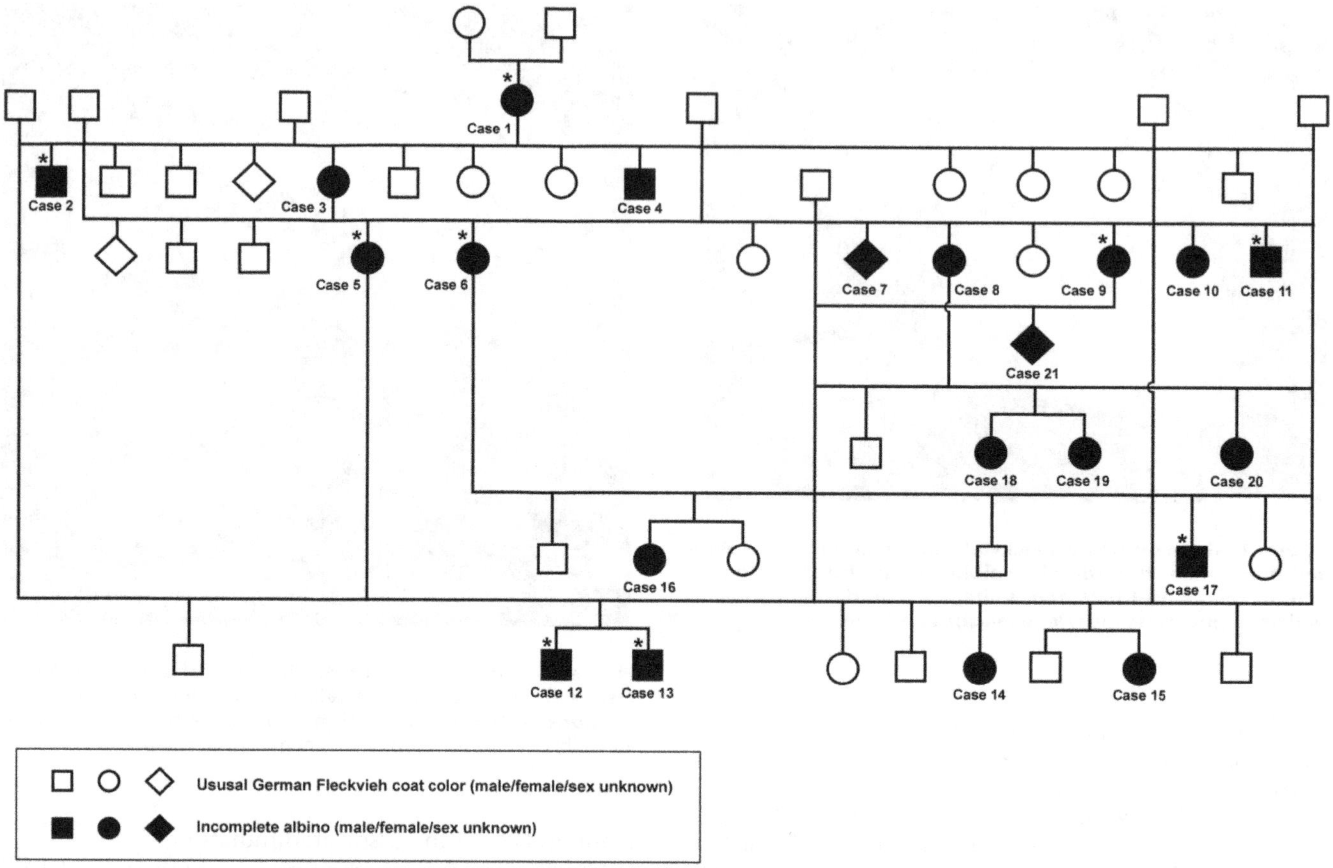

Figure 4. Pedigree of the German White Fleckvieh family resembling an incomplete albino phenotype. The founder animal for all white animals is Case 1. All animals marked with a star were examined on the farm and genotyped for the c.629G>T and g.32387485A>G mutations. Not all spotted progeny are depicted in the pedigree. With exception of Case 13 and Case 17, all white animals marked with a star were genotyped using the *bovine* high density Illumina beadchip.

order to evaluate possible effects on *MITF* expression through mutations in the binding sites of *SOX10* and *PAX3*, we analyzed the *MITF* M-form promoter region for all previously reported binding sites of *SOX10* and *PAX3* [9,13]. Both genes, *SOX10* and *PAX3* act directly and synergistically to activate the *MITF* promoter. Mutations in the binding sites of the *MITF* promoter can abolish transcriptional activation of *MITF* [13,14]. We detected eight putative *SOX10* and two putative *PAX3* binding sites after screening approximately 1 kb of the bovine reference sequence Btau 5.2 upstream of the 5′end of *MITF* transcription start site. Therefore, we sequenced a 581 bp amplicon containing the putative eight *SOX10* and the two putative *PAX3* binding sites. Mutation screening revealed a g.32387485A>G SNP at position −212 of the putative *SOX10* binding site 7/8. However, this binding site showed only minor effects on transcriptional activity in co-transfection assays with HeLa cells [13]. The mutant G allele appeared generally common in Fleckvieh and even more frequently distributed among German White Fleckvieh. Eight of the nine German White Fleckvieh cattle and two of the spotted German Fleckvieh cattle were homozygous for the G allele (Table 2). At the putative *PAX3* binding sites, we could not detect any mutations.

Discussion

In German White Fleckvieh, a perfect cosegregation was demonstrated for a missense mutation affecting the DNA binding domain of *MITF*. Function of protein domains was shown in detail for transcription factor TFEB [15] which shares critically conserved residues with MITF and other bHLH-Zip proteins [16,17]. Arginine210 seems to be necessary to contact the phosphate backbone of DNA and to build a hydrogen bond to an N-terminal glutamine. In German White Fleckvieh, the p.210R>I substitution probably disrupts both functions as the strong basic amino acid arginine is replaced by the non-polare isoleucine. In humans, the Tietz syndrome is characterized by a missense mutation (N210K) [18] or a 3-bp in-frame deletion (DelR217) [7,8]. In the semi-dominant oak ridge mouse mutant ($Mitf^{mi-or}$), the corresponding arginine is replaced by lysine (R216K) which affects the DNA binding domain [19]. In mice, further semi-dominant mutations affecting the DNA binding domain of MITF were seen in the $Mitf^{mi}$, $Mitf^{mi-wh}$, $Mitf^{mi-b}$, $Mitf^{mi-H}$, $Mitf^{mi-enu5}$, $Mitf^{mi-bcc2}$ and $Mitf^{mi-ew}$ mutations [9]. The $Mitf^{mi}$ mutation in the mouse is identical to the human DelR217 mutation. It is worth to mention that the bovine R210I and the human DelR217 and N210K mutations lead to more similar phenotypes than the murine mutations in this critical region. In humans and cattle, the mutations cause a dominant-negative effect with no variable expressivity. Humans and cattle, both are born white and sensorineural hearing loss was always bilateral [6–9,18]. In contrast to humans, cattle show heterochromia irides and this could be caused by the substitution of the non-polare isoleucine amino acid. In mice however, the trait is transmitted in a semi-

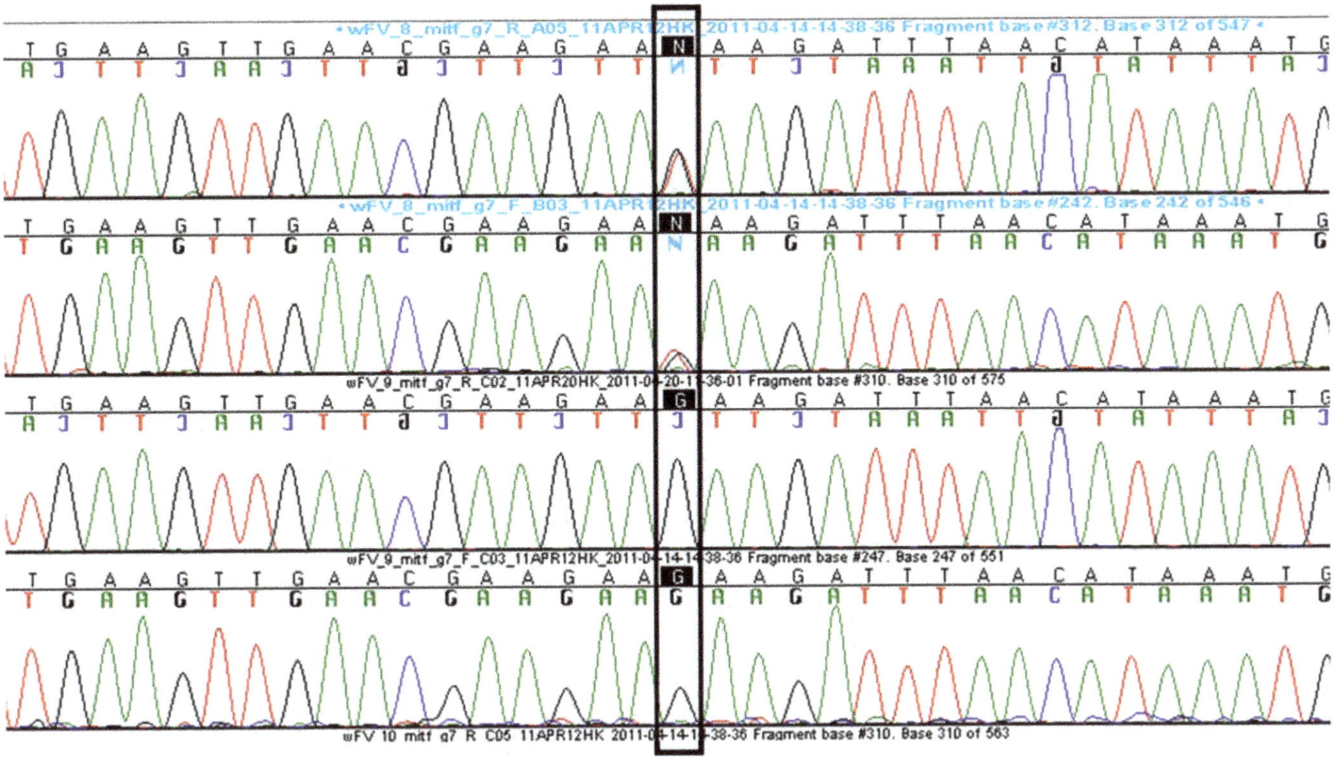

Figure 5. Sequences of exon 7 of the *MITF* M-form of a dominant German White Fleckvieh and a spotted German Fleckvieh animal. Base pairs in boxes demonstrate the c.629G>T mutation causing the Tietz-like-syndrome in German White Fleckvieh. The first row shows the forward and the second row the reverse sequence of an affected animal with the heterozygous G/T genotype, the third and fourth row contain the forward and the reverse sequence of a spotted German Fleckvieh animal with the homozygous G/G wildtype.

dominant or recessive fashion and phenotypes differ from human WS2A and TS [9] as well as the German White Fleckvieh reported here. In heterozygous mice, white spotting and/or color dilution is observed and in some cases reduced iris pigment. In the homozygous condition, microphthalmia or even absent eyes, osteopetrosis and in some inner ear defects and reduced fertility have been noted [9]. In humans with WS2A or TS and in addition, in German White Fleckvieh, neither eye defects nor osteopetrosis have been found.

The homozygous genotype of the mutation of the putative *SOX10* binding site 7/8 was not specific for the German White Fleckvieh and thus, an effect on the white phenotype can be ruled out. However, this *MITF* promoter mutation could be associated with the distribution of the white coat color in spotted German

Table 1. Protein sequence alignment of the MITF basic helix-loop-helix (bHLH) domain in vertebrate species.

Species/Breed	Protein identifier	Protein sequence
German White Fleckvieh		SEARALAKERQKKDNHNLIERR/RFNINDRIKELGTLIPKSNDPDMRWNKGTILKASV
Cow	ENSBTAP00000053693	SEARALAKERQKKDNHNLIERRRFNINDRIKELGTLIPKSNDPDMRWNKGTILKASV
Human	ENSP00000295600	********************** R **********************************
Mouse	ENSMUSP00000044938	********************** R **********************************
Rat	ENSRNOP00000044350	********************** R **********************************
Dog	ENSCAFP00000009730	********************** R **********************************
Horse	ENSECAP00000004487	********************** R **********************************
Dolphin	ENSTTRP00000006690	********************** R **********************************
Elefant	ENSLAFP00000017388	********************** R **********************************
Kangaroo rat	ENSDORP00000003119	********************** R **********************************
Chicken	ENSGALP00000012434	********************** R **********************************
Frog	ENSXETP00000000313	********************** R **********************************
Lion's cove	BAD69632	A*V******************* R **********************************

Table 2. Genotype and allele frequencies in German White Fleckvieh and German Fleckvieh genotyped for the g.32387485A>G *MITF* promoter mutation.

Breed	n	Coat color	Number of animals			Allele frequency
			G/G	G/A	A/A	G
German White Fleckvieh	'	white	8	1	-	0.947
German Fleckvieh related with German White Fleckvieh	6	spotted	2	3	1	0.583

Fleckvieh because the bovine reference sequence was from an animal of the Hereford breed.

In conclusion, we have identified the mutation responsible for a Tietz-like-syndrome in cattle. This is the first time that an unambiguous mutation in the *MITF* gene is identified in non-human and non-rodent mammals. The German White Fleckvieh is a useful large animal model to study human Tietz syndrome and the MITF transcription factor network. This study highlights the strength of trait mapping using high density SNP arrays in domestic animals, particularly with regard to one or a few founder animals for the target trait.

Materials and Methods

Ethics statement

All animal work has been conducted according to the national and international guidelines for animal welfare. The study has been approved by the Lower Saxony state veterinary office Niedersächsisches Landesamt für Verbraucherschutz und Lebensmittelsicherheit, Oldenburg, Germany, and registered under the approval ID 33.42502-05-04A247.

Animals

The genome-wide association study (GWAS) included genomic DNA samples of seven white and 79 spotted German Fleckvieh whereof five samples of the spotted German Fleckvieh were from the same herd as the German White Fleckvieh. From the seven white animals, three animals were males and four females. In controls, females and males were at the same proportions. DNA samples of nine German White Fleckvieh, six German Fleckvieh related with German White Fleckvieh, 89 German Fleckvieh unrelated with German White Fleckvieh and 288 animals from nine other breeds and German Fleckvieh x Red Holstein crossbred animals were used to test the *MITF* c.629G>T mutation. For cDNA analysis, hair root samples of two white males and one spotted female were used.

On the farm where the German White Fleckvieh had been detected, only the female white animals were used for breeding, whereas all bull calves were used for fattening without siring offspring. Therefore, all white animals had a white mother and a normally spotted German Fleckvieh sire (Figure 4). In total, six female colour variants gave birth to 20 white animals and 24 spotted offspring. Matings among spotted descendants with German Fleckvieh sires did not result in white offspring. The ratio of white to spotted offspring from the six white dams used for breeding was close to the 1:1 ratio expected for a monogenic autosomal dominant mode of inheritance. All other modes of inheritance are unlikely. The colour variant of the founder cow appears to be caused by a spontaneous mutation as both parents were normally spotted and other white offspring from the parents of the founder dam had not been reported.

Genotyping and genome-wide association analysis

DNA from seven dominant white German Fleckvieh (cases) and 79 spotted German Fleckvieh cattle (controls) randomly sampled from the whole German Fleckvieh cattle population were genotyped using the *bovine* Illumina high density beadchip with 774,660 single nucleotide polymorphisms (SNPs). Quality control for genotyping was performed using two duplicates. Consistency of genotyping was >0.999. After filtering for a minor allele frequency >0.05 and genotyping rate >0.99, 585,047 SNPs were left for a genome-wide association study (GWAS) among cases and controls. GWAS was performed using Tassel, version 3.0 (URL:http://www.maizegenetics.net/index.php?option = com_content&task = view&id = 89&Itemid = 119). A general model was employed to control for the data structure in GWAS. The fixed effects in the model included sex and the first eight principal components. Principal components were estimated using TASSEL and a pruned set of SNPs. A sliding window size of 50 SNPs, window shift steps of five SNPs and a pairwise correlation (r^2)<0.2 were used for generating this set of 56,535 SNPs. In order to test the consistency of the model, the first four, first six or first ten principal components were employed in additional models. The association results were consistent among the different models and therefore, data from these models are not shown. Genome-wide significance was ascertained through a Bonferroni correction for the number of SNPs tested. Association of haplotypes with the dominant white phenotype was tested using the procedure HAPLOTYPE of SAS/Genetics (Statistical Analysis System, version 9.2, Cary, NC, USA, 2011, http://support.sas.com/documentation /cdl_main/index.html).

DNA sequence analysis

Genomic DNA was isolated from frozen EDTA stabilized blood samples using an in-house desalting method. For identifying DNA polymorphisms within the bovine *MITF* gene (Gene ID: 407219), the putative exons of the *MITF* gene were determined by comparative alignment of the bovine genomic sequence ((NC_007320.4, 157513 bp–618513 bp) versus the known bovine mRNA isoform M (NM_001001150) and the eight human *MITF* mRNA isoform sequences (NM_000248.3, NM_001184967.1, NM_001184968.1, NM_006722.2, NM_198158.1, NM_00198159.1, NM_00198177.1 and NM_00198178.1) using Spidey (http://www.ncbi.nlm.nih.gov/blast/). For sequence analysis, primer pairs for all identified exons and adjacent intronic regions were designed using PRIMER3 software (http://frodo.wi.mit.edu/cgi-bin/primer3/primer3_www.cgi).

For mutation analysis of the *MITF* M-form promoter the previously reported murine *SOX10* and *PAX3* binding sites were identified by searching their core sequences [9] in the bovine reference sequence Btau 5.2 upstream of the 5′end of the putative *MITF* transcription site. Primer pairs were designed for a 581 bp amplicon that contained all previously reported binding sites for *SOX10* (sites S1–S8) and *PAX3* (sites P1–P2) [9].

PCR was carried out in 30 µl containing 10 ng genomic DNA according to the standard protocol advised by the manufacturer of the *Taq* DNA polymerase (Qbiogene Heidelberg, Germany). The subsequent sequencing of the PCR products was performed using the ABI BigDye Terminator v3.1 sequencing kit (Life Technologies, Darmstadt, Germany). The products were analyzed on an automated ABI 3500 capillary sequencer (Life Technologies).

cDNA sequence analysis

RNA was extracted from hair root cells using the RNeasy Universal Tissue kit (Qiagen, Hilden, Germany). The following cDNA synthesis was carried out in a 20 µl reaction volumes using Maxima First strand cDNA synthesis kit (Fermentas, St. Leon-Rot, Germany). The open reading frame of *MITF* was generated with two amplicons. In addition, specific primer pairs were designed to amplify the predicted different *MITF* isoforms (Table S2). The RT amplicons were directly sequenced using the PCR primer pairs for sequencing. Sequencing was performed using the BigDye Terminator v3.1 sequencing kit (Life Technologies). The products were analyzed on an ABI 3500 capillary sequencer (Life Technologies).

SNP detection using the ABI SNP detection system

Primer pairs and probes for the *MITF* c.629G>T SNP were designed using the Custom Taqman SNP genotyping assay service (Table S2). MGB probes were dye-labelled with FAM and VIC, respectively. Genotyping was performed in 12.0 µl reaction volumes containing 6.0 µl SensiMix DNA Kit (Quantace, London, UK), 0.3125 µl 40×Assay (Applied Biosystems, Darmstadt, Germany) and 1.5 µl genomic DNA on an ABI 7300 sequence detection system (Life Technologies). Reaction conditions for a two step PCR were set using ABI instructions. Test samples were run in single reactions, controls for homozygous T/T and G/T genotypes were run in duplex on every analyzed plate. DNA samples of dominant white cattle were used as heterozygous controls while the homozygous T/T genotypes were generated by cloning a heterozygous Mitf_Ex7_M-form amplicon using the Qiagen PCR cloning kit (Qiagen). Clones containing the strand with the mutated base T were confirmed by sequencing.

All new sequence data and polymorphisms from this study have been submitted to the EMBL/GenBank Data Libraries.

Supporting Information

Figure S1 Manhattan plot of the $-\log_{10}$ P-values for the genome-wide association analysis of the dominant white phenotype in German Fleckvieh from a general model analysis using TASSEL, version 3.0. The highest $-\log_{10}$ p-values (254) were obtained for bovine chromosome 22 at 33 and 36 Mb.

Figure S2 *In silico* identified bovine *MITF* isoforms using bovine genomic *MITF* gene sequences (Gene ID: 407219), bovine mRNA sequences of the *MITF* isoform M (NM_001001150) and all eight human *MITF* mRNA isoform sequences (NM_000248.3, NM_001184967.1, NM_001184968.1, NM_006722.2, NM_198158.1, NM_00198159.1, NM_00198177.1 and NM_00198178.1).

Table S1 Haplotype frequencies and their standard errors (SE) for all animals, German White Fleckvieh (GWF) and controls and haplotype-trait association with χ^2- and P-values. The founder dam haplotye conforms to G-A-A.

Table S2 Primer pairs used for sequencing the bovine *MITF* gene and mutation detection, amplicon size and annealing temperature (AT) for the amplicons.

Table S3 Number of animals (n) per breed, their coat color and genotype for the c.629G>T *MITF* mutation.

Acknowledgments

The authors thank the breeders for sending samples and Heike Klippert-Hasberg and Stefan Neander for their expert technical assistance.

Author Contributions

Conceived and designed the experiments: OD UP. Performed the experiments: UP BL OD SM. Analyzed the data: OD UP. Contributed reagents/materials/analysis tools: OD VS AT JCE JR. Wrote the paper: OD UP BT. Performed clinical and ophthalmogical examinations in animals: JCE BL JR. Tested hearing loss in animals: AT VT.

References

1. Leipold HW, Huston K (1968) Incomplete albinism and heterochromia irides in Herefords. J Hered 59: 3–8.
2. Leipold HW, Huston K (1969) Histopathology of incomplete albinism and heterochromia irides in the Herefords. Cornell vet 59: 69–75.
3. Leipold HW, Huston K (1968) Dominant incomplete albinism of cattle. J Hered 59: 223–224.
4. Rak SG, Distl O (2005) Congenital sensorineural deafness in dogs: a molecular genetic approach toward unravelling the responsible genes. Vet J 169: 188–196.
5. Tassabehji M, Newton VE, Read AP (1994) Waardenburg syndrome type 2 caused by mutations in the human microphthalmia (MITF) gene. Nat Genet 8: 251–255.
6. Tietz W (1963) A syndrome of deaf-mutism associated with albinism showing dominant autosomal inheritance. Am J Hum Genet 15: 259–264.
7. Amiel J, Watkon PM, Tassabehji M, Read AP, Winter RM (1998) Mutation of the MITF gene in albinism-deafness syndrome (Tietz syndrome). Clin Dysmorphol 7: 17–20.
8. Smith SD, Kelley PM, Kenyon JB, Hoover DJ (2000) Tietz syndrome (hypopigmentation/deafness) caused by mutation of MITF. Med Genet 37: 446–448.
9. Steingrímsson E, Copeland NG, Jenkins NA (2004) Melanocytes and the microphthalmia transcription factor network. Annu Rev Genet 38: 365–411.
10. Bradbury PJ, Zhang Z, Kroon DE, Casstevens TM, Ramdoss Y, et al. (2007) TASSEL: software for association mapping of complex traits in diverse samples. Bioinformatics 19: 2633–2635.
11. Zhang Z, Ersoz E, Lai CQ, Todhunter RJ, Tiwari HK, et al. (2010) Mixed linear model approach adapted for genome-wide association studies. Nat Genet 42: 355–360.
12. Moore KJ (1995) Insight into the microphthalmia gene. Trends Genet 11: 442–448.
13. Bondurand N, Pingault V, Goerich DE, Lemort N, Sock E, et al. (2000) Interaction among SOX10, PAX3 and MITF, three genes altered in Waardenburg syndrome. Hum Mol Genet 9: 1907–1917.
14. Potterf SB, Furumura M, Dunn KJ, Arnheiter H, Pavan WJ (2000) Transcription factor hierarchy in Waardenburg syndrome: regulation of MITF expression by SOX10 and PAX3. Hum Genet 107: 1–6.
15. Fisher DE, Parent LA, Sharp PA (1993) High affinity DNA-binding Myc analogs: recognition by an alpha helix. Cell 72: 467–476.
16. Ferré-D'Amaré AR, Prendergast GC, Ziff EB, Burley SK (1993) Recognition by Max of its cognate DNA through a dimeric b/HLH/Z domain. Nature 363: 38–45.
17. Lüscher B, Larsson LG (1999) The basic region/helix-loop-helix/leucine zipper domain of Myc proto-oncoproteins: function and regulation. Oncogene 18: 2955–2966.
18. Izumi K, Kohta T, Kimura Y, Ishida S, Takahashi T, et al. (2008) Tietz syndrome: unique phenotype specific to mutations of MITF nuclear localization signal. Clin Genet 74: 93–95.
19. Steingrímsson E, Moore KJ, Lamoreux ML, Ferré-D'Amaré AR, Burley SK, et al. (1994) Molecular basis of mouse microphthalmia (mi) mutations helps explain their developmental and phenotypic consequences. Nat Genet 8: 256–263.

5

Simultaneous Screening of Multiple Mutations by Invader Assay Improves Molecular Diagnosis of Hereditary Hearing Loss

Shin-ichi Usami[1]*, Shin-ya Nishio[1], Makoto Nagano[2], Satoko Abe[2], Toshikazu Yamaguchi[2], the Deafness Gene Study Consortium[¶]

1 Department of Otorhinolaryngology, Shinshu University School of Medicine, Asahi, Matsumoto, Japan, **2** Department of Clinical Genomics, Biomedical Laboratories, Inc., Matoba, Kawagoe-shi, Saitama, Japan

Abstract

Although etiological studies have shown genetic disorders to be a common cause of congenital/early-onset sensorineural hearing loss, there have been no detailed multicenter studies based on genetic testing. In the present report, 264 Japanese patients with bilateral sensorineural hearing loss from 33 ENT departments nationwide participated. For these patients, we first applied the Invader assay for screening 47 known mutations of 13 known deafness genes, followed by direct sequencing as necessary. A total of 78 (29.5%) subjects had at least one deafness gene mutation. Mutations were more frequently found in the patients with congenital or early-onset hearing loss, i.e., in those with an awareness age of 0–6 years, mutations were significantly higher (41.8%) than in patients with an older age of awareness (16.0%). Among the 13 genes, mutations in *GJB2* and *SLC26A4* were mainly found in congenital or early-onset patients, in contrast with mitochondrial mutations (12S rRNA m.1555A>G, tRNA(Leu(UUR)) m.3243A>G), which were predominantly found in older-onset patients. The present method of simultaneous screening of multiple deafness mutations by Invader assay followed by direct sequencing will enable us to detect deafness mutations in an efficient and practical manner for clinical use.

Editor: Francesc Palau, Instituto de Ciencia de Materiales de Madrid - Instituto de Biomedicina de Valencia, Spain

Funding: This work was supported by the (then) Ministry of Health and Welfare, Japan (http://www.mhlw.go.jp/english/) (S.U.) and a Grant-in-Aid for Scientific Research from the (then) Ministry of Education, Science and Culture of Japan (http://www.mext.go.jp/english/) (S.U.). The funders had no role in study design, data collection and analysis, decision to publish, or preparation of the manuscript.

Competing Interests: The authors have read the journal's policy and have the following conflicts. The authors did not receive funding from the Department of Clinical Genomics, Biomedical Laboratories, Inc. They felt that for genetic analysis of patients with hearing impairment in which many gene/gene mutations are involved, Invader Assay is the appropriate choice. However, for patent reasons, the authors cannot develop this method independently. The development of this method was therefore performed in collaboration with Biomedical Laboratories. This relationship had no influence on results and the direct sequencing results were all double checked for accuracy. Although Invader Assay is more efficient, if a method other than Invader Assay had been used, the results would have been identical.

* E-mail: usami@shinshu-u.ac.jp

¶ Membership of the Deafness Gene Study Consortium is provided in the Acknowledgments.

Introduction

From a series of etiological studies, 60–70% of childhood hearing loss has been estimated to be of genetic etiology, with the rest due to environmental causes, including newborn delivery trouble, acoustic trauma, ototoxic drug use, and prenatal/postnatal infection [1]. However, until now, there has been no multicenter study based on genetic testing. Along with early discovery of hearing loss by newborn hearing screening programs and subsequent intervention programs, much attention has been paid to the determination of the hearing loss etiology. Therefore, genetic testing has become more important for highly accurate diagnosis, prediction of severity of hearing loss, estimation of associated abnormalities, selection of appropriate habilitation options, prevention of hearing loss, and better genetic counseling. Although more than one hundred loci have been mapped and 46 genes reported to be responsible for hereditary hearing loss (Hereditary Hearing Homepage; http://webh01.ua.ac.be/hhh/), many may cause similar phenotypes without any abnormality other than hearing loss. This genetic heterogeneity has made clinical application difficult, in spite of the considerable advances in discovery of deafness genes. We have previously established a screening strategy focusing on recurrent mutations and demonstrated its benefits for clinical application [2]. We carried out the current multicenter study to determine 1) whether the simultaneous screening of the multiple deafness mutations by Invader assay is applicable for clinical use, 2) whether the genetic etiology is truly prevalent among hearing loss patients and 3) whether genetic causes differ by ages.

Materials and Methods

Subjects and clinical status

As summarized in Table 1, two hundred sixty-four Japanese patients with bilateral sensorineural hearing loss from 33 ENT departments nationwide participated in the present study. We first applied the Invader assay for screening forty-seven known mutations of 13 known deafness genes, followed by direct sequencing as necessary.

Table 1. Clinical features of subjects in this study.

	Total (n = 264)	*Early onset (n = 141)*	*Late onset (n = 100)*
Severity of HL			
normal - moderate	148	58	78
severe - profound	95	70	21
unknown	21	13	1
Inheritance			
AD or Mitochondrial	38	9	24
AR or Sporadic	119	69	42
unknown	107	63	34
Other clinical features			
inner ear malformations	52	37	10
EVA	30	22	4
goiter	8	4	3
diabetes mellitus	14	3	11

HL: Hearing loss.
AD: Autosomal dominant.
AR: Autosomal recessive.
EVA: Enlarged vestibular aqueduct.

Hearing loss was evaluated using pure-tone audiometry (PTA) classified by a pure-tone average over 500, 1000, 2000 and 4000 Hz in the better hearing ears. For children who were unable to be tested by PTA, we used an average over 500, 1000, 2000 Hz in either auditory steady-stem response (ASSR) or conditioned oriented reflex audiometry (COR), or the response threshold (dB) from auditory brainstem response (ABR). Computed tomography (CT) scans were performed to check for congenital inner ear anomalies.

Status of hearing loss in the 264 patients was: mild (21–40 dB) in 39 patients (14.7%), moderate (41–70 dB) in 84 (31.8%), severe (71–94 dB) in 39 (14.8%) and profound (>95 dB) in 56 patients (21.2%). Twenty-four subjects were classified as having normal hearing due to a specific audiogram with hearing loss only in the high or low frequency portions. With regard to onset age (the age of awareness), 141 patients had early onset deafness (below 6 y.o.), 100 had late onset deafness, and the rest had unknown onset ages.

The inheritance composition of the subjects was as follows: 38 subjects from autosomal dominant or mitochondrial inherited families (two or more generations affected); 119 subjects from autosomal recessive families (parents with normal hearing and two or more affected siblings) or subjects with sporadic deafness (also compatible with recessive inheritance or non-genetic hearing loss). None of the patients had an X-linked pattern of inheritance. The numbers of patients with other manifestations were inner ear malformations (52), enlarged vestibular aqueduct (EVA) (30), goiter (8), and diabetes mellitus (14). None of the patients had typical clinical features of Usher syndrome or BOR syndrome.

All subjects gave prior informed consent for participation in the project and the Ethical Committee of Shinshu University as well as the relevant bodies of the participating institutions of the Deafness Gene Study Consortium approved the study.

Invader assay

Invader technology is convenient for mutation genotyping, offering a simple diagnostic platform to detect single nucleotide changes with high specificity and sensitivity from unamplified genomic DNA.

We applied the Invader assay for screening forty-seven known mutations of 13 known deafness genes [*GJB2*(NM_004004.5), *SLC26A4*(NM_000441.1), *COCH*(NM_001135058.1), *KCNQ4*(NM_172163.2), *MYO7A*(NM_000260.3), *TECTA*(NM_005422.2), *CRYM* (NM_001888.3), *POU3F4*(NM_000307.3), *EYA1*(NM_172060.2), mitochondrial 12 s ribosomal RNA, mitochondrial tRNA(Leu), mitochondrial tRNA(Ser), and mitochondrial tRNA(Lys)] (Table 2). Mutations were selected on the basis of a mutation/gene database established in the Japanese deafness population. The detailed methodological protocol was described elsewhere [2]. In brief, 1.2 ul of primary probe/Invader oligonucleotides mixture (containing 0.5 umol/l wild type primary probes, 0.5 umol/l mutant primary probe, 0.05 umol/l Invader oligonucleotide, and 10 mmol/l MOPS) were poured into each well of 384-well plates. Fluorescent resonance energy transfer (FRET)/Cleavase mixture (Third Wave Technologies, Madison, WI) was added to the probe/Invader oligonucleotide-containing plates. Then, 3 ul of 5–100 fmol/l synthetic target oligonucleotides (positive control), 10 ug/ml yeast tRNA (no target control), and denatured genomic DNA samples (>15 ng/ul) were added. Next, 6 ul of mineral oil (Sigma, St. Louis, MO) were overlayed into all reaction wells and incubated at 63°C for 4 hour. After incubation fluorescence was measured by a Cyto Fluor 4000 fluorescent micro plate reader (Applied Biosystems, Foster CA). The heteroplasmy rate for mitochondrial mutations was quantified by detection of fluorescently labeled and digested PCR products through a fluorescence imaging system [2].

Direct sequencing

Dominant mutations and mitochondrial mutations are themselves diagnostic criteria for molecular diagnosis. But a hallmark of recessive mutations, in *GJB2* and *SLC26A4* for example, is the detection of two mutations in the paternal and maternal alleles. In this study, direct sequencing was further carried out as follows: 1) *GJB2* mutation analysis for all subjects, because the authors wanted to clarify whether the number of mutations on the invader panel are enough (saturated) or not. 2) *SLC26A4* mutation analysis for all the subjects with EVA, 3) *SLC26A4* mutation analysis for heterozygous patients for these genes. DNA fragments containing the entire coding region were sequenced as described elsewhere [3,4].

Results

The mutations found by Invader assay and direct sequencing in this study are summarized in Table 2 and 3.

Invader Assay

A total of 74 (28.0%) hearing-impaired subjects (n = 264) were found to have at least one deafness gene mutation. Among the deafness genes situated on the present diagnostic panel, mutations were most frequently found in the *GJB2* gene. Screening of *GJB2* showed mutations of one or both alleles of the gene in 43 (43/264; 16.2%) samples from the subjects, of which 13 cases had only a single mutation, and 30 cases were compound heterozygotes or homozygotes, confirmed by segregation analysis (Table 4). The most common mutation was c.235delC, accounting for nearly 67% (29/43) of all *GJB2* mutated patients. On the other hand, the *GJB2*: c.35delG mutation, which is known to be the most common mutation in Caucasian or other ethnic populations, was not found in this group. The second most common group of *GJB2* mutations consisted of p.[G45E; Y136X], p.V37I, and c.299_300del. These mutations were detected in more than 5 patients each, and their allele frequencies were relatively high. Three mutations (p.T86R, p.R143W, and c.176_191del) were observed in more than one

Table 2. Mutation list of Invader based genetic screening test.

Gene	*Exon*	*Codon location*	*Nucleotide change*	*Frequency of mutant alleles (n = 528)*	*Number of patients with mutations (n = 264)*
GJB2	exon 2	p.L79fs	c.235delC	43 (8.1%)	29 (10.9%)
GJB2	exon 2	p.V37I	c.109G>A	7 (1.3%)	6 (2.3%)
GJB2	exon 2	p.[G45E; Y136X]	c.[134G>A; 408C>A]	10 (1.9%)	10 (3.8%)
GJB2	exon 2	p.G59fs	c.176_191del	3 (0.6%)	3 (1.1%)
GJB2	exon 2	p.R143W	c.427C>T	4 (0.8%)	4 (1.5%)
GJB2	exon 2	p.H100fs	c.299_300del	5 (0.9%)	5 (1.9%)
GJB2	exon 2	p.T123N	c.368C>A	4 (0.8%)	4 (1.5%)
GJB2	exon 2	p.T86R	c.257C>G	1 (0.2%)	1 (0.4%)
GJB2	exon 2	p.F191L	c.570T>C	0	0
GJB2	exon 2	p.I71T	c.212T>C	0	0
GJB2	exon 2	p.A49V	c.146C>T	0	0
GJB2	exon 2	p.G12fs	c.35delG	0	0
SLC26A4	exon 19	p.H723R	c.2168A>G	22 (4.1%)	17 (6.4%)
SLC26A4	int 7/exon 8	splice site	c.919-2A>G	2 (0.4%)	2 (0.8%)
SLC26A4	exon 7	p.T410M	c.1229C>T	4 (0.8%)	3 (1.1%)
SLC26A4	exon 7	p.V306fs	c.917insG	0	0
SLC26A4	exon 19	p.T721M	c.2162C>T	0	0
SLC26A4	exon 8/int 8	splice site	c.1001+1G>A	0	0
SLC26A4	exon 9	p.A372V	c.1115C>T	0	0
SLC26A4	exon 5	p.M147V	c.439A>G	1 (0.2%)	1 (0.4%)
SLC26A4	int 5/exon 6	splice site	c.601-1G>A	0	0
SLC26A4	exon 9	p.K369E	c.1105A>G	1 (0.2%)	1 (0.4%)
SLC26A4	exon 15	p.S551fs	c.1652insT	1 (0.2%)	1 (0.4%)
SLC26A4	exon 15	p.C565Y	c.1693G>A	0	0
SLC26A4	exon 17	p.S666F	c.1997C>T	0	0
SLC26A4	exon 19	p.E704fs	2111ins GCTGG	1 (0.2%)	1 (0.4%)
SLC26A4	exon 4	p.L108fs	c.322delC	0	0
SLC26A4	exon 4	p.P123S	c.367C>T	0	0
SLC26A4	exon 10	p.N392Y	c.1174A>T	0	0
SLC26A4	exon 17	p.S610X	c.1829C>A	0	0
SLC26A4	exon 17	p.S657N	c.1970G>A	0	0
EYA1	exon 12	p.D396G	c.1187A>G	0	0
EYA1	exon 8	p.R264X	c.790C>T	0	0
EYA1	exon 7	p.Y193X	c.579C>G	0	0
COCH	exon 5	p.A119T	c.441G>A	0	0
KCNQ4	exon 5	p.W276S	c.827G>C	0	0
MYO7A	exon22	p.A886fs	c.2656_2664del	0	0
TECTA	exon 16	p.R1773X	c.5318C>T	0	0
TECTA	exon 20	p.R2121H	c.6063G>A	0	0
Mitochondrial 12S rRNA			m.1555A>G	-	5 (1.9%)
Mitochondrial tRNALeu			m.3243A>G	-	6 (2.3%)
Mitochondrial tRNASer			m.7445A>G	-	0
Mitochondrial tRNALys			m.8296 A>G	-	0
CRYM	exon 8	p.K314T	c.941 A>C	0	0
CRYM	exon 8	p.X315Y	c.945 A>T	0	0

Table 3. Mutation list found by direct sequencing analysis.

Gene	*Exon*	*Codon location*	*Nucleotide change*	*Frequency of mutant alleles (n = 528)*	*Number of patients with mutations (n = 264)*
GJB2	exon 2	p.T8M	c.23C>G	1 (0.2%)	1 (0.4%)
GJB2	exon 2	p.K12fs	c.35insG	1 (0.2%)	1 (0.4%)
GJB2	exon 2	p.F106Y	c.317T>A	1 (0.2%)	1 (0.4%)
GJB2	exon 2	p.A171fs	c.511insAACG	2 (0.4%)	2 (0.8%)
GJB2	exon 2	p.C174S	c.522G>C	1 (0.2%)	1 (0.4%)
SLC26A4	exon 14	p.S532I	c.1595G>T	2 (0.4%)	2 (0.8%)
SLC26A4	exon 16	p.R581S	c.1743G>C	1 (0.2%)	1 (0.4%)
SLC26A4	exon 17	p.V659L	c.1975G>C	2 (0.4%)	2 (0.8%)
SLC26A4	exon 10	p.L407fs	c.1219delCT	1 (0.2%)	1 (0.4%)
SLC26A4	exon 15/int 15	splice site	c.1931+5 G>A	5 (0.9%)	4 (1.5%)

patient. p.F191L, p.I71T, p.A49V and c.35delG mutations were not found. One pair of p.[G45E; Y136X] mutations was detected among 10 persons in a heterozygous state. Subsequent parental DNA segregation study through direct sequencing indicated two mutations were in *cis*. The p.T123N mutation was found in 4 subjects but, based on our recent study, is not likely to be a pathologic mutation [5].

The second most frequent gene with mutations was the *SLC26A4* gene (23/264; 8.7%). Five cases were homozygotes of p.H723R, one was a homozygote of p.T410M, 3 were compound heterozygotes, and 14 had only one mutation of *SLC26A4* (Table 4). Of the 19 *SLC26A4* mutations, 12 (c.917insG, p.T721M, c.1001+1G>A, p.A372V, c.601-1G>A, p.C565Y, p.S666F, c.322delC, p.P123S, p.N392Y, p.S610X, and p.S657N) were not found in any samples, but the remaining 7 *SLC26A4* mutations were confirmed in more than one subject. Especially, the p.H723R mutation was found to be in high allele frequency (4.1%). All of the patients with *SLC26A4* mutations had EVA, which has been demonstrated to be a result of the mutations of this gene. *SLC26A4* mutations were detected by Invader assay in 63.6% of the patients with EVA.

Mitochondrial m.1555A>G mutations were found in 1.9% (5/264) of the patients and the m.3243A>G mutation was identified in 2.3% (6/264).

Mutations in nine deafness genes (*COCH*, *KCNQ4*, *MYO7A*, *TECTA*, *CRYM*, *POU3F4*, *EYA1*, mitochondrial tRNA(Lys) m.8296A>G, mitochondrial tRNA(Ser) m.7445A>G) were not identified in any patients (Table 2).

Notably, 4 subjects were found to have double gene mutations. Two cases were *SLC26A4* compound heterozygous or homozygous mutations with a *GJB2* heterozygous mutation. One case was a compound heterozygous of *GJB2* with a *SLC26A4* heterozygous mutation and the remaining case was a *GJB2*

Table 4. Diagnostic efficiency of Invader assay alone and Invader assay and direct sequencing.

	Total (n = 264)	*Early onset (n = 141)*	*Late onset (n = 100)*
Invader assay alone			
GJB2 homozygote/compound heterozygote	30 (11.4%)	29 (20.6%)	1 (1.0%)
GJB2 heterozygote	13 (4.9%)	7 (5.0%)	6 (6.0%)
SLC26A4 homozygote/compound heterozygote	9 (3.4%)	9 (6.4%)	0 (0%)
SLC26A4 heterozygote	14 (5.3%)	10 (27.1%)	2 (2.0%)
Mitochondria A1555G	5 (1.9%)	2 (1.4%)	2 (2.0%)
Mitochondria A3243G	6 (2.2%)	1 (0.7%)	5 (5.0%)
Total	74 (28.0%)*	55 (39.0%)*	16 (16.0%)
Invader assay and direct sequencing			
GJB2 homozygote/compound heterozygote	33 (12.5%)	31 (21.9%)	2 (2.0%)
GJB2 heterozygote	13 (4.9%)	7 (5.0%)	5 (5.0%)
SLC26A4 homozygote/compound heterozygote	18 (6.8%)	18 (12.7%)	0 (0%)
SLC26A4 heterozygote	7 (2.7%)	4 (2.8%)	2 (2.0%)
Mitochondria A1555G	5 (1.9%)	2 (1.4%)	2 (2.0%)
Mitochondria A3243G	6 (2.2%)	1 (0.7%)	5 (5.0%)
Total	78 (29.5%)**	59 (41.8%)**	16 (16.0%)

*Three cases carried double mutations (cases 1 to 3 in Table 5).
**Four cases carried double mutations shown in Table 5.

Table 5. Double mutation cases found in simultaneous mutation screening.

Genotype	*Patients Number*
GJB2:p.[V37I];[V37I]; Mitochondria m.1555A>G	1 (0.4%)
GJB2:c.[235delC];p.[R143W]; *SLC26A4*:p.[M147V]	1 (0.4%)
GJB2:p.[V37I]; *SLC26A4*:p.[H723R];[H723R]	1 (0.4%)
GJB2:p.[F106Y]; *SLC26A4*:p.[H723R]; c.[1931+5G>A]	1 (0.4%)
Total	4 (1.5%)

homozygous mutation with a mitochondrial 1555A>G mutation (Table 5).

The detection rate of mutations was 40.4% for the patients with congenital or early-onset hearing loss, i.e. in those with an awareness age of 0~6 years. The rate in congenital hearing loss patients also increased when restricting to the patients with moderate or more severe hearing loss (>50 dB; 40.7%) or severe hearing loss (>70 dB; 44.3%) (Fig. 1). In contrast, the detection rate was only 16.0% in the patients with an older age of onset/awareness (Fig. 1). Among the 13 included genes, mutations is *GJB2* and *SLC26A4* were mainly found in congenital patients or early-onset patients, in contrast with mitochondrial mutations, such as 12S rRNA m.1555A>G or tRNA(Leu(UUR)) m.3243A>G, which were predominantly found in older-onset patients (Table 4). The p.V37I mutation in the *GJB2* gene was also found in older-onset patients (data not shown).

With regard to the relationship between radiographic findings and genetic testing, the mutation detection rate was elevated when restricting to the patients with inner ear anomaly (50.0%) and EVA (63.6%) (Fig. 2).

Direct sequencing

Direct sequencing identified 9 mutations in 15 cases which were not included in the Invader assay panel and improved the mutation detection/diagnostic rate obtained by Invader assay analysis (28.0%/18.6%) to 29.5%/22.7%. (Fig. 1). Combining direct sequencing with invader screening enhanced the diagnostic rate notably but not the mutation detection rate. In detail, direct sequencing identified additional mutations in three cases with single *GJB2* mutations by Invader assay that were finally diagnosed as compound heterozygous mutations of *GJB2* (p.[T86R]; c.[511insAACG], p[T8M];[V37I] and c.[35insG];[235delC]).

In 7 cases only a single *SLC26A4* mutation was found by invader assay, and additional mutations were found by direct sequencing (two cases of p.[H723R];c[1931+5G>A] and one each cases of p.[R581S];[H723R], p.[V659L];[H723R], p.[S532I]; c.[2111insG-CTGG], p.[T410M]; c.[1931+5G>A] and p.[K396E];[S532I]). Two cases carried EVA but without any mutations found in Invader assay, c[1931+5G>A]; [1931+5G>A] and p.[V659L];c[1219 delCT] compound heterozygous mutations were found by direct sequencing. With the combination of Invader assay and direct sequencing, and restriction to patients with EVA, the mutation detection rate was elevated to 17/22 cases (77.3%, Fig. 2). Fifteen of them carried homozygous or compound heterozygous *SLC26A4* mutations.

Discussion

We previously reported that simultaneous detection of common deafness gene mutations has excellent sensitivity and accuracy [2]. In this study, using samples from patients at 33 institutions nationwide from northern to southern Japan, we confirmed that the Invader assay based on the Japanese deafness gene mutation database works efficiently in the clinical base to detect the responsible gene mutations from the patients with

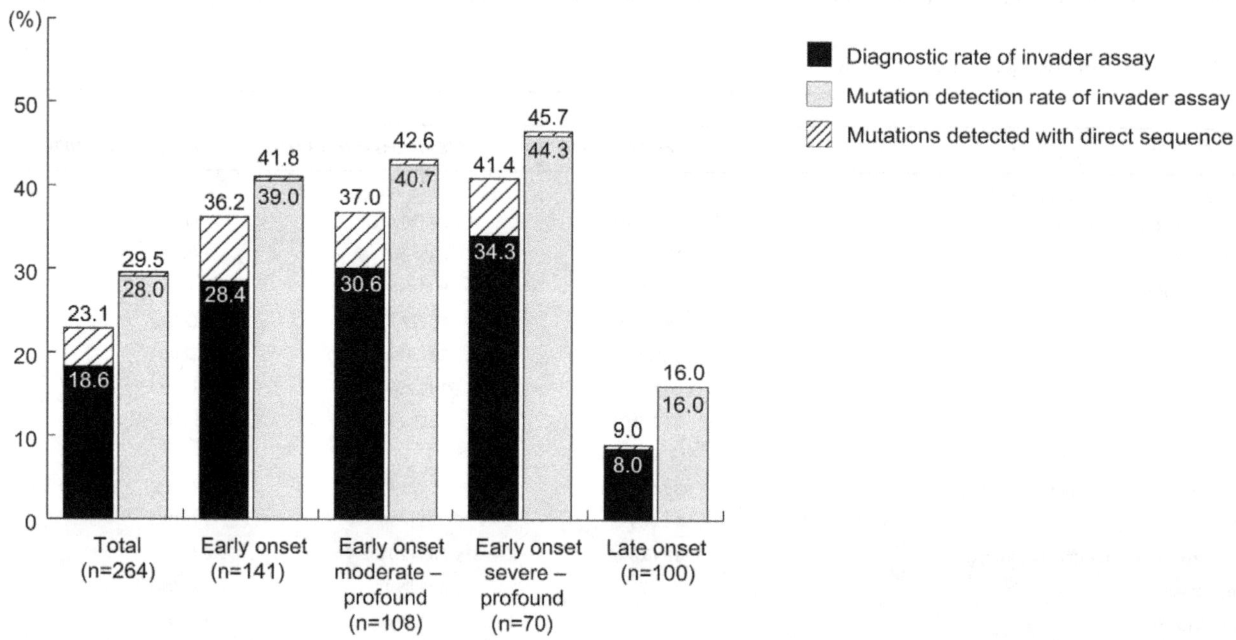

Figure 1. Detection rate by onset/awareness age and severity of hearing loss. Diagnostic rates and detection rates of this simultaneous multiple mutations screening and direct sequencing for biallelic mutations in autosominal recessive genes or mitochondrial mutations increased when restricted to congenital/early-onset hearing loss, and moderate or severe hearing loss. Combined direct sequence and invader screening enhanced the diagnostic rate but not the mutation detection rate.

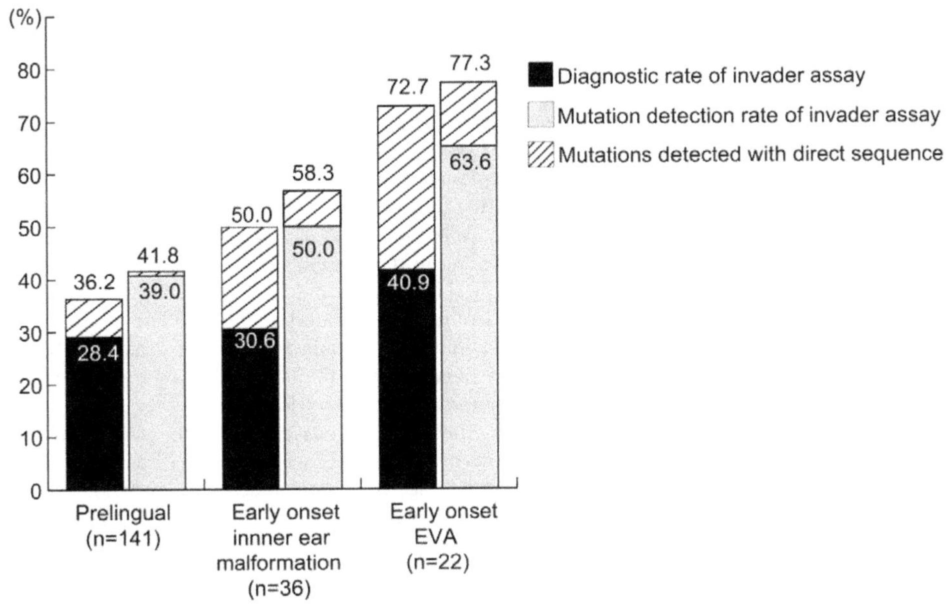

Figure 2. Radiographic findings and detection rate. Detection rate was elevated when subjects were restricted to those with inner ear anomaly or EVA. Combined direct sequence and invader screening enhanced the diagnostic rate but not the mutation detection rate.

various onset/awareness ages. We detected mutations in 29.5% overall, and the 41.8% detection rate for congenital or early onset sensorineural hearing loss was especially remarkable. A series of epidemiological studies have demonstrated that genetic disorders are common causes of congenital deafness and it is estimated that 60–70% of the etiology may be caused by genetic factors [1]. Genetic testing is crucial to diagnose the etiology, but more than 100 genes are estimated to be involved and such genetic heterogeneicty has hampered the genetic testing for deafness as a routine clinical test. The present detection rate; i.e., 41.8%, is a strikingly good rate for a clinical application, and it is expected that clinical deafness mutation screening will greatly improve medical management and facilitate extensive genetic counseling for hearing impairment. Additional direct sequencing, as well as a new version of the screening panel which includes novel identified mutations, will likely improve the detection rate. For the older ages of onset, the detection rate was comparatively low (16.0%). Probably this is due to the panel mainly including responsible genes for congenital deafness but not the responsible genes for late onset hearing loss. An alternative explanation may be that environmental factors may be involved in this group of deafness patients.

The present study confirmed that mutations in three genes, *GJB2*, *SLC26A4*, and the mitochondrial 12 s rRNA, are so far the major known causes of hereditary hearing loss nationwide in Japanese [6], and thus much attention should be paid to these genes when performing genetic testing of hearing loss patients.

The most frequently found were mutations in the *GJB2* gene. This gene is so far the most common responsible gene for congenital deafness worldwide [7]. The detection rates (17.4% for all, 27.0% for congenital) are in accordance with our previous data of 15% in the overall deafness population and 25% in congenital deafness patients [5]. The mutation spectrum found in this study is also in accordance with our previous results [2,4,5]. In *GJB2* screening, 46 (17.4%) samples from deafness subjects had mutations of one or both alleles of the *GJB2* gene. As expected from the above reports, the c.235delC mutation was found to be the most prevalent mutation in our screening, accounting for 10.9% (29 of 264) of the hearing-impaired persons. Fourteen patients were c.235delC homozygotes and 11 were compound heterozygotes having c.235delC, confirmed by segregation analysis, and 4 patients were c.235delC heterozygotes without a second mutation. Direct sequencing identified novel mutations (p.T8M, c.35insG, p.F106Y, p.C174S and c.512insAACG) in the patients with a single mutation detected by Invader assay (Table 3).

Many benefits of *GJB2* gene genetic testing have been pointed out. There have been general rules that inactivating mutations (deletion mutations and stop mutations) show more severe phenotypes compared to those caused by non-inactivating mutations (missense mutations) [5,8,9]. As well as a highly accurate diagnosis, these genotype-phenotype correlation data could provide prognostic information to help decide the strategy of intervention with hearing, i.e., whether a child should receive cochlear implantation or hearing aids. For the patients with severe phenotypes who have *GJB2* mutations, genetic information would aid decision-making regarding cochlear implantation, because their hearing loss is of cochlear origin and they therefore are good candidates for implantation. In fact, cochlear implantation has resulted in remarkable improvement in auditory skills and development of speech production for patients with profound hearing loss associated with *GJB2* mutations [10].

In the *SLC26A4* gene, 7 cases were homozygotes, 11 cases were compound heterozygotes, and 7 cases had only one mutation (Table 4). Of the 19 *SLC26A4* mutations, 12 were not found in any samples, but the remaining 7 mutations were all confirmed in more than one patient. Especially, the p.H723R mutation was found to be in high allele frequency (4.1%). Direct sequencing identified novel mutations (c.1931+5G>A, p.S532I, p.R581S, p.V659L) in the patients with a single mutation by Invader assay and c.1219delCT mutation in a patient with EVA (Table 3).

As in our previous study [2], *SLC26A4* mutations were found only in the patients with EVA, suggesting a phenotype of hearing loss with EVA can be a diagnostic indicator of this category of disease.

Fluctuation and progressiveness of hearing loss are characteristic of hearing loss associated with EVA [11,12] and the early detection of *SLC26A4* mutations enables prediction of these clinical symptoms. Genetic testing is also useful in estimating associated abnormalities (goiter), selection of appropriate habilitation options, and better genetic counseling. In some cases, goiter is evident during the teen years [12]. In this study, 8 patients had hearing loss and goiter and 4 of them carried homozygous or compound heterozygous *SLC26A4* mutations.

In recessive mutations such as *GJB2* and *SLC26A4*, detection of two mutations in the paternal and maternal alleles is a hallmark. In the present "two step" screening method Invader assay is first performed followed by direct sequencing. As seen in Figs. 1 and 2, most of the mutations were successfully detected by the first Invader screening and the additional direct sequencing improved the "diagnostic" rate. This is very important to find the first mutation for identifying the responsible gene and the results indicate this screening is technically efficient. Difficult cases of a heterozygous state without a second mutation are also seen [4,5,13,14]. As previously reported, in a substantial proportion of patients our Invader techniques and additional direct sequencing revealed only one mutant *GJB2* or *SLC26A4* allele causing deafness by recessive pattern. We believe that there is one more occult mutation somewhere because the frequency of heterozygous patients was much higher than that of mutation frequency in the control population. Another explanation may be the high frequency of carriers in the population. But given the carrier frequency in normal controls, the number of heterozygous deafness cases was greater than would be expected. Second mutations may be present in the same gene or genes in the same chromosomal region. Recent statistical analysis has shown that one allele mutation of *GJB2* and *SLC26A4* is more likely to be a pathological status than a carrier status [15] and indeed, patients with one *SLC26A4* mutation are associated with EVA, therefore it is strongly likely that there is a second mutation within this gene. Another possibility is that mutations in the regulatory region may be involved in phenotypic expression [16].

The m.1555A>G mutation in the mitochondrial 12SrRNA gene, which was found in 5 4 subjects, was mainly found in those with older onset age. This mutation has been reported to be associated with aminoglycoside injection and found in 3% of the patients who visited the outpatient clinic [17,18]. The current findings are compatible with our previous report that this mutation is a frequently encountered cause for postlingual deafness in patients who received cochlear implantation [18]. This mutation was also found in the congenital or early onset age group as well, in line with our previous study [2]. It is likely that there is a considerably large high-risk population worldwide and a rapid screening method as well as careful counseling should be established to prevent aminoglycoside-induced hearing loss in this group.

The m.3243A>G mutation in the tRNA(Leu (UUR)) gene was found in 6 patients in the older-onset group. This mutation was first reported at a high frequently in the patients with clinical manifestations of MELAS [19], and has also been found in diabetes mellitus patients [20]. It is known to be commonly associated with hearing loss patients (especially with diabetes mellitus) [21]. The hearing loss is adult onset, symmetric high frequency involved [22]. In this study, all 6 patients with this mutation were associated with diabetes mellitus and progressive hearing loss. Five patients had maternally inherited hearing loss (the mother also had hearing loss), but one subject was a sporadic case (the mother did not have hearing loss from the anamnestic evaluation) and therefore is unlikely to be a mitochondrial candidate from clinical evaluation. The present multigene screening is also unexpectedly efficient for such atypical cases.

Heteroplasmy is one of the significant factors determining the expression of mitochondrial disease. The Invader assay is comparatively accurate at detecting the heteroplasmic rate [2], and the present two patients with the 3243 mutation showed 3% and 24% heteroplasmic rates.

In contrast to the three genes discussed above, mutations of the *COCH, KCNQ4, MYO7A, TECTA, CRYM, POU3F4 and EYA1* genes were not found in the present deaf subjects in line with our previous study [2]. This is likely due to them being very rare and usually independent mutations found in only one family. Although analysis for these mutations should be performed to identify the molecular nature of deafness as the first deafness screening step, a different strategy may be necessary for screening for them.

In conclusion, the simultaneous examination of the multiple deafness mutations by Invader assay followed by direct sequencing if necessary, will enable us to detect deafness mutations in an efficient and practical manner for clinical use. This screening strategy will facilitate more precise clinical genetic diagnosis, appropriate genetic counseling and proper medical management for auditory disorders. Against this background, since 2008 the Ministry of Health and Welfare of Japan has allowed this screening to be performed as an advanced medical technology.

A Japanese summary of this article has been provided as Supporting Information (Japanese summary S1).

Supporting Information

Japanese Summary S1 Simultaneous Screening of Multiple Mutations by Invader Assay. The present method of simultaneous screening of multiple deafness mutations by Invader assay followed by direct sequencing will enable us to detect deafness mutations in an efficient and practical manner for clinical use.

Acknowledgments

We thank the participants of the Deafness Gene Study Consortium: Drs. Norihito Takeichi and Satoshi Fukuda (Hokkaido University), Drs. Atsushi Namba and Hideichi Shinkawa (Hirosaki University), Drs. Yumiko Kobayashi and Hiroaki Sato (Iwate Medical University), Drs. Tetsuaki Kawase and Toshimitsu Kobayashi (Tohoku University), Drs. Tomoo Watanabe, Tsukasa Ito and Masaru Aoyagi (Yamagata University), Drs. Hiroshi Ogawa and Koichi Omori (Fukushima Medical University), Drs. Kotaro Ishikawa and Keiichi Ichimura (Jichi Medical University), Drs. Kyoko Nagai and Nobuhiko Furuya (Gunma University), Drs. Shuntaro Shigihara, Yasuyuki Nomura and Minoru Ikeda (Nihon University School), Drs. Tetsuo Ikezono and Toshiaki Yagi (Nippon Medical School), Dr. Shunichi Tomiyama (Nippon Medical School Tama Nagayama Hospital), Drs. Hiromi Kojima, Yuika Sakurai and Hiroshi Moriyama (Jikei University), Dr. Kozo Kumakawa (Toranomon Hospital), Drs. Hajime Sano and Makito Okamoto (Kitasato University), Dr. Satoshi Iwasaki (Hamamatsu Medical University), Dr. Kazuhiko Takeuchi (Mie University), Dr. Masako Nakai (Shiga Medical Center for Children), Drs. Masahiko Higashikawa and Hiroshi Takenaka (Osaka Medical College), Drs. Yuko Saito, Masafumi Sakagami (Hyogo College of Medicine), Dr. Yasushi Naito (Kobe City Medical Center General Hospital), Drs. Keiji Fujihara, Akihiro Sakai and Noboru Yamanaka (Wakayama Medical University), Drs. Kunihiro Fukushima, and Kazunori Nishizaki (Okayama University), Drs. Kazuma Sugahara and Hiroshi Yamashita (Yamaguchi University), Drs. Naoto Hato and Kiyofumi Gyo (Ehime University), Drs. Yasuhiro Kakazu and Shizuo Komune (Kyushu University), Drs. Mayumi Sugamura and Takashi Nakagawa (Fukuoka University), Dr. Haruo Takahashi (Nagasaki University), Dr. Yukihiko Kanda (Kanda ENT Clinic), Drs. Hirokazu Kawano and Tetsuya Tono (Miyazaki Medical College), Drs. Ikuyo Miyanohara andYuichi Kurono (Kagoshima University), Drs. Akira Ganaha and Mikio Suzuki (Ryukyus University), for providing samples of their patients. We also thank A. C. Apple-Mathews for help in preparing the manuscript.

Author Contributions

Conceived and designed the experiments: SU. Performed the experiments: SN MN SA TY. Analyzed the data: SN MN SA TY. Contributed reagents/materials/analysis tools: SN MN SA TY. Wrote the paper: SU. Collection of DNA samples and clinical data: The Deafness Gene Study Consortium.

References

1. Morton CC, Nance WE (2006) Newborn hearing screening: a silent revolution. N Engl J Med 354: 2151–2164.
2. Abe S, Yamaguchi T, Usami S (2007) Application of deafness diagnostic screening panel based on deafness mutation/gene database using Invader Assay. Genetic Testing 11(3): 333–340.
3. Usami S, Abe S, Weston MD, Shinkawa H, Van Camp G, et al. (1999) Non-syndromic hearing loss associated with enlarged vestibular aqueduct is caused by PDS mutations. Hum Genet 104: 188–192.
4. Ohtsuka A, Yuge I, Kimura S, Namba A, Abe S, et al. (2003) GJB2 deafness gene shows a specific spectrum of mutations in Japan, including a frequent founder mutation. Hum Genet 112: 329–333.
5. Tsukada K, Nishio S, Usami S (2010) A large cohort study of GJB2 mutations in Japanese hearing loss patients. Clin Genet 78: 464–470.
6. Usami S, Wagatsuma M, Fukuoka H, Suzuki H, Tsukada K, et al. (2008) The responsible genes in Japanese deafness patients and clinical application using Invader assay. Acta Otolaryngol 128: 446–454.
7. Smith RJ, Bale JF, Jr., White KR (2005) Sensorineural hearing loss in children. Lancet 365: 879–890. Review.
8. Snoeckx RL, Huygen PLM, Feldmann D, Marlin S, Denoyelle F, et al. (2005) GJB2 mutations and degree of hearing loss: a multicenter study. Am J Hum Genet 77: 945–957.
9. Oguchi T, Ohtsuka A, Hashimoto S, Oshima A, Abe S, et al. (2005) Clinical features of patients with GJB2 (connexin 26) mutations: severity of hearing loss is correlated with genotypes and protein expression patterns. J Hum Genet 50: 76–83.
10. Fukushima K, Sugata K, Kasai N, Fukuda S, Nagayasu R, et al. (2002) Better speech performance in cochlear implant patients with GJB2-related deafness. Int J Pediatr Otorhinolaryngol 62: 151–157.
11. Abe S, Usami S, Shinkawa H (1997) Three familial cases of hearing loss associated with enlargement of the vestibular aqueduct. Ann Otol Rhinol Laryngol 106: 1063–1069.
12. Suzuki H, Oshima A, Tsukamoto K, Abe S, Kumakawa K, et al. (2000) Clinical characteristics and genotype-phenotype correlation of hearing loss patients with SLC26A4 mutations. Acta Otolaryngol 127: 1292–1297.
13. Azaiez H, Chamberlin GP, Fischer SM, Welp CL, Prasad SD, et al. (2004) GJB2: the spectrum of deafness-causing allele variants and their phenotype. Hum Mutat 24: 305–311.
14. Tsukamoto K, Suzuki H, Harada D, Namba A, Abe S, et al. (2003) Distribution and frequencies of PDS (SLC26A4) mutations in Pendred syndrome and nonsyndromic hearing loss associated with enlarged vestibular aqueduct: a unique spectrum of mutations in Japanese. Eur J Hum Genet 11: 916–922.
15. Kimberling WJ (2005) Estimation of the frequency of occult mutations for an autosomal recessive disease in the presence of genetic heterogeneity: application to genetic hearing loss disorders. Hum Mutat 26: 462–470.
16. Yang T, Vidarsson H, Rodrigo-Blomqvist S, Rosengren SS, Enerback S, et al. (2007) Transcriptional control of SLC26A4 is involved in Pendred syndrome and nonsyndromic enlargement of vestibular aqueduct (DFNB4). Am J Hum Genet Jun; 80(6): 1055–1063.
17. Usami S, Abe S, Kasai M, Shinkawa H, Moeller B, et al. (1997) Genetic and clinical features of sensorineural hearing loss associated with the 1555 mitochondrial mutation. Laryngoscope 107: 483–490.
18. Usami S, Abe S, Akita J, Namba A, Shinkawa H, et al. (2000) Prevalence of mitochondrial gene mutations among hearing impaired patients. J Med Genet 37: 38–40.
19. Goto Y, Nonaka I, Horai S (1990) A mutation in the tRNA(Leu)(UUR) gene associated with the MELAS subgroup of mitochondrial encephalomyopathies. Nature Dec 13;348(6302): 651–653.
20. Kadowaki T, Kadowaki H, Mori Y, Tobe K, Sakuta R, et al. (1994) A subtype of diabetes mellitus associated with a mutation of mitochondrial DNA. N Engl J Med Apr 7;330(14): 962–968.
21. den Ouweland JM, Lemkes HH, Ruitenbeek W, Sandkuijl LA, de Vijlder MF, et al. (1992) Mutation in mitochondrial tRNA(Leu)(UUR) gene in a large pedigree with maternally transmitted type II diabetes mellitus and deafness. Nat Genet 1992 Aug;1(5): 368–371.
22. Oshima T, Ueda N, Ikeda K, Abe K, Takasaka T (1996) Bilateral sensorineural hearing loss associated with the point mutation in mitochondrial genome. Laryngoscope Jan; 106(1 Pt 1): 43–48.

6

Failure of Fluid Absorption in the Endolymphatic Sac Initiates Cochlear Enlargement that Leads to Deafness in Mice Lacking *Pendrin* Expression

Hyoung-Mi Kim, Philine Wangemann*

Anatomy and Physiology Department, Kansas State University, Manhattan, Kansas, United States of America

Abstract

Mutations of *SLC26A4* are among the most prevalent causes of hereditary deafness. Deafness in the corresponding mouse model, *Slc26a4*$^{-/-}$, results from an abnormally enlarged cochlear lumen. The goal of this study was to determine whether the cochlear enlargement originates with defective cochlear fluid transport or with a malfunction of fluid transport in the connected compartments, which are the vestibular labyrinth and the endolymphatic sac. Embryonic inner ears from *Slc26a4*$^{+/-}$ and *Slc26a4*$^{-/-}$ mice were examined by confocal microscopy *ex vivo* or after 2 days of organ culture. Culture allowed observations of intact, ligated or partially resected inner ears. Cochlear lumen formation was found to begin at the base of the cochlea between embryonic day (E) 13.5 and 14.5. Enlargement was immediately evident in *Slc26a4*$^{-/-}$ compared to *Slc26a4*$^{+/-}$ mice. In *Slc26a4*$^{+/-}$ and *Slc26a4*$^{-/-}$ mice, separation of the cochlea from the vestibular labyrinth by ligation at E14.5 resulted in a reduced cochlear lumen. Resection of the endolymphatic sacs at E14.5 led to an enlarged cochlear lumen in *Slc26a4*$^{+/-}$ mice but caused no further enlargement of the already enlarged cochlear lumen in *Slc26a4*$^{-/-}$ mice. Ligation or resection performed later, at E17.5, did not alter the cochlea lumen. In conclusion, the data suggest that cochlear lumen formation is initiated by fluid secretion in the vestibular labyrinth and temporarily controlled by fluid absorption in the endolymphatic sac. Failure of fluid absorption in the endolymphatic sac due to lack of *Slc26a4* expression appears to initiate cochlear enlargement in mice, and possibly humans, lacking functional *Slc26a4* expression.

Editor: Noam Cohen, Hospital of the University of Pennsylvania, United States of America

Funding: NIH R01 DC01098; NIH R01 DC00212; NIH P20 RR017686; SMILE-Kansas State University. The funders had no role in study design, data collection and analysis, decision to publish, or preparation of the manuscript.

Competing Interests: The authors have declared that no competing interests exist.

* E-mail: wange@vet.ksu.edu

Introduction

Mutations of *SLC26A4* are worldwide among the most prevalent causes of deafness [1,2,3,4]. Particularly in Chinese populations, mutations of *SLC26A4* are found in as many as 13.7% of deaf subjects [5]. Phenotypes associated with mutations of *SLC26A4* include deafness at birth as well as fluctuating hearing loss that progresses toward deafness during childhood [6,7,8]. The compatibility of *SLC26A4* mutations with hearing, although limited to early childhood, provides the imperative to investigate the etiology of *SLC26A4* related deafness with the ultimate goal to develop strategies to preserve hearing in afflicted individuals. Toward this goal, the first mouse model, *Slc26a4*$^{-/-}$ (formerly named *Pds*$^{-/-}$), had been developed [9]. Studies using this mouse model have mainly focused on the postnatal development since normal mice acquire hearing during the second postnatal week and since most human patients lose hearing during early childhood. Three synergistic pathophysiological pathways have so far been delineated.

1) Lack of pendrin, the protein coded for by the gene *Slc26a4*, leads to a ~10-fold enlargement of scala media [9,10]. Scala media, is an endolymph-filled luminal space that is lined by the cochlear epithelium, which includes both the sensory hair cells as well as stria vascularis (Fig. 1A). Stria vascularis secretes K^+ into endolymph and generates the endocochlear potential that provides the majority of the driving force for the sensory transduction, which occurs in the hair cells. Enlargement of scala media leads to hampered cell-to-cell communication and disruption of development toward hearing [10].

2) The enlargement of scala media forces stria vascularis in the postnatal cochlea to elevate rates of K^+ secretion in order to maintain a normal endolymphatic K^+ concentration [11]. Oxidative stress ensues from increased transport and leads to a loss of the K^+ channel *Kcnj10*, which generates the endocochlear potential [12,13,14]. Loss of *Kcnj10* leads to a loss of the endocochlear potential and thereby of the driving force necessary for hearing.

3) The enlargement of scala media and the associated elevated rates of K^+ secretion lead to an enhanced metabolic acid production by marginal cells of stria vascularis that is partially released into endolymph. Acid release into endolymph in conjunction with a loss of pendrin-mediated HCO_3^- secretion lead to a luminal acidification by ~0.3 pH-units [12]. Acid-mediated inhibition of Ca^{2+} absorption results in a ~100-fold elevation in the endolymphatic Ca^{2+} concentration in *Slc26a4*$^{-/-}$ mice compared to *Slc26a4*$^{+/-}$ mice [12]. Excessive Ca^{2+} concentrations in endolymph impair sensory transduction by damaging outer hair cells through excessive Ca^{2+} influx via the apical transduction channel and subsequent cellular Ca^{2+} overload [9,15].

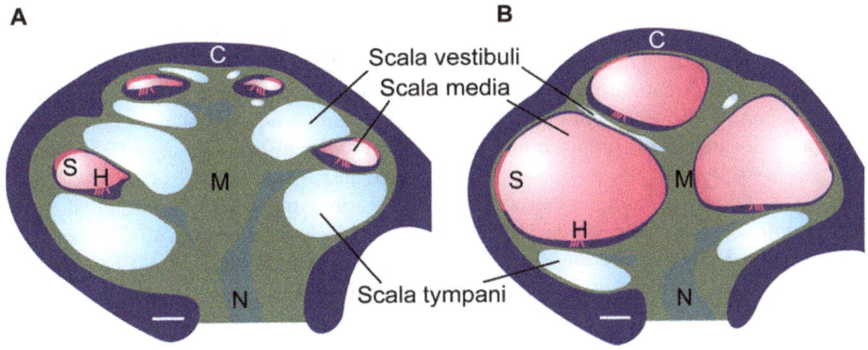

Figure 1. Schematic diagram of the cochlea. A) Diagram based on a cochlea obtained from an E18.5 *Slc26a4*$^{+/-}$ mouse. B) Diagram based on a cochlea obtained from an E18.5 *Slc26a4*$^{-/-}$ mouse, see Fig. 3. Abbreviations: C, otic capsule; S, stria vascularis; H, sensory hair cells; M, modiolus; N, cochlear nerve. Note, that spaces occupied by mesenchymal cell (green) are compressed in *Slc26a4*$^{-/-}$ mice. Particular, fibrocytes in the modiolus (M) and between the otic capsule (C) and stria vascularis (S) are displaced.

From these studies in the mouse model, it is evident that the enlargement of scala media is a key event in the etiology of deafness. Most likely, the enlargement is due to a dysfunction of epithelial fluid transport, since *Slc26a4* codes for pendrin, which is an epithelial anion exchanger and since the enlargement occurs shortly after the onset of expression [9]. Conceptually, the enlargement could be the result of a net increase in fluid secretion or decrease in absorption. Pendrin itself does not mediate net solute transport, since it transports anions with a stoichiometry of 1:1 [16]. Whether and how pendrin contributes to fluid secretion or absorption is unknown. This question is complicated by two issues:

First, virtually nothing is known about ion and fluid transport in the embryonic cochlea, which is when the enlargement develops. The adult ion composition, characterized by a high K^+ concentration and low Na^+ and Ca^{2+} concentrations, is established during postnatal development [12,17,18]. This means that investigations of ion transport in the postnatal cochlea cannot be extrapolated to the early embryonic stage when the cochlear lumen first develops.

Second, the epithelial enlargement in *Slc26a4*$^{-/-}$ mice is not limited to the cochlea. The vestibular labyrinth and the endolymphatic sac are prominently enlarged, too [9]. Interestingly, these compartments are connected to the cochlea and each contains pendrin-expressing epithelial cells. The role of pendrin in fluid transport may be different in the different compartments and it is conceivable that one compartment 'pumps up' or 'drains' the others. Thus, the goal of the present study was to determine the onset of cochlear enlargement and to investigate whether the enlargement of the cochlea in *Slc26a4*$^{-/-}$ mice is due to a local cochlear dysfunction or whether the cochlear enlargement is caused by dysfunction of the adjacent vestibular labyrinth or endolymphatic sac.

Methods

Animals

A colony of *Slc26a4*$^{-/-}$ and *Slc26a4*$^{+/-}$ mice was maintained at Kansas State University. Pairs of *Slc26a4*$^{+/-}$ dams and *Slc26a4*$^{-/-}$ sires were housed together. Litters sizes averaged 5.1 pups with *Slc26a4*$^{+/-}$ and *Slc26a4*$^{-/-}$ offspring in the Mendelian ratio of 50.1 to 49.9. The gestational period was 21 days. Genetic drift was limited by occasional back-crossing to the original strain, 129SvEvTac, that is maintained by Taconic, Germantown, NY. The colony was maintained free of known and suspected murine pathogens. Serologic tests (Radil, Columbia, MO), that were consistently and repeatedly negative, included the following antibodies: EDIM (Epizootic diarrhea of infant mice virus - a mouse rotavirus), TMEV (Theiler's murine encephalomyelitis virus - mouse poliovirus, strain GDVII), MHV (Mouse hepatitis virus - a mouse coronavirus), MVM (Minute virus of mice - a mouse parvovirus), MNV (Murine norovirus - a mouse calicivirus), M. pulmonis (Mycoplasma pulmonis – the agent of murine mycoplasmosis), MPV (a mouse parvovirus), Parvo NS-1 (a conserved recombinant parvoviral protein, rNS1) and Sendai (Sendai virus – a type 1 paramyxovirus).

Slc26a4$^{+/-}$ and *Slc26a4*$^{-/-}$ mice ranging from E11.5 to P7 were used for the present study. Time-pregnant dams were deeply anesthetized with 4% tri-bromo-ethanol and sacrificed by decapitation after harvesting embryos by sterile laparotomy. Gestational age was counted from the day, when a vaginal plug was detected. This day was set to embryonic (E) day 0.5 (E0.5). Gestational age, however, was verified, and in rare cases corrected, by evaluating gross morphological features including limbs, digits, and appearance of the pinna and auditory meatus [19,20]. Neonatal mice (P0-P3) were anesthetized by a combination of i.p. injection of 0.013 ml/g body weight of 4% tri-bromo-ethanol and rapid cooling on an ice slush. Older mice (P5-P7) were anesthetized solely by i.p. injection of 0.013 ml/g body weight of 4% tri-bromo-ethanol. Embryos and postnatal mice were sacrificed by decapitation. All procedures involving animals were approved by the Institutional Animal Care and Use Committee of Kansas State University (IACUC#: 2613).

Organ culture

Procedures for organ culture were adapted with modifications from methods developed by Dr. Thomas van de Water [21]. Embryos were harvested at E14.5 and E17.5. Otocysts were isolated in sterile NaCl solution maintained at 4°C. NaCl solution contained (in mM) 150 NaCl, 5 HEPES, 3.6 KCl, 1 $CaCl_2$, 1 $MgCl_2$ and 5 glucose, pH 7.4. The cranium was opened medially and otocysts were isolated after removal of the cerebrum.

Otocysts were left intact or altered either by ligation of the vestibular labyrinth or by resection of the endolymphatic sac. One otocyst from each embryo was left intact and the other was altered to facilitate paired comparisons. In one set of experiments, the cochlea was isolated from the vestibular labyrinth by ligation. Otocysts were isolated and tied at the base of the cochlea with a braided silk surgical suture (size 10-0, Deknatel, Queens Village, NY). After tying off the cochlea, the vestibular part of the otocyst, including the endolymphatic sac, was cut away from the isolated cochlear preparation. In another set of experiments, the endolymphatic sac was removed by resection. The endolymphatic sac was carefully peeled off the otocyst. Great care was taken in this set of experiments to not injure the endolymphatic sac, particularly the distal end, which is located in the posterior cranial fossa within the dura.

Otocysts, altered or intact, were maintained in organ culture for two days. Otocysts were placed into 12-well plates (Cat# 353503, Fisher, St. Louis, MO), submersed in DMEM/F-12 media (Cat# 12500-062, Invitrogen, Carlsbad, CA) supplemented with 10% fetal bovine serum (Cat# 30-2020, ATCC, Waldorf, MD) and 1% penicillin-streptomycin (Cat# 15140-122, Invitrogen) and incubated at 37°C in a humidified atmosphere enriched with 5% CO_2 (HeraCell 240, Heraeus, Germany). Media was changed every 24 hrs.

Confocal immunocytochemistry

Freshly isolated or cultured otocysts were fixed at 4°C for 2 hrs in a solution containing (in mM) 150 NaCl, 3.6 KCl, 5 HEPES, 1 $CaCl_2$, 1 $MgCl_2$ and 5 glucose, pH 7.4 and 4% paraformaldehyde. Fixed otocysts were processed through a sucrose gradient (10% and 20%, each 20 min, followed by 30% overnight, all at 4°C), infiltrated with polyethylene glycol (Cat# 72592-B, Electron Microscopy Sciences, Hatfield, PA) and cryo-sectioned (12 μm, CM3050S, Leica, Germany). Serial sections throughout the entire cochlea were obtained from embryos between ages E11.5 and E14.5 and mid-modiolar sections of the cochlea were obtained from embryos between ages E15.5 and E18.5 and from neonates aged P3.

Sections mounted on charged slides (Cat#22-230-900, Fisher) were blocked for 1 hr with 5% bovine serum albumin (BSA) in PBS-TX containing (in mM) 137 NaCl, 2.7 KCl, 10.1 Na_2HPO_4, 1.8 KH_2PO_4, pH 7.4, and 0.2% Triton-X-100. For morphological observations, sections were stained for actin filaments (Alexa488 conjugated phalloidin, Invitrogen) and for nuclei (DAPI, Invitrogen). Slides were incubated for 1 hr at room temperature with phalloidin and DAPI diluted with PBS-TX at 1:40 and 1:1,000, respectively. For immunocytochemistry, slides were incubated overnight at 4°C with primary antibody (rabbit anti-Na^+/K^+ ATPase 1 alpha subunit, Novus Biologicals, Littleton, CO) diluted 1:200 with PBS-TX containing 1–3% BSA. Slides were washed three times in PBS-TX and incubated for 1 hr at room temperature with secondary antibody (Alexa594 conjugated goat-anti-rabbit (Invitrogen) diluted 1:1,000 with PBS-TX containing 1–3% BSA. Stains for actin filaments (Alexa488 conjugat-

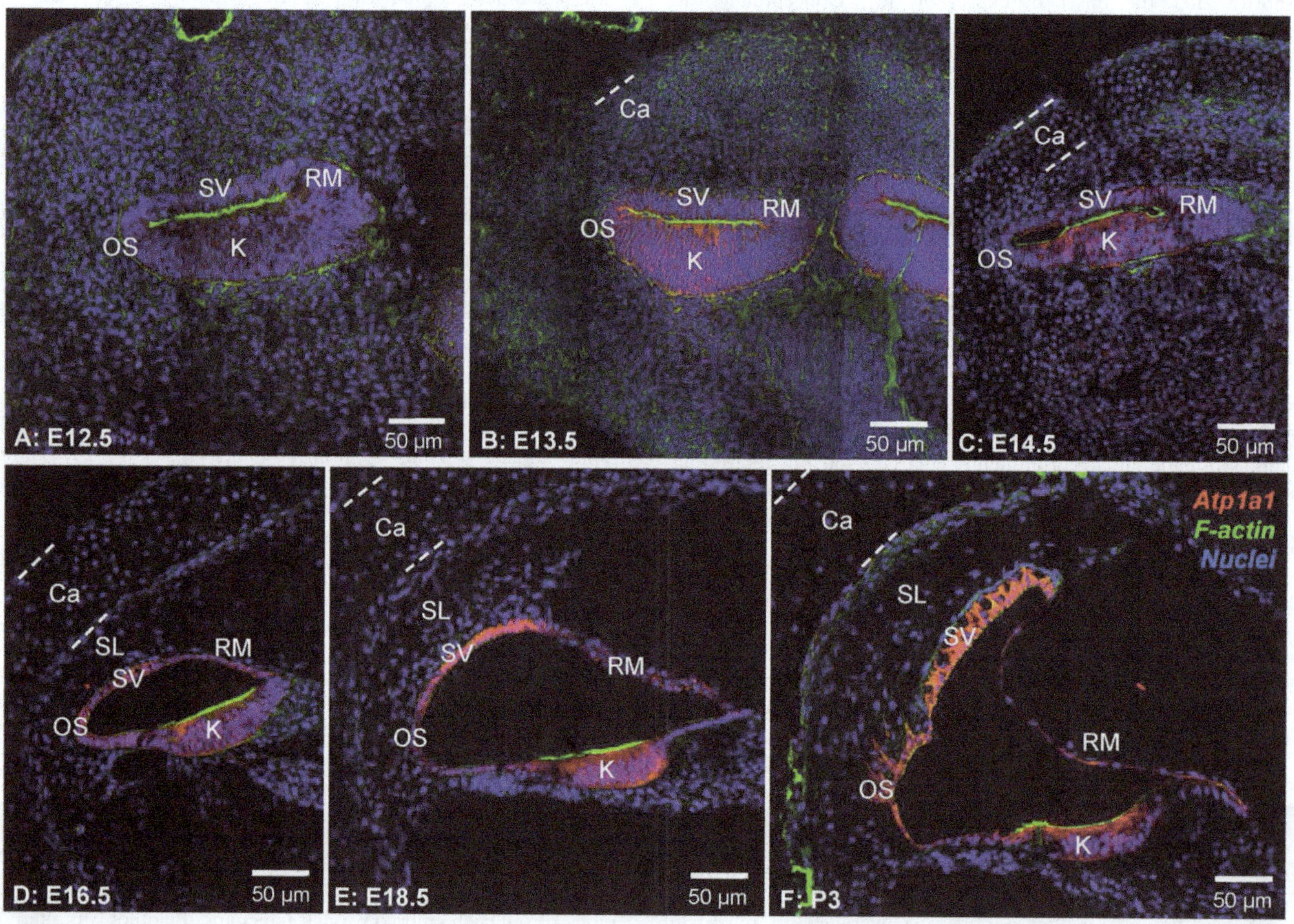

Figure 2. Cochlear development from E12.5 to P3 in *Slc26a4*$^{+/-}$ mice. Na^+/K^+ ATPase (red) was visualized by immunocytochemistry. F-actin (green) and nuclei (blue) were labeled. A-F: Six different stages of development ranging from E12.5 to P3 are shown. Abbreviations: SV, stria vascularis; OS, outer sulcus; K, Kölliker's organ; RM, Reissner's membrane; Ca, otic capsule; SL, spiral ligament. The thickness of the otic capsule is marked by dashed lines.

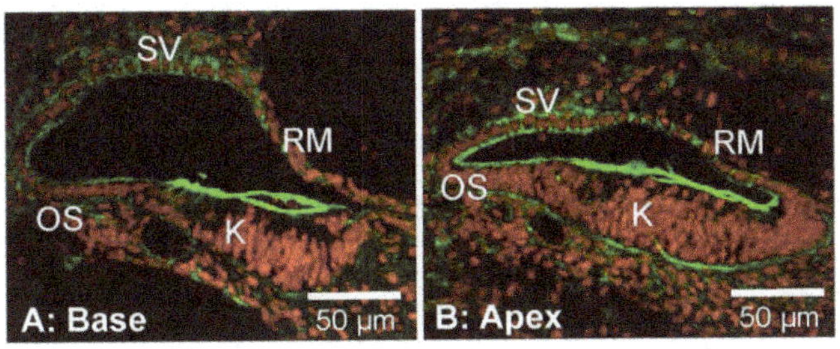

Figure 3. Cochlear lumen formation progressed from the base to the apex. A: Base of the cochlea. B: Apex of the same cochlea. F-actin (green) and nuclei (red) were labeled. Abbreviations: SV, stria vascularis; OS, outer sulcus; K, Kölliker's organ; RM, Reissner's membrane.

ed phalloidin (Invitrogen) and for nuclei (DAPI) were added to the secondary antibody at dilutions 1:40 and 1:1,000, respectively. After staining, slides were washed three times with PBS-TX, cover-slipped with FluorSave (Calbiochem, La Jolla, CA) and observed by confocal laser scanning microscopy (LSM 510 Meta, Carl Zeiss, Göttingen, Germany). The size of the cochlear lumen was evaluated by digital area measurements using image analysis software (Carl Zeiss).

Statistics

Data are generally presented as average ± sem with n being the number of animals. Data acquired in paired experiments using littermates were evaluated by paired t-test. Significance was assumed when $p<0.05$.

Results

Cochlear lumen formation

In a first set of experiments, we determined the onset of lumen formation in the cochlea. Inner ears ranging from embryonic (E) day E12.5 to postnatal (P) day P3 were sectioned and examined by confocal microscopy. At E12.5 and E13.5, the cochlear duct consisted of a closed epithelial tube (Fig. 2). Köllikers organ, the precursor of the organ of Corti, was evident on the basal side of

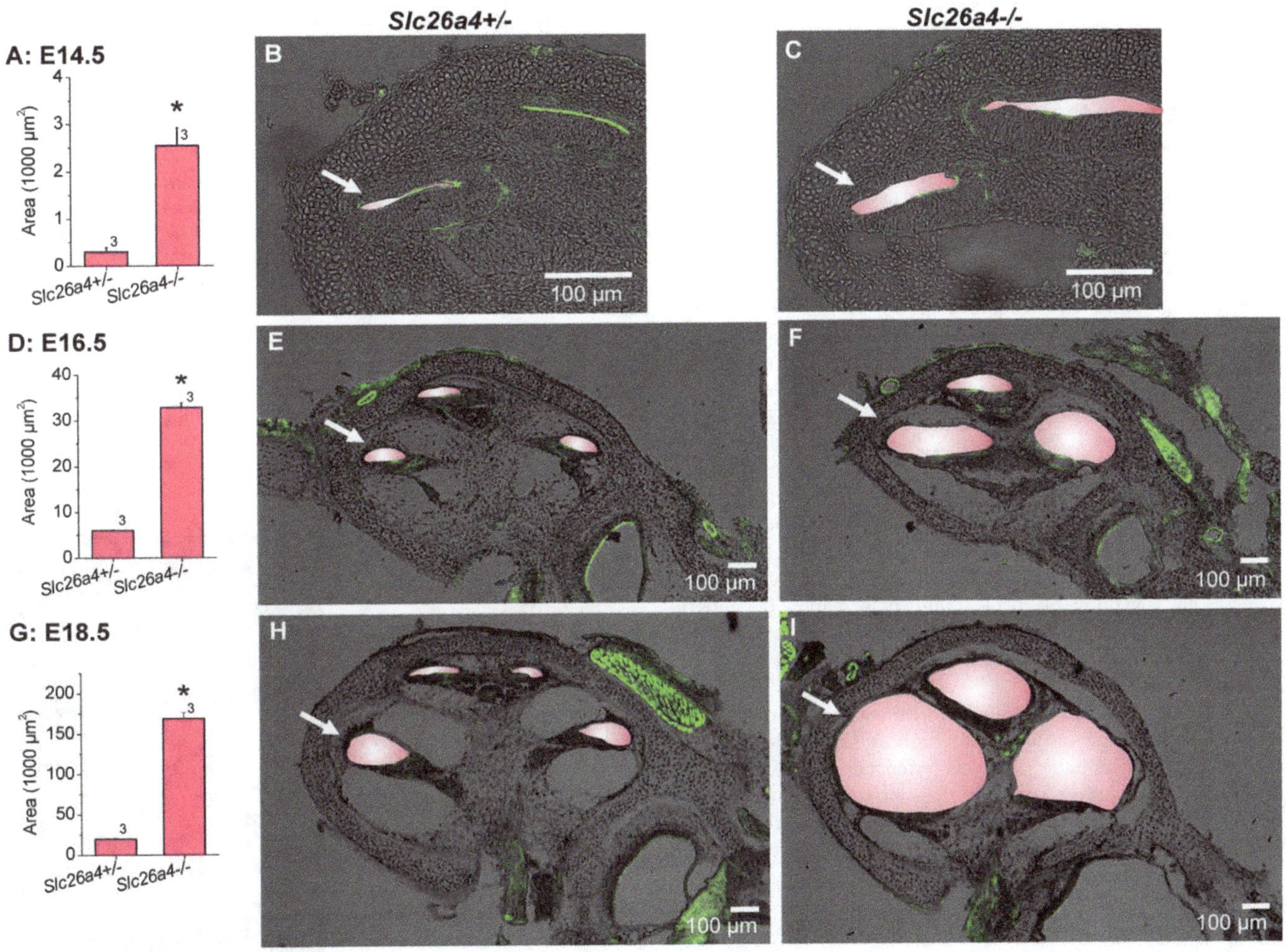

Figure 4. Cochlear lumen formation in *Slc26a4*$^{+/-}$ and *Slc26a4*$^{-/-}$ mice. A, D and G: Luminal area measurements of cross-section #1 in cochleae obtained from E14.5, E16.5 and E18.5 littermates, respectively. The number next to the bars represents the N number of animals. Significant differences are marked (*). B and C, cochlear cross-sections of E14.5 *Slc26a4*$^{+/-}$ and *Slc26a4*$^{-/-}$ littermates. E and F, cochlear cross-sections of E16.5 *Slc26a4*$^{+/-}$ and *Slc26a4*$^{-/-}$ littermates. H and I, cochlear cross-sections of E18.5 *Slc26a4*$^{+/-}$ and *Slc26a4*$^{-/-}$ littermates. Scala media was highlighted in pink. Images without the pink overlay are available in Figure S1 (Supporting information). Arrows point to cross-section #1, which was used for digital area measurements. F-actin (green) was labeled. Cochlear cross-sections were imaged by laser-scanning microscopy.

the epithelial tube as a multilayered epithelium with an actin-rich region near the apical membrane. Köllikers organ was clearly distinct from the precursors of stria vascularis, outer sulcus and Reissner's membrane. At E13.5, the otic capsule was beginning to form. At E14.5, a clear distinction became evident between chondrocytes comprising the otic capsule and mesenchymal cells surrounding the cochlear epithelium. Further, the cochlear epithelium began to form a lumen. Around E16.5, the characteristic triangular cross section of the cochlea began to develop. At E18.5, stria vascularis began to differentiate from a monolayer to the multi-layered architecture including the characteristic vascularization. Lumen formation progressed from the base to the apex of the cochlea (Fig. 3).

Cochlear enlargement occurs prior to cochlear *Slc26a4* expression

In a second set of experiments, we compared the onset of cochlear lumen formation in *Slc26a4*$^{+/-}$ and *Slc26a4*$^{-/-}$ mice and monitored the progression of the enlargement between E14.5 and ~P4.5. Lumen formation at E14.5 was advanced in *Slc26a4*$^{-/-}$ mice compared to *Slc26a4*$^{+/-}$ littermates (Fig. 4). The cochlear lumen increased with development in *Slc26a4*$^{+/-}$ and *Slc26a4*$^{-/-}$ mice (Fig. 5). The ratio between the luminal size in *Slc26a4*$^{+/-}$ and *Slc26a4*$^{-/-}$ increase from factor 6 at E16.5 to factor 12 at E18.5.

Fluid secretion in the vestibular labyrinth 'pumps up' the cochlea during lumen formation

In a third series of experiments, we determined whether the vestibular labyrinth contributes to cochlear lumen formation. Embryonic inner ears were harvested at E14.5, which is at the onset of lumen formation, and later, at E17.5. The endolymphatic sac was removed and the cochlea was separated from the vestibular labyrinth by ligation (Fig. 6). To ensure complete isolation of the cochlea from the vestibular labyrinth, the latter was removed micro-surgically after ligation. Ligated and non-ligated inner ears were maintained in organ culture for two days, then sectioned and examined by confocal microscopy. Scala media of inner ears harvested at E14.5 from *Slc26a4*$^{+/-}$ mice was found to be significantly smaller in ligated compared to non-ligated preparations (Fig. 7). Similar observations were made in inner ears harvested at E14.5 from *Slc26a4*$^{-/-}$ mice. In contrast, no difference in the size of scala media was found between ligated and non-ligated inner ears harvested at E17.5. These observations suggest that the onset of cochlear lumen formation depends in *Slc26a4*$^{+/-}$ and *Slc26a4*$^{-/-}$ mice on fluid secretion by the vestibular labyrinth. This dependency is transient and was found to be lost at E17.5.

Ligation of the vestibular labyrinth can be expected to isolate the cochlea from the vestibular labyrinth and the endolymphatic sac. The endolymphatic sac was removed in this series of experiments to avoid variations in the preparations due to injury of this extremely fragile structure. The question, whether the endolymphatic sac affects the cochlear lumen was addressed in the next series of experiments.

Fluid absorption in the endolymphatic sac 'drains' the cochlea during lumen formation

In a fourth series of experiments, we determined whether the endolymphatic sac contributes to cochlear lumen formation. Embryonic inner ears were again harvested at E14.5 and E17.5. Great care was taken to not injure the endolymphatic sac during dissection. The endolymphatic sac was then removed by manual resection (Fig. 8). Resected and non-resected inner ears were maintained in organ culture for two day, then sectioned and examined by confocal microscopy. The cochlear lumen of inner ears harvested at E14.5 from *Slc26a4*$^{+/-}$ mice was found to be

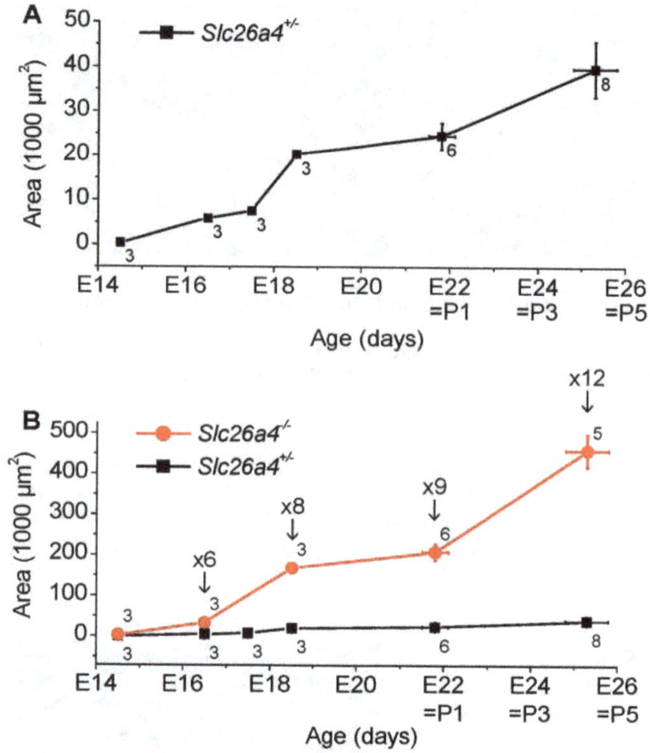

Figure 5. Cochlear lumen development in *Slc26a4*$^{+/-}$ and *Slc26a4*$^{-/-}$ mice. A, lumen development in *Slc26a4*$^{+/-}$ mice. B, lumen development in *Slc26a4*$^{-/-}$ mice. Numbers next to symbols represent the N number of *Slc26a4*$^{+/-}$ and *Slc26a4*$^{-/-}$ littermates. Figure preceded by 'x' indicate the factor between measurements in *Slc26a4*$^{+/-}$ and *Slc26a4*$^{-/-}$ littermates.

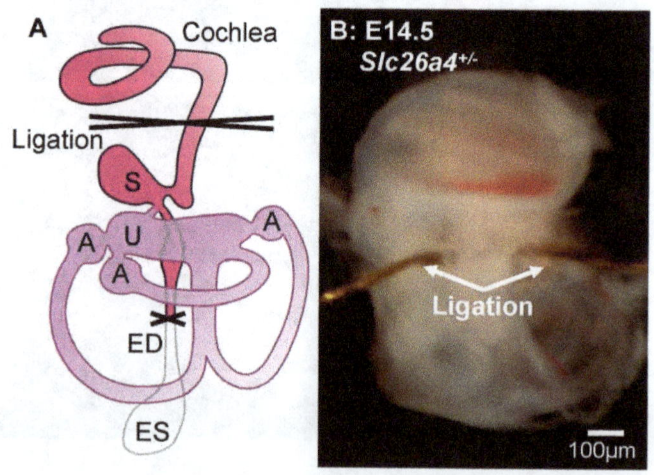

Figure 6. Isolation of the cochlea from the vestibular labyrinth by ligation. A: Diagram of the inner ear. Abbreviations: S, saccule; U, utricle; A, Ampulla; ED, endolymphatic duct; ES, endolymphatic sac. B: Photograph of a ligated inner ear obtained from an E14.5 *Slc26a4*$^{+/-}$ mouse.

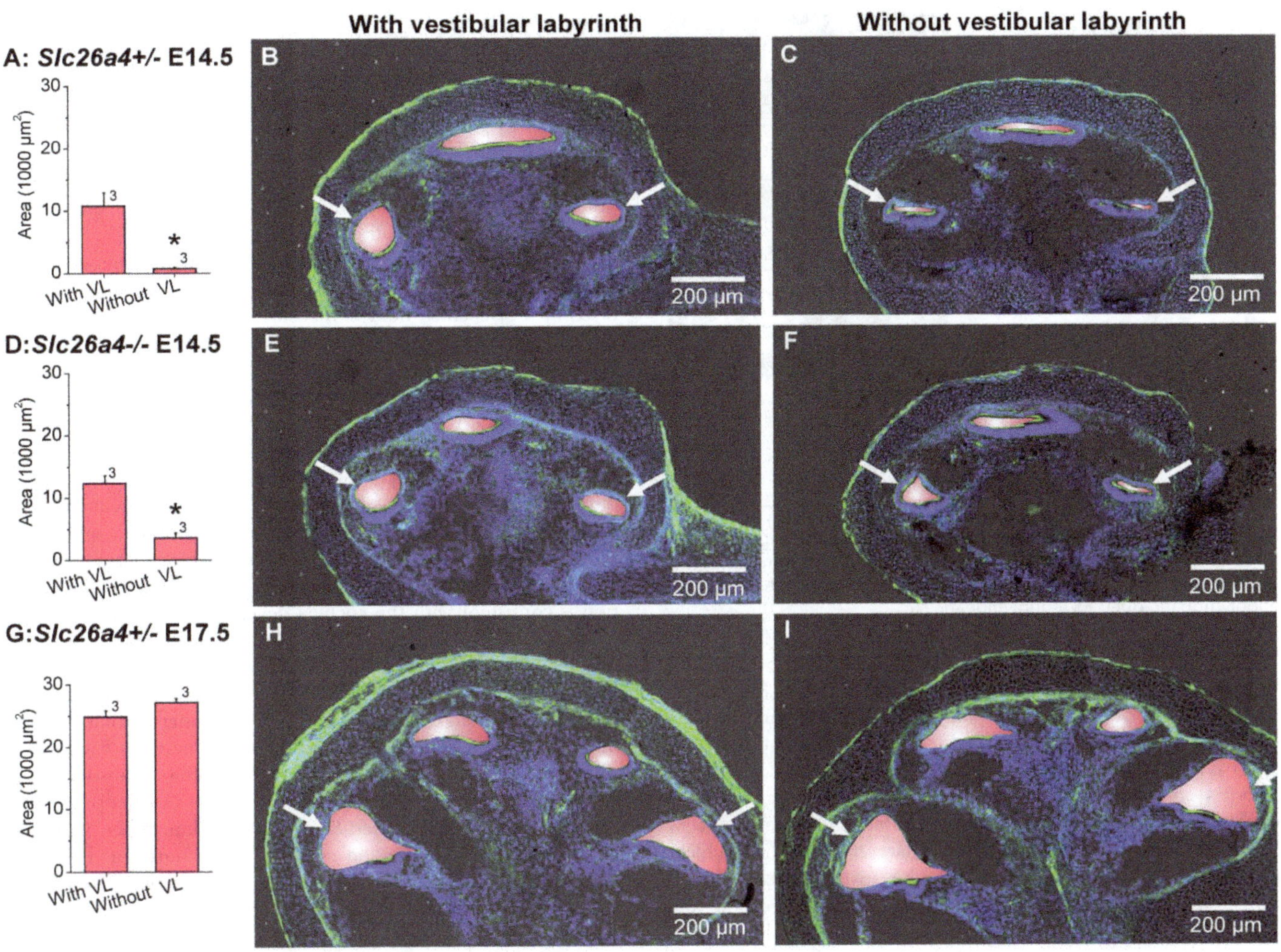

Figure 7. Fluid secretion in the vestibular labyrinth 'pumps up' the cochlea during lumen formation. A, D and G: Luminal area measurements (average of the two basal cross-sections) in cochleae with and without vestibular labyrinth. Cochleae were harvested at E14.5 and E17.5 from *Slc26a4*$^{+/-}$ and *Slc26a4*$^{-/-}$ mice and maintained two days in organ culture. The number next to the bars represents the N number of animals. Significant differences are marked (*). B and C, cochlear cross-sections of E14.5 *Slc26a4*$^{+/-}$ mice with and without vestibular labyrinth. E and F, cochlear cross-sections of E14.5 *Slc26a4*$^{-/-}$ mice with and without vestibular labyrinth. H and I, cochlear cross-sections of E17.5 *Slc26a4*$^{+/-}$ mice with and without vestibular labyrinth. Scala media was highlighted in pink. Images without the pink overlay are available in Figure S1 (Supporting information). F-actin (green) and nuclei (blue) were labeled. Cochlear cross-sections were imaged by laser-scanning microscopy. Arrows point to the two basal cross-sections, which were used for digital area measurements.

significantly larger in resected compared to non-resected inner ears (Fig. 9). In contrast, the cochlear lumen of inner ears harvested at E14.5 from *Slc26a4*$^{-/-}$ mice was enlarged and no difference was apparent between resected and non-resected inner ears. Further, no difference in the cochlear lumina were found between resected and non-resected inner ears harvested at E17.5. These observations suggest that the onset of cochlear lumen formation is controlled in *Slc26a4*$^{+/-}$ mice by fluid absorption in the endolymphatic sac. This control is transient and found to be lost at E17.5. The observed enlargement in *Slc26a4*$^{-/-}$ suggests that loss of *Slc26a4* expression impairs fluid absorption in the endolymphatic sac.

Discussion

The most salient findings of this study are 1) that lumen formation begins between E13.5 and E14.5 at the base of the cochlea, 2) that the cochlea lumen is transiently, prior to E17.5, controlled by fluid secretion in the vestibular labyrinth and absorption in the endolymphatic sac and 3) that loss of pendrin expression leads to an enlargement of the cochlear lumen that is similar to the enlargement caused by resection of the endolymphatic sac.

The inner ear develops from an invagination of the ectoderm that forms a vesicular otocyst [22]. At ~E10.5, two protrusions begin to extend from the otocyst; one forms the cochlea and the other forms the endolymphatic sac. While the protrusions elongate and coil, in case of the cochlea, the center of the otocyst reorganizes into the vestibular labyrinth. Pendrin is an anion exchanger that is prominently expressed in the cochlea, the vestibular labyrinth and the endolymphatic sac. In the postnatal cochlea, pendrin is expressed in a spiraling sheet of outer sulcus and spindle cells located in the lateral wall [14]. In the vestibular labyrinth, pendrin is expressed in sheets of transitional cells that surround sensory cell patches, and in the endolymphatic sac, pendrin is expressed in mitochondrial-rich cells that are

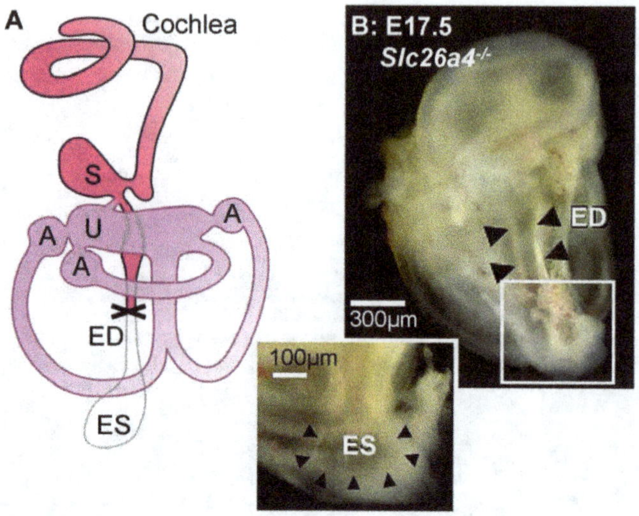

Figure 8. Resection of the endolymphatic sac. A: Diagram of the inner ear. B: Photograph of an inner ear obtained from an E17.5 *Slc26a4*$^{-/-}$ mouse. Abbreviations: S, saccule; U, utricle; A, Ampulla; ED, endolymphatic duct; ES, endolymphatic sac.

interspersed among the principal ribosomal-rich cells [11,14,23]. The onset of pendrin expression differs among the different compartments of the inner ear. In the endolymphatic sac the onset is at E13 and in the vestibular labyrinth and the cochlea at E15 [24]. A dysfunction of fluid transport due to a lack of pendrin expression can be expected to occur after but is not likely to occur before the onset of expression. The enlargement of the cochlear lumen at E14.5 is therefore unlikely due to local cochlear fluid transport. The relationship been the onset of expression and the onset of cochlear enlargement suggests an involvement of the endolymphatic sac. A reduction in fluid absorption in the endolymphatic sac presents a conceivable reason for the enlargement of the cochlear lumen. This view is supported by the finding that resection of the endolymphatic sac in *Slc26a4*$^{+/-}$ mice led to an enlargement similar to that observed in *Slc26a4*$^{-/-}$ mice.

The concept that the endolymphatic sac is engaged in fluid absorption is not new although a direct, *in vitro*, demonstration of fluid absorption is so far lacking. Indirect evidence for an absorptive function comes from the observation that anoxia leads to a rise in the luminal Na^+ and Cl^- concentrations [25,26] and that obliteration of the endolymphatic sac in adult guinea pigs to an enlargement of the cochlear lumen [27]. Investigations of the endolymphatic sac are hampered by the difficulty of access and the heterogeneity of the epithelium, which consists principally of ribosome-rich cells with interspersed mitochondrial-rich cells [28]. Nevertheless, a number of ion transporters have been identified. These include apical Na^+ channels [29,30], apical H^+ ATPase subunits [23,31,32], basolateral Na^+/K^+ ATPases [33], basolateral Na^+/H^+ exchangers [34,35] and apical as well as basolateral Cl^-/HCO_3^- exchangers including pendrin [11,23,31]. The epithelium generates a lumen-positive transepithelial potential that is sensitive to inhibition of Na^+ channels, H^+ ATPase, Cl^-/HCO_3^- exchangers, Na^+/H^+ exchangers and carbonic anhydrase [25,36]. It is intriguing to speculate that the heterogenic epithelium of the endolymphatic sac resembles a frog skin in that it engages in H^+ ATPase-driven Na^+ reabsorption. Frog skin is comprised of principal cells equipped with apical Na^+ channels and mitochondria-rich cells equipped with an apical H^+ ATPase and a Cl^-/HCO_3^- exchanger. Highly effective Na^+ absorption is powered by the H^+ ATPase, which generates a current that drives Na^+ absorption through the Na^+ channels [37]. The role of the Cl^-/HCO_3^- exchangers is this model is to export HCO_3^- that is generated by carbonic anhydrase in the process of generating H^+ as substrate for the H^+ ATPase (Fig. 10). Lack of the Cl^-/HCO_3^- exchanger pendrin would inhibit H^+ production by carbonic anhydrase through product-inhibition and a reduce the current that drives Na^+ reabsorption.

The observation that resection of the endolymphatic sac caused an enlargement at E14.5, but not at E17.5, is intriguing. The loss of control of cochlea fluid homeostasis by the endolymphatic sac may be the result of the maturation of local cochlear fluid homeostasis. Further, the capacity for Na^+ reabsorption in the endolymphatic sac may be higher at E14.5 than at E17. Support for this hypothesis comes from the finding that numbers of mRNA copies coding for the three subunits of the Na^+ channel ENaC decline from P2 to P6 of early postnatal development, which is ~4 days after E17 [29]. It is conceivable that this decline can be extrapolated to the embryonic phase of development.

Lumen formation was observed in the cochlea to progress from base to apex. A base-to-apex gradient in developmental maturation is consistent with the cochlea developing from an elongating protrusion of the otocyst, which implies that cells near the base are developmentally more mature than cells at the apex. Cochlear lumen formation could thus be due to a base-to-apex progressing onset of local fluid transport. Alternatively, lumen formation could be aided by the vestibular labyrinth, which matures earlier than the cochlea. For example, the onset of mechanotransduction in vestibular hair cells is at E17, which is ~4 days earlier than in the cochlea [38,39]. The observation that ligation of the vestibular labyrinth caused a reduction of the cochlear lumen at E14.5 but not at E17.5 suggests that cochlear lumen formation is transiently aided by fluid secretion in the vestibular labyrinth. Fluid secretion in the embryonic cochlea or vestibular labyrinth is poorly understood. Mechanism of ion transport, that are well established in the postnatal cochlea, cannot be extrapolated to the embryonic stage since the adult ion composition of the luminal fluid, which is characterized by a high K^+ concentration and low Na^+ and Ca^{2+} concentrations, is established only during postnatal development [12,17,18]. Nevertheless, the observation that ligation of the vestibular labyrinth led to a reduction in the cochlear lumen in *Slc26a4*$^{+/-}$ and *Slc26a4*$^{-/-}$ mice suggests that pendrin does not play a major role in fluid secretion in the embryonic vestibular labyrinth.

Studies in *Slc26a4*$^{-/-}$ mice have provided a basis to understand the spectrum of phenotypes seen in human patients that range from deafness at birth to deafness during childhood. Mice lacking pendrin have been shown to develop a ~10-fold enlargement of the cochlear lumen. This enlargement forms during embryonic development and persists throughout postnatal life [9,10,14].

During the developmental phase, the enlargement may disrupt cell-to-cell signaling that is necessary for the development of hearing. Gap junction mediated signaling between epithelial cells, for example, may be compromised by increased diffusional distances that are inherent to stretched epithelial cells enclosing an enlarged lumen (Fig. 1B). The importance of gap junction mediated cell signaling is underlined by the fact that loss-of-function mutations of the gap junction protein connexin 26 cause deafness at birth. Coincidentally, mutations of connexin 26 are the most frequent cause for non-syndromic hearing loss in children [40,41]. Further, the enlargement may disrupt signaling between mesenchymal and epithelial cells as shown in the early postnatal cochlea where mesenchymal cells generate thyroid hormone by

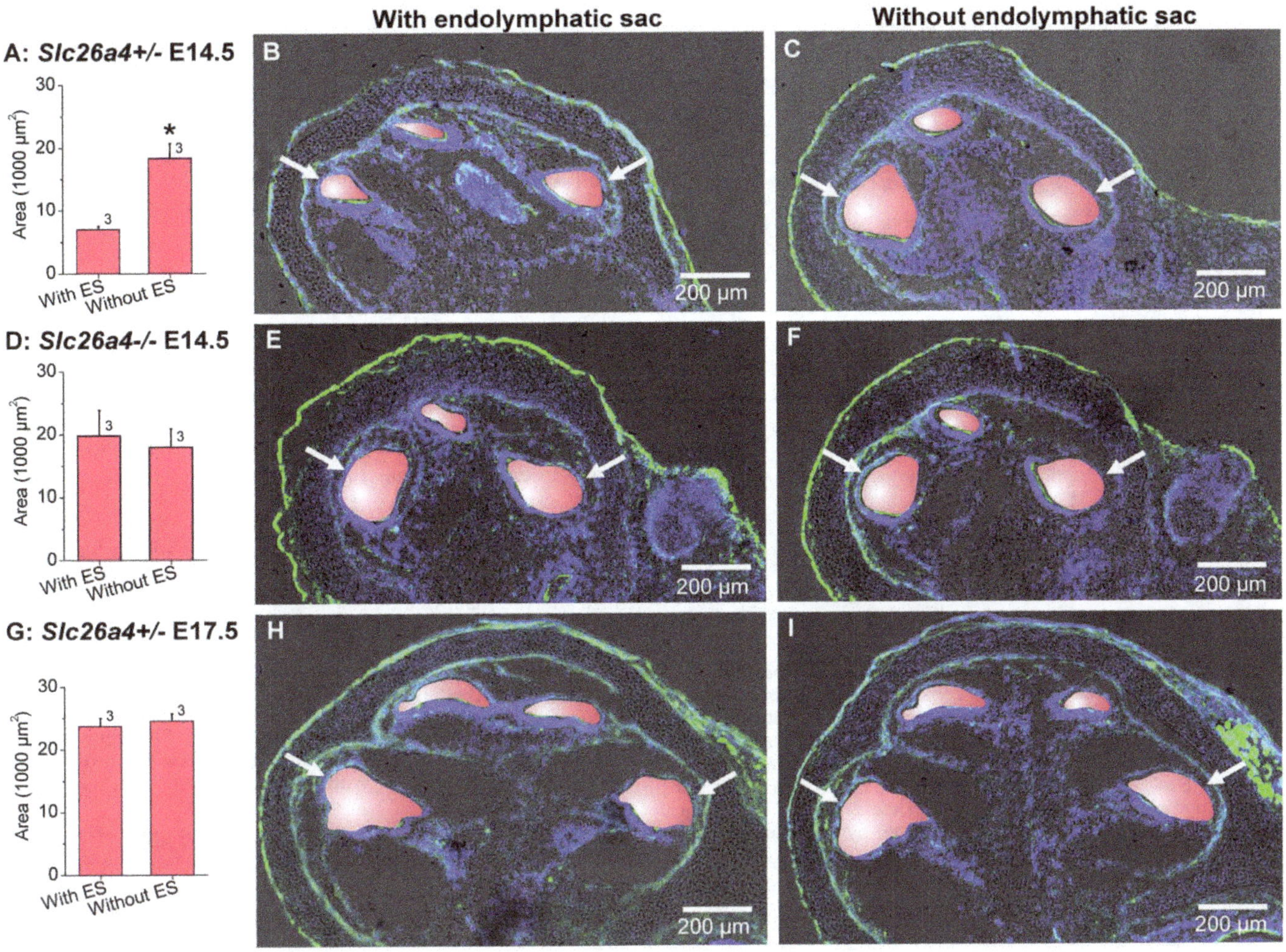

Figure 9. Fluid absorption in the endolymphatic sac 'drains' the cochlea during lumen formation. A, D and G: Luminal area measurements (average of the two basal cross-sections) in cochleae with and without endolymphatic sac. Cochleae were harvested at E14.5 and E17.5 from *Slc26a4*$^{+/-}$ and *Slc26a4*$^{-/-}$ mice and maintained two days in organ culture. The number next to the bars represents the N number of animals. Significant differences are marked (*). B and C, cochlear cross-sections of E14.5 *Slc26a4*$^{+/-}$ mice with and without endolymphatic sac. E and F, cochlear cross-sections of E14.5 *Slc26a4*$^{-/-}$ mice with and without endolymphatic sac. H and I, cochlear cross-sections of E17.5 *Slc26a4*$^{+/-}$ mice with and without endolymphatic sac. Scala media was highlighted in pink. Images without the pink overlay are available in Figure S1 (Supporting information). F-actin (green) and nuclei (blue) were labeled. Cochlear cross-sections were imaged by laser-scanning microscopy. Arrows point to the two basal cross-sections, which were used for digital area measurements.

conversion of the prohormone to the hormone and epithelial cells bear the thyroid hormone receptors that control proper maturation of the cochlea [42,43,44,45]. The enlargement of the cochlea lumen in *Slc26a4*$^{-/-}$ mice displaces mesenchymal cells and thereby disrupts cell signaling, which leads to local cochlear hypothyroidism during the early postnatal phase of development [10]. Taken together, cell-to-cell signaling is critically important during development of the cochlea. The enlargement appears to disrupt critical cell-to-cell signaling mechanisms at multiple stages, thereby disrupt proper development and account for deafness at birth in mice and possibly human patients.

Many human patients bearing loss-of-function mutations of *SLC26A4* are born hearing, which suggests that cochlear development in humans may to some extent escape the detriment of hampered cell-to-cell signaling during early development. The majority of patients bearing mutations of *SLC26A4* lose hearing during early childhood - often after a period of fluctuating hearing loss that progresses toward deafness [8,46]. Based on studies in the *Slc26a4*$^{-/-}$ mouse model, fluctuating hearing loss may be due to oscillations of a negative feedback system that oscillates and generates fluctuations in the endocochlear potential and thereby in the driving force on which hearing depends. This feedback loop is comprised of reactive oxygen species (ROS) generated by marginal cells of stria vascularis as a byproduct of elevated rates of K^+ secretion and the ROS-sensitive K^+ channel *KCNJ10* that generates the endocochlear potential and supplies K^+ to the marginal cells [12,13]. The ROS-induced loss of *KCNJ10* abolishes the endocochlear potential and hearing and the associated reduction in K^+ flux to marginal cells would limit K^+ secretion, reduce ROS production, allow restoration of *KCNJ10* expression, restoration of the endocochlear potential and restoration of hearing. This feedback loop may oscillate and thereby generate fluctuating hearing loss. Irreversible deafness would ensue, when endolymphatic Ca^{2+} concentrations rise and hair cells succumb to Ca^{2+} overload [9,12].

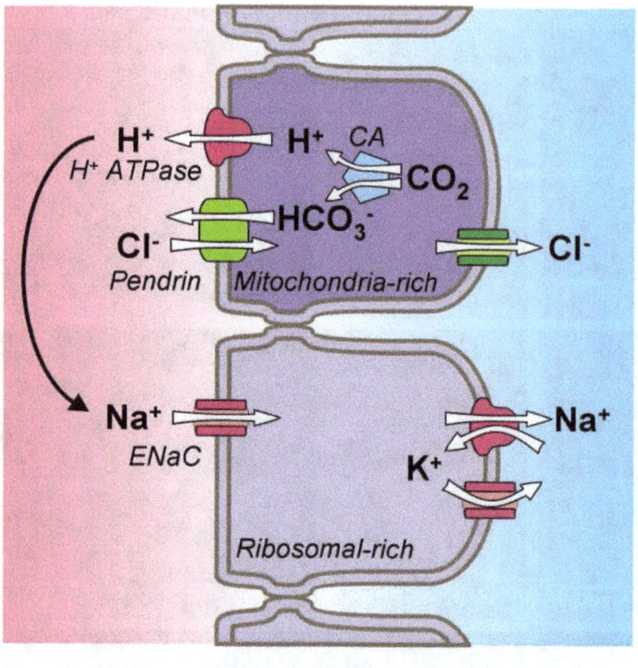

Figure 10. Diagram of ion transport in the endolymphatic sac. The endolymphatic sac epithelium consists mainly of ribosomal-rich cells that are interspersed by mitochondrial-rich cells. Mitochondrial-rich cells express H^+ ATPase and the Cl^-/HCO_3^- exchanger pendrin in their apical membrane. Ribosomal-rich cells express Na^+ channels including ENaC. A current generated by the H^+ ATPase drives Na^+ reabsorption via Na^+ channels. The role of the Cl^-/HCO_3^- exchanger pendrin is to export HCO_3^- that is generated by carbonic anhydrase (CA) in the reaction that leads to the generation of H^+.

In summary, the present study demonstrates that a lack of functional *Slc26a4* expression leads to a failure of fluid absorption in the endolymphatic sac that initiate cochlear enlargement in mice, and possibly humans. It is conceivable that deafness in mice, and possible humans, is a direct consequence of the cochlear enlargement and inherent disruption of cell signaling and cochlear ion homeostasis.

Supporting Information

Figure S1 Cochlear lumen formation in *Slc26a4+/−* and *Slc26a4−/−* mice. These images correspond to Fig. 4 in the main manuscript.

Figure S2 Fluid secretion in the vestibular labyrinth 'pumps up' the cochlea during lumen formation. These images correspond to Fig. 7 in the main manuscript.

Figure S3 Fluid absorption in the endolymphatic sac 'drains' the cochlea during lumen formation. These images correspond to Fig. 9 in the main manuscript.

Author Contributions

Conceived and designed the experiments: HMK PW. Performed the experiments: HMK. Analyzed the data: HMK PW. Contributed reagents/materials/analysis tools: PW. Wrote the paper: PW.

References

1. Fraser GR (1965) Association of congenital deafness with goitre (Pendred's syndrome) a study of 207 families. Ann Hum Genet 28: 201–249.
2. Reardon W, Coffey R, Phelps PD, Luxon LM, Stephens D, et al. (1997) Pendred syndrome–100 years of underascertainment? QJM 90: 443–447.
3. Park HJ, Shaukat S, Liu XZ, Hahn SH, Naz S, et al. (2003) Origins and frequencies of SLC26A4 (PDS) mutations in east and south Asians: global implications for the epidemiology of deafness. J Med Genet 40: 242–248.
4. Albert S, Blons H, Jonard L, Feldmann D, Chauvin P, et al. (2006) SLC26A4 gene is frequently involved in nonsyndromic hearing impairment with enlarged vestibular aqueduct in Caucasian populations. Eur J Hum Genet 14: 773–779.
5. Yuan Y, You Y, Huang D, Cui J, Wang Y, et al. (2009) Comprehensive molecular etiology analysis of nonsyndromic hearing impairment from typical areas in China. J Transl Med 7: 79–(epub).
6. Luxon LM, Cohen M, Coffey RA, Phelps PD, Britton KE, et al. (2003) Neuro-otological findings in Pendred syndrome. Int J Audiol 42: 82–88.
7. Colvin IB, Beale T, Harrop-Griffiths K (2006) Long-term follow-up of hearing loss in children and young adults with enlarged vestibular aqueducts: relationship to radiologic findings and Pendred syndrome diagnosis. Laryngoscope 116: 2027–2036.
8. Choi BY, Stewart AK, Madeo AC, Pryor SP, Lenhard S, et al. (2009) Hypo-Functional SLC26A4 variants associated with nonsyndromic hearing loss and enlargement of the vestibular aqueduct: Genotype-phenotype correlation or coincidental polymorphisms? Hum Mutat 30: 599–608.
9. Everett LA, Belyantseva IA, Noben-Trauth K, Cantos R, Chen A, et al. (2001) Targeted disruption of mouse Pds provides insight about the inner-ear defects encountered in Pendred syndrome. Hum Mol Genet 10: 153–161.
10. Wangemann P, Kim HM, Billings S, Nakaya K, Li X, et al. (2009) Developmental delays consistent with cochlear hypothyroidism contribute to failure to develop hearing in mice lacking Slc26a4/pendrin expression. Am J Physiol Renal Physiol 297(5): F1435–47.
11. Royaux IE, Belyantseva IA, Wu T, Kachar B, Everett LA, et al. (2003) Localization and functional studies of pendrin in the mouse inner ear provide insight about the etiology of deafness in pendred syndrome. J Assoc Res Otolaryngol 4: 394–404.
12. Wangemann P, Nakaya K, Wu T, Maganti R, Itza EM, et al. (2007) Loss of cochlear HCO_3^- secretion causes deafness via endolymphatic acidification and inhibition of Ca^{2+} reabsorption in a Pendred syndrome mouse model. Am J Physiol Renal Physiol 292: 1345–1353.
13. Singh R, Wangemann P (2008) Free radical stress mediated loss of Kcnj10 protein expression in stria vascularis contributes to deafness in Pendred syndrome mouse model. Am J Physiol Renal Physiol 294: F139–F148.
14. Wangemann P, Itza EM, Albrecht B, Wu T, Jabba SV, et al. (2004) Loss of KCNJ10 protein expression abolishes endocochlear potential and causes deafness in Pendred syndrome mouse model. BMC Medicine 2: 30.
15. Wangemann P (2006) Supporting sensory transduction: cochlear fluid homeostasis and the endocochlear potential. J Physiol 576: 11–21.
16. Shcheynikov N, Yang D, Wang Y, Zeng W, Karniski LP, et al. (2008) The Slc26a4 transporter functions as an electroneutral $Cl^-/I^-/HCO_3^-$ exchanger: role of Slc26a4 and Slc26a6 in I^- and HCO_3^- secretion and in regulation of CFTR in the parotid duct. J Physiol 586: 3813–3824.
17. Nakaya K, Harbidge DG, Wangemann P, Schultz BD, Green E, et al. (2007) Lack of pendrin HCO_3^- transport elevates vestibular endolymphatic $[Ca^{2+}]$ by inhibition of acid-sensitive TRPV5 and TRPV6. AmJ Physiol Renal Physiol 292: 1314–1321.
18. Yamasaki M, Komune S, Shimozono M, Matsuda K, Haruta A (2000) Development of monovalent ions in the endolymph in mouse cochlea. ORL J Otorhinolaryngol Relat Spec 62: 241–246.
19. Theiler K (1972) The house mouse. Springer Verlag.
20. Rugh R (1968) The mouse: Its reproduction and development. Burgess Publishing Company.
21. Van De Water TR, Ruben RJ (1973) Quantification of the "in vitro" development of the mouse embryo inner ear. Ann Otol Rhinol Laryngol 82: Suppl-21.
22. Mansour SL, Schoenwolf GC (2005) Morphogenesis of the inner ear. In: Kelley MW, Wu D, Popper AN, Fay RR, eds. Springer Handbook of Auditory Research: Development of the inner ear Springer. pp 43–84.
23. Dou H, Xu J, Wang Z, Smith AN, Soleimani M, et al. (2004) Co-expression of pendrin, vacuolar H^+-ATPase alpha4-subunit and carbonic anhydrase II in epithelial cells of the murine endolymphatic sac. J Histochem Cytochem 52: 1377–1384.
24. Everett LA, Morsli H, Wu DK, Green ED (1999) Expression pattern of the mouse ortholog of the Pendred's syndrome gene (Pds) suggests a key role for pendrin in the inner ear. Proc Natl Acad Sci USA 96: 9727–9732.

25. Mori N, Ninoyu O, Morgenstern C (1987) Cation transport in the ampulla of the semicircular canal and in the endolymphatic sac. Arch Otorhinolaryngol 244: 61–55.
26. Amano H, Orsulakova A, Morgenstern C (1983) Intracellular and extracellular ion current of the endolymphatic sac. Arch Otorhinolaryngol 237: 273–277.
27. Kimura RS (1967) Experimental blockage of the endolymphatic duct and sac and its effect on the inner ear of the guinea pig. A study on endolymphatic hydrops. Ann Otol Rhinol Laryngol 76: 664–687.
28. Lundquist PG, Kimura R, Wersäll J (1964) Ultrastructural organization of the epithelial lining in the endolymphatic duct and sac in the guinea pig. Acta Otolaryngol 57: 65–80.
29. Grunder S, Muller A, Ruppersberg JP (2001) Developmental and cellular expression pattern of epithelial sodium channel alpha, beta and gamma subunits in the inner ear of the rat. Eur J Neurosci 13: 641–648.
30. Mori N, Wu D (1996) Low-amiloride-affinity Na^+ channel in the epithelial cells isolated from the endolymphatic sac of guinea-pigs. Pflugers Arch 433: 58–64.
31. Stankovic KM, Brown D, Alper SL, Adams JC (1997) Localization of pH regulating proteins H^+ATPase and Cl^-/HCO_3^- exchanger in the guinea pig inner ear. Hear Res 114: 21–34.
32. Karet FE, Finberg KE, Nelson RD, Nayir A, Mocan H, et al. (1999) Mutations in the gene encoding B1 subunit of H^+-ATPase cause renal tubular acidosis with sensorineural deafness. Nat Genet 21: 84–90.
33. ten Cate WJ, Curtis LM, Rarey KE (1994) Na,K-ATPase subunit isoform expression in the guinea pig endolymphatic sac. ORL J Otorhinolaryngol Relat Spec 56: 257–262.
34. Son EJ, Moon IS, Kim SH, Kim SJ, Choi JY (2009) Interferon-gamma suppresses Na^+-H^+ exchanger in cultured human endolymphatic sac epithelial cells. J Cell Biochem 107: 965–972.
35. Wu D, Mori N (1998) Evidence for the presence of a Na^+-H^+ exchanger in the endolymphatic sac epithelium of guinea-pigs. Pflugers Arch 436: 182–188.
36. Couloigner V, Loiseau A, Sterkers O, Amiel C, Ferrary E (1998) Effect of locally applied drugs on the endolymphatic sac potential. Laryngoscope 108: 592–598.
37. Harvey BJ (1992) Energization of sodium absorption by the H^+-ATPase pump in mitochondria-rich cells of frog skin. J ExpBiol 172: 289–309.
38. Geleoc GS, Holt JR (2003) Developmental acquisition of sensory transduction in hair cells of the mouse inner ear. Nat Neurosci 6: 1019–1020.
39. Lelli A, Asai Y, Forge A, Holt JR, Geleoc GS (2009) Tonotopic gradient in the developmental acquisition of sensory transduction in outer hair cells of the mouse cochlea. J Neurophysiol 101: 2961–2973.
40. Kelsell DP, Dunlop J, Stevens HP, Lench NJ, Liang JN, et al. (1997) Connexin 26 mutations in hereditary non-syndromic sensorineural deafness. Nature 387: 80–83.
41. Del Castillo I, Moreno-Pelayo MA, Del Castillo FJ, Brownstein Z, Marlin S, et al. (2003) Prevalence and evolutionary origins of the del(GJB6-D13S1830) mutation in the DFNB1 locus in hearing-impaired subjects: a multicenter study. Am J Hum Genet 73: 1452–1458.
42. Rueda J, Prieto JJ, Cantos R, Sala ML, Merchan JA (2003) Hypothyroidism prevents developmental neuronal loss during auditory organ development. Neurosci Res 45: 401–408.
43. Deol MS (1973) An experimental approach to the understanding and treatment of hereditary syndromes with congenital deafness and hypothyroidism. J Med Genet 10: 235–242.
44. Campos-Barros A, Amma LL, Faris JS, Shailam R, Kelley MW, et al. (2000) Type 2 iodothyronine deiodinase expression in the cochlea before the onset of hearing. Proc Natl Acad Sci USA 97: 1287–1292.
45. Ng L, Hernandez A, He W, Ren T, Srinivas M, et al. (2008) A protective role for type 3 deiodinase, a thyroid hormone-inactivating enzyme, in cochlear development and auditory function. Endocrinology 150: 1952–1560.
46. Suzuki H, Oshima A, Tsukamoto K, Abe S, Kumakawa K, et al. (2007) Clinical characteristics and genotype-phenotype correlation of hearing loss patients with SLC26A4 mutations. Acta Otolaryngol 127: 1292–1297.

7

Prevalence and Clinical Features of Hearing Loss Patients with *CDH23* Mutations

Maiko Miyagawa, Shin-ya Nishio, Shin-ichi Usami*

Department of Otorhinolaryngology, Shinshu University School of Medicine, Matsumoto, Japan

Abstract

Screening for gene mutations in *CDH23*, which has many exons, has lagged even though it is likely to be an important cause for hearing loss patients. To assess the importance of *CDH23* mutations in non-syndromic hearing loss, two-step screening was applied and clinical characteristics of the patients with *CDH23* mutations were examined in this study. As a first screening, we performed Sanger sequencing using 304 probands compatible with recessive inheritance to find the pathologic mutations. Twenty-six possible mutations were detected to be pathologic in the first screening. For the second screening, using the probes for these 26 mutations, a large cohort of probands (n = 1396) was screened using Taqman amplification-based mutation analysis followed by Sanger sequencing. The hearing loss in a total of 52 families (10 homozygous, 13 compound heterogygous, and 29 heterozygous) was found to be caused by the *CDH23* mutations. The majority of the patients showed congenital, high frequency involved, progressive hearing loss. Interestingly, some particular mutations cause late onset moderate hearing loss. The present study is the first to demonstrate the prevalence of *CDH23* mutations among non-syndromic hearing loss patients and indicated that mutations of the *CDH23* gene are an important cause of non-syndromic hearing loss.

Editor: Iris Schrijver, Stanford University School of Medicine, United States of America

Funding: This study was supported by a Health and Labour Sciences Research Grant for Comprehensive Research on Disability Health and Welfare from the Ministry of Health, Labour and Welfare of Japan (http://www.mhlw.go.jp/english/) (SU), by the Acute Profound Deafness Research Committee of the Ministry of Health, Labour and Welfare of Japan (http://www.mhlw.go.jp/english/) (SU), by a Health and Labour Sciences Research Grant for Research on Specific Diseases (Vestibular Disorders) from the Japanese Ministry of Health, Labour and Welfare (http://www.mhlw.go.jp/english/) (SU), and by a Grant-in-Aid for Scientific Research from the Ministry of Education, Science and Culture of Japan (http://www.mext.go.jp/english/) (SU). The funders had no role in study design, data collection and analysis, decision to publish, or preparation of the manuscript.

Competing Interests: The authors have declared that no competing interests exist.

* E-mail: usami@shinshu-u.ac.jp

Introduction

Mutations in the *CDH23* (NM_22124) gene are known to be responsible for both Usher syndrome type ID (USH1D) and non-syndromic hearing loss (DFNB12) [1,2]. Molecular confirmation of *CDH23* mutations has become important in the diagnosis of these conditions.

This gene encodes cadherin 23, a protein of 3354 amino acids with 27 extracellular (EC) domains, a single transmembrane domain and a short cytoplasmic domain. Cadherin-specific amino acid motifs such as DRE, DXNDN, and DXD, that are highly conserved in sequence and spacing and required for cadherin dimerization and calcium binding were found in each extracelluar domain [3].

The cadherin 23 protein is known to be an important composition of the tip link that maintains the arrangement of streocilia [4].

More than 50 mutations have been reported for the Usher phenotype (USH1D) and 24 mutations reported for the non-syndromic hearing loss phenotype (DFNB12) [1,2,5–7]. As suggested by genotype–phenotype correlation study, Usher 1D, which has congenital profound hearing impairment, vestibular dysfunction, and retinitis pigmentosa, is usually associated with nonsense mutations, whereas DFNB12, which has a milder phenotype, is associated with missense mutations [1,2,5–8].

We previously reported that four pathologic mutations were identified in 5 out of 64 Japanese families compatible with autosomal recessive inheritance, suggesting that *CDH23*-caused deafness may be commonly found among non-syndromic hearing loss patients [6]. *GJB2* has been shown to be a common gene involved in congenital hearing impairment. *SLC26A4* is also frequently involved among those patients. *GJB2* and *SLC26A4* are comparatively small making Sanger sequencing relatively easy. The latter is also associated with the typical inner ear anomaly, enlarged vestibular aqueduct. Therefore, screening is relatively easy and many studies have focused on just these two genes. Clinical molecular diagnosis has been dramatically improved for these genes. However, screening strategy of other hearing loss genes is difficult and Sanger sequencing of the candidate genes, such as *CDH23*, with many exons is time consuming. Consequently, only a few reports are available for the mutation spectrum of *CDH23*.

In the present study, we performed Sanger sequencing using 304 patients whose pedigrees are compatible with recessive inheritance to find additional pathologic mutations. Also, to find the novel pathologic mutations and to clarify the frequency and clinical characteristics of patients with *CDH23* mutations, a large cohort of probands from unrelated families (n = 1396) was screened using TaqMan amplification-based mutation analysis of the variants observed in the initial 304 patients.

Table 1. Possible pathologic variants found in this study.

Amino acid change	Nucleotide change	EXON	Domain	Evolutionary conservation	The highly conserved calcium -binding elements	Number in probands (n = 1396)			Allele frequency in patients (in 2792 allele)	Allele frequency in control (in 384 allele)	Allele frequency in HL patients based on a Next generation sequencing database (in 432 allele)	Allele frequency in controls based on a Next generation sequencing database (in 144 allele)	PolyPhen 2 score*	SIFT Score*	Reference
						homozygote	compound heterozygote	heterozygote							
p.P240L	c.719C>T	7	EC3	7	-	7	12	19	1.612	0.260	0.63	0.67	0.999	0.06	Wagatsuma et al.
p.R301Q	c.902G>A	9	EC3	7	DRE	-	3	-	0.107	0.260	0	0	1.000	0	Wagatsuma et al.
p.E956K	c.2866G>A	25	EC9	7	DRE	-	1	2	0.107	0	0.21	0	1.000	0.04	this study
p.T1368M	c.4103C>T	32	EC13	7	-	-	1	-	0.036	0	0	0	1.000	0	this study
p.R1417W	c.4249C>T	35	EC13	5	-	1	-	2	0.143	0	0.25	0	0.998	0.19	Wagatsuma et al.
p.D1626A	c.4877A>C	39	EC15	7	DXNDN	-	1	-	0.036	0	0	0	0.999	0.01	this study
p.Q1716P	c.5147A>C	39	EC16	7	-	-	3	-	0.107	0	0	0	0.957	0.3	Wagatsuma et al.
p.R2029W	c.6085C>T	46	EC19	7	DRE	2	2	6	0.430	0	0	0	0.999	0.01	Wagatsuma et al.
p.N2287K	c.6861T>G	50	EC21	7	DXNDN	-	2	-	0.072	0	0	0	0.971	0	this study
p.E2438K	c.7312G>A	52	EC23	6	-	-	1	-	0.036	0	0	0	0.986	1	this study

*Computer analysis to predict the effect of missense variants on *CDH23* protein function was performed with Sorting Intolerant from Tolerant (SIFT; http://sift.jcvi.org/), and Polymorphism Phenotyping (PolyPhen2;http://genetics.bwh.harvard.edu/pph2/).

Table 2. Variants with uncertain pathogenicity found in this study.

Amino acid change	Nucleotide change	EXON	Domain	Evolutionary conservation	The highly conserved calcium -binding elements	Number in probands (n = 1396)			Allele frequency in patients (in 2792 allele)	Allele frequency in control (in 384 allele)	Allele frequency in HL patients based on a Next generation sequencing database (in 432 allele)	Allele frequency in controls based on a Next generation sequencing database (in 144 allele)	PolyPhen 2 score***	SIFT Score***	Reference
						homozygote	compound heterozygote	heterozygote							
p.D160N	c.478G>A	4	EC2	7	DXD	-	-	2	0.072	0.260	0	0	1.000	0	this study
p.V803I	c.2407G>A	23	EC8	7	-	-	-	3	0.107	0	0	0	0.761	0.41	this study
p.S1415I	c.4244G>T	35	EC13	7	-	-	-	1	0.036	0	0	0	0.840	0.06	this study
p.A1443G *	c.4328C>G	35	EC14	7	-	1*	-	2	0.143	0	0.2	0	0.944	0.06	this study
p.R1588W **	c.4762C>T	38	EC15	7	-	4**	-	18	0.931	0.260	2.22	0	1.000	0.01	Wagatsuma et al.
p.V1711I	c.5131G>A	40	EC16	7	-	-	-	2	0.072	0	0	0	0.970	0.12	Wagatsuma et al.
p.V1807M	c.5419G>A	42	EC17	5	-	-	1	-	N/A	0.260	0	0	0.054	0.22	this study
p.S1876N	c.5627G>A	43	EC18	5	-	-	-	6	0.215	0	0	0	0.981	0.26	Wagatsuma et al.
p.V1908I	c.5722G>A	44	EC9	5	-	-	-	12	0.430	0.260	1.09	0.53	0.948	1	Wagatsuma et al.
p.A2130V	c.6389C>T	48	EC20	6	-	-	-	1	0.036	0	0	0	0.999	0.24	this study
p.R2171C	c.6511C>T	48	EC20	7	DXNDNR	-	-	1	0.036	0.521	0	0	0.999	0.11	Wagatsuma et al.
p.Q2227P	c.6680A>C	48	EC21	6	-	-	-	1	0.036	0.260	0	0	0.930	0.2	Wagatsuma et al.
p.L2473P	c.7418T>C	53	EC23	7	-	-	-	1	0.036	0	0	0	0.999	0	Wagatsuma et al.
p.I2669V	c.8005A>G	56	EC25	5	-	-	-	1	0.036	0	0	0	0.134	0.7	Wagatsuma et al.
p.F2801V	c.8401T>G	59	EC26	5	-	-	-	1	0.036	0.781	1.52	1.27	0.800	0.01	Wagatsuma et al.
p.G2912S	c.8734G>A	61	EC27	7	-	-	-	1	0.036	0	0.23	0	0.996	0	this study
p.R3175C	c.9523C>T	68	CYTO	7	-	-	-	1	0.036	0.260	0	0	0.886	0.01	Wagatsuma et al.

*not confirmed by segregation study.
**one normal hearing subject with homozygotes.
***Computer analysis to predict the effect of missense variants on *CDH23* protein function was performed with Sorting Intolerant from Tolerant (SIFT; http://sift.jcvi.org/), and Polymorphism Phenotyping (PolyPhen2;http://genetics.bwh.harvard.edu/pph2/).
N/A: TaqMan probe not available.

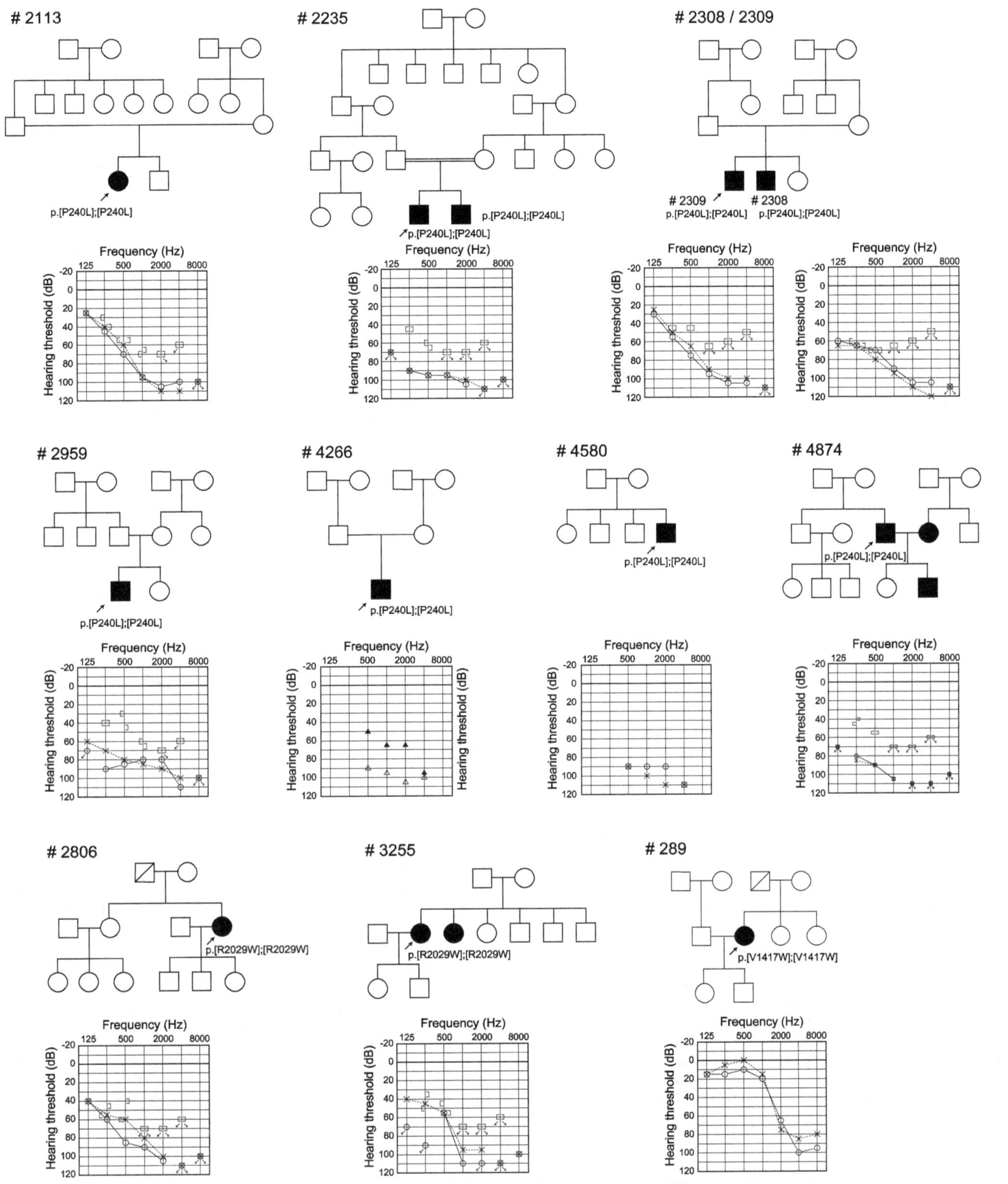

Figure 1. Pedigrees, mutations, and audiograms of the patients with homozygous *CDH23* mutations.

Results

The first screening using 304 Japanese probands compatible with autosomal recessive inheritance identified 26 candidates for disease causing mutations. These include four previously reported pathologic mutations: p.P240L, p.R301Q, p.Q1716P, and p.R2029W, as well as 6 possible pathologic variants in the coding region of *CDH23*. All of the mutations were missense mutations.

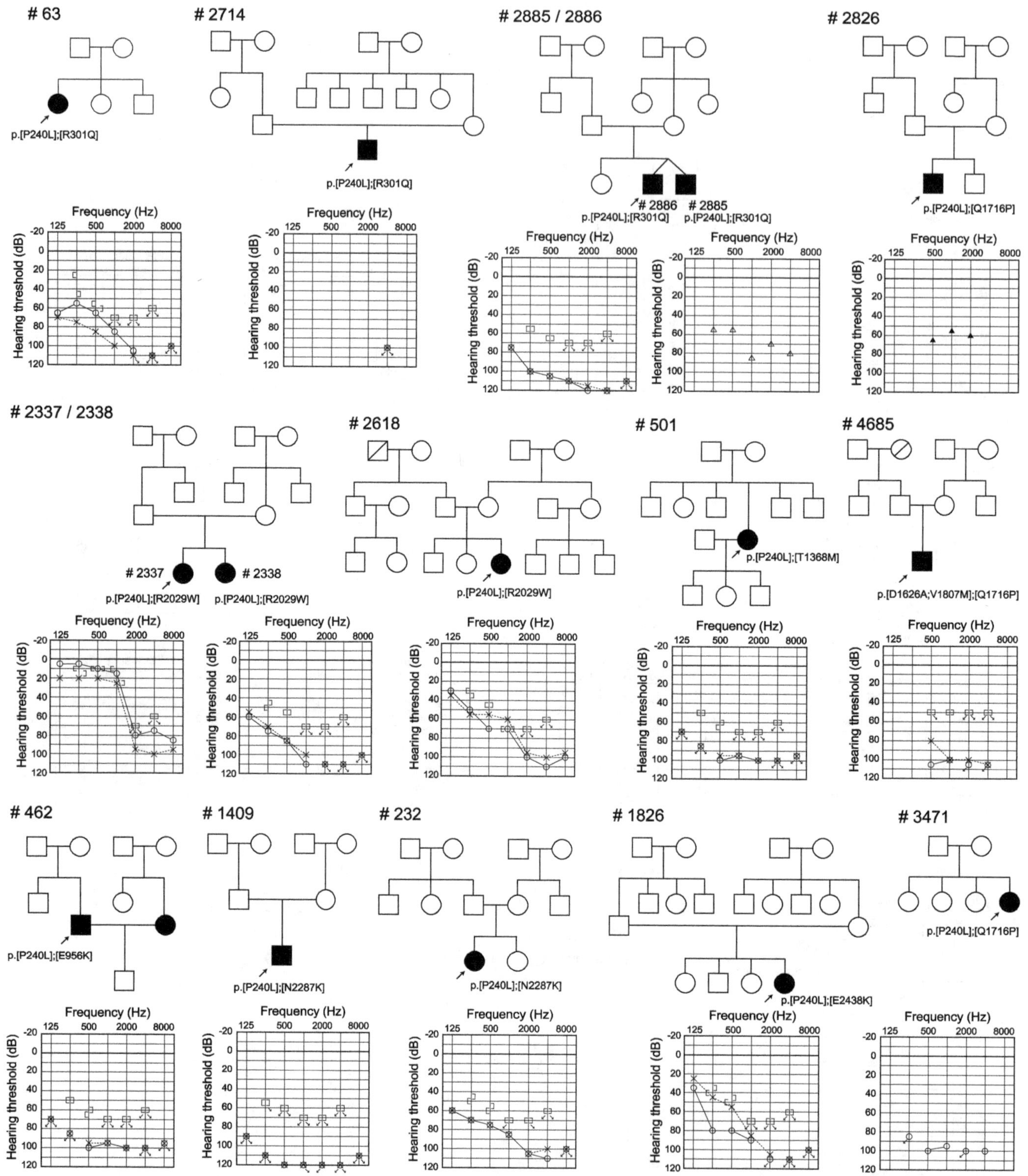

Figure 2. Pedigrees, mutations, and audiograms of the patients with compound heterozygous *CDH23* mutations.

The following second screening based on TaqMan assay followed by Sanger sequencing confirmed 10 "possibly pathologic" mutations (Table 1) and 17 variants with uncertain pathogenicity (Table 2) in a large cohort of the patients. "Possible pathologic" mutations were defined as 1) mutations found to be homozygotes or compound heterozygotes (and determined by segregation study), 2) variants which were not found or were very few in 192 control subjects, 3) amino acids that were well-conserved among various species, 4) compatible with next generation sequencing database, and 5) compatible with the predicted effect

Table 3. Details of phenotype and genotype of 11 patients in 10 families with homozygous *CDH23* mutation.

Sample No	relationship	Amino acid Change	Hereditary form	Threshold* (Rt)(dB)	Threshold* (Lt)(dB)	severity	Residual hearing in the lower frequencies** (dB)	Hearing in the higher frequencies*** (dB)	Age	Age of awareness	Progres-siveness	Hearing aid/ cochlear implant	Vertigo	Tinnitus
#2113		p.[P240L]; [P240L]	sporadic	91.3	90	severe	44.2	104.2	12	6	+	HA	–	–
#2235		p.[P240L]; [P240L]	AR	97.5	96.3	profound	85.0	104.2	22	0	–	HA	–	–
#2308		p.[P240L]; [P240L]	AR	88.8	95	severe	67.5	110.0	11	0****	–	HA	–	–
#2309	sibling of #2308	p.[P240L]; [P240L]	AR	92.5	86.3	severe	50.0	105.0	9	0****	–	HA	–	–
#2959		p.[P240L]; [P240L]	sporadic	81.3	85	severe	75.8	96.7	8	0****	–	HA	–	–
#4266		p.[P240L]; [P240L]	sporadic	96.3	96.3	severe	70.0	91.3	3	0****	+	CI	–	–
#4580		p.[P240L]; [P240L]	sporadic	102.5	97.5	profound	88.3	106.7	1	0****	–	CI	–	N/A
#4874		p.[P240L]; [P240L]	sporadic	102.5	102.5	profound	80.8	106.7	38	2	+	HA	–	–
#2806		p.[R2029W]; [R2029W]	sporadic	92.5	80	severe	56.7	104.2	53	48	+	HA	–	+
#3255		p.[R2029W]; [R2029W]	AR	96.3	85	severe	59.2	104.2	71	60	+	HA	–	+
#289		p.[V1417W]; [V1417W]	sporadic	31.3	26.3	mild	10.0	85.0	34	14	+	HA	–	–

*average of 500, 1000, 2000 and 4000 Hz.
**average of 125, 250, and 500 Hz.
***average of 2000, 4000, and 8000 Hz.
****found by newborn hearing screening.

Table 4. Details of phenotype and genotype of 15 patients in 13 families with compound heterozygous *CDH23* mutation.

Sample No	relationship	Amino acid Change	Hereditary form	Threshold* (Rt)(dB)	Threshold* (Lt)(dB)	severity	Residual hearing in the lower frequencies** (dB)	Hearing in the higher frequencies*** (dB)	Age	Age of awareness	Progres-siveness	Hearing aid/ cochlear implant	Vertigo	Tinnitus
#63		p.[P240L]; [R301Q]	sporadic	85	98.8	severe	69.2	105.8	27	0	–	HA	–	+
#2714		p.[P240L]; [R301Q]	sporadic	97.5	97.5	profound	71.7	105.0	2	0****	+	HA	–	–
#2885		p.[P240L]; [R301Q]	AR	90	108.7	profound	55.0	75.0	13	3	+	CI	–	–
#2886	sibling of #2885	p.[P240L]; [R301Q]	AR	115	110	profound	93.3	115.8	13	2	+	CI	–	–
#2337		p.[P240L]; [R2029W]	AR	30	41.3	mild	13.3	88.3	13	11	+	HA	–	+
#2338	sibling of #2337	p.[P240L]; [R2029W]	AR	103.8	98.8	profound	71.7	106.7	8	2	+	HA	–	–
#2618		p.[P240L]; [R2029W]	sporadic	77.5	67.5	moderate	49.2	100.0	8	3	+	CI	–	–
#2826		p.[P240L]; [Q1716P]	sporadic	91.3	95	profound	66.7	112.5	6	0	+	HA	–	–
#3471		p.[P240L]; [Q1716P]	sporadic	97.5	97.5	profound	92.5	100.0	4	0	–	CI	–	–
#462		p.[P240L]; [E956K]	sporadic	97.5	97.3	profound	84.2	98.3	38	10	–	HA	–	–
#501		p.[P240L]; [T1368M]	sporadic	>90	>90	profound	N/A	N/A	68	44	+	HA	+	+
#1409		p.[P240L]; [N2287K]	sporadic	120	120	profound	107.5	123.3	17	0	+	HA	–	–
#232		p.[P240L]; [N2287K]	sporadic	87.5	86.3	severe	67.5	104.2	15	0	–	HA	–	+
#1826		p.[P240L]; [E2438K]	sporadic	91.3	106.3	severe	70.8	105.8	11	3	+	HA	–	–
#4685		p.[D1626A; V1807M]; [Q1716P]	sporadic	97.5	103.8	severe	96.3	105.0	1	0*	–	CI	–	N/A

*average of 500, 1000, 2000 and 4000 Hz.
**average of 125, 250, and 500 Hz.
***average of 2000, 4000, and 8000 Hz.
****found by newborn hearing screening.

Table 5. Details of phenotype and genotype of 29 patients with heterozygous *CDH23* mutation.

Sample No relationship	Amino acid Change	Hereditary form	Threshold* (Rt)(dB)	Threshold* (Lt)(dB)	severity	Residual hearing in the lower frequencies** (dB)	Hearing in the higher frequencies*** (dB)	Age	Age of awareness	Progressiveness	Hearing aid/ cochlear implant	Vertigo	Tinnitus
#334	p.[P240L];[-]	AD	96.25	83.75	severe	63.3	96.7	23	0	+	HA	N/A	+
#340	p.[P240L];[-]	sporadic	>90	>90	profound	N/A	N/A	54	14	+	HA	N/A	N/A
#569	p.[P240L];[-]	sporadic	86.25	90	severe	75.0	98.3	26	3	+	HA	−	−
#653	p.[P240L];[-]	sporadic	53.75	57.5	moderate	44.2	71.7	36	33	+	HA	−	+
#754	p.[P240L];[-]	sporadic	110	101.25	profound	87.5	104.2	57	0	+	HA	N/A	N/A
#1039	p.[P240L];[-]	sporadic	48.75	56.25	moderate	33.3	74.2	76	76	−	HA	+	−
#1598	p.[P240L];[-]	sporadic	56.25	10	unilateral	34.2	41.7	60	49	−	−	+	+
#1807	p.[P240L];[-]	sporadic	110	8.75	unilateral	50.8	60.0	50	9	−	−	−	−
#1846	p.[P240L];[-]	AD	100	96.25	profound	83.3	98.3	62	6	+	HA	+	+
#2159	p.[P240L];[-]	AR	67.5	66.25	moderate	60.0	69.2	10	65	+	HA	−	−
#2374	p.[P240L];[-]	AR	86.25	90	severe	78.3	78.3	5	0	−	HA	−	−
#2835	p.[P240L];[-]	sporadic	85	91.25	severe	65.8	101.7	12	3	+	HA	+	−
#3492	p.[P240L];[-]	AD	103.75	103.75	profound	88.8	107.5	1	0	−	HA	−	−
#3499	p.[P240L];[-]	AD	96.25	110	severe	84.2	105.8	57	50	−	CI	−	+
#3761	p.[P240L];[-]	AR	32.5	40	mild	43.3	75.8	71	0	−	−	−	+
#4040	p.[P240L];[-]	AR	S/O	S/O	profound	S/O	S/O	2	0	+	HA	−	−
#4159	p.[P240L];[-]	AR	97.5	71.25	severe	71.7	95.0	38	38	+	HA	+	+
#4313	p.[P240L];[-]	AD/Mit	130	102.5	profound	107.5	116.7	6	0	−	CI	−	−
#4615	p.[P240L];[-]	sporadic	90	90	profound	90.0	90.0	0	0****	−	CI	−	−
#265	p.[E956K];[-]	sporadic	110	6.25	unilateral	57.5	59.2	16	0	−	−	−	−
#3116	p.[E956K];[-]	AD	47.5	53.75	moderate	58.3	40.8	63	N/A	+	HA	−	+
#280	p.[R1417W];[-]	sporadic	110	6.25	unilateral	50.0	55.8	8	3	−	−	N/A	N/A
#2649	p.[R1417W];[-]	sporadic	95	110	profound	87.5	105.0	11	0	+	CI	−	N/A
#1131	p.[R2029W];[-]	sporadic	73.75	72.5	severe	55.0	93.3	24	17	+	HA	−	−
#1539	p.[R2029W];[-]	AD	53.75	110	moderate	70.0	83.3	71	60	+	HA	−	+
#1618	p.[R2029W];[-]	sporadic	26.25	61.25	mild	31.7	60.8	67	N/A	−	−	−	+
#1919	p.[R2029W];[-]	AD	38.75	36.25	mild	20.8	75.0	25	3	+	−	N/A	N/A
#2271	p.[R2029W];[-]	AD	58.75	62.5	moderate	41.7	50.0	6	N/A	N/A	HA	N/A	N/A
#4138	p.[R2029W];[-]	AR	71.25	53.75	moderate	50.8	65.8	10	3	+	HA	+	−

*average of 500, 1000, 2000 and 4000 Hz.
**average of 125, 250, and 500 Hz.
***average of 2000, 4000, and 8000 Hz.
****found by newborn hearing screening.

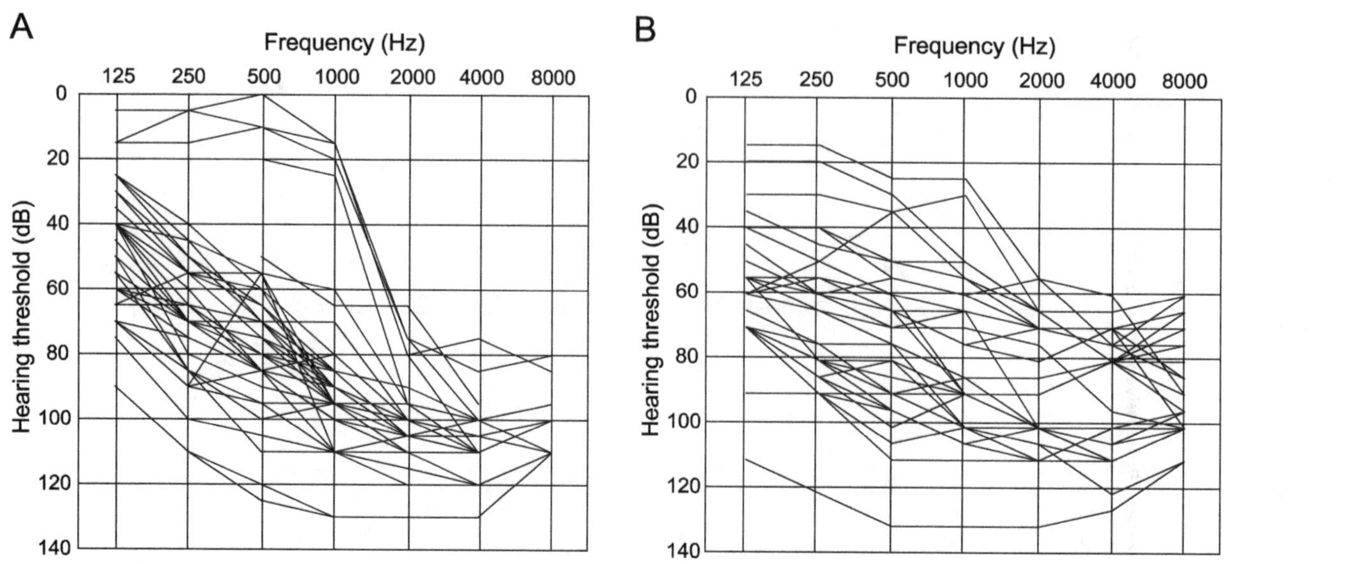

Figure 3. Overlapping audiograms of the patients with *CDH 23* mutations. A: patients with hearing loss caused by the *CDH23* mutations (homozygous or compound heterozygous cases), B: patients potentially caused by the *CDH23* mutations (heterozygous cases).

of missense mutations on *CDH23* protein function. Results of the compatibility of the next generation sequence database, the SIFT and PolyPhen2 score for prediction are shown in Tables 1 and 2.

The 17 variants found as heterozygous and therefore with uncertain pathogenicity did not fulfill all the above criteria. For example, p.A1443G was uncertain because DNA samples from family members were not available and we could not confirm its pathogenicity by segregation study. p.R1588W was found to be homozygous in 4 patients and heterozygous in 16 patients, but only 1 was found in 384 control alleles. However, a member of the patient's family (#2841) showed normal hearing instead of being homozygous. Also p.V803I, p.V1807M and p.I2669V are obscure from the functional prediction analysis.

In one family (#4685), three mutation were found in proband and two of them were found in same allele p.[D16126A;V1807M] confirmed by segregation analysis.

As p.V1807M predicted to have no effect on *CDH23* structure, p.D1626A might be a pathogenic mutation.

For 10 possible pathologic mutations, amino acids were well-conserved among various species, including *Homo sapiens, P. troglodytes, B. traurus, M. musculus, R. norvegicus, G. gallus*, and *D. rario.* Many mutations (5 out of 10 possible pathologic mutations, 2 out of 17 uncertain variants) were found in DRE, DXNDN, and DXD motif (Table 1 and 2). Ten possible pathologic mutations were found to be either homozygotes (n = 11, Table 3, Fig. 1) or compound heterozygotes (n = 15) (Table 4, Fig. 2). Twenty-nine patients were found to be heterozygous without a second mutation (Table 5).

Tables 3 and 4 summarize 23 families with hearing loss caused by the *CDH23* mutations (homozygous or compound heterozygous cases) and Table 5 summarizes 29 families with hearing loss potentially caused by the *CDH23* mutations (heterozygous cases). The frequency was 1.6% (23/1396) or 2.1% (29/1396) of the overall hearing loss population. When restricted to patients compatible with recessive inheritance, the frequency was increased to 2.5% (23/919) or 3.2% (29/919). Table 3, 4 and 5 also summarize clinical characteristics including hereditary form, hearing threshold, severity, residual hearing in the lower frequencies, hearing in the higher frequencies, onset age (age of awareness), progressiveness of hearing loss, use of hearing aid/ cochlear implantation, visual impairment, and vestibular symptoms. The ages of these patients were from 1 to 71 years. Age of onset (awareness of hearing loss) ranged from congenital to 60 years old, though the majority was congenital or early onset. There were some correlations between genotype and phenotype (onset age). The patients associated with p.P240L showed congenital and severe hearing loss regardless of whether associated with one more mutation, whereas the patients with p.R2029W or p.T1368M showed late-onset moderate hearing loss (Tables 3 and 4). Concerning type of hearing loss, the majority of the patients had some residual hearing in the lower frequencies, and overlapping audiograms showed characteristic high frequency involved hearing loss (Fig. 3). The majority of the patients showed progressive nature of hearing loss evaluated by serial audiogram (Fig. 4). No patients had associated visual impairment or vestibular symptoms (Tables 3, 4 and 5). Seven patients received cochlear implantation due to the insufficient amplification of hearing aids (Tables 3, 4 and 5).

Discussion

Mutations in the *CDH23* gene are known to be responsible for both Usher syndrome type ID (USH1D) as well as non-syndromic hearing loss (DFNB12), and molecular confirmation of *CDH23* mutations is clinically important for diagnosis of these conditions. However, clinical application of the detection of *CDH23* mutations has lagged because of the size of the gene. Especially for DFNB12, which is not associated with visual impairment, screening is comparatively difficult, and therefore, little is known about frequencies among the hearing loss population as well as clinical characteristics.

In this study, we have applied two-step screening and identified a significant number of novel pathologic mutations of *CDH23* responsible for non-syndromic hearing loss in a large cohort of patients. All of the possible pathologic mutations identified in this study (Table 1) were missense mutations, being consistent with previous reports that DFNB12 patients associated with missense mutations have milder hearing impairment than in USH1D, which is associated with nonsense, splice-site, or frameshift

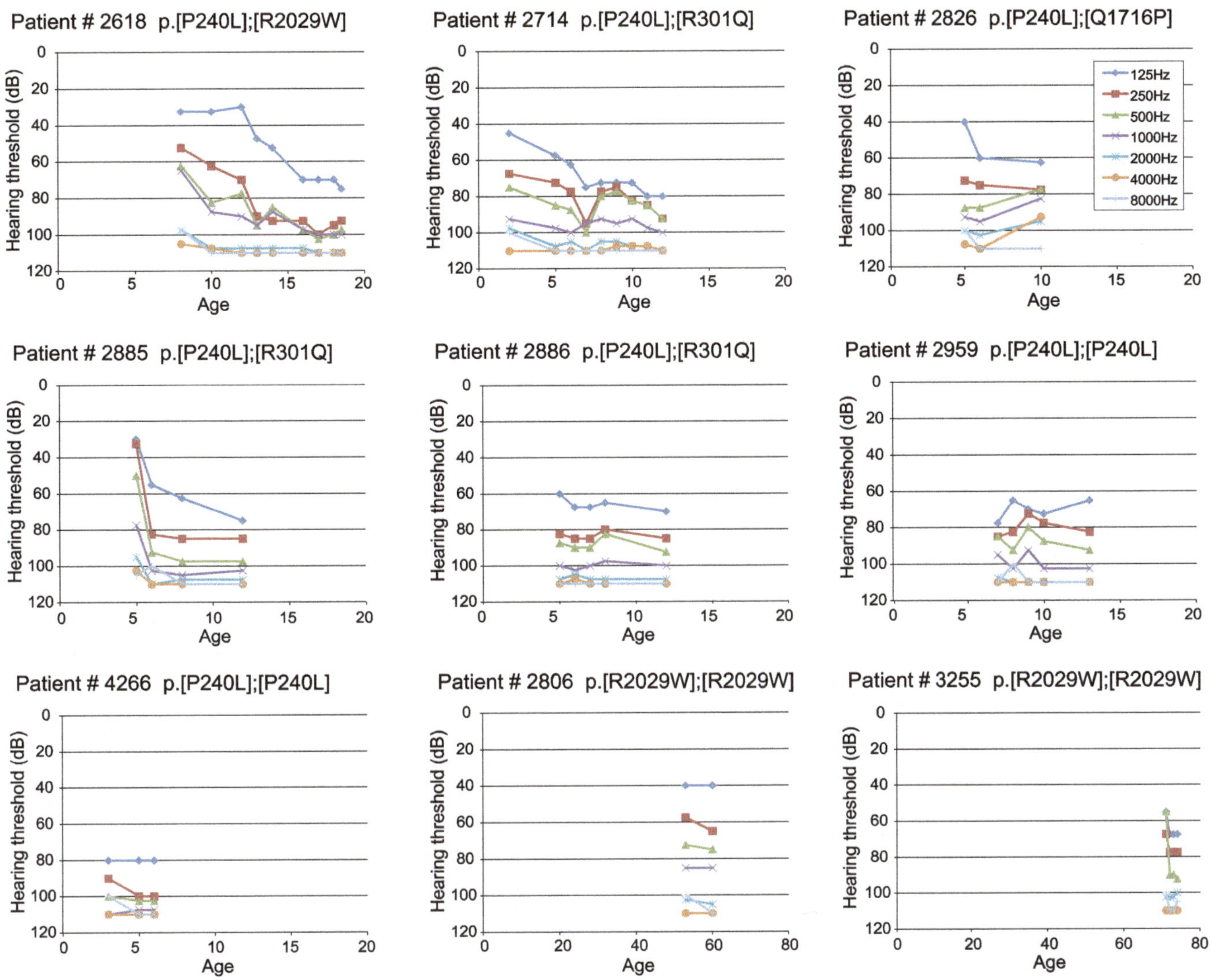

Figure 4. Hearing progression of the patients with *CDH23* mutations. Note that the high frequency portion was already worsened, and the low frequency portion was deteriorated by ages.

mutations [2,5–7]. None had visual impairment, also supporting this rule. That the majority was found in the EC domain with only one exception found in the cytoplasmic domain, was also in line with the previous reports on DFNB12 [2,5–7]. Of these 26 mutations, five out of 10 possible pathologic mutations were found in DRE, DXNDN, and DXD motifs, which are thought to be important for calcium binding property. These highly conserved EC calcium binding motifs are thought to be essential for linearization, rigidification, and dimerization of the cadherin molecules [9,10]. And the results of computer analysis to predict the impact of amino acid change, all of 10 possible pathologic mutations predicted to cause a severe damage for protein function of *CDH23*.

As a result, 26 patients (from 23 families) had two mutations (in a homozygous or compound heterozygous state), and met criteria for recessive inheritance. A hallmark of recessive mutations is the detection of two mutations in the paternal and maternal alleles and the parents having normal hearing. As seen in previous mutation screening reports, including those for *CDH23* [6,7] as well as *GJB2* and *SLC26A4* [11,12], we encountered a significant number of heterozygous cases without a second mutation even after direct sequencing of the coding region of the gene. Possible explanations are: 1) the existence of a second mutation in the intron or regulatory region of *CDH23*, which has not been explored, 2) the observed mutations are rare polymorphisms, 3) the screening method fails to detect the second mutation, and 4) an additional modulatory gene may contribute to hearing loss (for example, *PCDH15*). Although we have not reached the final conclusion, it is most likely that these heterozygous cases are also related to *CDH23* mutations because: 1) allele frequencies are found to be higher in the hearing loss group (Table 2), and 2) the phenotype is similar to that of the patients with two mutations. As shown in Fig. 3, overlapping audiograms of the patients with only one mutation was similar to that with the patients with two mutations (high frequency involved sensorineural hearing loss with residual hearing at the lower frequencies).

Based on the frequencies of 3.7% (including heterozygous cases) of the hearing loss population and 5.7% (including heterozygous cases) of the recessive inherited cases in this study, we confirmed that mutations of *CDH23* are an important cause for nonsyndromic hearing loss and should be borne in mind next to *GJB2* or *SLC26A4* screening. This study revealed that p.P240L account for nearly 43.3%(45/104) of all *CDH23* mutated families in Japan. Common mutations, such as c.35delG or c.235delC in *GJB2* or p.H723R in the *SLC26A4* gene, have been reported in many recessive deafness genes, and usually they are population-specific [12–14]. It is an interesting question whether p.P240L is frequent because of a founder effect or mutational hot spot, but the existence of such a common mutation makes mutation screening easier. Additional frequent mutations found in this study together with TaqMan procedures will facilitate genetic testing for deafness patients.

Concerning mutation spectrum, as in our previous report [6], the *CDH23* mutation spectrum in Japanese is very different from that found in Caucasians and may be representative of those in Eastern Asian populations. Its elucidation is expected to facilitate the molecular diagnosis of DFNB12 and USH1D. It has also been known that prevalent *GJB2* mutations are highly ethnic-specific (see The connexin-deafness homepage; http://davinci.crg.es/deafness/): c.35delG is common in the Caucasoid population, c.167delT was reported as prevalent in Ashkenazi Jews, p.R143W in a restricted village in Africa, and c.235delC in East Asian populations. A series of studies proved a founder effect for these frequent mutations [11,15].

In the present study, using a large cohort of patients, clinical characteristics (onset age, progression, audiograms) of patients with *CDH23* mutations were clarified.

Concerning genotype/phenotype correlations, hearing of the patients with p.[P240L];[P240L] is worse than in those with the other mutations, and tends to be congenital and severe. In contrast, the patients with p.[R2029W];[R2029W] showed a milder phenotype of middle age onset. Overlapping audiograms showed typical high frequency involved sensorineural hearing loss with residual hearing at the lower frequencies.

Concerning age of onset (awareness of hearing loss), the majority was congenital or early onset. But rather later-onset was seen in three patients (#2806, 3255, 501), and they were associated with some particular mutations (p.R2029W and p.T1368M). Their phenotype was rather mild and gradually progressive. It is interesting to note that their phenotype was similar to presbycusis. Actually, *CDH23* mutations have been reported as responsible for age-related hearing loss in mice [16,17].

Progressive nature of hearing loss and the presence of residual hearing are particular phenotypic features of the patients with *CDH23* mutations. Our previous genetic analysis for the patients with high frequency involved hearing loss successfully identified *CDH23* mutations [18]. Seven patients received cochlear implantation and showed good performance after implantation. For the patients with residual hearing, newly developed cochlear implantation; EAS (Electric Acoustic Stimulation) is a good therapeutic option and therefore much attention should be paid to the etiology when considering individual intervention, i.e., regular cochlear implantation or EAS. Genetic testing will be very important prognostic information together with various hearing tests.

In conclusion, a large cohort study using Taqman amplification-based mutation analysis indicated that mutations of the *CDH23* gene are important causes of non-syndromic hearing loss. A mutation screening strategy using TaqMan assay based on the ethnic-specific frequent mutations is a powerful and effective method for such a large gene. Clinical characteristics of patients with *CDH23* mutations is that hearing loss is progressive, high frequency involved sensorineural hearing loss with residual hearing in the lower frequencies. Most cases are congenital but care is needed because some patients show presbycusis-like hearing loss. Cochlear implantation (including EAS) is a good therapeutic intervention for the patients with *CDH23* mutations.

Materials and Methods

To identify additional pathologic *CDH23* mutations, two-step screening was applied in this study. Subjects from independent families were collected from 33 ENT departments nationwide in Japan. All subjects gave prior informed consent for participation in the project, which was approved by the ethical committee of each hospital. Genomic DNA was isolated from peripheral blood by DNeasy Blood and Tissue Kit (QIAGEN, Düsseldorf, Germany) according to the manufacturer's procedure.

First screening (Direct sequencing)

First, we sequenced the *CDH23* gene in 304 Japanese non-syndromic sensorineural hearing loss probands (including our previously reported 64 samples [6]) compatible with autosomal recessive inheritance or sporadic cases. None of the subjects had any other associated neurological signs, vestibular or visual dysfunction. Sanger sequencing was applied to these samples to find mutations responsible for deafness. Detailed procedures were described in our previous report [6]. 26 candidates for disease causing mutations were collected according to the following criteria; 1) non-synonymous variants, and 2) allele carrier rates were less than 2% in control subjects.

Second screening (TaqMan genotyping assay based screening and Direct sequencing)

For the second screening, probes of these 26 mutations selected in the first screening was applied for a custom TaqMan® SNP Genotyping Assays (Applied Biosystems, Foster City, CA) [19]. 1396 probands of sensorineural hearing loss patients including 304 probands used in the first screening were used for the second assay. Of them, 1347 had bilateral sensorineural hearing loss and 49 had unilateral sensorineural hearing loss. The inheritance composition of the subjects was as follows: 298 subjects from autosomal dominant or maternally inherited families (two or more generations affected); 919 subjects from autosomal recessive families (parents with normal hearing and two or more affected siblings) or subjects with sporadic deafness (compatible with recessive inheritance or non-genetic hearing loss); the rest had unknown inheritance mode. After TaqMan assay, Sanger sequencing was performed: 1) to confirm these mutations found in TaqMan genotyping assays, 2) to confirm whether mutations were homozygotes or heterozygote, and 3) in cases found in heterozygous state, direct sequencing of the coding region of the *CDH23* was performed.

Controls

The control group consisted of 192 unrelated Japanese individuals without any noticeable hearing loss evaluated by auditory testing.

Next generation sequencing and computer analysis

To elucidate the allele frequency of 26 mutations, comparison was made between allele frequency found in 216 deafness patients and 72 controls based on a next generation sequencing database that is currently being established at Shinshu University (unpublished). In brief, exome sequencing was performed with SureSelect target DNA enrichment (Agilent Technologies, Santa Clara, CA) and Illumina GAIIx sequencing (Illumina, San Diego, CA) according to the manufacturers' procedures. In the SureSelect library, 76 already reported genes responsible for sensorineural hearing loss and syndromic hearing loss were contained. After base calling, sequence results were aligned with a bowtie program [20] and allele frequencies of each *CDH23* mutation in patients and the control population were calculated. Computer analysis to predict the effect of missense variants on *CDH23* protein function was performed with Sorting Intolerant from Tolerant (SIFT; http://sift.jcvi.org/), and Polymorphism Phenotyping (PolyPhen2; http://genetics.bwh.harvard.edu/pph2/) [21,22].

Acknowledgments

We thank Dr. William J Kimberling for helpful comments. We would also like to thank A. C. Apple-Mathews for help in preparing the manuscript.

Author Contributions

Conceived and designed the experiments: SU. Performed the experiments: MM SN. Analyzed the data: MM SN. Wrote the paper: MM SU.

References

1. Bolz H, von Brederlow B, Ramírez A, Bryda EC, Kutsche K, et al. (2001) Mutation of *CDH23*, encoding a new member of the cadherin gene family, causes Usher syndrome type 1D. Nat Genet 27: 108–112.
2. Bork JM, Peters LM, Riazuddin S, Bernstein SL, Ahmed ZM, et al. (2001) Usher syndrome 1D and nonsyndromic autosomal recessive deafness DFNB12 are caused by allelic mutations of the novel cadherin-like gene *CDH23*. Am J Hum Genet 68: 26–37.
3. Rowlands TM, Symonds JM, Farookhi R, Blaschuk OW (2000) Cadherins: crucial regulators of structure and function in reproductive tissues. Rev Reprod 5: 53–61.
4. Muller U (2008) Cadherins and mechanotransduction by hair cells. Curr Opin Cell Biol 20: 557–566.
5. Astuto LM, Bork JM, Weston MD, Askew JW, Fields RR, et al. (2002) *CDH23* mutation and phenotype heterogeneity: a profile of 107 diverse families with Usher syndrome and nonsyndromic deafness. Am J Hum Genet 71: 262–275.
6. Wagatsuma M, Kitoh R, Suzuki H, Fukuoka H, Takumi Y, et al. (2007) Distribution and frequencies of *CDH23* mutations in Japanese patients with non-syndromic hearing loss. Clin Genet 72: 339–344.
7. Oshima A, Jaijo T, Aller E, Millan JM, Carney C, et al. (2008) Mutation profile of the *CDH23* gene in 56 probands with Usher syndrome type I. Hum Mutat 29: E37–46.
8. McHugh RK, Friedman RA (2006) Genetics of hearing loss: Allelism and modifier genes produce a phenotypic continuum. Anat Rec A Discov Mol Cell Evol Biol 288: 370–381.
9. Nagar B, Overduin M, Ikura M, Rini JM (1996) Structural basis of calcium-induced E-cadherin rigidification and dimerization. Nature 380: 360–364.
10. Angst BD, Marcozzi C, Magee AI (2001) The cadherin superfamily: diversity in form and function. J Cell Sci 114: 629–641.
11. Tsukada K, Nishio S, Usami S (2010) A large cohort study of *GJB2* mutations in Japanese hearing loss patients. Clin Genet 78: 464–470.
12. Tsukamoto K, Suzuki H, Harada D, Namba A, Abe S, et al. (2003) Distribution and frequencies of PDS (*SLC26A4*) mutations in Pendred syndrome and nonsyndromic hearing loss associated with enlarged vestibular aqueduct: a unique spectrum of mutations in Japanese. Eur J Hum Genet 11: 916–922.
13. Park HJ, Shaukat S, Liu XZ, Hahn SH, Naz S, et al. (2003) Origins and frequencies of *SLC26A4* (PDS) mutations in east and south Asians: global implications for the epidemiology of deafness. J Med Genet 40: 242–248.
14. Usami S, Wagatsuma M, Fukuoka H, Suzuki H, Tsukada K, et al. (2008) The responsible genes in Japanese deafness patients and clinical application using Invader assay. Acta Otolaryngol 128: 446–454.
15. Van Laer L, Coucke P, Mueller RF, Caethoven G, Flothmann K, et al. (2001) A common founder for the 35delG *GJB2* gene mutation in connexin 26 hearing impairment. J Med Genet 38: 515–518.
16. Johnson KR, Erway LC, Cook SA, Willott JF, Zheng QY (1997) A major gene affecting age-related hearing loss in C57BL/6J mice. Hear Res 114: 83–92.
17. Zheng QY, Yan D, Ouyang XM, Du LL, Yu H, et al. (2005) Digenic inheritance of deafness caused by mutations in genes encoding cadherin 23 and protocadherin 15 in mice and humans. Hum Mol Genet 14: 103–111.
18. Usami S, Miyagawa M, Suzuki N, Moteki H, Nishio S, et al. (2010) Genetic background of candidates for EAS (Electric-Acoustic Stimulation). Audiologidal Medicine 8: 28–32.
19. de Kok JB, Wiegerinck ET, Giesendorf BA, Swinkels DW (2002) Rapid genotyping of single nucleotide polymorphisms using novel minor groove binding DNA oligonucleotides (MGB probes). Hum Mutat 19: 554–559.
20. Langmead B, Trapnell C, Pop M, Salzberg SL (2009) Ultrafast and memory-efficient alignment of short DNA sequences to the human genome. Genome Biol 10: R25.
21. Kumar P, Henikoff S, Ng PC (2009) Predicting the effects of coding non-synonymous variants on protein function using the SIFT algorithm. Nat Protoc 4: 1073–1081.
22. Adzhubei IA, Schmidt S, Peshkin L, Ramensky VE, Gerasimova A, et al. (2010) A method and server for predicting damaging missense mutations. Nat Methods 7: 248–249.

8

Common Molecular Etiologies are Rare in Nonsyndromic Tibetan Chinese Patients with Hearing Impairment

Yongyi Yuan[1,3], Xun Zhang[2], Shasha Huang[1], Lujie Zuo[1,2], Guozheng Zhang[1,2], Yueshuai Song[1], Guojian Wang[1,3], Hongtian Wang[1], Deliang Huang[1]*, Dongyi Han[1]*, Pu Dai[1,3]*

1 Department of Otolaryngology, PLA General Hospital, Beijing, People's Republic of China, **2** Department of Otolaryngology, 3rd hospital of Hebei Medical University, Shijiazhuang, Hebei Province, People's Republic of China, **3** Department of Otolaryngology, Hainan Branch of PLA General Hospital, Sanya, People's Republic of China

Abstract

Background: Thirty thousand infants are born every year with congenital hearing impairment in mainland China. Racial and regional factors are important in clinical diagnosis of genetic deafness. However, molecular etiology of hearing impairment in the Tibetan Chinese population living in the Tibetan Plateau has not been investigated. To provide appropriate genetic testing and counseling to Tibetan families, we investigated molecular etiology of nonsyndromic deafness in this population.

Methods: A total of 114 unrelated deaf Tibetan children from the Tibet Autonomous Region were enrolled. Five prominent deafness-related genes, *GJB2*, *SLC26A4*, *GJB6*, *POU3F4*, and mtDNA *12S rRNA*, were analyzed. Inner ear development was evaluated by temporal CT. A total of 106 Tibetan hearing normal individuals were included as genetic controls. For radiological comparison, 120 patients, mainly of Han ethnicity, with sensorineural hearing loss were analyzed by temporal CT.

Results: None of the Tibetan patients carried diallelic *GJB2* or *SLC26A4* mutations. Two patients with a history of aminoglycoside usage carried homogeneous mtDNA *12S rRNA* A1555G mutation. Two controls were homozygous for *12S rRNA* A1555G. There were no mutations in *GJB6* or *POU3F4*. A diagnosis of inner ear malformation was made in 20.18% of the Tibetan patients and 21.67% of the Han deaf group. Enlarged vestibular aqueduct, the most common inner ear deformity, was not found in theTibetan patients, but was seen in 18.33% of the Han patients. Common molecular etiologies, *GJB2* and *SLC26A4* mutations, were rare in the Tibetan Chinese deaf population.

Conclusion: The mutation spectrum of hearing loss differs significantly between Chinese Tibetan patients and Han patients. The incidence of inner ear malformation in Tibetans is almost as high as that in Han deaf patients, but the types of malformation vary greatly. Hypoxia and special environment in plateau may be one cause of developmental inner ear deformity in this population.

Editor: Iris Schrijver, Stanford University School of Medicine, United States of America

Funding: This work was supported by Chinese National Nature Science Foundation Research Grant (30572015, 30728030, 31071109), State 863 High Technology R&D Key Project of China(SQ2010AA0221634001) and grant from the Minister of Science and Technology (2012BAI09B02) to Dr. Pu Dai, Chinese National Nature Science Foundation Research Grant (30801285) and Beijing Nova programme (2009B34) to Dr. Yongyi Yuan, Chinese National Nature Science Foundation Research Grant (81000415) and Beijing Nova programme (2010B081) to Dr. Guojian Wang. The funders had no role in study design, data collection and analysis, decision to publish, or preparation of the manuscript.

Competing Interests: The authors have declared that no competing interests exist.

* E-mail: daipu301@vip.sina.com (PD); hdy301@263.net (D. Han); huangdl301@sina.com (D. Huang)

These authors contributed equally to this work.

Introduction

Hereditary hearing loss is a genetically heterogeneous disorder in humans, with an incidence rate of approximately 1 in 1000 children [1]. Nonsyndromic deafness accounts for 60–70% of inherited hearing impairment cases and involves 114 loci and 66 different genes with autosomal dominant (DFNA), autosomal recessive (DNFB), X-linked (DFN), and maternal inheritance patterns [2].

In China, there are 27.80 million people with hearing and speech disabilities; of these, 20.04 million have simple hearing disability [3], with genetic factors accounting for about 55% of the Chinese deaf population of Han ethnicity [3–4]. Worldwide, the most common causes of nonsyndromic autosomal recessive hearing loss are mutations in connexin 26, a gap-junction protein encoded by the GJB2 gene [5–13]. Defects in *SLC26A4*, which encodes the anion (chloride/iodide, chloride/bicarbonate) transporter Pendrin, can cause nonsyndromic DFNB4 deafness with enlargement of the vestibular aqueduct (EVA) and Pendred syndrome [14,15]. A mutation of *SLC26A4* mutation is the second most common cause of deafness in China [4]. Although the majority of cases of hereditary hearing loss are caused by nuclear gene defects, it has become clear that mutations in mitochondrial DNA (mtDNA) can also cause nonsyndromic hearing loss. The best studied mutations related to aminoglycoside suscepterblity are A1555G and C1494T in the mitochondrial *12S rRNA* gene [16–

18]. Nonsyndromic inherited hearing impairment caused by mutations in *GJB2*, *SLC26A4*, or mtDNA *12S rRNA* typical accounts for 33.8% of the cases of deafness in areas of China [4].

China is a multiethnic country. Tibetans live mainly on the Tibetan Plateau, an area of southwest China with an average altitude of 4000 m above sea level, making it one of the highest region in the world. High-altitude hypoxia (reduced inspired oxygen tension owing to decreased barometric pressure) exerts severe physiological stress on the human body. Populations living on the Tibetan Plateau exhibit unique circulatory, respiratory, and hematological adaptations to life at high altitude, and these responses have been well characterized physiologically. Recent studies of the genetics associated with high-altitude adaptation have facilitated the genotype–phenotype studies necessary to confirm the role of selection-determined candidate genes and gene regions involved in adaptation to altitude [19,20]. Although hearing and vestibular disorders at high altitude have been reported since 1938, the etiologies of these disorders are still unknown. The mechanisms by which the auditory system adapts to high altitude have not been elucidated in detail, and the molecular etiology of hereditary hearing loss in populations on the Tibetan Plateau remains unknown.

In the present study, we comprehensively analyzed five prominent deafness-related genes, *i.e.*, *GJB2*, *SLC26A4*, mtDNA *12S rRNA*, *GJB6*, and *POU3F4*, in 114 Tibetan patients from unrelated families in the Tibetan Plateau who experienced early-onset, nonsyndromic hearing impairment, to investigate the molecular etiology of hereditary hearing loss in this region. All of the patients underwent temporal computed tomography (CT) to evaluate inner ear development. In addition, detailed genotype and phenotype analyses were performed in the Tibetan hearing loss patients.

Materials and Methods

Patients and DNA samples

A total of 114 Tibetan deaf subjects from unrelated families were included in this study. They were all from Lhasa Special Education School, which is the only special education school in Tibet Autonomous Region. This cohort consisted of 57 males and 57 females ranging in age from 8 to 21 years, with an average age of 12.10±2.75 years. The study protocol was approved by the ethics committee of the Chinese PLA General Hospital. Written informed consent was obtained from all subjects or their parents prior to blood sampling. Parents were interviewed with regard to age at onset, family history, mother's health during pregnancy, and patient's clinical history, including infection, possible head or brain injury, and the use of aminoglycoside antibiotics.

All subjects showed moderate to profound bilateral sensorineural hearing impairment on audiograms. Careful medical examinations revealed no clinical features other than hearing impairment. None of the Tibetan patients with hearing impairment in our study showed any sign of vestibular dysfunction in their case history. Using a commercially available DNA extraction kit (Watson Biotechnologies Inc., Shanghai, China), DNA was extracted from the peripheral blood leukocytes of the 114 patients with nonsyndromic hearing loss and the 106 region- and ethnicity-matched controls with normal hearing.

Mutational analysis

For all patients, the *GJB2* coding region plus approximately 50 bp of the flanking intron regions and the mitochondrial *12S rRNA* gene (nt611 to nt2007) were amplified by PCR, followed by sequence analysis using the Big Dye sequencing protocol with an ABI 3100 Genetic Analyzer and analysis software v.3.7 NT (Applied Biosystems, Foster City, CA), according to the manufacturer's protocol. Patients with a monoallelic *GJB2* coding region mutation were further tested for the *GJB2* IVS1+1G>A mutation or defects in exon 1 and the promoter of *GJB2*. The specific promoter region of *GJB2* includes 128 bp.The basal promoter,-exon 1 and donor splice site of GJB2 gene can be found in GenBank (accession number U43932.1); the *GJB6* 309-kb deletion; and the mutations of the entire *GJB6* coding region. The presence of the 309-kb *GJB6* deletion was analyzed by PCR [15,16]. A positive control (provided by Balin Wu, Department of Laboratory Medicine, Children's Hospital Boston and Harvard Medical School, Boston, MA) was used to detect *GJB6* gene deletions.

The exons of *SLC26A4* of all 114 patients were sequenced individually, starting with the frequently mutated exons, until two mutant alleles were identified. The patients verified with an inner ear malformation on a temporal bone CT scan were further tested for a POU3F4 gene mutation.

Similarly, the *GJB2*, *SLC26A4*, and mtDNA *12S rRNA* genes from 106 Tibetan controls with normal hearing were sequenced to determine the presence of mutations and exon variants. As no *POU3F4* variants, with the exception of two silent mutations, were found in the individuals with hearing loss, *POU3F4* was not sequenced in the control group.

CT scan

All 114 patients were examined by temporal bone CT for diagnosis of EVA or other inner ear malformations, at the General Hospital of Tibet Military District. The diagnosis of EVA was based on a diameter of >1.5 mm at the midpoint between the common crus and the external aperture. For radiological comparison, the temporal CT results in 120 patients, mainly of Han ethnicity, with sensorineural hearing loss were analyzed at the Genetic Testing Center for Deafness of PLA General Hospital.

Results

Among the 114 cases included in this study, 88 had prelingual hearing loss, including 56 cases of congenital hearing loss. Eight cases showed postlingual hearing loss, with an average age of onset of 2.97±1.37 years. The age of onset was unclear in the remaining 18 cases. Thirteen cases (8 prelingual and 5 postlingual), with an average age of onset of 2.01±1.18 years, had a clear history of aminoglycoside administration. Patients with no history of aminoglycoside usage showed a significantly earlier average age of onset (0.92±1.03 years; $P<0.001$).

GJB2 gene mutations

Sequence analysis of the *GJB2* gene indicated that none of the Tibetan patients carried two pathogenic mutations. Only two Tibetan patients carried a confirmed *GJB2* heterozygous pathogenic mutation, c.235delC and c.299_300delAT mutation, respectively (Table 1). One Han patient carried a heterozygous c.235delC mutation.

The allele frequency of p.R127H, classified as a pathogenic *GJB2* mutation, was significantly higher in the patient group than in the control group ($P<0.05$), indicating that p.R127H may be a mutation in the Chinese Tibetan hearing loss population. However, all 15 patients with the p.R127H mutation were heterozygotes. The pathogenic *GJB2* mutation p.R32H was carried by a control subject, but was not found in the patients. An unclassified variant, p.T123N, had been counted as a mutation in a previous Japanese study, but as a polymorphism in studies

Table 1. Genotypes of GJB2 gene in Tibetan patients with hearing loss and Tibetan controls.

Allele 1			Allele 2			numbers found in patients	numbers found in controls
Nucleotide Change	**Consequence or amino acid change**	**Category**	**Nucleotide change**	**Consequence or amino acid Change**	**Category**		
c.235delC	Frameshift TM2	Pathogenic				1	0
c.299_300delAT	Frameshift IC2	Pathogenic				1	0
c.341A>G	p.E114G IC2	Polymorphism	c.79G>A, c.341A>G	p.V27I,p.E114G	Polymorphism	1	0
c.79G>A	p.V27I	Polymorphism	c.79G>A, c.341A>G	p.V27I,p.E114G	Polymorphism	3	1
c.79G>A, c.341A>G	p.V27I,p.E114G	Polymorphism	-			15	24
c.79G>A, c.341A>G	p.V27I,p.E114G	Polymorphism	c.79G>A, c.341A>G	p.V27I,p.E114G	Polymorphism	2	1
c.341A>G	p.E114G	Polymorphism				1	0
c.79G>A	p.V27I TM1	Polymorphism				15	16
c.79G>A	p.V27I	Polymorphism	c.79G>A	p.V27I	Polymorphism	1	3
c.79G>A	p.V27I	Polymorphism	c.380G>A	p.R127H	Pathogenic	3	0
c.79G>A	p.V27I	Polymorphism	c.368C>A	p.T123N IC2	Polymorphism	0	2
c.380G>A	p.R127H IC2	Pathogenic	c.79G>A, c.341A>G	p.V27I,p.E114G	Polymorphism	6	0
c.380G>A	p.R127H	Pathogenic	c.457G>A	p.V153I TM3	Polymorphism	1	0
c.380G>A	p.R127H	Pathogenic				5	0
c.109G>A	[c]p.V37I, TM1	[c]See note				1	0
c.109G>A	[c]p.V37I	[c]See note	c.380G>A	p.R127H	Pathogenic	1	0
c.608T>C	p.I203T TM4	Polymorphism				1	2
c.95G>A	p.R32H TM1	Pathogenic				0	1
c.438C>T	p.F146F TM3	Polymorphism				2	1

TM, transmembrane domain; EC, extracellular domain; IC, intracellular domain.
Note: p.V37I is controversy variant, see the discussion.

performed in Taiwan and Turkey [12,21,22]. We found two p.T123N alleles in our Tibetan control subjects, but none in the Tibetan patient group (P>0.05), suggesting that it may be a neutral variant. The frequency of p.V37I was higher in the deaf group than in the controls in the present study, but the difference was not significant (P>0.05). The p.V37I variant was considered a pathogenic mutation in Japanese, Iranian, Korean, Moroccan, Malay, Israeli, Australian, and Italian studies [12,23–30], but was reported as a variant in African-American, Caribbean Hispanic, French, Chinese, and Thai individuals with hearing impairment [31–34]. There was no significant difference in the allele frequency of p.V153I, classified previously as a polymorphism [2], between the Tibetan patient group and the controls in the present study (P>0.05), and we regarded it as a polymorphism. The p.V27I, p.E114G, and p.I203T variants were polymorphisms in the Chinese populations of Han [13] and Tibetan ethnicity. The *GJB2* IVS1+1G to A mutation was not detected in patients with a heterozygous *GJB2* mutation, and no novel nucleotide alterations were identified in the Tibetan hearing loss patients or control subjects.

SLC26A4 gene mutations

Six nucleotide changes in the *SLC26A4* gene were verified through sequencing of all 20 exons of the gene from 114 Tibetan patients (Table 2). None of the Tibetan patients carried an *SLC26A4* mutation on two alleles. Four patients exhibited the heterozygous c.1826T>G (p.V609G) variant. In addition, four c.1826T>G heterozygotes were verified in the control group. As there was no significant difference between the patient and control groups, we considered this a polymorphism in the Tibetan population, although Pryor et al. classified it as a mutation in 2005 [2]. The IVS13+9 C>T variant was first reported as a splice site mutation by Yong et al. in 2001 [35]. The IVS13+9 C>T variant was carried by one patient in the heterozygous state in our study population, and it did not predict a gain or loss of a splice site when analyzed using the Neural Network Splice Site Prediction Tool NNSPLICE0.9 (available at http://www.fruitfly.org/seq_tools/splice.html). Therefore, we considered this to be a benign variant.

Two patients carried novel unclassified missense variants of *SLC26A4*, c.757A>G (p.I253V) and c.1522A>G (p.T508A), respectively. We found four p.I253V heterozygotes, but no p.T508A carriers in the control group. The frequency of p.I253V was higher in the control group than in the patient group (P>0.05). No p.I253V allele was found in 100 normally hearing individuals of Han ethnicity (unpublished data). Thus, we considered it to be a polymorphism typical of the Tibetan Chinese population.

Both c.273A>T (p.G91G) and c.753C>T (p.L251L) are silent variants of *SLC26A4*. The intron18-56delCAAA was considered to be an intron variant.

Table 2. Genotypes and phenotype of SLC26A4 gene in Tibetan patients with hearing loss.

Allele 1			Allele 2			numbers found in patients	Temporal bone CT scan phenotype
Nucleotide Change	Amino acid change	Category	Nucleotide change	Amino acid change	Category		
c. 1826T>G	p.V609G	Polymorphism	intron18-56delCAAA		intron variant	1	hypoplastic cochlea, enlargement of IAC
c. 1826T>G	p.V609G	Polymorphism	intron18-56delCAAA		intron variant	3	nl
c.273A>T	p.G91G	Silent variant	.			1	Stenosis of IAC
c.753C>T	p.L251L	Silent variant				1	nl
c.757A>G	p.I253V	Polymorphism				1	hypoplastic cochleavestibular and semicircular canals
c.1522A>G	p.T508A	Less likely be Pathogenic or exon variant				1	nl
IVS13+9C>T	aberrant splicing	intron variant				1	nl

nl, normal; EVA, enlarged vestibular aqueduct; IVS7, intravening sequence 7 (intron 7); IVS13, intravening sequence 13 (intron 13);IVS15, intravening sequence 15 (intron 15);IVS18, intravening sequence 18 (intron 18);IAC,internal auditory canal.

MtDNA 12S rRNA gene mutations

Two Tibetan patients and two normal hearing Tibetan controls carried a homogeneous mtDNA *12S rRNA* A1555G mutation. Neither the C1494T mutation nor any other *12S rRNA* mutation associated with hearing impairment, including nucleotide changes at positions 961 and 1095, were found in the Tibetan patient or control groups.

POU3F4 mutations

No *POU3F4* mutations, with the exception of the two polymorphisms 708A>G (E236E) and 710G>C (E236E), were identified in the 23 patients with inner ear malformation.

Temporal bone CT scan

Nine types of inner ear malformations were verified on temporal bone CT scans in 23 Tibetan patients (a total of 37 ears) (Table 3). The frequency of inner ear malformation in the Tibetan hearing-loss patients was 20.18% (23/114). EVA, the most common type of inner ear malformation in China reported in previous studies, was not detected in the Tibetan deafness patients in the present study. The results of temporal CT in 120 patients, mainly of Han ethnicity, with sensorineural hearing loss revealed that 21.67% (26/120) had an inner ear malformation, 18.33% (22/120) had EVA, and only 3.33% (4/120) showed other types of inner ear malformations, including hypoplastic cochlea, hypoplastic vestibular aqueduct, incomplete partition type I, and common cavity (Fig. 1).

Discussion

According to the second nationwide survey of the disabled Chinese population performed in 2006, there were 27.80 million people with hearing and speech disabilities in China. The number of Chinese with hearing disability alone is 20.04 million, representing 1.54% of the population (20.04 million/1300 million). The percentage of the population with hearing disability in the Tibet Autonomous Region is 1.65% [36]. More than 92% of the whole population in the Tibet Autonomous Region is Tibetan, and 93.4% of the patients in our study population were Tibetan. Despite a similar incidence of moderate to profound sensorineural hearing loss in the Tibetan and Chinese populations, the molecular etiology in Tibetan patients appeared differ markedly from that in the Chinese population as a whole based on the present results. We found no homozygous or compound heterozygous mutations of the *GJB2* or *SLC26A4* gene. The mtDNA *12S rRNA* A1555G homogeneous mutation and the use of aminoglycoside antibiotics were responsible for hearing loss in 1.75% (2/114) of the Tibetan patients. In typical areas of China, *GJB2* gene mutations account for the etiology in about 18.31% of patients with hearing loss, *SLC26A4* mutations account for about 13.73%, and the *12S rRNA* A1555G mutation accounts for 1.76% [4]. There is no significant difference in the *12S rRNA* A1555G mutation rate between the Tibetan patients with hearing impairment and the patients mainly of Han ethnicity.

The pathogenicity of the *GJB2* p.V37I mutation is controversial. In a multicenter study, p.V37I was shown to be associated with mild to moderate hearing impairment (median, 25–40 dB) [37]. Our recent study indicated p.V37I had an allele frequency of 6.7% (185/2744) in a Han patient group (excluding all cases with two clearly pathogenic mutations), and this was significantly higher than that in a control population (2.8%, 17/602; $P=0.0003$) [13], supporting Wu's suggestion that p.V37I should be reassigned from an allele variant to a pathogenic mutation [38]. In the present study, the frequency of p.V37I was higher in Tibetan patients with hearing loss than in ethnicity-matched controls, but the difference was not significant ($P>0.05$). Since our sample size was still too small to reach a confident statistical conclusion.and only two of our Tibetan patients carried *GJB2* p.V37I (table 1), our results didn't support that p.V37I was pathogenic in Tibetan Chinese patients. Alternative explanation may be another unknown mutation associated with the V37I mutation is responsible for the etiology of Tibetan Chinese patients with hearing loss.

POU3F4 has been identified only for the Locus DFN3. The clinical features of DFN3 often include mixed progressive hearing loss, temporal bone anomalies, and stapes fixation [39–41]. *POU3F4* belongs to a subfamily of transcription factors characterized by two conserved DNA-binding domains, a POU and a HOX domain, containing a helix-turn-helix structural DNA-binding motif. Several reports have described *POU3F4* mutations in patients with hearing loss and temporal bone abnormalities [42]. Temporal bone CT scans of DFN3 patients as well as the *Pou3f4* knockout inner ear phenotypes have suggested that most of

Table 3. Temporal bone CT Scan Phenotype in Chinese Tibetan patients with hearing loss.

	Phenotype	numbers found in patients	Numbers of ears found in patients
a	incomplete partition type I	1	1
b	common cavity deforrmity	[c]1	1
c	malformation of inner ears including cochlea,vestibular and semicircular canals	10	18
d	malformation of cochlea and enlargement of internal auditory canals	1	2
e	narrow internal auditory canal	3	6
f	malformation of vestibular and semicircular canals	5	6
g	malformation of semicircular canals	1	1
h	malformation of cochlea	1	1
i	ossification of the inner ear	1	1
j	enlarged vestibular aqueduct	0	0

Note:One patient shows common cavity deforrmity in the right ear and incomplete partition type I in the left ear.

the inner ear malformations were in structures derived from the mesenchyme [43,44]. However, no variants or mutations were found in Tibetan patients recruited in this study with inner ear malformation.A series of transcription factors, including Pax2, Six, Eya1, Dlx, Hmx2–3, GATA3, RA, Otx1–2, IGF-1, and Tbx1, are related to the development of the mammalian otic capsule, and defects in these factors were reported to cause inner ear deformities in mice [45–54]. As the phenotype and genotype correlations for these genes in human patients with inner ear malformation are not clear, we did not screen for these genes in our patients.

The inner ear malformations in our Tibetan patients were diverse and severe. EVA, the most common inner ear deformity, was not found in our cases. This radiological finding was consistent with the genetic analyses, as no diallelic mutations were found in the open reading frame of *SLC26A4*. A novel *SLC26A4* variant,

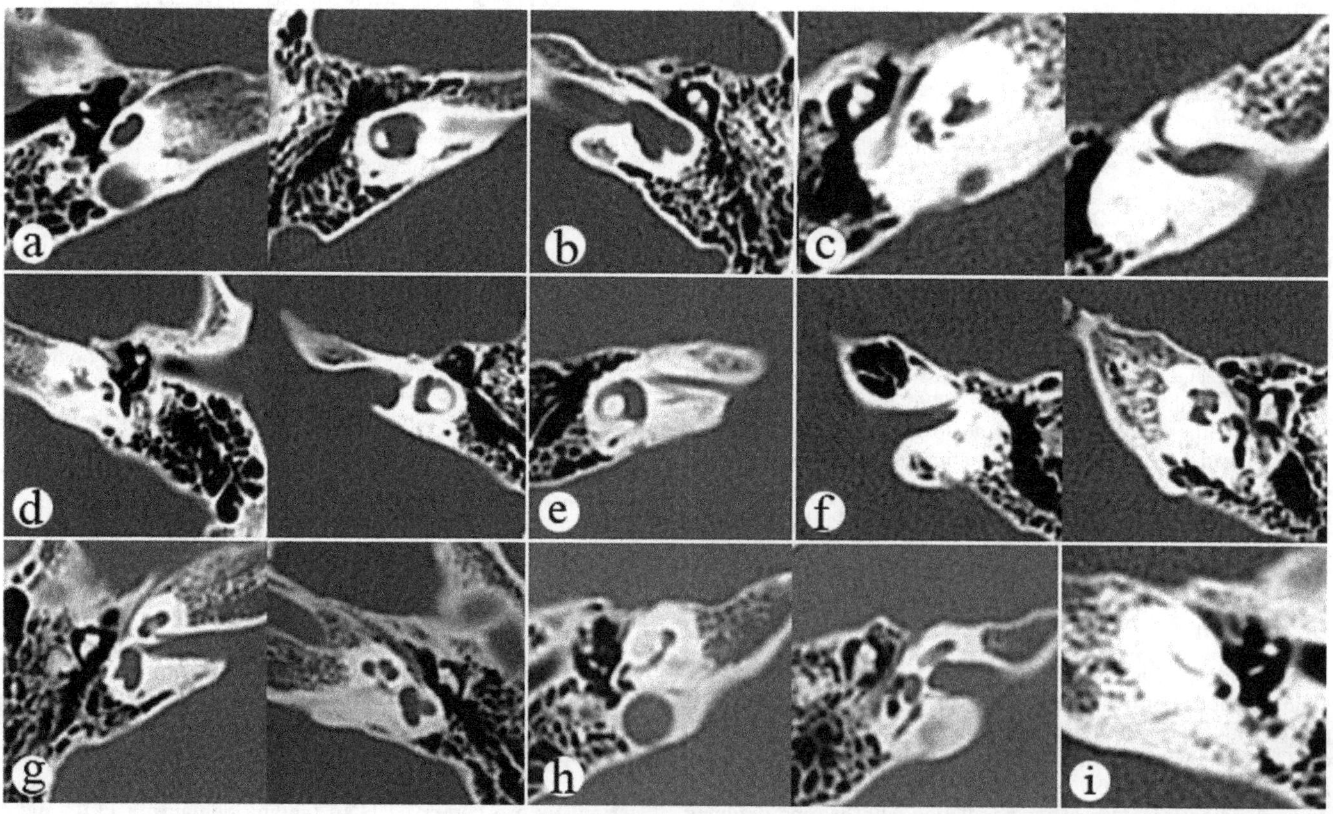

Figure 1. CT images of inner ear malformation in Tibetan patients with hearing impairment. a. incomplete partition type I **b.** common cavity deforrmity **c.** malformation of inner ears including cochlea,vestibular and semicircular canals **d.** malformation of cochlea and enlargement of internal auditory canals **e.** narrow internal auditory canal **f.** malformation of vestibular and semicircular canals **g.** malformation of semicircular canals **h.** malformation of cochlea **i.** ossification of the inner ear.

p.T508A, was identified in the Tibetan patient group. The location of this amino acid in an evolutionarily conserved region implies that its substitution may result in a structurally and/or functionally different protein. We then carried a SIFT analysis on *SLC26A4* p.T508A variant.The SIFT score was 0.17 and the SIFT prediction result was that the amino acid change was tolerated,- which indicated it may be only a variant or be less likely a pathogenic mutation.There are two types of inner ear malformation: osseous labyrinth deformity and membranous labyrinth deformity. We assessed only the osseous labyrinth shape by high-resolution temporal bone CT. Magnetic resonance imaging (MRI) and water image of the inner ear may be valuable for assessment of membranous labyrinth deformity. However, we did not perform these two radiological examinations and could not evaluate the membranous labyrinth. Whether malformation of vestibular and/ or semicircular canals can cause hearing-related phenotypes is not certain, but imbalances of the ion environment in the cochlea as well as structural abnormalities can result in hearing impairment. Hearing loss caused by EVA is an example of a pathology with normal cochlear structure, but with a suggested cochlear ion imbalance.

To our knowledge, there have been no previous studies of the genetic etiology of hearing loss in Tibetan patients. The distinct mutational spectrum of common hearing-related genes in the Tibetan patients compared with typical patients in other areas of China may be explained by ethnic and regional factors. According to archeological data, the Tibetan Plateau was first populated approximately 25,000 years ago. Compared with low-altitude populations, the populations indigenous to the high-altitude zones possess unique physiological characteristics [55]. Some of the environmental hardships at high altitudes include, but are not limited to, decreased ambient oxygen tension, increased solar radiation, extreme diurnal ranges in temperature, arid climate, and poor soil quality. The incidence of congenital heart disease including patent ductus arteriosus,ventricular septal defect,ventricular septal defect, atrial septal defect and valvular insufficiency in the Tibetan plateau is 0.615%.It is higher than that in lower altitude areas in China,which is 0.31% in Chengdu from Sichuang Province, 0.239% in Hefei from Anhui Province and 0.28% in Fuzhou from Fujian Province,respectively [56]. And with the increase of altitude in the same province,the incidence of congenital heart disease is increasing,which indicated that anoxia in high altitude area was regarded as one of the enviromental factors related with congenital heart disease [57]. Several studies have shown that Tibetan populations have lower hemoglobin concentrations than lowland Chinese populations [58]. Related studies have explored the heritability of specific altitude-related phenotypes, such as arterial oxygen saturation and hemoglobin concentration [58–60]. One heritability study concluded that there is a major autosomal dominant locus for high oxygen saturation, and Tibetan women carrying this high oxygen-saturation allele had higher offspring survival than those with a low oxygen-saturation allele [59]. In addition, positively selected haplotypes of EGLN1 and PPARA were significantly associated with the decreased hemoglobin phenotype unique to this highland population [20]. The genetic evidence for high-altitude adaptation in Tibet suggests that epigenetic regulation may play a greater role in the physiopathological process in Tibetans, although this has yet to be confirmed. High-altitude hypoxia exerts severe physiological stress on the human body, including embryonic auditory organ development.

Conclusion

The results of the present study indicate that the mutation spectrum of Tibetan Chinese patients with hearing loss is significantly different from that seen in patients of Han ethnicity. The incidence of inner ear malformation in the Tibetan Chinese population is almost as high as that in Chinese Han patients, but the types of malformation vary greatly in the Tibetan population. The most common inner ear deformity, enlarged vestibular aqueduct (EVA), is rare in the Chinese Tibetan hearing-loss population. Hypoxia may be one of the causes for the development of inner ear deformity, but further studies are required to determine the genetic etiology of hearing loss in Tibetan patients.

Acknowledgments

We thank the professional editors from Textcheck for English check of our manuscript. For a certificate, please see: http://www.textcheck.com/certificate/1XyxQd.

Author Contributions

Conceived and designed the experiments: PD D. Huang D. Han. Performed the experiments: SH LZ GZ GW YS. Analyzed the data: YY XZ. Contributed reagents/materials/analysis tools: HW. Wrote the paper: YY.

References

1. Cohen MM, Gorlin RJ (1995) Epidemiology, etiology and genetic patterns. In: Gorlin RJ, Toriello HV, Cohen MM, eds. Hereditary hearing loss and its snydromes, Oxford University Press, Oxford. pp 9–21.
2. Hereditary Hearing Loss website. Available: http://hereditaryhearingloss.org/main.aspx?c=.HHH&n=86162 Accessed 2011 Dec 3.
3. Han DY (2010) Strengthen the research on prevention and treatment of sensorineural hearing loss in China. Zhonghua Er Bi Yan Hou Tou Jing Wai Ke Za Zhi 45(4): 265–268.
4. Yuan Y, You Y, Huang D, Cui J, Wang Y, et al. (2009) Comprehensive molecular etiology analysis of nonsyndromic hearing impairment from typical areas in China. J Transl Med 7: 79(1–12).
5. Estivill X, Fortina P, Surrey S, Rabionet R, Melchionda S, et al. (1998) Connexin-26 mutations in sporadic and inherited sensorineural deafness. Lancet 351: 394–398.
6. Lench N, Houseman M, Newton V, Van Camp G, Mueller R (1998) Connexin-26 mutations in sporadic non-syndromal sensorineural deafness. Lancet 351: 415.
7. Morell RJ, Kim HJ, Hood LJ, Goforth L, Friderici K, et al. (1998) Mutations in the connexin 26 gene (*GJB2*) among Ashkenazi Jews with nonsyndromic recessive deafness. N Engl J Med 339: 1500–1505.
8. Park HJ, Hahn SH, Chun YM, Park K, Kim HN (2000) Connexin26 mutations associated with nonsyndromic hearing loss. Laryngoscope 110: 1535–1538.
9. Rabionet R, Zelante L, Lopez-Bigas N, D'Agruma L, Melchionda S, et al. (2000) Molecular basis of childhood deafness resulting from mutations in the *GJB2* (connexin 26) gene. Hum Genet 106: 40–44.
10. Wilcox SA, Saunders K, Osborn AH, Arnold A, Wunderlich J, et al. (2000) High frequency hearing loss correlated with mutations in the GJB2 gene. Hum Genet 106: 399–405.
11. Gabriel H, Kupsch P, Sudendey J, Winterhager E, Jahnke K, et al. (2001) Mutations in the connexin26/GJB2 gene are the most common event in non-syndromic hearing loss among the German population. Hum Mutat 17: 521–522.
12. Ohtsuka A, Yuge I, Kimura S, Namba A, Abe S, et al. (2003) *GJB2* deafness gene shows a specific spectrum of mutations in Japan, including a frequent founder mutation. Hum Genet 112: 329–333.
13. Dai P, Yu F, Han B, Wang G, Li Q, et al. (2009) GJB2 mutation spectrum in 2063 Chinese patients with nonsyndromic hearing impairment. J Transl Med 7: 26(1–12).
14. Everett LA, Morsli H, Wu DK, Green ED (1999) Expression pattern of the mouse ortholog of the Pendred's syndrome gene (Pds) suggests a key role for pendrin in the inner ear. Proc Natl Acad Sci USA 96: 9727–9732.
15. Royaux IE, Suzuki K, Mori A, Katoh R, Everett LA, et al. (2000) Pendrin, the protein encoded by the Pendred syndrome gene (PDS), is an apical porter of iodide in the thyroid and is regulated by thyroglobulin in FRTL-5 cells. Endocrinology 141: 839–845.

16. Fischel-Ghodsian N (1998) Mitochondrial genetics and hearing loss: the missing link between genotype and phenotype. Proc Soc Exp Biol Med 218: 1–6.
17. Hutchin TP, Cortopassi GA (2000) Mitochondrial defects and hearing loss. Cell Mol Life Sci 57: 1927–1937.
18. Zhao H, Li R, Wang Q, Yan Q, Deng JH, et al. (2004) Maternally inherited aminoglycoside-induced and nonsyndromic deafness is associated with the novel C1494T mutation in the mitochondrial 12S rRNA gene in a large Chinese family. Am J Hum Genet 74: 139–152.
19. Beall CM (2007) Two routes to functional adaptation: Tibetan and Andean high-altitude natives. Proc Natl Acad Sci U S A 104(suppl. 1): 8655–8660.
20. Simonson TS, Yang Y, Huff CD, Yun H, Qin G, et al. (2010) Genetic evidence for high-altitude adaptation in Tibet. Science 329(5987): 72–75.
21. Hwa HL, Ko TM, Hsu CJ, Huang CH, Chiang YL, et al. (2003) Mutation spectrum of the connexin 26 (GJB2) gene in Taiwanese patients with prelingual deafness. Genet Med 5: 161–165.
22. Bonyadi M, Esmaeili M, Abhari M, Lotfi A (2009) Mutation analysis of familial GJB2-related deafness in Iranian Azeri Turkish patients. Genet Test Mol Biomarkers 13(5): 689–692.
23. Tsukada K, Nishio S, Usami S (2010) A large cohort study of GJB2 mutations in Japanese hearing loss patients. Clin Genet 78(5): 464–470.
24. Mahdieh N, Rabbani B, Shirkavand A, Bagherian H, Movahed ZS, et al. (2011) Impact of Consanguineous Marriages in GJB2-Related Hearing Loss in the Iranian Population: A Report of a Novel Variant. Genet Test Mol Biomarkers 15(7–8): 489–493.
25. Han SH, Park HJ, Kang EJ, Ryu JS, Lee A, et al. (2008) Carrier frequency of GJB2 (connexin-26) mutations causing inherited deafness in the Korean population. J Hum Genet 53(11–12): 1022–1028.
26. Abidi O, Boulouiz R, Nahili H, Bakhouch K, Wakrim L, et al. (2008) Carrier frequencies of mutations/polymorphisms in the connexin 26 gene (GJB2) in the Moroccan population. Genet Test 12(4): 569–574.
27. Ruszymah BH, Wahida IF, Zakinah Y, Zahari Z, Norazlinda MD, et al. (2005) Congenital deafness: high prevalence of a V37I mutation in the GJB2 gene among deaf school children in Alor Setar. Med J Malaysia 60(3): 269–274.
28. Zlotogora J, Carasquillo M, Barges S, Shalev SA, Hujerat Y, et al. (2006) High incidence of deafness from three frequent connexin 26 mutations in an isolated community. Genet Test 10(1): 40–43.
29. Dahl HH, Tobin SE, Poulakis Z, Rickards FW, Xu X, et al. (2006) The contribution of GJB2 mutations to slight or mild hearing loss in Australian elementary school children. J Med Genet 43(11): 850–855.
30. Gualandi E, Ravani A, Berto A, Burdo S, Trevisi P, et al. (2004) Occurrence of del(GIB6-D13S1830) mutation in Italian non-syndromic hearing loss patients carrying a single GJB2 mutated allele. Acta Otolaryngol Suppl 552: 29–34.
31. Samanich J, Lowes C, Burk R, Shanske S, Lu J, et al. (2007) Mutations in GJB2, GJB6, and mitochondrial DNA are rare in African American and Caribbean Hispanic individuals with hearing impairment. Am J Med Genet A143A(8): 830–838.
32. Shi GZ, Gong LX, Xu XH, Nie WY, Lin Q, et al. (2004) GJB2 gene mutations in newborns with non-syndromic hearing impairment in Northern China. Hear Res 197(1–2): 19–23.
33. Wattanasirichaigoon D, Limwongse C, Jariengprasert C, Yenchitsomanus PT, Tocharoenthanaphol C, et al. (2004) High prevalence of V37I genetic variant in the connexin-26 (GJB2) gene among non-syndromic hearing-impaired and control Thai individuals. Clin Genet 66(5): 452–460.
34. Roux AF, Pallares-Ruiz N, Vielle A, Faugère V, Templin C, et al. (2004) Molecular epidemiology of DFNB1 deafness in France. BMC Med Genet 5: 5.
35. Yong AM, Goh SS, Zhao Y, Eng PH, Koh LK, et al. (2001) Two Chinese families with Pendred's syndrome–radiological imaging of the ear and molecular analysis of the pendrin gene. J Clin Endocrinol Metab 86(8): 3907–3911.
36. Office of the 2nd nationwide survey of the disabled Chinese population (2007) Handbook of major data on the 2nd nationwide survey of the disabled Chinese population. Beijing: HuaXia publishing company. 2 p, 38 p.
37. Snoeckx RL, Huygen PL, Feldmann D, Marlin S, Denoyelle F, et al. (2005) GJB2 mutations and degree of hearing loss: a multicenter study. Am J Hum Genet 77: 945–957.
38. Wu BL, Lindeman N, Lip V, Adams A, Amato RS, et al. (2002) Effectiveness of sequencing connexin 26(GJB2) in familial or sporadic childhood deafness referred for molecular diagnostic testing. Genet Med 4: 279–288.
39. Stankovic KM, Hennessey AM, Herrmann B, Mankarious LA (2010) Cochlear implantation in children with congenital X-linked deafness due to novel mutations in POU3F4 gene. Ann Otol Rhinol Laryngol 119(12): 815–822.
40. Li J, Cheng J, Lu Y, Lu Y, Chen A, et al. (2010) Identification of a novel mutation in POU3F4 for prenatal diagnosis in a Chinese family with X-linked nonsyndromic hearing loss. J Genet Genomics 37(12): 787–793.
41. Han B, Cheng J, Yang SZ, Cao JY, Shen WD, et al. (2009) Phenotype and genotype analysis of a Chinese family with prelingual X-linked hereditary hearing impairment. Chin Med J (Engl) 122(7): 830–833.
42. Lee HK, Lee SH, Lee KY, Lim EJ, Choi SY, et al. (2009) Novel POU3F4 mutations and clinical features of DFN3 patients with cochlear implants. Clin Genet 75(6): 572–575.
43. Minowa O, Ikeda K, Sugitani Y, Oshima T, Nakai S, et al. (1999) Altered cochlear fibrocytes in a mouse model of DFN3 nonsyndromic deafness. Science 285: 1408–1411.
44. Phippard D, Heydemann A, Lechner M, Lu L, Lee D, et al. (1998) Changes in the subcellular localization of the Brn4 gene product precede mesenchymal remodeling of the otic capsule. Hear Res 120: 77–85.
45. Burton Q, Cole LK, Mulheisen M, Chang W, Wu DK (2004) The role of Pax2 in mouse inner ear development. Dev Biol 272: 161–175.
46. Ozaki H, Nakamura K, Funahashi J, Ikeda K, Yamada G, et al. (2004) Six1 controls patterning of the mouse otic vesicle. Development 131: 551–562.
47. Xu PX, Adams J, Peters H, Brown MC, Heaney S, et al. (1999) Eya1 - deficient mice lack ears and kidneys and show abnormal apoptosis of organ pripordia. Nat Genet 23: 113–117.
48. Merlo GR, Paleari L, Mantero S, Zerega B, Adamska M, et al. (2002) The Dlx5 homebox gene is essential for vestibular morphogenesis in the mouse embryo through a BMP - mediated pathway[J]. Dev Bilo 248: 157–169.
49. Wang W, Chan EK, Baron S, Van de Water T, Lufkin T (2001) Hmx2 homeobox gene control of murine vestibular morphogenesis. Development 128(24): 5017–5029.
50. Karis A, Pata I, van Doorninck JH, Grosveld F, de Zeeuw CI, et al. (2001) Transcription factor GATA- 3 alters pathway selection of oliv ochochlear neurons and affects morphogenesis of the ear. J Comp Neurol 429: 615–630.
51. Romand R, Niederreither K, Abu-Abed S, Petkovich M, Fraulob V, et al. (2004) Complementary expression patterns of retinoid acid - synthesizing and - metabolizing enzymes in pre - natal mouse inner ear structures. Gene Expr Patterns 4: 123–133.
52. Morsli H, Tuorto F, Choo D, Postiglione MP, Simeone A, et al. (2005) Otx1 and Otx2 activities are required for the normal development of the mouse inner ear. Development 126: 2235–2343.
53. Camarero G, Villar MA, Contreras J, Fernández-Moreno C, Pichel JG, et al. (2002) Cochlear abnormalities in insulin-like growth factor-1 mouse mutants. Hear Res 170: 2–11.
54. Moraes F, Nóvoa A, Jerome-Majewska LA, Papaioannou VE, Mallo M (2005) Tbx1 is required for proper neural crest migration and to stabilize spatial patterns during middle and inner ear development. Mech Dev 122: 199–212.
55. Niermeyer S, Zamdio S, Moore LG (2001) The People. In: HTaS RB, ed. High Altitude: An exploration of Human Adaptation. New York: Marcel Dekker, Inc.
56. Wang J, Wang ZN, Li SZ, Wang LJ, Chen ZD, et al. (2002) Examination on congenital heart disease for 6500 students. Tibet's Science and Technology 1: 12–14.
57. Liu RC, Wu TY, Ge RL (1982) Survey on congenital heart disease in Qinghai Plateau. Chin J Cardiol 1 0: 241–242.
58. Beall CM, Brittenham GM, Strohl KP, Blangero J, Williams-Blangero S, et al. (1998) Hemoglobin concentration of high-altitude Tibetans and Bolivian Aymara. Am J Phys Anthropol 106: 385–400.
59. Beall CM, Blangero J, Williams-Blangero S, Goldstein MC (1994) Major gene for percent of oxygen saturation of arterial hemoglobin in Tibetan highlanders. Am J Phys Anthropol 95: 271–276.
60. Beall CM, Strohl KP, Blangero J, Williams-Blangero S, Decker MJ, et al. (1997) Quantitative genetic analysis of arterial oxygen saturation in Tibetan highlanders. Hum Biol 69: 597–604.

9

Whole-Exome Sequencing Efficiently Detects Rare Mutations in Autosomal Recessive Nonsyndromic Hearing Loss

Oscar Diaz-Horta[1], Duygu Duman[2], Joseph Foster II[1], Aslı Sırmacı[1], Michael Gonzalez[1], Nejat Mahdieh, Nikou Fotouhi[4], Mortaza Bonyadi[4], Filiz Başak Cengiz[2], Ibis Menendez[1], Rick H. Ulloa[1], Yvonne J. K. Edwards[1], Stephan Züchner[1], Susan Blanton[1], Mustafa Tekin[1]*

1 John P. Hussman Institute for Human Genomics and the Dr. John T. Macdonald Department of Human Genetics, University of Miami Miller School of Medicine, Miami, Florida, United States of America, **2** Division of Pediatric Genetics, Ankara University School of Medicine, Ankara, Turkey, **3** Growth and Development Research Center, Tehran University of Medical Sciences, Tehran, Iran, **4** Faculty of Natural Sciences, Center of Excellence for Biodiversity, University of Tabriz, Tabriz, Iran

Abstract

Identification of the pathogenic mutations underlying autosomal recessive nonsyndromic hearing loss (ARNSHL) is difficult, since causative mutations in 39 different genes have so far been reported. After excluding mutations in the most common ARNSHL gene, *GJB2*, via Sanger sequencing, we performed whole-exome sequencing (WES) in 30 individuals from 20 unrelated multiplex consanguineous families with ARNSHL. Agilent SureSelect Human All Exon 50 Mb kits and an Illumina Hiseq2000 instrument were used. An average of 93%, 84% and 73% of bases were covered to 1X, 10X and 20X within the ARNSHL-related coding RefSeq exons, respectively. Uncovered regions with WES included those that are not targeted by the exome capture kit and regions with high GC content. Twelve homozygous mutations in known deafness genes, of which eight are novel, were identified in 12 families: *MYO15A*-p.Q1425X, -p.S1481P, -p.A1551D; *LOXHD1*-p.R1494X, -p.E955X; *GIPC3*-p.H170N; *ILDR1*-p.Q274X; *MYO7A*-p.G2163S; *TECTA*-p.Y1737C; *TMC1*-p.S530X; *TMPRSS3*-p.F13Lfs*10; *TRIOBP*-p.R785Sfs*50. Each mutation was within a homozygous run documented via WES. Sanger sequencing confirmed co-segregation of the mutation with deafness in each family. Four rare heterozygous variants, predicted to be pathogenic, in known deafness genes were detected in 12 families where homozygous causative variants were already identified. Six heterozygous variants that had similar characteristics to those abovementioned variants were present in 15 ethnically-matched individuals with normal hearing. Our results show that rare causative mutations in known ARNSHL genes can be reliably identified via WES. The excess of heterozygous variants should be considered during search for causative mutations in ARNSHL genes, especially in small-sized families.

Editor: Andreas R. Janecke, Innsbruck Medical University, Austria

Funding: This study was supported by National Institutes of Health - National Institute on Deafness and Other Communication Disorders grant R01DC009645 to MT. The funders had no role in study design, data collection and analysis, decision to publish, or preparation of the manuscript.

Competing Interests: The authors have declared that no competing interests exist.

* E-mail: mtekin@med.miami.edu

Introduction

Hearing loss is one of the most common sensory disorders in humans. Genetic factors account for more than 50% of cases with congenital hearing loss where the majority exhibit autosomal recessive inheritance [1,2]. Identification of the responsible gene/mutation in affected families is difficult since there are 39 different genes involved in ARNSHL [3] (http://hereditaryhearingloss.org/). Except for mutations in *GJB2*, which are the cause in up to 50% of families with ARNSHL in some populations, most deafness mutations are private and are seen in only a single or few families [4]. Approximately 85% of disease-related mutations in Mendelian disorders have been found in the protein-coding regions (exons and splice sites), although this portion constitutes only approximately 1% of the human genome [5]. Many of ARNSHL genes consist of long and/or many exons making conventional genetic methods to screen for mutations extremely expensive and time-consuming (e.g. Sanger sequencing alone or in combination with genome wide SNP genotyping).Whole-exome sequencing (WES) has recently been introduced as an alternative approach to more traditional methods [6]. WES allows for a targeted enrichment and resequencing of nearly all exons of protein-coding genes. Exome sequences are analyzed to identify genetic variation at a base-pair resolution and survey the protein coding portion of the human genome. Accordingly, WES using next generation technologies provides a transformational approach for identifying causative mutations in Mendelian disorders. Different targeted genomic capture methods and massive parallel sequencing have been successfully applied to screen mutations in hereditary deafness in relatively small sets of families [7–9]. In the present work, we applied WES to ARNSHL in a set of 20 multiplex and consanguineous families. The systematic use of WES shows that this method is an effective mean to identify causative mutations in affected families.

Materials and Methods

Ethics Statement

This study was approved by the University of Miami Institutional Review Board (USA), Ankara University Medical School Ethics Committee (Turkey), and Growth and Development Research Ethics Committee (Iran). All participants provided written informed consent prior to enrollment. Written informed consent was obtained from the next of kin on the behalf of the minors/children participants involved in this study.

Subjects

Twenty families were included in this study based on the presence of both parental consanguinity and at least two members with hearing loss (Figure S1). Seventeen families were from Turkey and three were from Iran. Diagnosis of sensorineural hearing loss was established via standard audiometry in a sound-proofed room according to current clinical standards [10]. Clinical evaluation of all affected individuals by a geneticist and an ENT surgeon included a thorough physical examination and otoscopy. A high resolution CT scan of the temporal bone was obtained in one affected person in each family to look for inner ear anomalies. DNA was extracted from peripheral leukocytes of each member of the family via a phenol chloroform method. Samples were prescreened for mutations in *GJB2* (MIM 121011) via Sanger sequencing; none were identified in any of the 20 families. Either one or two affected members of each family underwent WES based on the availability of sufficient DNA.

Whole-Exome Sequencing

The SureSelect Human All Exon 50 Mb kit (Agilent) was used for in-solution enrichment of coding exons and flanking intronic sequences following the manufacturer's standard protocol. Adapter sequences for the Illumina Hiseq2000 were ligated and the enriched DNA samples were subjected to standard sample preparation for the Hiseq2000 instrument (Illumina). The Illumina CASAVA v1.8 pipeline was used to produce 99 bp sequence reads. BWA [11] was used to align sequence reads to the human reference genome (hg19) and variants were called using the GATK software package [12,13]. All variants were submitted to SeattleSeq134 for further characterization. Coverage analysis was performed on coding exons +/−2 bp of cDNA transcripts listed in the Human Gene Mutation Database (https://portal.biobase-international.com) of known ARNSHL genes, which is comprised of 115,447 bps and 782 exons. Positions of heterozygous and homozygous variants were used to determine the location and size of the homozygous blocks containing the mutations.

Sanger Sequencing

Candidate variants observed via WES were confirmed using conventional capillary sequencing. The primers were designed using Primer3, v. 0.4.0 (http://frodo.wi.mit.edu/). PCR reactions included 10–40 ng of genomic DNA with Taq DNA polymerase (Roche). Corresponding DNA fragments were amplified using a touch down protocol. PCR products were visualized on agarose gels, cleaned over Sephadex columns or with NucleoFast 96 PCR plates (Clontech) in accordance with the manufacturers' protocols. Sequence analysis was performed with the ABI PRISM Big Dye Terminator Cycle Sequencing V3.1 Ready Reaction Kit and the ABI PRISM 3730 DNA Analyzer (Applied Biosystems). Sequence traces were analyzed using the Sequencher 4.7 program (Gene Codes Corporation).

In silico Analysis of Identified Variants

The program Conseq was used to calculate conservation scores for the amino acid residue affected by the missense variants [14]. Scores ranged from 1–9, where a score of 9 represented a highly conserved residue. PolyPhen-2 [15] and SIFT [16] were used to predict the effect of reported missense changes on protein function.

Results

Exome Sequencing

On average, each exome in the 20 families had 97%, 81% and 66% of mappable bases of the Gencode defined exome represented by coverage of at least 1, 10 and 20 reads, respectively. Considering only the 39 selected ARNSHL-related genes the percentage of mappable bases was 93%, 84% and 73%, respectively (Fig. 1A). An average depth of 53.4 reads was achieved for all known ARNSHL genes. The average quality of single nucleotide variations and insertions or deletions (INDELs) was 798 and 1014, respectively. Uncovered regions (read depth <1) within the known ARNSHL genes were mostly limited to small segments (less than 200 bp) in seven genes (Fig. 1B and 1C), except for *PTPRQ* of which only four out of 39 exons were targeted. Poor coverage was associated with untargeted regions of the capture kit as well as with segments having an excessively high GC content (Fig. 1C).

Identification of ARNSHL Mutations

An average of 90,237 single nucleotide variations and 8,059 INDELs per sample were found prior to applying any filter. We utilized the Genomes Management Application (GEMapp), University of Miami Miller School of Medicine (https://secureforms.med.miami.edu/hihg/gem-app) for filtering of variants. We filtered the variants according to the inheritance model (autosomal recessive with both homozygous and compound heterozygous), the variant function class including missense, nonsense, splice sites, in-frame INDELs and frame-shift INDELs and for the following genes: *BSND, CDH23, CLDN14, COL11A2, DFNB31, ESPN, ESRRB, GIPC3, GJB2, GJB3, GJB6, GRXCR1, HGF, ILDR1, LHFPL5, LOXHD1, LRTOMT, MARVELD2, MSRB3, MYO15A, MYO3A, MYO6, MYO7A, OTOA, OTOF, PCDH15, PJVK, PTPRQ, RDX, SERPINB6, SLC26A4, STRC, TECTA, TMC1, TMIE, TMPRSS3, TPRN, TRIOBP,* and *USH1C*. We searched for variants that were not listed in dbSNP137, NHLBI (http://evs.gs.washington.edu/EVS/) or that had a minor allele frequency of less than 1% in these databases. Variants were also filtered for presence in less than five samples in our internal database that includes 1010 exomes, including 69 ethnicity matched unrelated samples. We did not use a filter for read depth and included even variants with 1×coverage because we were searching for homozygous variants. This simple filtering strategy rapidly extracted only 1 homozygous variant in one of the searched ARNSHL genes in 12 families. Subsequent Sanger sequencing confirmed co-segregation of the mutations with the phenotype (Table 1 and Figure S1). For the five missense mutations detected, estimated conservation and pathogenicity scores (Table 1) suggested that single amino acid changes were likely to be highly damaging to protein function. Moreover, all single amino acid changes were located within conserved domains of the protein (Table 1). In the affected members of the remaining families, we looked for homozygous haplotypes flanking *ESPN, GIPC3, TMIE, TPRN, PCDH15, MYO15A,* and *PTPRQ* which were not fully covered by WES. This analysis did not show homozygous runs in any family suggesting that autozygous

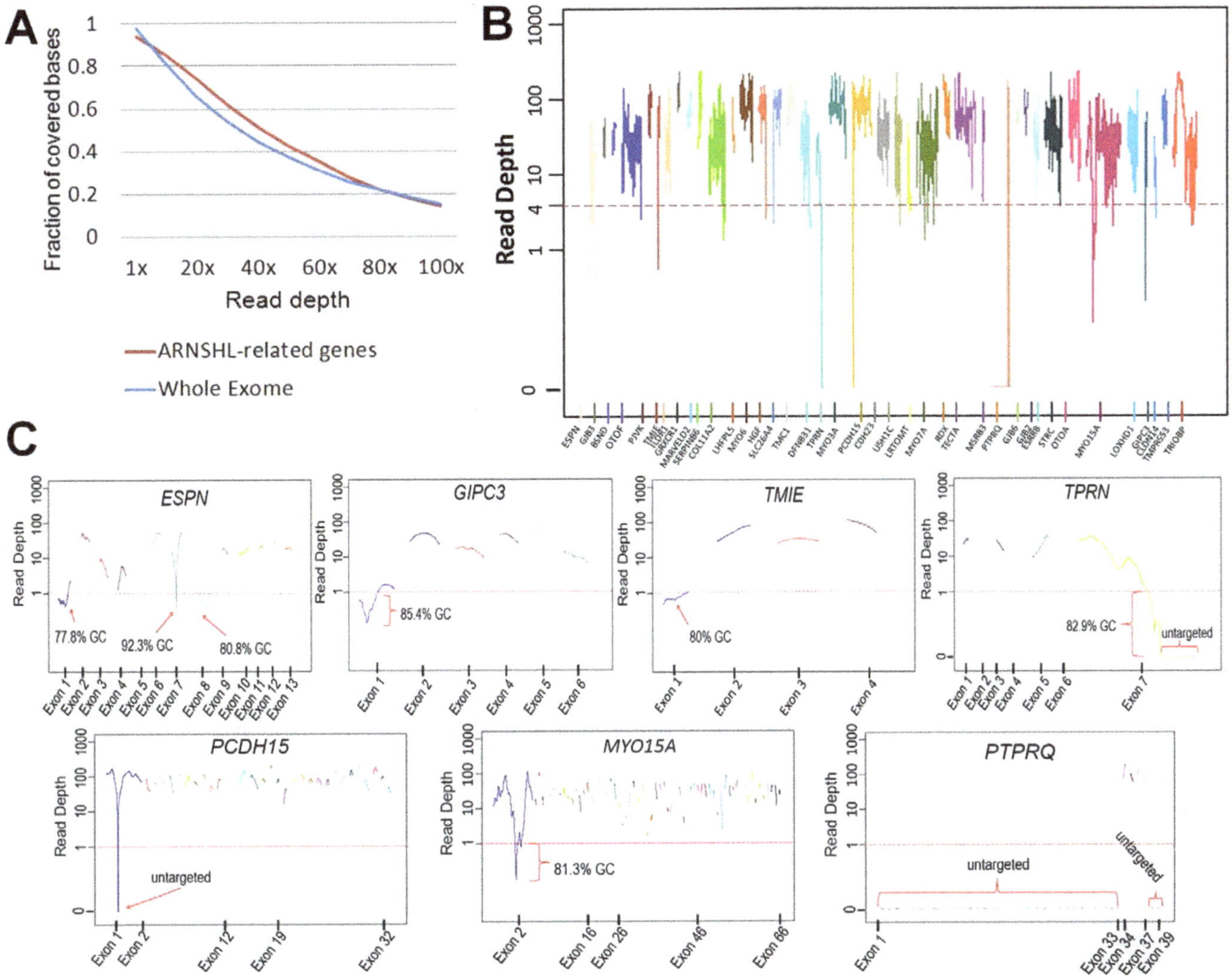

Figure 1. A) The exome coverage of the 39 ARNSHL genes. The plots are the average of the fraction of covered bases (Y-axis) and the read depth (X-axis) in the 20 families included in the study. B) Average sequence coverage (base 10 logarithmic scale) of ARNSHL genes. Exome sequencing results in a range of sequence coverage depth. C) Detailed uncovered segments of ARNSHL genes. Untargeted and high GC content sequences are indicated.

mutations in those genes are unlikely. As shown in Table S1, all identified mutations were within homozygous runs. Our work searching for novel deafness genes in other autozygous areas in the remaining families is ongoing.

During the analysis we also noticed an unexpectedly high frequency (four variants in 12 families) of heterozygous variants in known deafness genes in families where homozygous causative mutations were already identified (Table S2). Variants were selected based on a <1% frequency in the dbSNP137 database, high pathogenicity scores calculated by Polyphen-2 and SIFT and having at least 20X read depth. Using our internal WES database, the frequency of heterozygous variants (same criteria applied) in 39 ARNSHL genes were also determined in hearing individuals (n = 15) matched for ethnicity (Table S2). There were six heterozygous variants in 15 normal hearing individuals.

Discussion

WES allows for screening of mutations in a large number of genes at the same time and is cost effective compared to other genetic testing options when the number of genes is large. This is particularly true when the condition under study is extremely heterogeneous, as with ARNSHL. Although very small regions are not adequately covered, the present study indicates that our current WES protocol can reliably test most of the deafness genes. Limitations inherent in the processes of exome enrichment and amplification are evident mostly because of a high GC content (Fig. 1C) and because the SureSelect Human All Exon 50 Mb kit does not capture all the nucleotides of clinical interest. Most exons of *PTPRQ* in particular are not targeted by this exome capture kit. To overcome this, Sanger sequencing of the poorly targeted genes can be performed. If the study population includes multiplex and/or consanguineous families, such as those studied in this report, co-segregation of a haplotype flanking a known gene can be easily assessed with the WES data. We used the latter approach for the assessment of homozygosity around the uncovered regions. We previously showed that compound heterozygous mutations are detected in less than 5% of consanguineous families with deafness [3]. Thus, it is unlikely that the families in which we did not

Table 1. Mutations identified in the ARNSHL-related genes.

Family ID	# exomes sequenced	Origin	Gene	cDNA change[1]	Amino acid change[1]	Conseq Score	PolyPhen-2	SIFT	Affected Protein Domain	Reference
1	2	Turkey	*TRIOBP*	c.2355_2356delAG	p.R785Sfs*50	n/a	n/a	n/a	n/a	Novel
2	2	Turkey	*TMC1*	c.1589_1590delCT	p.S530X	n/a	n/a	n/a	n/a	[18]
3	1	Turkey	*LOXHD1*	c.4480C>T	p.R1494X	n/a	n/a	n/a	n/a	Novel
4	2	Turkey	*TMPRSS3*	c.36dupC	p.F13Lfs*10	n/a	n/a	n/a	n/a	Novel
5	1	Turkey	*MYO15A*	c.4441T>C	p.S1481P	4	1.000	0.01	Myosin Motor Domain	[19]
6	2	Turkey	*MYO15A*	c.4652C>A	p.A1551D	7	1.000	0.0	Myosin Motor Domain	Novel
7	1	Turkey	*MYO15A*	c.4273C>T	p.Q1425X	n/a	n/a	n/a	n/a	Novel
8	1	Turkey	*LOXHD1*	c.2863G>T	p.E955X	n/a	n/a	n/a	n/a	Novel
9	2	Turkey	*GIPC3*	c.508C>A	p.H170N	5	0.991	0.04	PDZ Domain	[20]
10	1	Iran	*ILDR1*	c.820C>T	p.Q274X	n/a	n/a	n/a	n/a	Novel
11	1	Iran	*MYO7A*	c.6487G>A	p.G2163S	9	1.000	0.0	FERM Central Domain	[21]
12	1	Iran	*TECTA*	c.5210A>G	p.Y1737C	7	0.999	0.0	C8 domain	Novel

[1]According to cDNA and protein sequences used for each gene in the HGMD.

identify a homozygous haplotype flanking the poorly covered regions harbor compound heterozygous mutations in these genes.

Our dataset allows us to perform an additional analysis that is relevant for the clinical usage of next-generation sequencing: since we have already found the cause of deafness in our 12 families, we can then look for other variants in the same genes that have the potential to be pathogenic. As shown in Table S2, four out of 12 families with hearing loss caused by homozygous mutations in known deafness genes also carried heterozygous variants that could potentially cause hearing loss in the homozygous state. Our subsequent analysis in 15 ethnically-matched hearing individuals revealed six similar variants, suggesting that this observation is not limited to families with deafness. Although these variants are predicted to damage the corresponding protein function, it is unlikely for most of them that they cause prelingual deafness because their frequencies are too high in both hearing and deaf families. They might have the potential to modify the phenotype or contribute to late onset hearing loss. It is important to recognize that there is an excess of heterozygous, rare, and predicted to be pathogenic variants in known deafness genes. This is especially relevant for simplex cases or small-sized families where co-segregation of the identified variant cannot be investigated in a large pedigree.

Our study corroborates the extreme heterogeneity of ARNSHL. Within the twenty family exome set, there was not a single recurrent mutation causing deafness. In addition, eight out of the 12 mutations in known deafness genes are novel (Table 1). These data also indicate the great potential that WES provides for the discovery of novel deafness genes. We can then concentrate on the remaining eight families to identify mutations in novel genes for ARNSHL.

As discussed in a recent review by Shearer and Smith, targeted genome enrichment (e.g. subsets of deafness-related genes) followed by massively parallel sequencing constitute an efficient strategy for deafness gene mutation screening [17]. Two independent studies screening more than 50 known deafness genes reported the identification of causative mutations in 5 out of 6 and 6 out of 11 families, respectively [8,9]. This approach has several advantages over WES including: a higher coverage (the reads are not "diluted" over more than 20,000 genes), and a significant lowering of costs (e.g. the lower the capture size the higher number of samples per HiSeq lane can be processed). However, custom enrichment has limitations, especially when considering that a minimum of 34% of deafness genes have yet to be discovered [17].Thus, if the causative mutation resides in novel genes, additional experiments will be required. In this sense, custom capture kits for deafness genes should be subject to periodical updates that may negatively influence their price. WES allows performing post *in silico* analysis as the stored data comprises the entire coding sequence of the genome.

In summary, we have successfully applied WES for mutation screening within ARNSHL-related genes. The high percentage of unsolved mutations in those genes indicates the great potential of novel gene discovery in consanguineous families utilizing whole exome enrichment methods and next generation sequencing.

Supporting Information

Figure S1 Pedigrees and electropherograms showing segregating mutations in known deafness genes. The levels of consanguinity are indicated; −/−: homozygous mutant; +/−: heterozygous; +/+: homozygous wild type.

Table S1 Size and location of the homozygous blocks containing the causative mutations in the studied families. Asterisks indicate families in which homozygous blocks were calculated by overlapping sequence data from two individuals.

Table S2 Heterozygous mutations in known deafness genes in affected families and hearing individuals. HGMD: Human Gene Mutation Database. [1]Minor allele frequency is from dbSNP137 database accessed on 10/17/2012. [2]Internal database allele frequency does not include the family on this table with a given variant.

Author Contributions

Conceived and designed the experiments: MT SZ SB. Performed the experiments: ODH DD JF AS. Analyzed the data: ODH MAG IM RHU YE MT. Contributed reagents/materials/analysis tools: NM NF MB FBC. Wrote the paper: ODH MT.

References

1. Friedman TB, Griffith AJ (2003) Human nonsyndromic sensorineural deafness. Annu Rev Genomics Hum Genet 4: 341–402.
2. Morton CC, Nance WE (2006) Newborn hearing screening–a silent revolution. N Engl J Med 354: 2151–2164.
3. Duman D, Sirmaci A, Cengiz FB, Ozdag H, Tekin M (2011) Screening of 38 genes identifies mutations in 62% of families with nonsyndromic deafness in Turkey. Genet Test Mol Biomarkers 15: 29–33.
4. Duman D, Tekin M (2012) Autosomal recessive nonsyndromic deafness genes: a review. Front Biosci 17: 2213–2236.
5. Teer JK, Mullikin JC (2010) Exome sequencing: the sweet spot before whole genomes. Hum Mol Genet 19: R145–151.
6. Ng SB, Turner EH, Robertson PD, Flygare SD, Bigham AW, et al. (2009) Targeted capture and massively parallel sequencing of 12 human exomes. Nature 461: 272–276.
7. Walsh T, Shahin H, Elkan-Miller T, Lee MK, Thornton AM, et al. (2010) Whole exome sequencing and homozygosity mapping identify mutation in the cell polarity protein GPSM2 as the cause of nonsyndromic hearing loss DFNB82. Am J Hum Genet 87: 90–94.
8. Brownstein Z, Friedman LM, Shahin H, Oron-Karni V, Kol N, et al. (2011) Targeted genomic capture and massively parallel sequencing to identify genes for hereditary hearing loss in middle eastern families. Genome Biol 12: R89.
9. Shearer AE, DeLuca AP, Hildebrand MS, Taylor KR, Gurrola J, 2nd, et al. (2010) Comprehensive genetic testing for hereditary hearing loss using massively parallel sequencing. Proc Natl Acad Sci U S A 107: 21104–21109.
10. American_National_Standards_Institute (2004) Methods for manual pure-tone threshold audiometry. New York.
11. Li H, Durbin R (2010) Fast and accurate long-read alignment with Burrows-Wheeler transform. Bioinformatics 26: 589–595.
12. McKenna A, Hanna M, Banks E, Sivachenko A, Cibulskis K, et al. (2010) The Genome Analysis Toolkit: a MapReduce framework for analyzing next-generation DNA sequencing data. Genome Res 20: 1297–1303.
13. DePristo MA, Banks E, Poplin R, Garimella KV, Maguire JR, et al. (2011) A framework for variation discovery and genotyping using next-generation DNA sequencing data. Nat Genet 43: 491–498.
14. Berezin C, Glaser F, Rosenberg J, Paz I, Pupko T, et al. (2004) ConSeq: the identification of functionally and structurally important residues in protein sequences. Bioinformatics 20: 1322–1324.
15. Adzhubei IA, Schmidt S, Peshkin L, Ramensky VE, Gerasimova A, et al. (2010) A method and server for predicting damaging missense mutations. Nat Methods 7: 248–249.
16. Kumar P, Henikoff S, Ng PC (2009) Predicting the effects of coding non-synonymous variants on protein function using the SIFT algorithm. Nat Protoc 4: 1073–1081.
17. Shearer AE, Smith RJ (2012) Genetics: advances in genetic testing for deafness. Curr Opin Pediatr.
18. Hildebrand MS, Kahrizi K, Bromhead CJ, Shearer AE, Webster JA, et al. (2010) Mutations in TMC1 are a common cause of DFNB7/11 hearing loss in the Iranian population. Ann Otol Rhinol Laryngol 119: 830–835.
19. Cengiz FB, Duman D, Sirmaci A, Tokgoz-Yilmaz S, Erbek S, et al. (2010) Recurrent and private MYO15A mutations are associated with deafness in the Turkish population. Genet Test Mol Biomarkers 14: 543–550.
20. Sirmaci A, Edwards YJ, Akay H, Tekin M (2012) Challenges in whole exome sequencing: an example from hereditary deafness. PLoS One 7: e32000.
21. Janecke AR, Meins M, Sadeghi M, Grundmann K, Apfelstedt-Sylla E, et al. (1999) Twelve novel myosin VIIA mutations in 34 patients with Usher syndrome type I: confirmation of genetic heterogeneity. Hum Mutat 13: 133–140.

10

CHD7 Mutational Analysis and Clinical Considerations for Auditory Rehabilitation in Deaf Patients with CHARGE Syndrome

Mee Hyun Song[1]ᵠ, Hyun-Ju Cho[2]ᵠ, Hee Keun Lee[2], Tae Jun Kwon[2], Won-Sang Lee[3], Sanghee Oh[3], Jinwoong Bok[4], Jae Young Choi[3], Un-Kyung Kim[2]*

1 Department of Otorhinolaryngology, Kwandong University College of Medicine, Goyang, South Korea, **2** Department of Biology, College of Natural Sciences, Kyungpook National University, Daegu, South Korea, **3** Department of Otorhinolaryngology, Yonsei University College of Medicine, Seoul, South Korea, **4** Department of Anatomy, BK 21 Project for Medical Science, Yonsei University College of Medicine, Seoul, South Korea

Abstract

Background: Otologic manifestations are one of the most consistent findings of CHARGE syndrome found in more than 90%. Since genetic analysis of the *CHD7* gene has rarely been performed in previous reports dealing with ear abnormalities, the genotypic spectrum of *CHD7* mutations was analyzed in deaf patients with CHARGE syndrome, and the clinical considerations concerning auditory rehabilitation were investigated.

Methods: Nine Korean patients with CHARGE syndrome showing profound hearing loss and semicircular canal aplasia were included. All 38 exons of *CHD7* were analyzed by direct sequencing. For splice site variations, *in silico* and exon-trapping analyses were performed to verify the pathogenicity of nucleotide variations. Clinical features and the outcome of auditory rehabilitation were also analyzed.

Results: Eight of 9 patients revealed alterations of the *CHD7* gene including 3 frameshift, 2 nonsense, 2 splice site, and 1 missense mutations. Five of 9 patients were clinically diagnosed as atypical CHARGE syndrome but demonstrated various mutations of the *CHD7* gene. One familial case showed intra-familial variability. Radiologic findings suggesting cochleovestibular nerve deficiency were identified in most of the patients. Of the 8 patients who underwent cochlear implantation, 5 patients demonstrated favorable outcome. Larger diameter of the cochleovestibular nerve on imaging and absence of severe mental retardation were factors related to better outcome after cochlear implantation rather than the type of *CHD7* mutations. Auditory brainstem implantation was performed in two patients who did not benefit from cochlear implantation.

Conclusions: Genetic analysis of the *CHD7* gene should be performed in cases with semicircular canal aplasia even when other typical features of CHARGE syndrome are absent. For auditory rehabilitation in CHARGE syndrome, cochlear implantation should be strongly recommended in selected cases with favorable prognostic factors. Auditory brainstem implantation may be a viable option in patients with CHARGE syndrome who have failed to benefit from cochlear implantation.

Editor: Francesc Palau, Instituto de Ciencia de Materiales de Madrid - Instituto de Biomedicina de Valencia, Spain

Funding: This study was supported by a grant of the Korea Healthcare Technology Research and Development Project, Ministry of Health & Welfare, Republic of Korea (A100367). The funders had no role in study design, data collection and analysis, decision to publish, or preparation of the manuscript.

Competing Interests: The authors have declared that no competing interests exist.

* E-mail: kimuk@knu.ac.kr

ᵠ These authors contributed equally to this work.

Introduction

CHARGE is an acronym describing a set of conditions including "C"oloboma of eye, "H"eart malformations, "A"tresia of choanae, "R"etardation in growth and development, "G"enital hypoplasia, and "E"ar anomalies. The combination of these anomalies was first reported by Hall and Hittner [1,2] in 1979 after which the acronym was proposed by Pagon *et al.* [3] in 1981. The diagnostic criteria proposed by Blake *et al.* [4] in 1998 and those updated by Verloes [5] emphasizing the importance of semicircular canal hypoplasia or aplasia are widely used today for the clinical diagnosis of CHARGE syndrome. The incidence of CHARGE syndrome is approximately 1/10,000 and most of the cases are sporadic although 17 familial cases have been reported to date [6]. The mode of inheritance is autosomal dominance with variable penetrance [6].

Haploinsufficiency of the *CHD7* gene has been identified as the molecular basis of CHARGE syndrome by Vissers *et al.* [7] in 2004. The *CHD7* gene located on chromosome 8q12.1 is 188 kb in size and consists of 37 coding and one non-coding exons [7]. The CHD7 protein comprised of 2,997 amino acids belongs to the chromodomain helicase DNA binding family, one of the four major families of ATP-dependent chromatin remodeling proteins. Approximately 60–70% of patients clinically diagnosed as CHARGE syndrome were found to have pathogenic mutations in the *CHD7* gene [8]. Truncating mutations including nonsense or frameshift mutations are the most frequently encountered forms of genetic alterations followed by splice site or missense mutations found in lower incidences [8]. Chromosomal abnormalities with or without involvement of the *CHD7* gene also have been reported to cause phenotypic features of CHARGE syndrome [9].

Among the various clinical manifestations of CHARGE syndrome, otologic symptoms and signs are one of the most consistent findings which are included as one of the major criteria in both Blake's and Verloes' clinical criteria [4,5]. Characteristic temporal bone anomalies are reported to be found in 98% of *CHD7* mutation positive cases along with external ear malformations and hearing loss also found in more than 90% [8,9]. Analysis of temporal bone computed tomography (CT) findings has revealed aplasia or hypoplasia of the semicircular canal, cochlear dysplasia, atresia of bony cochlear nerve canal (BCNC), oval window atresia, ossicular malformations as common characteristics of CHARGE syndrome [10]. Although mild semicircular canal dysplasia is one of the most commonly seen inner ear anomalies, complete aplasia of the semicircular canals with relatively intact cochlear structures is a very rare condition. Since CHARGE syndrome manifests a variety of different conditions that may overlap other syndromes such as velocardiofacial syndrome or Noonan syndrome, aplasia of the semicircular canals may be a decisive clue in suspecting CHARGE syndrome leading to molecular analysis of the *CHD7*gene [11,12].

Considering that hearing loss of variable degrees is present in most of the cases with CHARGE syndrome, auditory rehabilitation is another important factor in the management of these patients. It has been reported that early auditory rehabilitation is especially important in patients with multiple disabilities for adequate development of communication skills [13]. In CHARGE syndrome patients with severe to profound hearing loss, cochlear implantation (CI) has resulted in variable outcomes because of concomitant multiple handicaps and anatomical factors such as cochlear nerve aplasia [14,15]. Most of the patients with CHARGE syndrome achieve limited auditory benefit and improved attentiveness and responsiveness following CI but open-set speech perception is acquired in very rare cases [14,16,17].

Although there have been many reports concerning otologic manifestations and auditory rehabilitation in CHARGE syndrome, molecular analysis of the *CHD7* gene was not performed in most of the reports [14,16,17]. Genetic analysis is especially important in CHARGE syndrome considering that this disorder shares many features with other syndromes which may lead to incorrect diagnosis and that some patients with mutations in the *CHD7* gene manifest only mild symptoms as seen in familial cases of CHARGE syndrome [6]. Therefore, in this study, we have performed *CHD7* mutational analysis in Korean patients with CHARGE syndrome presenting with profound hearing loss and typical inner ear malformations in order to broaden the genotypic spectrum of CHARGE syndrome. The clinical features were also analyzed with emphasis on auditory rehabilitation including CI and auditory brainstem implantation. In addition, factors that may influence the outcome of auditory rehabilitation in these patients were further investigated.

Materials and Methods

Subjects

Among the patients who were enrolled in the auditory rehabilitation program at Severance Hospital, nine patients with profound sensorineural hearing loss showing semicircular canal aplasia on the temporal bone CT were included in this study. Eight of 9 patients received CI for auditory rehabilitation, and two children underwent subsequent auditory brainstem implantation because no sound perception was possible using a CI. There were 6 males and 3 females; and the ages of the patients at the time of CI ranged from 14 months to 20 years (mean: 6.2 years). One patient aged 15 years was recommended to receive CI but the parents have refused surgery. Combined disabilities and other medical conditions were reviewed and further evaluations including ophthalmologic examination and echocardiography were performed. Written informed consent was obtained from participating individuals, and this study was approved by the Institutional Review Board of the Yonsei University College of Medicine.

Genetic analysis

From the peripheral blood of 9 subjects, genomic DNA was extracted using a FlexiGene DNA extraction kit (Qiagen, Hilden, Germany). All 38 exons and flanking intronic sequences of *CHD7* were amplified by polymerase chain reaction (PCR) and the quality of the PCR products were examined by electrophoresis on 2% agarose gels. The sequences of the primers and PCR conditions are provided in Table S1. Each fragment was purified and subsequently sequenced using ABI PRISM Big Dye Terminator Cycle Sequencing Kit (V3.1) and an ABI PRISM3130XL DNA analyzer (Applied Biosystems, Foster City, CA, USA). ABI Sequencing Analysis (v.5.0) and Lasergene-SeqMan software were used for the data analysis. For the identified missense variation, the presence of the variant was evaluated in 100 unrelated Korean subjects who showed normal audiograms. For chromosomal analysis, leukocytes from the peripheral blood were cultured and Giemsa staining of the chromosomes of cells arrested in metaphase was performed for karyotyping.

Exon trapping analysis

For the two splice site variations, *in silico* splice site prediction was analyzed to identify any possible effects of the variation on the native splicing process. Three online applications were used for each variation (FruitFly; www.fruitfly.org/seq_tools/splice.html, NetGene2; www.cbs.dtu.dk/services/NetGene2 and Human Splicing Finder; www.umd.be/SSF) and the significance was indicated by a score.

For *in vitro* splicing assay, mini-gene system vector was constructed, and the basement vector pSPL3 was kindly provided by Dr. Thomas v. O. Hansen. DNA sequences containing one or two exons adjacent to the splice site variations and the ~300-bp flanking intronic sequences were amplified from the genomic DNA of patients having heterozygous variations and inserted into the pSPL3 vector (Table S2). After vector sequencing to isolate wild type and mutant constructions, the isolated vectors and a mock pSPL3 vector were transfected into HeLa cells using FuGENE HD Transfection Reagent (Roche Diagnostics GmbH, Mannheim, Germany). The transfected cells were lysed 48 hrs after the tranfection and total RNA was extracted using the RNeasy Mini Kit (Qiagen, Hilden, Germany). With 1 μg of RNA, first strand cDNA was synthesized by reverse transcription using oligo-$(dT)_{16}$ primer and High Capacity cDNA Reverse Transcription Kit (Applied Biosystems, Foster City, CA, USA). Using 1 μl of cDNA as template, PCR amplification was performed with pSPL3 vector specific primers SD6 and SA2, and the size of the generated mock, normal, and mutant type PCR fragments were compared on 2% of agarose gels. The sequence of PCR products were confirmed with direct sequencing or vector sequencing after TA cloning to isolate various fragments.

Diagnostic criteria for CHARGE syndrome

The criteria proposed by Verloes [5] were applied for clinical diagnosis of CHARGE syndrome (Table 1).The three major signs included coloboma, choanal atresia, and semicircular canal hypoplasia and the minor signs included rhombencephalic dysfunction, hypothalamo-hypophyseal dysfunction, abnormal middle or external ear, malformation of mediastinal organs, and mental retardation. CHARGE syndrome was classified into typical, partial/incomplete, or atypical according to the number of major or minor signs present.

Radiologic evaluations

The temporal bone CT scan was performed with a 16 multidetector row CT scanner (Somatom Sensation 16; Siemens, Erlangen, Germany) using a standard temporal bone protocol. Contiguous 0.7-mm scans of the temporal bone were acquired in the axial plane and reformatted coronally with 1.0-mm increments. CT images were performed, digitally stored, and displayed by using the Picture Archiving Communication System (PACS) (Centricity; GE Healthcare, Milwaukee, WI).

Magnetic resonance imaging (MRI) was acquired by using a 3.0-T (Achieva; Philips Medical Systems, Best, the Netherlands) or 1.5-T system (Intera; Philips Medical Systems, Best, the Netherlands) with a six-channel sensitivity encoding (SENSE) head coil. The targeted parasagittal scan perpendicular to the long axis of the internal auditory canal was obtained with T2-weighted three-dimensional (3-D) turbo spin-echo (TSE) sequence with driven equilibrium RF reset pulse (DRIVE), following routine MR sequences with spin-echo T1- and T2-weighted images. The sequence parameters for the T2-weighted 3-D FSE sequence with DRIVE were as follows: repetition time (TR)/echo time (TE) = 1500/200 ms, 256 acquisition/256 reconstruction, 15-cm field of view, 1.5-mm section thickness with a 0.75-mm overlap, number of acquisitions = 2, and the scan time was less than 5 minutes.

Audiologic tests and evaluation of speech performances

Audiologic tests including pure tone audiometry, auditory brainstem response, otoacoustic emission were performed before undergoing CI. Overall auditory performances were evaluated by categories of auditory performance (CAP) [18]. Speech evaluations were performed preoperatively and 1, 3, 6, 12, 18, 24 months after either CI or auditory brainstem implantation.

Results

Mutations of the CHD7 gene

CHD7 mutations were identified in 8 of 9 patients showing characteristics of CHARGE syndrome (Table 2). Six mutations were found in the coding sequence while two were intronic variations suspected of splice site mutations. The mutations in the coding sequence included 3 frameshift mutations causing truncation of the protein, 2 nonsense mutations, and 1 missense mutation. The missense mutation was not found in 100 unrelated normal controls. The region of the protein containing the missense mutation, p.R2065S, was identified as highly conserved in various vertebrate species (Figure S1). In one family, the sibling of the proband (Patient 1) identified as having a frameshift mutation of the *CHD7* gene demonstrated the same mutation, whereas no mutation was found in their parents. Five of the 8 mutations identified in this study were novel mutations of the *CHD7* gene. None of these novel mutations were listed in the 1000 genome sequencing data. The *CHD7* gene was not mutated in one patient diagnosed as typical CHARGE syndrome. No chromosomal abnormalities were identified in any of the patients.

In silico splice site prediction and in vitro splicing assay

The two intronic variations of the *CHD7* gene located adjacent to the splice site were analyzed further by *in silico* splice site prediction programs and *in vitro* splicing assay to assess whether these variants alter the splicing of pre-mRNA. Three different splice site prediction programs were tested and the results are shown in Table S3. One variation (c.5210+5G>C) was predicted as a loss of strength of native splice donor site in all three prediction programs. The other variation (c.5405-7G>A) resulted in appearance of a new cryptic splice site in two of the prediction programs.

Further study with *in vitro* splicing assay using pSPL3 mini-gene system demonstrated alternative splicing more clearly and supported the prediction results. The variation c.5210+5G>C caused exon skipping as a result of splice donor site deterioration and c.5405-7G>A introduced a 5-bp intronic sequence by activation of a cryptic acceptor site (Figures S2, S3).

Clinical diagnosis of CHARGE syndrome

The diagnostic criteria proposed by Verloes [5] were applied for the diagnosis of CHARGE syndrome (Table 3). Of nine patients, four patients were diagnosed as typical CHARGE syndrome, while five were categorized as atypical CHARGE syndrome. Because of the inclusion criteria of this study, one major (semicircular canal aplasia) and one minor criteria (rhomence-

Table 1. Diagnostic criteria by Verloes.

Criteria	Definition
Major	Typical CHARGE
1. Coloboma (iris or choroid, with or without microphthalmia)	3 major signs
2. Atresia of choanae	2/3 major + 2/5 minor
3. Hypoplastic semicircular canals	Partial/incomplete CHARGE
Minor	2/3 major + 1/5 minor
1. Rhombencephalic dysfunction (brainstem dysfunctions, cranial nerve VII to XII palsies and neurosensory deafness)	Atypical CHARGE
2. Hypothalamo-hypophyseal dysfunction (including GH and gonadotrophin deficiencies)	2/3 major + 0/5 minor
3. Abnormal middle or external ear	1/3 major + 3/5 minor
4. Malformation of mediastinal organs (heart, esophagus)	
5. Mental retardation	

Table 2. Genetic analysis of Korean patients with CHARGE syndrome.

Patient No.	Clinical diagnosis	Mutation (Nucleotide)	Mutation (Protein)	Type	In-vitro splicing assay	In-silico assay	Ref
1	Typical	c.921–922delAG	p.G308AfsX9	Frameshift			(20)
2	Atypical	c.7331T>A	p.L2444X	Nonsense			Novel
3	Atypical	c.6193C>A	p.R2065S	Missense			Novel
4	Atypical	c.6832insC	p.T2278HfsX3	Frameshift			Novel
5	Atypical	c.5210+5G>C		Splice site	Exon 23 skipping	Deterioration of splicing donor site	Novel
6	Typical	c.222delG	p.Q74HfsX9	Frameshift			Novel
7	Typical	c.5405-7G>A		Splice site	Insertion of 5bp at cryptic acceptor site	New cryptic splicing site	(20–21)
8	Typical	-	-	-			
9	Atypical	c.1465C>T	p.Q489X	Nonsense			(20)

phalic dysfunction; sensorineural hearing loss) were met in all patients. Coloboma was identified in three patients at sites including optic disc (Patients 6 and 8) and chorioretina (Patient 7). One of the patients with coloboma (Patient 7) was blind whereas the other two patients demonstrated preserved vision. Malformations of the mediastinal organs were found in 6 of 9 patients. Five had cardiac anomalies; two patients showed patent ductus arteriosis and 3 patients demonstrated subaortic septal hypertrophy with tricuspid and mitral regurgitation, endocardiac cushion defect, and ventricular septal defect, respectively. Foregut duplication requiring surgical resection was identified in one patient (Patient 1). External ear defects including the characteristic cup-shaped deformity of the auricles were shown in three patients, two of whom also exhibited middle ear defects such as oval window atresia and ossicular deformities. Unilateral incomplete facial palsy, one of rhomencephalic dysfunctions, was shown in three patients.

Table 3. Clinical diagnosis of CHARGE syndrome.

Criteria	Patient No. 1	2	3	4	5	6	7	8	9
Major									
Coloboma						+	+	+	
Choanal atresia	+								
Semicircular canal aplasia	+	+	+	+	+	+	+	+	+
Minor									
Rhomencephalic dysfunction	+	+	+	+	+	+	+	+	+
Hypothalamohypophyseal dysfunction	+		+	+	+	+	+	+	+
Abnormal middle/external ear	+	+		+		+			+
Malformation of mediastinal organs	+	+		+	+	+	+		
Mental retardation	+		+		+	+	+	+	
Others									
Urogenital anomalies								+	+
Cleft palate/lip				+					
Limb abnormalities									+
Facial dysmorphia						+			
CHARGE syndrome (Verloes)	Typ	Atyp	Atyp	Atyp	Atyp	Typ	Typ	Typ	Atyp

According to the criteria proposed by Verloes [5], hypothalamohypophyseal dysfunction which corresponds to the previous "R" or "G" of CHARGE acronym can be diagnosed only when growth hormone or gonadotrophin deficiencies are demonstrated. Since not all of the patients in this study performed endocrinological laboratory tests, hypothalamohypophyseal dysfunction was considered to be present when definite retardation of development was demonstrated on objective developmental tests. However, genital abnormalities were not included as hypothalamohypophyseal dysfunction in this study to eliminate the male preference in the diagnosis of CHARGE syndrome.

In the familial case (Patient 1), the proband was diagnosed as typical CHARGE syndrome demonstrating features such as choanal atresia, laryngomalacia, foregut duplication, and myasthenia gravis in addition to the sensorineural hearing loss and inner ear malformations. The parents who did not carry any detectable mutations of the *CHD7* gene showed normal hearing on pure tone audiometry (data not shown) without any clinical features of CHARGE syndrome, and the other family members also did not have any subjective hearing loss although they were not audiologically tested (Fig. 1A). The sibling who carried the same frameshift mutation as the proband revealed unilateral profound sensorineural hearing loss and normal hearing on the contralateral side (Fig. 1B). On temporal bone CT, the sibling of Patient 1 revealed slightly dilated but present semicircular canals with slightly hypoplastic cochlea and normal sized internal auditory canals on the affected side, and normal inner ear structures on the contralateral side with normal hearing (Fig. 1C). In contrast, Patient 1 with bilateral congenital deafness demonstrated complete absence of all semicircular canals as well as hypoplastic cochlea and narrow internal auditory canals bilaterally (Fig. 1D). Atrial septal defect was present in the sibling, whereas no cardiac defect was found in Patient 1.

Radiologic findings

Temporal bone CT of the patients revealed typical findings of the cochlea and vestibule (Table 4). Complete aplasia of all three semicircular canals and cochlear anomalies consistent with cochlear hypoplasia were identified in all patients (Fig. 2A, 2B). All but one patient exhibited narrow internal auditory canals, and

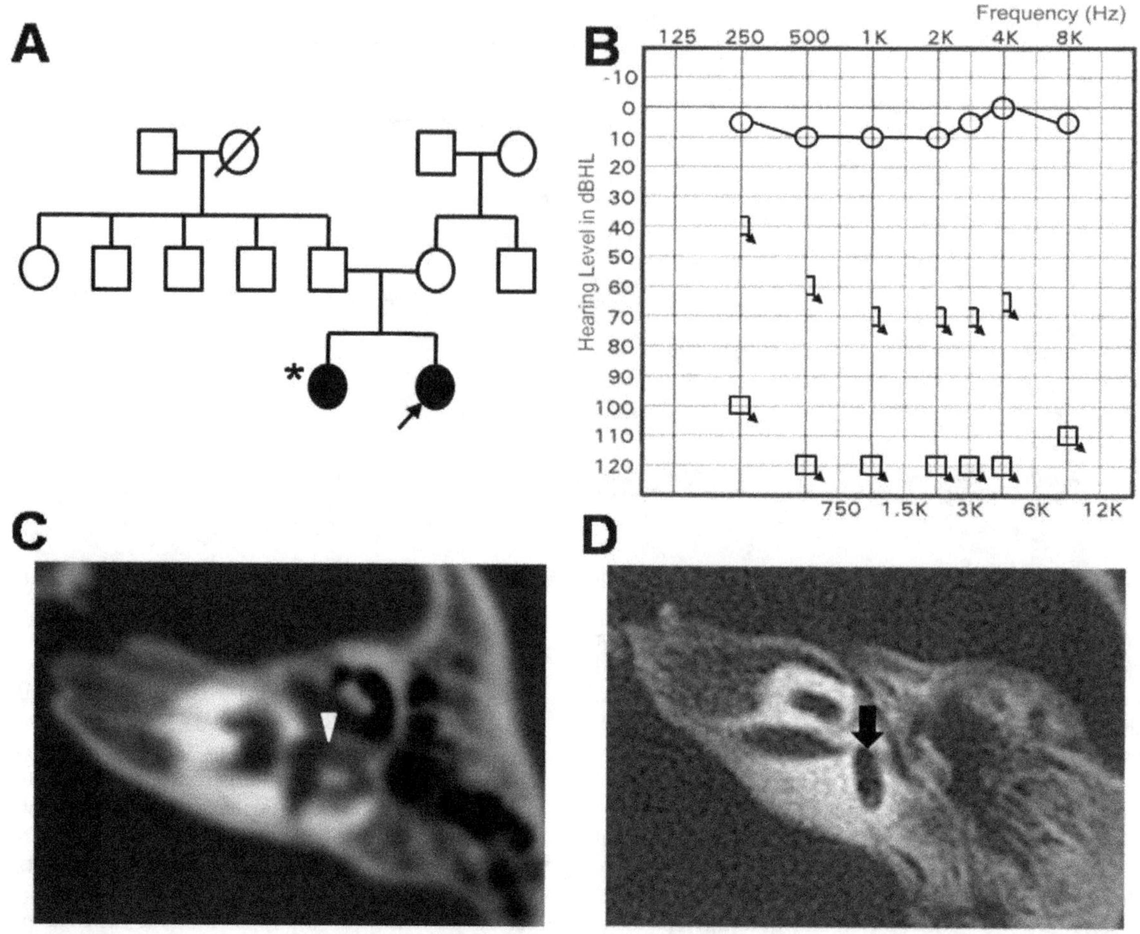

Figure 1. Pedigree and clinical findings of familial case of CHARGE syndrome (Patient 1). (A) Pedigree shows that only two siblings are affected by deafness either bilaterally (Patient 1; proband marked by black arrow) or unilaterally (sister of Patient 1 marked by asterisk). (B) The sister of Patient 1 demonstrated unilateral deafness on pure tone audiometry. (C) Temporal bone CT of the sister of Patient 1 with unilateral deafness showed slightly dilated but present semicircular canals (white arrowhead) with mild cochlear abnormality and normal sized internal auditory canal on the affected side. (D) Temporal bone CT of Patient 1 with bilateral congenital deafness demonstrated complete absence of all semicircular canals (black arrow).

the bony cochlear nerve canal (BCNC) was obliterated in 7 patients (Fig. 2B). Deformities of the incus and stapes were identified in 6 patients, and most of these patients had combined oval window atresia (Fig. 2B, 2D). Complete bony obliteration of the round window was shown in only one patient (Fig. 2C).

On parasagittal view of temporal MRI, the cochleovestibular nerve (CVN) was identified at the cerebellopontine angle and within the internal auditory canal in 5 of 7 patients whose images were available for review (Table 4). Because of narrow internal auditory canals, individual branching of the CVN into the cochlear nerve and superior/inferior vestibular nerves that is usually identified on parasagittal images of MRI could not be distinguished in most of the patients. When the size of the CVN was compared to that of the facial nerve on MRI, the diameter of the CVN was equal to or larger than the facial nerve in 2 cases and smaller in 3 cases (Fig. 3).

Audiologic data and outcome of auditory rehabilitation

All of the patients demonstrated profound sensorineural hearing loss showing no response on auditory brainstem response test. Auditory performances evaluated at the time of initial visit were CAP 0 in all patients except for one who showed response to speech sounds (CAP 2) using hearing aids (Table 5).

CI was performed in 8 of 9 patients (Table 5). After at least 12 months of follow-up, 5 of 8 patients including one typical and four atypical CHARGE patients demonstrated significant improvement in auditory performances ranging from CAP 4 to 6 (Fig. 4). Among these patients showing good outcome, one patient aged 20 years (Patient 2) who exhibited residual hearing of CAP 2 preoperatively, improved to CAP 5 after 16 months following CI. Another patient with typical CHARGE syndrome (Patient 1) showed good outcome of CAP 6 after 2 years following CI, and the bisyllabic word identification improved from 0% to 70% without visual cues. One patient (Patient 6) showed suboptimal results after CI only reaching CAP 2 after 18 months postoperative to CI. In two patients, no sound detection could be achieved despite continued rehabilitation for more than 2 years following CI. Consequently, auditory brainstem implantation was performed in these two patients, following which improvements in auditory perception were perceived (Fig. 4).

No single factor seemed to be correlated with the outcome of auditory rehabilitation after CI in the patients. Although 3 of 4 patients diagnosed with typical CHARGE syndrome demonstrated poor outcome following CI (Patients 6, 7, and 8), Patient 1 was the best performer of all patients included in this study.

Table 4. Radiologic findings of patients with CHARGE syndrome.

Patient No.	Age* (Y;M)	Sex	Cochlea	Vestibule	Middle ear	Facial canal	IAC	BCNC	Nerve component on MRI
1	3	F	Cochlear hypoplasia	SCC aplasia	ME opacification, incus/ stapes deformity	-	Narrow	Patent	CVN>FN
2	20;8	M	Cochlear hypoplasia	SCC aplasia	OW atresia, incus/stapes deformity	LS, TS	Narrow	Obliterated	CVN = FN
3	4;7	M	Cochlear hypoplasia	SCC aplasia	-	LS	Narrow	Patent	FN>CVN
4	2;5	M	Cochlear hypoplasia	SCC aplasia	ME opacification, incus/ stapes deformity, ankylosis, OW atresia??	-	Narrow	Obliterated	FN>CVN
5	2;4	M	Cochlear hypoplasia	SCC aplasia	-	-	Normal	Obliterated	NA
6	1;2	F	Cochlear hypoplasia	SCC aplasia	OW atresia, RW atresia, incus/stapes deformity	LS	Narrow	Obliterated	FN only
7	2	F	Cochlear hypoplasia	SCC aplasia	-	LS	Narrow	Obliterated	FN only
8	4;7	M	Cochlear hypoplasia	SCC aplasia	OW atresia, incus/stapes deformity	LS	Narrow	Obliterated	FN>CVN
9	15**	M	Cochlear hypoplasia	SCC aplasia	OW atresia, incus/stapes deformity	LS	Narrow	Obliterated	NA

*Age at cochlear implantation;
**age at initial visit; IAC: internal auditory canal; BCNC: bony cochlear nerve canal; IP-II: incomplete partition type II; SCC: semicircular canal, ME: middle ear, CVN: cochleovestibular nerve, FN: facial nerve; OW: oval window, RW: round window, LS: labyrinthine segment, TS: tympanic segment; NA; not available.

Nevertheless, the three typical CHARGE patients (Patients 6, 7, and 8) all demonstrated coloboma, which may be related to poor prognosis after CI in CHARGE syndrome. The type of mutations of *CHD7* was not correlated with outcome. On radiologic evaluation, obliteration of BCNC was not a factor relevant to outcome, while MRI findings demonstrating no visible CVN or very thin CVN compared to the facial nerve at the cerebello-pontine angle were more suggestive of poorer outcome. In

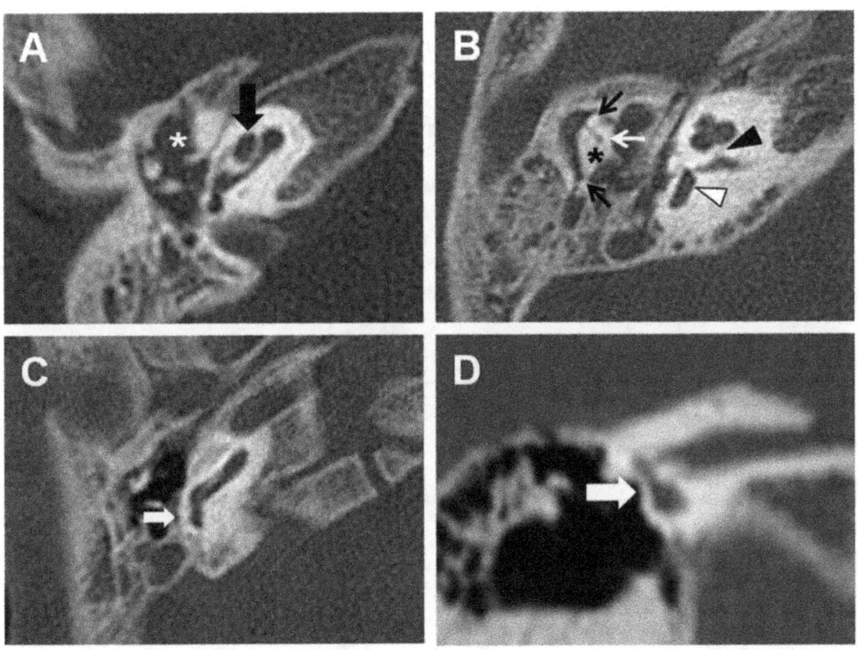

Figure 2. Computed tomography findings of inner ear anomalies typically seen in patients with CHARGE syndrome. (A) Cochlear hypoplasia is shown by a black arrow (Patient 1). (B) Bony cochlear nerve canal is obliterated (black arrowhead) and complete aplasia of the semicircular canals is seen (white arrowhead). The incus is dysmorphic and slightly rotated state (asterisk). Ankylosis between the incus and malleus (white arrow) and between the ossicles and epitympanic bone (black arrows) is shown (Patient 4). (C) Bony obliteration of the round window is seen (small white arrow) (Patient 6). (D) Oval window atresia is seen on the coronal image (large white arrow) (Patient 2).

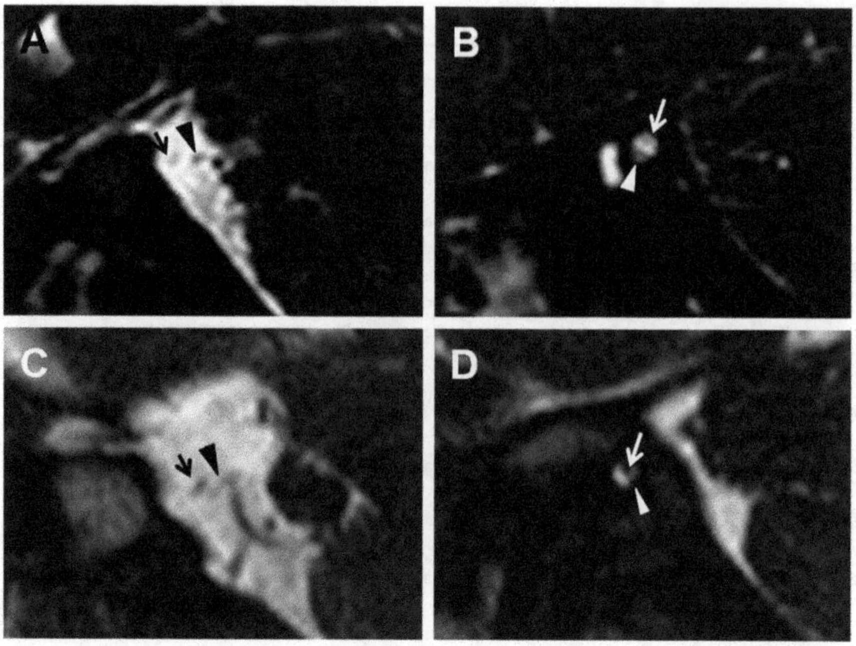

Figure 3. The parasagittal images of temporal MRI in patients with CHARGE syndrome. (A–B) The cochleovestibular nerve (arrowheads) is larger in diameter than the facial nerve (arrows) at the cerebellopontine angle (A) and within the internal auditory canal (B) in Patient 1. (C–D) The cochleovestibular nerve (arrowheads) is smaller in diameter than the facial nerve (arrows) at the cerebellopontine angle (C) and within the internal auditory canal (D) in Patient 4.

addition, two patients who could not achieve any sound detection after CI both had severe combined disabilities such as blindness (Patient 7) and severe mental retardation (Patient 8), which seems to be associated with poor outcome after CI.

Discussion

Five novel mutations and three previously reported mutations of the *CHD7* gene was identified in Korean patients with CHARGE syndrome presenting with profound hearing loss and typical inner ear anomalies. None of the mutations overlapped the previously reported mutations of the *CHD7* gene found in Korean patients [19]. The mutation rate was 89%, higher than previously reported despite inclusion of many patients with atypical CHARGE syndrome [8]. As Verloes [5] has emphasized, we believe that complete aplasia of the semicircular canals is a very specific finding that strongly suggests the presence of *CHD7* mutations even if other characteristic signs of CHARGE syndrome are missing. In comparison to the clinical features seen in *CHD7* mutation positive cohort in previous studies, the incidence of choanal atresia (13%) and coloboma (38%) were relatively lower in this report, which may be a finding more specific to the Korean population [6,19].

Various types of mutations were encountered regardless of clinical diagnosis as typical or atypical CHARGE syndrome. Truncating mutations including nonsense and frameshift mutations were most commonly detected (63%), similar to the previous reports [8]. The patient who carried a missense mutation of the *CHD7* gene presented with the mildest symptoms demonstrating only mild developmental delay and mental retardation without any classical features of CHARGE syndrome other than hearing loss and semicircular canal aplasia. Three mutations identified in this study were previously reported; however, the phenotypes of

Table 5. Auditory rehabilitation in Patients with CHARGE syndrome.

Patient No.	Age at CI (ABI)	Clinical diagnosis	CI site (ABI site)	CI Device	Pre-op CAP	Post-CI CAP	Post-ABI CAP	F/U after CI (after ABI)
1	3	Typical	R	Clarion 90K	0	6		2;8
2	20;8	Atypical	R	MedEl Pulsar	2	5		2;3
3	4;7	Atypical	R	Nucleus CI24R	0	4		3
4	2;5	Atypical	R	Nucleus CI24R	0	4		1;1
5	2;4	Atypical	R	Nucleus Freedom	0	4		2;4
6	1;2	Typical	R	Clarion 90K	0	2		1;6
7	2 (5;10)	Typical	R (R)	Clarion CII	0	0	1	4;7 (2)
8	4;7 (7;5)	Typical	L (L)	Clarion 90K	0	0	2	2;9 (0;1)
9	15**	Atypical	-		0	-	-	-

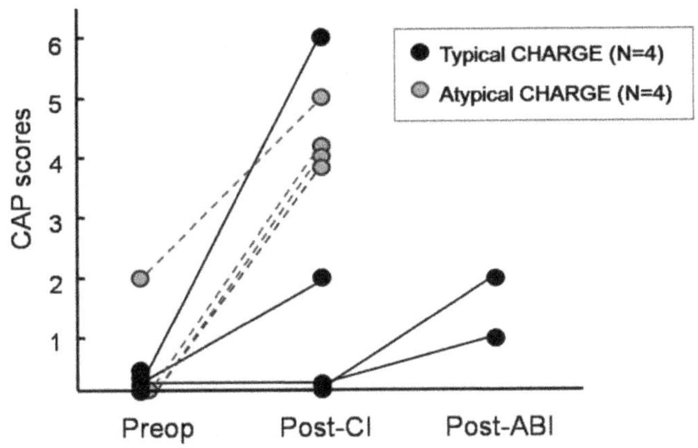

Figure 4. The improvement of auditory performance after cochlear implantation (CI) and auditory brainstem implantation (ABI) in patients with typical or atypical CHARGE syndrome.

patients having the same mutations differed considerably (Table S4) [20,21]. No mutation was found in one patient diagnosed of typical CHARGE syndrome by direct sequencing of the 5′ UTR and coding region of the *CHD7* gene. There may be small intragenic deletions or mutations in the upstream regulatory region of the *CHD7* gene, or it is possible that a different gene responsible for other syndromes with similar phenotypes as CHARGE syndrome may be involved.

To date, 17 cases of molecularly confirmed familial CHARGE syndrome have been reported, which include seven sib-pairs, three monozygotic twin pairs, and seven two-generation families [6]. This study presents another familial case of CHARGE syndrome in which a sib-pair carried the same frameshift mutation causing truncation of the *CHD7* gene. Since no mutation was found in their parents, de novo mutation or germline mosaicism was suspected. The sister of the proband had hearing loss and semicircular canal aplasia only on one side unlike the proband who was diagnosed with typical CHARGE syndrome and bilateral ear abnormalities, demonstrating the intra-familial variability of CHARGE syndrome and also expanding the phenotypic spectrum of mildly affected patients.

Radiologic analysis of patients with typical and atypical CHARGE syndrome revealed that narrowing of the internal auditory canals and obliteration of the BCNC were also common findings in addition to aplasia of the semicircular canals typically seen in CHARGE syndrome. These findings have great clinical significance because of their correlation with CVN deficiency, which may lead to poor outcomes after CI [15,22]. Indeed, CVN hypoplasia or aplasia was identified in all of our patients who underwent temporal MRI. Other than the anatomical factors, it is known that combined disabilities such as developmental delay, mental retardation, and blindness often seen in CHARGE syndrome act as hindering factors for proper auditory and speech developments [13].

Most of the previous studies dealing with the auditory outcome after CI or auditory brainstem implantation in CHARGE syndrome rely on clinical diagnosis only and did not perform genetic analysis of the *CHD7* gene [14,16]. Since CHARGE syndrome is a clinically complex disorder, mutational analysis of the *CHD7* gene allows molecular confirmation of the diagnosis and also enables inclusion of mildly affected patients showing only few clinical features of CHARGE syndrome. Following CI, a wide range of auditory improvement was encountered from no sound perception to open-set speech discrimination without visual cues in our patients with CHARGE syndrome. The type of mutation of the *CHD7* gene did not demonstrate clear correlation with the prognosis after CI. Despite the presence of narrow internal auditory canals and obliterated BCNC, which may be considered as a contraindication to CI, the outcomes of CI were promising in majority of our patients [23]. In our opinion, CI should be recommended in CHARGE patients with profound hearing loss even if CVN deficiency or BCNC obliteration is present on imaging, especially when the size of the CVN is larger than or equal to that of the facial nerve on parasagittal view of MRI and severe mental retardation is not present.

In two patients with CHARGE syndrome who failed to perceive any sound stimulation with a CI, auditory brainstem implantation was performed and early results show increased attentiveness and responsiveness despite limited improvement in auditory perception. Auditory brainstem implantation in nontumor patients has shown promising outcomes recently, and we believe that auditory brainstem implantation is a viable option in patients with CHARGE syndrome in cases of failed stimulation after CI [24,25]. Nevertheless, considering the difficulties in the pitch ranking process after auditory brainstem implantation in children that can be further complicated by the additional disabilities of CHARGE patients, long and strenuous rehabilitation may be warranted in these patients. Therefore, the parents must be counseled carefully and informed about the variability of outcome and the auditory rehabilitation process after CI or auditory brainstem implantation in patients with CHARGE syndrome.

In conclusion, 8 mutations of the *CHD7* gene including 5 novel mutations were identified in Korean patients with CHARGE syndrome showing semicircular canal aplasia and profound hearing loss, which will broaden the genotypic and phenotypic spectrum of CHARGE syndrome. Genetic analysis of the *CHD7* gene should be performed in cases with semicircular canal aplasia considering the high mutation rate even when the other typical features of CHARGE syndrome are not present. CI should be recommended in patients with CHARGE syndrome when the size of the CVN is larger than or equal to that of the facial nerve on MRI and mental retardation is not severe, since favorable outcome is expected in these cases. Auditory brainstem implantation may be considered in patients with CHARGE syndrome who have failed to benefit from CI.

Supporting Information

Figure S1 Multiple sequence alignment of the CHD7 protein orthologs. CHD7 amino acid sequences of various vertebrate species are aligned using the Clustal W2 program (http://www.ebi.ac.uk/Tools/msa/clustalw2/). The region containing the novel missense mutation, p.R2065S (indicated as an asterisk), is highly conserved in vertebrates.

Figure S2 Exon-trapping analysis of the novel splice site variation, c.5210+5G>C. For the c.5210+5G>C variation, exons 22 and 23 of *CHD7* were introduced into the pSPL3 vector and analyzed by the *in vitro* splicing assay. For the wild type, normal 623-bp mRNA was identified. For the mutant type, 463-bp mRNA variant was seen together with the normal 623-bp mRNA (A). When sequencing analysis was performed, the normal 623-bp mRNA demonstrated both exons 22 and 23 between the pSPL3 exons (B), whereas the short 463-bp mRNA variant identified in the mutant type contained only exon 22 (C). SM, standard marker; WT, wild-type; MT, mutant type; N, negative.

Figure S3 Exon-trapping analysis of splice site variation, c.5405-7G>A. For the c.5405-7G>A variation, exon 26 of

CHD7 was introduced into the pSPL3 vector and analyzed by the *in vitro* splicing assay. For the wild type, normal 393-bp mRNA was identified, while the mutant type demonstrated only the 398-bp mRNA variant (A). Sequencing analysis of the wild type mRNA revealed exon 26 of *CHD7* between the pSPL3 exons (B), but the mutant mRNA variant sized 398-bp contained an additional 5-bp intronic sequence upstream of exon 26 (C). SM, standard marker; WT, wild-type; MT, mutant type; N, negative.

Table S1 Primers and PCR conditions used for *CHD7* sequencing analysis.

Table S2 Splicing variants for *in vitro* splicing assay. * The exon directly associated with the splice variation is presented in bold. Exon 22 of Patient 5 is closely located to exon 23 and was inserted into the pSPL3 vector together. Restriction enzyme recognition sites of the primer sequences are underlined.

Table S3 *In silico* analysis through splice site prediction programs. * Values in bold represent scores of the new splice site that is introduced by the intronic variation.

Table S4 Comparison of the clinical features of patients with CHARGE syndrome who have the same mutations of the *CHD7* gene. Of the three mutations identified in this study that had previously been reported, clinical features were provided for only two patients in the previous reports. TE: tracheoesophageal.

Author Contributions

Conceived and designed the experiments: MHS JB JYC U-KK. Performed the experiments: H-JC HKL TJK. Analyzed the data: MHS H-JC TJK W-SL JYC. Contributed reagents/materials/analysis tools: MHS W-SL SO JYC. Wrote the paper: MHS H-JC U-KK.

References

1. Hall BD (1979) Choanal atresia and associated multiple anomalies. J Pediatr 95: 395–398.
2. Hittner HM, Hirsch NJ, Kreh GM, Rudolph AJ (1979) Colobomatous microphthalmia, heart disease, hearing loss, and mental retardation--a syndrome. J Pediatr Ophthalmol Strabismus 16: 122–128.
3. Pagon RA, Graham JM, Zonana J, Yong SL (1981) Coloboma, congenital heart disease, and choanal atresia with multiple anomalies: CHARGE association. J Pediatr 99: 223–227.
4. Blake KD, Davenport SL, Hall BD, Hefner MA, Pagon RA, et al. (1998) CHARGE association: an update and review for the primary pediatrician. Clin Pediatr (Phila) 37: 159–173.
5. Verloes A (2005) Updated diagnostic criteria for CHARGE syndrome: a proposal. Am J Med Genet A 133A: 306–308.
6. Bergman JE, Janssen N, Hoefsloot LH, Jongmans MC, Hofstra RM, et al. (2011) CHD7 mutations and CHARGE syndrome: the clinical implications of an expanding phenotype. J Med Genet.
7. Vissers LE, van Ravenswaaij CM, Admiraal R, Hurst JA, de Vries BB, et al. (2004) Mutations in a new member of the chromodomain gene family cause CHARGE syndrome. Nat Genet 36: 955–957.
8. Zentner GE, Layman WS, Martin DM, Scacheri PC (2010) Molecular and phenotypic aspects of CHD7 mutation in CHARGE syndrome. Am J Med Genet A 152A: 674–686.
9. Sanlaville D, Verloes A (2007) CHARGE syndrome: an update. Eur J Hum Genet 15: 389–399.
10. Morimoto AK, Wiggins RH, 3rd, Hudgins PA, Hedlund GL, Hamilton B, et al. (2006) Absent semicircular canals in CHARGE syndrome: radiologic spectrum of findings. AJNR Am J Neuroradiol 27: 1663–1671.
11. Jyonouchi S, McDonald-McGinn DM, Bale S, Zackai EH, Sullivan KE (2009) CHARGE (coloboma, heart defect, atresia choanae, retarded growth and development, genital hypoplasia, ear anomalies/deafness) syndrome and chromosome 22q11.2 deletion syndrome: a comparison of immunologic and nonimmunologic phenotypic features. Pediatrics 123: e871–877.
12. Jongmans M, Sistermans EA, Rikken A, Nillesen WM, Tamminga R, et al. (2005) Genotypic and phenotypic characterization of Noonan syndrome: new data and review of the literature. Am J Med Genet A 134A: 165–170.
13. Berrettini S, Forli F, Genovese E, Santarelli R, Arslan E, et al. (2008) Cochlear implantation in deaf children with associated disabilities: challenges and outcomes. Int J Audiol 47: 199–208.
14. Lanson BG, Green JE, Roland JT, Lalwani AK, Waltzman SB (2007) Cochlear implantation in Children with CHARGE syndrome: therapeutic decisions and outcomes. Laryngoscope 117: 1260–1266.
15. Papsin BC (2005) Cochlear implantation in children with anomalous cochleovestibular anatomy. Laryngoscope 115: 1–26.
16. Arndt S, Laszig R, Beck R, Schild C, Maier W, et al. (2010) Spectrum of hearing disorders and their management in children with CHARGE syndrome. Otol Neurotol 31: 67–73.
17. Warren FM, 3rd, Wiggins RH, 3rd, Pitt C, Harnsberger HR, Shelton C (2010) Apparent cochlear nerve aplasia: to implant or not to implant? Otol Neurotol 31: 1088–1094.
18. Archbold S, Lutman ME, Marshall DH (1995) Categories of Auditory Performance. Ann Otol Rhinol Laryngol Suppl 166: 312–314.
19. Lee YW, Kim SC, Shin YL, Kim JW, Hong HS, et al. (2009) Clinical and genetic analysis of the CHD7 gene in Korean patients with CHARGE syndrome. Clin Genet 75: 290–293.
20. Jongmans MC, Admiraal RJ, van der Donk KP, Vissers LE, Baas AF, et al. (2006) CHARGE syndrome: the phenotypic spectrum of mutations in the CHD7 gene. J Med Genet 43: 306–314.
21. Aramaki M, Udaka T, Kosaki R, Makita Y, Okamoto N, et al. (2006) Phenotypic spectrum of CHARGE syndrome with CHD7 mutations. J Pediatr 148: 410–414.
22. Glastonbury CM, Davidson HC, Harnsberger HR, Butler J, Kertesz TR, et al. (2002) Imaging findings of cochlear nerve deficiency. AJNR Am J Neuroradiol 23: 635–643.
23. Shelton C, Luxford WM, Tonokawa LL, Lo WW, House WF (1989) The narrow internal auditory canal in children: a contraindication to cochlear implants. Otolaryngol Head Neck Surg 100: 227–231.
24. Sennaroglu L, Ziyal I, Atas A, Sennaroglu G, Yucel E, et al. (2009) Preliminary results of auditory brainstem implantation in prelingually deaf children with inner ear malformations including severe stenosis of the cochlear aperture and aplasia of the cochlear nerve. Otol Neurotol 30: 708–715.
25. Colletti V, Carner M, Miorelli V, Guida M, Colletti L, et al. (2005) Auditory brainstem implant (ABI): new frontiers in adults and children. Otolaryngol Head Neck Surg 133: 126–138.

11

Hearing Loss in Stranded Odontocete Dolphins and Whales

David Mann[1,2]*, Mandy Hill-Cook[3], Charles Manire[2¤a], Danielle Greenhow[1], Eric Montie[1], Jessica Powell[1,2¤b], Randall Wells[1,4], Gordon Bauer[2,5], Petra Cunningham-Smith[2], Robert Lingenfelser[6], Robert DiGiovanni Jr.[7], Abigale Stone[8], Micah Brodsky[9], Robert Stevens[9], George Kieffer[10], Paul Hoetjes[11]

1 College of Marine Science, University of South Florida, St. Petersburg, Florida, United States of America, **2** Mote Marine Laboratory, Sarasota, Florida, United States of America, **3** Department of Biology, Portland State University, Portland, Oregon, United States of America, **4** Chicago Zoological Society, c/o Mote Marine Laboratory, Sarasota, Florida, United States of America, **5** Division of Social Sciences, New College of Florida, Sarasota, Florida, United States of America, **6** Marine Mammal Conservancy, Key Largo, Florida, United States of America, **7** Riverhead Foundation for Marine Research and Preservation, Riverhead, New York, United States of America, **8** Clearwater Marine Aquarium, Clearwater, Florida, United States of America, **9** Dolphins Plus, Key Largo, Florida, United States of America, **10** Southern Caribbean Cetacean Network (SCCN), Bapor Kibra, Curaçao, Netherlands Antilles, **11** Department of Environment and Nature, Willemstad, Curaçao, Netherlands Antilles

Abstract

The causes of dolphin and whale stranding can often be difficult to determine. Because toothed whales rely on echolocation for orientation and feeding, hearing deficits could lead to stranding. We report on the results of auditory evoked potential measurements from eight species of odontocete cetaceans that were found stranded or severely entangled in fishing gear during the period 2004 through 2009. Approximately 57% of the bottlenose dolphins and 36% of the rough-toothed dolphins had significant hearing deficits with a reduction in sensitivity equivalent to severe (70–90 dB) or profound (>90 dB) hearing loss in humans. The only stranded short-finned pilot whale examined had profound hearing loss. No impairments were detected in seven Risso's dolphins from three different stranding events, two pygmy killer whales, one Atlantic spotted dolphin, one spinner dolphin, or a juvenile Gervais' beaked whale. Hearing impairment could play a significant role in some cetacean stranding events, and the hearing of all cetaceans in rehabilitation should be tested.

Editor: Andrew Iwaniuk, University of Lethbridge, Canada

Funding: Funding was provided by National Oceanographic and Atmospheric Administration (NOAA) Ocean Acoustics program for equipment and the Office of Naval Research (ONR) for pilot whale testing. The funders had no role in study design, data collection and analysis, decision to publish, or preparation of the manuscript.

Competing Interests: The authors have declared that no competing interests exist.

* E-mail: dmann@marine.usf.edu

¤a Current address: Atlantis Resort, Paradise Island, Bahamas
¤b Current address: Southeast Regional Office, National Oceanic and Atmospheric Administration (NOAA) Fisheries Service, St. Petersburg, Florida, United States of America

Introduction

Odontocete cetaceans (the toothed whales) use high frequency echolocation sounds for navigation and foraging and are well-known for possessing high frequency hearing abilities [1–2]. Many species strand in coastal areas, as individuals or sometimes in large mass stranding events [3]. The causes of dolphin and whale stranding are often difficult to determine. Here we show profound high-frequency hearing loss in three species of cetaceans that had stranded, which suggests that hearing impairment could be a causative factor for some stranding events.

Hearing measurements in captive cetaceans are often performed with behavioral conditioning, where the dolphin is trained to press a response paddle or vocalize when it hears a test signal [1,4–6]. Behavioral hearing tests cannot be easily performed on stranded cetaceans. Stranded dolphins often reside in rehabilitation facilities for short periods of time, and training of stranded dolphins that are likely to be returned to the wild is discouraged by federal wildlife management agencies. Auditory evoked potential (AEP) methods, which are commonly used to measure hearing in human infants [7], have been used to measure hearing in captive and wild cetaceans [8–10]. AEPs provide a rapid means to assess hearing and yield comparable results to behavioral measures [11–14]. A further advantage is that AEPs provide the means to screen free-ranging populations of cetaceans if individuals are able to be handled briefly.

Results

Severe (~70–90 dB loss) to profound (>90 dB loss) hearing loss was found in four out of seven (57%) of the stranded bottlenose dolphins (*Tursiops truncatus*) and 5 out of 14 (36%) rough-toothed dolphins (*Steno bredanensis*) examined in this study (definitions based on [15]) (Table 1; detailed information on each animal can be found in Table S1). This finding is in stark contrast to results of population-level hearing evaluations of bottlenose dolphin in Sarasota Bay, Florida, during capture-release health assessments [16] that have shown a general absence of hearing loss across more than 60 dolphins of a variety of ages and both sexes [17]. Profound hearing loss was also found in one stranded short-finned pilot whale (*Globicephala macrorhynchus*). No hearing loss was found in stranded Rissos's dolphins (*Grampus griseus*) from three different stranding events, two pygmy killer whales (*Feresa attenuata*) from a single stranding event, an Atlantic spotted dolphin (*Stenella frontalis*), and a spinner dolphin (*Stenella longirostris*; Table 1). The hearing of the Risso's dolphins were similar to the hearing measured from a stranded Risso's dolphin previously reported [18]. The audiograms of species with normal hearing will be reported elsewhere.

The audiograms of two stranded bottlenose dolphins are shown in Figure 1 to illustrate the degree of hearing loss that has been measured in stranded dolphins; in the case of the dolphin named "Castaway" there was at least 105 dB loss at 80 kHz and no auditory evoked potentials were detected at any frequency tested from 10 kHz to 120 kHz. In the rough-toothed dolphin named "Dancer", no response was seen to the loudest tone pips that could be generated (137–153 dB re 1 μPa SPL), but an evoked potential could be seen in response to a click at high sound levels (154 dB re 1 μPa_{peak}) (Figure 2). This audiogram shows at least 70 dB hearing loss in a rough-toothed dolphin (Figure 2). There was no statistical relationship between dolphin age group and hearing loss (Fisher Exact Test $p = 1.000$), when including all dolphins and grouping calves and subadults, because of the low sample size of calves (Table 2). However, none of the calves showed hearing loss, but 42% of the subadults had hearing loss. Five of the dolphins with profound hearing loss were males and five were females.

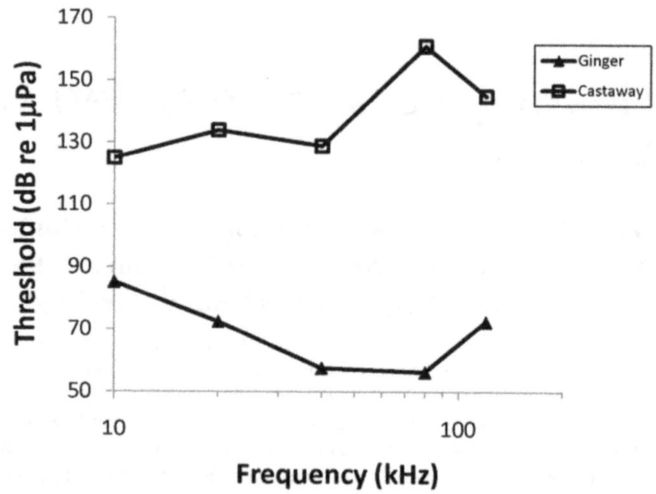

Figure 1. Audiogram of MML0807 (Ginger; filled triangles), a juvenile bottlenose dolphin with normal hearing, and MML FB303 (Castaway; open squares), an adult bottlenose dolphin with hearing loss. For Castaway, no response was detected at any frequency indicating that there was at least 40–100 dB hearing loss across all frequencies tested, and no response could be detected in response to click trains at 164 dB_{peak} re 1 μPa.

Discussion

There are five main contributing factors to hearing loss in mammals: intense chronic noise, transient intense noise (e.g. explosions), age-related hearing loss (presbycusis), congenital hearing impairment, and ototoxic drug treatment [19]. We do not know the noise exposure history of any of these dolphins. Based on the locations of stranding, it is possible that some of them have been exposed to chronic noise from boating and shipping, while for others this is unlikely. Experiments with odontocetes have shown that high levels of exposure are needed to induce temporary threshold shifts [20–24]. One of the stranded bottlenose dolphins (Caesar II) with high frequency hearing loss was assumed to be relatively old based on his lack of teeth, which can wear down and/or fall out with age. Age-related hearing loss has been reported in some captive dolphins [25-28], but not commonly in wild dolphins [17]. It is possible that wild dolphins with hearing loss have lower survival than dolphins with normal hearing.

It is likely that hearing loss was congenital in some of these stranding cases, especially two of the rough-toothed dolphins (Dancer and Vixen), which were estimated to each be approximately two years old at the time of stranding. Congenital hearing impairment in humans is not uncommon. In one study, 113 out of 52508 (about 2 out of 1,000) newborns screened in Texas had hearing loss [7]. In addition to genetic factors related to hearing loss, one extremely important, unexplored mechanism may be the impacts of chemical pollution on hearing. Cetaceans, particularly odontocetes, have been shown to accumulate very high levels of polychlorinated biphenyls (or PCBs), which can be maternally transferred to offspring [29–30]. Evidence from studies with rats suggests that these chemicals may affect how hearing develops. In fact, it has been shown that developmental exposure of rats to PCBs results in severe hearing loss [31]. It is not known how these or other contaminants might affect ear development in cetaceans.

Some odontocetes have social systems with strong mother-calf bonds where the mother can support the calf for years through lactation [32]. While dolphins rely heavily on echolocation for navigation and foraging, it is possible that a dependent calf with congenital hearing loss could survive with the help of its mother for a long period. Once it is weaned, however, it would not be able to forage successfully on its own. Indeed, both of the young rough-

Table 1. Summary of odontocete audiogram results.

Species	Common Name	Number Stranded Animals Tested	Number with Hearing Loss
Steno bredanensis	Rough-toothed dolphin	14	5
Tursiops truncatus	Bottlenose dolphin	7*	4*
Grampus griseus	Risso's dolphin	7	0
Feresa attenuata	Pygmy killer whale	2	0
Stenella longirostris	Spinner dolphin	1	0
Stenella frontalis	Atlantic spotted dolphin	1	0
Globicephala macrorhynchus	Short-finned pilot whale	1	1
Mesoplodon europaeus [13]	Beaked whale	1	0

*One bottlenose dolphin (Filly) became entangled in fishing gear and was rescued. This dolphin had high frequency hearing loss.

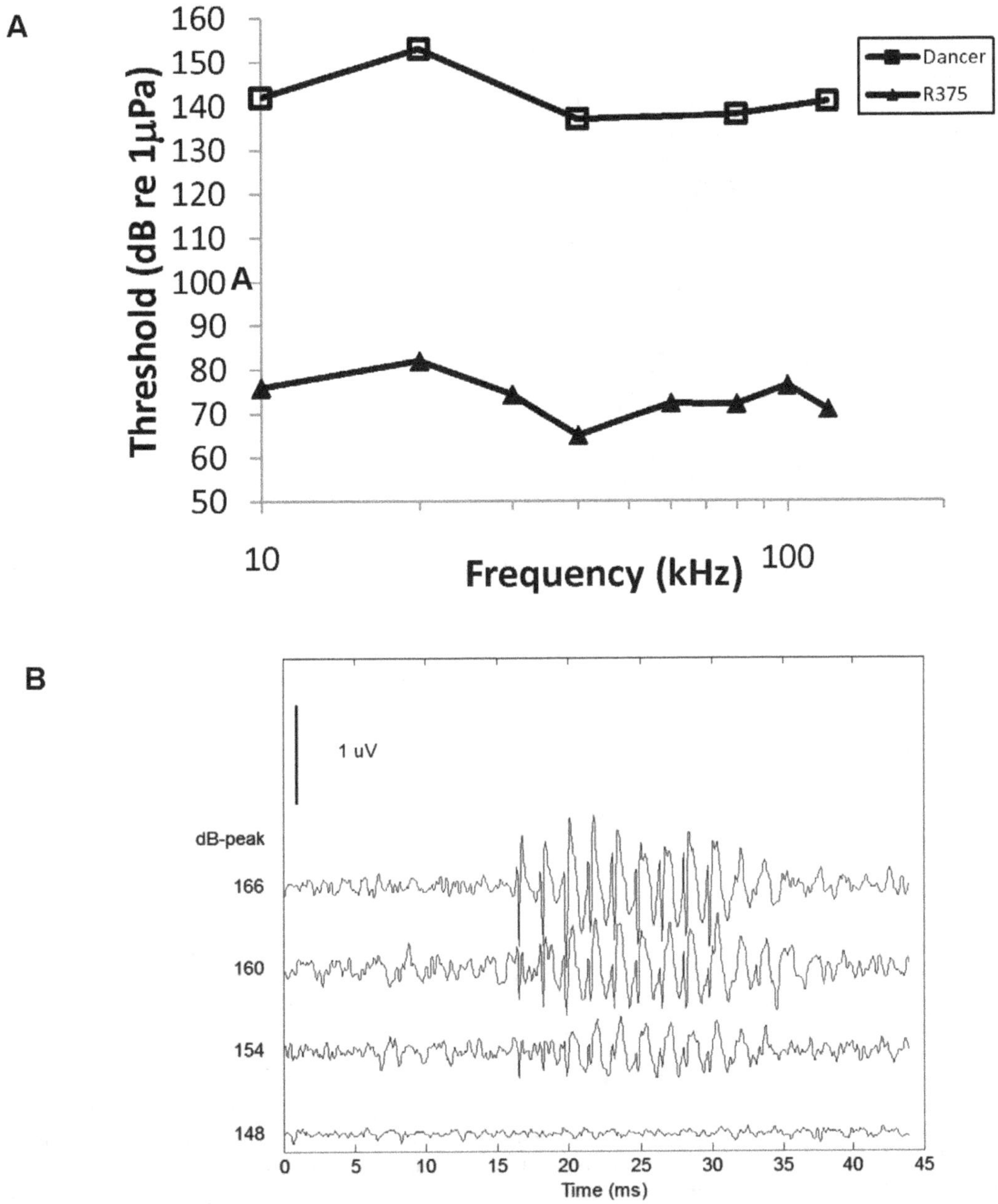

Figure 2. Results of hearing tests on two stranded rough-toothed dolphins. A. Audiogram of R375 (filled triangles), a normal hearing rough-toothed dolphin, and highest level tested for Dancer (open squares) rough-toothed (open squares) for which no response was detected at any frequency). For Dancer, there was at least a 70 dB hearing loss across all frequencies tested. B. Click-train (600 Hz click rate) evoked potential traces from the hearing-impaired rough-toothed dolphin (Dancer) at four stimulus levels. The click train sound starts at 15 ms. The lowest level detected was about 154 dB_{peak} re 1 μPa.

Table 2. Summary of hearing loss for all dolphins by age category.

	Normal	Hearing Loss	Total
Adult	13	5	18
Subadult	7	5	12
Calf	5	0	5

toothed dolphins that stranded were found to have consumed sponges, possibly indicating an inability to catch squid and fishes (Figure 3). A previous case of a deaf bottlenose dolphin, which was captured in the wild, was reported healthy at the time of capture, which suggests that it is possible for a deaf dolphin to survive in a social group [25].

Many of the stranded dolphins in this study were being treated for various infections with antibiotics and antifungals, including the oral administration of gentamicin sulfate and itraconazole and intramuscular injections of amikacin sulfate. Aminoglycoside antibiotics, including gentamicin and amikacin, are known to cause cochlear hair cell death in mammals [33]. This mechanism

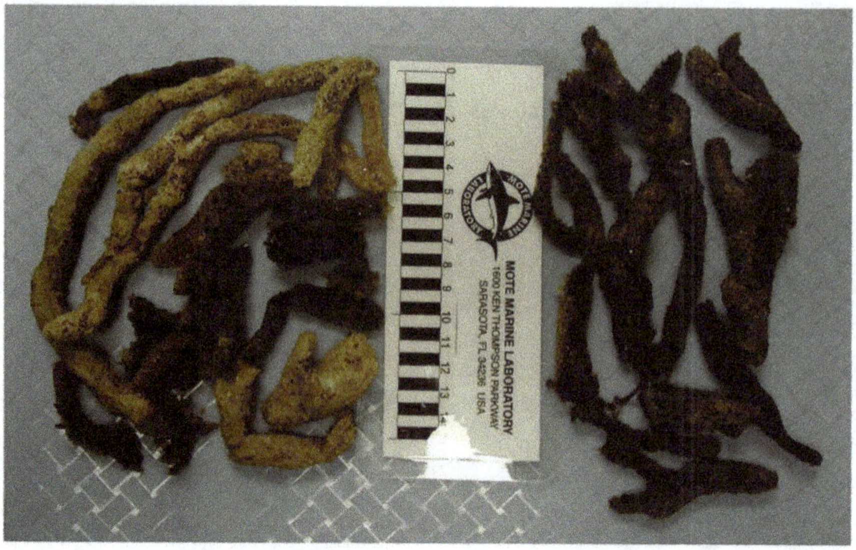

Figure 3. Image of sponges removed from the stomach of Vixen, a stranded rough-toothed dolphin with profound hearing loss.

has been suggested as a potential cause of hearing loss in captive marine mammals [27]. While drug administration cannot be ruled out as a cause of hearing loss, it is unlikely as some of the hearing tests were conducted soon after stranding. In addition, dolphins that showed hearing loss were treated with similar drug dosages as other animals that did not show hearing deficits. Hearing tests were conducted both before and after drug treatment with five Risso's dolphins, none of which showed an effect on hearing. In future stranding events, it is crucial that hearing measurements be performed both before and after any drug treatment. Rehabilitation will not be successful if drug treatments result in significant high frequency hearing loss. One recent report of aspergillosis in a stranded harbor porpoise showed infection of the otic region [34]. The high incidence of hearing impairment in stranded odontocetes also prompts us to argue that hearing screening should be part of the standard veterinary examination of stranded cetaceans.

Methods

All research was approved by the IACUC of the University of South Florida and Mote Marine Laboratory with permit authorization from NOAA. Hearing tests were conducted under NOAA permits #932-1489-06 (letter Sep 1, 2004) for *Steno bredanensis* at MML; #932-1489-06 (letter Apr 08, 2005) for *Grampus griseus* Riverhead Foundation; #932-1489-06 (letter April 20, 2005) for *S. bredanensis* at Marine Mammal Conservancy; #932-1489-08 (letter Aug 24, 2005) for *S. bredanensis* at Gulf World; #932-1489-08 (letter Aug 14, 2005) for *Grampus griseus* at MML; #1053-1825-00 (Nov 21, 2006) for all other dolphins. Hearing tests were conducted either in the water or on land, depending on the situation at the stranding facility (e.g., whether handlers could stand in the holding tanks or pens, or the number of other animals in the holding tanks). In all cases, a jawphone consisting of an ITC-1042 piezoceramic transducer embedded in a RTV silicone suction cup was placed on the lower jaw fat pad to deliver sound stimuli. Sound levels were calibrated underwater by measuring the sound 10 cm from the jawphone in a free field using a Reson TC4032 hydrophone. These underwater calibrations were used as the calibrations for the in-air tests. Background noise levels in test tanks were typically <45 dB re 1 $\mu Pa^2/Hz$ at frequencies above 20 kHz. Noise levels in field test locations, which were shallow beaches (Florida Bay at the Marine Mammal Conservancy and the Caribbean Sea at Curacao Seaquarium), were about 85 dB re 1 $\mu Pa^2/Hz$ at frequencies above 20 kHz.

Evoked potentials were measured in response to amplitude modulated (AM) tone pips. The AM rate was either 600 Hz or 1000 Hz, as these rates were found to yield large evoked potentials. Click evoked potentials were also measured for some dolphins. Clicks were generated by sending a 0.1 ms square wave into the transducer, which generated a click with a peak frequency of approximately 80–120 kHz. Evoked potentials were measured in response to click trains delivered at 600 Hz and 1000 Hz. All signals were generated by a Tucker-Davis Technologies (TDT) RX6 real-time processor with a 260 kHz sample rate.

Silver chloride electrodes embedded in suction cups were used to measure evoked potentials after 10,000× amplification through a differential amplifier (TDT HS4-DB4). The recording electrode was placed about 5–10 cm behind the blowhole, and a reference electrode was placed approximately 40 cm behind the blowhole. The ground electrode was placed in the water for in-water tests, or on the back of the dolphin for in-air tests.

Evoked potentials were averaged in response to up to 1000 presentations of the acoustic stimulus (TDT BioSig software). Fewer presentations were used when a response at one level was apparent. AEP signals were analyzed in a custom MATLAB program (BSlab) which performed a 2441-point FFT (resulting in a 10 Hz resolution) and measured the signal-to-noise ratio at the modulation frequency of the AM signals. A signal was considered to be present if the AEP signal was at least 3 dB above the background noise (either measured from 12 adjacent frequency bins, or from a portion of the signal in which sound was not presented). This is equivalent to the F-test with an alpha of at least 0.01 [35]. The threshold was defined as the lowest signal level that yielded a detectable AEP at the sound modulation frequency.

Supporting Information

Table S1 Summary of odontocete audiogram results. One bottlenose dolphin, MML0701 (Filly), became entangled in fishing gear and was rescued. MML = Mote Marine Laboratory; MMC = Marine Mammal Conservancy; CMA = Clearwater Marine Aquarium; Riverhead = Riverhead Foundation; Curacao =

Curacao Seaquarium. Dolphins with severe to profound hearing loss are also indicated in bold type.

Acknowledgments

We thank T. Rowles, T. Spradlin, B. Mase-Guthrie, K. Baker, A. Sloan, E. Tuohy-Sheen of NOAA for help with coordinating hearing tests and providing stranding information, B. Losch and D. Colbert for help in testing at Gulf World, J. Reynolds for arranging testing with the pilot whale in Curacao, and countless volunteers that helped with each dolphin and whale stranding.

Author Contributions

Conceived and designed the experiments: DAM MHC CM EM RW GB. Performed the experiments: DAM MHC CM DG EM JP PCS RL RDJ AS MB RS GK PCH. Analyzed the data: DAM MHC DG EM JP. Contributed reagents/materials/analysis tools: CM RW PCS RL RDJ AS MB RS GK PCH. Wrote the paper: DAM MHC CM DG EM JP RW GB MB.

References

1. Johnson CS (1967) Sound detection thresholds in marine mammals. In: Tavolga W, ed. Marine bio-acoustics. New York: Pergamon volume 2: 247–260.
2. Au W (1993) The Sonar of Dolphins. New York: Springer-Verlag. 277 p.
3. Odell D (1987) The mystery of marine mammal strandings. Cetus 7: 2–6.
4. Hall JD, Johnson CS (1972) Auditory thresholds of a killer whale *Orcinus orca*. Linneaus. J Acoust Soc Am 51: 515–517.
5. FT Awbrey FT, JA Thomas JA, Kastelein RA (1988) Low frequency underwater hearing sensitivity in belugas (*Dephinapterus leucas*). J Acoust Soc Am 84: 2273–2275.
6. Kastelein RA, Hagedoorn M, Au WWL, de Haan D (2003) Audiogram of a striped dolphin (*Stenella coeruleoalba*). J Acoust Soc Am 113: 1130–1137.
7. Finitzo T, Albright K, O'Neal J (1998) The newborn with hearing loss: detection in the nursery. Pediatrics 102: 1452–1460.
8. Popov VV, Supin AY (1990) Auditory brainstem responses in characterization of dolphin hearing. J Comp Physiol A 166: 385–393.
9. Supin AY, Popov VV (1995) Envelope-following response and modulation transfer function in the dolphin's auditory system. Hear Res 92: 38–46.
10. Dolphin WF, Au WW, Nachtigall PE, Pawloski J (1995) Modulation rate transfer functions to low-frequency carriers in three species of cetaceans. J Comp Physiol A 177: 235–245.
11. Szymanski MD, Bain DE, Kiehl K, Pennington S, Wong S, et al. (1999) Killer whale (*Orcinus orca*) hearing: Auditory brainstem response and behavioral audiograms. J Acoust Soc Am 106: 1134–1141.
12. Yuen MML, Nachtigall PE, Breese M, Supin AY (2005) Behavioral and auditory evoked potential audiograms of a false killer whale (*Pseudorca crassidens*). J Acoust Soc Am 118: 2688–2695.
13. Cook MLH, Varela RA, Goldstein JD, McCulloch SD, Bossart GD, et al. (2006) Beaked whale auditory evoked potential hearing measurements. J Comp Phys A 192: 489–495.
14. Houser DS, Finneran JJ (2006) A comparison of underwater hearing sensitivity in bottlenose dolphins (*Tursiops truncatus*) determined by electrophysiological and behavioral methods. J Acoust Soc Am 120: 1713–1722.
15. Clark JG (1981) Uses and abuses of hearing loss classification. ASHA 23: 493–500.
16. Wells RS, Rhinehart HL, Hansen LJ, Sweeney JC, Townsend FI, et al. (2004) Bottlenose dolphins as marine ecosystem sentinels: Developing a health monitoring system. EcoHealth 1: 246–254.
17. Cook MLH (2006) Behavioral and Auditory Evoked Potential (AEP) Hearing Measurements in Odontocete Cetaceans. Ph.D. Thesis, University of South Florida. 123 p.
18. Nachtigall PE, Yuen MML, Mooney TA, Taylor KA (2005) Hearing measurements from a stranded infant Risso's dolphin, *Grampus griseus*. J Exp Biol 208: 4181–4188.
19. Tarter SK, Robins TG (1990) Chronic noise exposure, high-frequency hearing loss, and hypertension among automotive assembly works. J Occupat Med 32: 685–689.
20. Finneran JJ, Schlundt CE, Dear R (2002) Temporary shift in masked hearing thresholds in odontocetes after exposure to single underwater impulses from a seismic watergun. J Acoust Soc Am 111: 2929–2940.
21. Nachtigall PE, Pawloski JL, Au WWL (2003) Temporary threshold shifts and recovery following noise exposure in the Atlantic bottlenose dolphin *Tursiops truncatus*. J Acoust Soc Am 113: 3425–3429.
22. Nachtigall PE, Supin AY, Pawloski JL, Au WWL (2004) Temporary threshold shifts after noise exposure in the bottlenose dolphin *Tursiops truncatus* measured using auditory evoked potentials. Mar Mamm Sci 20: 673–687.
23. Finneran JJ, Carder DA, Schlundt CE, Ridgway SH (2005) Temporary threshold shift in bottlenose dolphins (*Tursiops truncatus*) exposed to mid-frequency tones. J Acoust Soc Am 118: 2696–2705.
24. Lucke K, Siebert U, Lepper PA, Blanchet MA (2009) Temporary shift in masked hearing thresholds in a harbor porpoise (*Phocoena phocoena*) after exposure to seismic airgun stimuli. J Acoust Soc Am 125: 4060–4070.
25. Ridgway SH, Carder DA (1997) Hearing deficits measured in some *Tursiops truncatus*, and discovery of a deaf/mute dolphin. J Acoust Soc Am 101: 590–594.
26. Brill RL, Moore PWB (2001) Assessment of dolphin (*Tursiops truncatus*) auditory sensitivity and hearing loss using jawphones. J Acoust Soc Am 109: 1717–1722.
27. Houser DS, Finneran JJ (2006) Variation in the hearing sensitivity of a dolphin population obtained through the use of evoked potential audiometry. J Acoust Soc Am 120: 4090–4099.
28. Houser DS, Gomez-Rubio A, Finneran JJ (2008) Evoked potential audiometry of 13 Pacific bottlenose dolphins (*Tursiops truncatus gilli*). Mar Mamm Sci 24: 28–41.
29. Ross PS, Ellis GM, Ikonomou MG, Barrett-Lennard LG, Addison RF (2000) High PCB concentrations in free-ranging Pacific killer whales, Orcinus orca: effects of age, sex and dietary preference. Mar Pollut Bull 40: 504–15.
30. Wells RS, Tornero V, Borrell A, Aguilar A, Rowles TK, et al. (2005) Integrating life-history and reproductive success data to examine potential relationships with organochlorine compounds for bottlenose dolphins (Tursiops truncatus) in Sarasota Bay, Florida. Sci Total Environ 349: 106.
31. Goldey ES, Crofton KM (1998) Thyroxine replacement attenuates hypothyroxinemia, hearing loss, and motor deficits following developmental exposure to Aroclor 1254 in rats. Toxic Sci 45: 94–105.
32. Brodie PF (1969) Duration of lactation in Cetacea: An indicator of required learning? Amer Mid Nat 82: 312–314.
33. Matz GJ, Lerner SA (1980) Aminoglycoside ototoxicity. Am J Otolaryng 1: 169–180.
34. Prahl S, Jepson PD, Sanchez-Hanke M, Deaville R, Sibert U (2010) Aspergillosis in the middle ear of a harbour porpoise (*Phocoena phocoena*): a case report. Mycoses, doi:10.1111/j.1439-0507.2010.01863.x pages 1-5.
35. Dobie RA, Wilson MJ (1996) A comparison of t test, F test, and coherence methods of detecting steady-state auditory evoked potentials, distortion-product otoacoustic emissions, or other sinusoids. J Acoust Soc Am 100: 2236–2246.

12

Inner Ear Morphology is Perturbed in Two Novel Mouse Models of Recessive Deafness

Kerry A. Miller[1]*, Louise H. Williams[1], Elizabeth Rose[2], Michael Kuiper[3], Hans-Henrik M. Dahl[1,4,5], Shehnaaz S. M. Manji[1,2,5]

1 Genetic Hearing Research, Murdoch Childrens Research Institute, Royal Children's Hospital, Melbourne, Victoria, Australia, **2** Department of Otolaryngology, University of Melbourne, Royal Victorian Eye and Ear Hospital, Melbourne, Victoria, Australia, **3** Victorian Life Sciences Computation Initiative, University of Melbourne, Melbourne, Victoria, Australia, **4** Department of Paediatrics, University of Melbourne, Melbourne, Victoria, Australia, **5** The HEARing CRC, Audiology, Hearing and Speech Sciences, University of Melbourne, Melbourne, Victoria, Australia

Abstract

Human *MYO7A* mutations can cause a variety of conditions involving the inner ear. These include dominant and recessive non-syndromic hearing loss and syndromic conditions such as Usher syndrome. Mouse models of deafness allow us to investigate functional pathways involved in normal and abnormal hearing processes. We present two novel mouse models with mutations in the *Myo7a* gene with distinct phenotypes. The mutation in $Myo7a^{I487N/I487N}$ *ewaso* is located within the head motor domain of Myo7a. Mice exhibit a profound hearing loss and manifest behaviour associated with a vestibular defect. A mutation located in the linker region between the coiled-coil and the first MyTH4 domains of the protein is responsible in $Myo7a^{F947I/F947I}$ *dumbo*. These mice show a less severe hearing loss than in $Myo7a^{I487N/I487N}$ *ewaso*; their hearing loss threshold is elevated at 4 weeks old, and progressively worsens with age. These mice show no obvious signs of vestibular dysfunction, although scanning electron microscopy reveals a mild phenotype in vestibular stereocilia bundles. The $Myo7a^{F947I/F947I}$ *dumbo* strain is therefore the first reported *Myo7a* mouse model without an overt vestibular phenotype; a possible model for human DFNB2 deafness. Understanding the molecular basis of these newly identified mutations will provide knowledge into the complex genetic pathways involved in the maintenance of hearing, and will provide insight into recessively inherited sensorineural hearing loss in humans.

Editor: Tiansen Li, National Eye Institute, United States of America

Funding: This work was supported by NHMRC grants #284550 and #436944, J. & J. Calvert-Jones and the Victorian Government's Operational Infrastructure Support (OIS) Program. The authors acknowledge the financial support from the HEARing CRC, established and supported under the Australian Government's Cooperative Research Centers Program. The funders had no role in study design, data collection and analysis, decision to publish, or preparation of the manuscript.

Competing Interests: The authors have declared that no competing interests exist.

* E-mail: kerry.miller@mcri.edu.au

Introduction

A fully functional auditory system is required by humans to communicate and to perceive the surrounding environment. Disruption of this system, and the closely associated vestibular system, can lead to severe impairments to an individual's hearing and balance, and can be attributed to genetic and/or environmental factors. A highly heterogeneous trait, hearing loss is the most prevalent congenital sensory defect, where 1 in 500 newborns suffer from a considerable hearing impairment [1]. A moderate to severe hearing impairment can have a significant impact on speech, language and general development, incurring lifelong social, educational and economic costs [2]. Hearing loss can also be associated with additional clinical abnormalities, as seen in Pendred and Usher syndromes [3–5]. However in 70% of cases inherited hearing loss is non-syndromic, presenting as the only clinical feature [1], and in 80% of these cases is inherited in an autosomal recessive mode [6].

The mammalian ear is a highly complex and diverse organ. This is reflected in the extreme heterogeneity of inherited deafness. To date, 70 autosomal recessive loci have been mapped and 40 genes identified (http://hereditaryhearingloss.org), but there may be as many as 200 genes that contribute to this condition [7]. Several members of the myosin gene family have been implicated in hearing loss, including *MYO7A*, where mutations in humans are responsible for causing non-syndromic dominant (DFNA11; [8,9]) and recessive (DFNB2; [10,11]) deafness and the deaf-blindness condition Usher Syndrome type 1B (USH1B; [12–14]). Therefore it is evident that different mutations in *MYO7A* lead to differing phenotypic outcomes. The myosin motor superfamily of proteins consists of more than 20 distinct classes that regulate many cellular processes including the regulation of actin filament tension and cargo transportation [15,16]. Myo7a is an unconventional myosin consisting of an N-terminal motor head domain that enables movement along actin filaments, and a neck and tail domain [1,15]. It has a relatively restricted pattern of expression, detected in the testis, retina, lung, kidney and hair cells of the inner ear [17–19]. Mutations in this gene are reported to cause structural defects of the protein and consequently, auditory dysfunction [20].

Mouse models of disease provide insights into complex mammalian developmental and genetic pathways [21]. As the mammalian cochlea is highly conserved across species, mouse models are often used in the identification of genes involved in hearing loss and in the study of auditory processes and clinical features of genetic deafness [22–25].

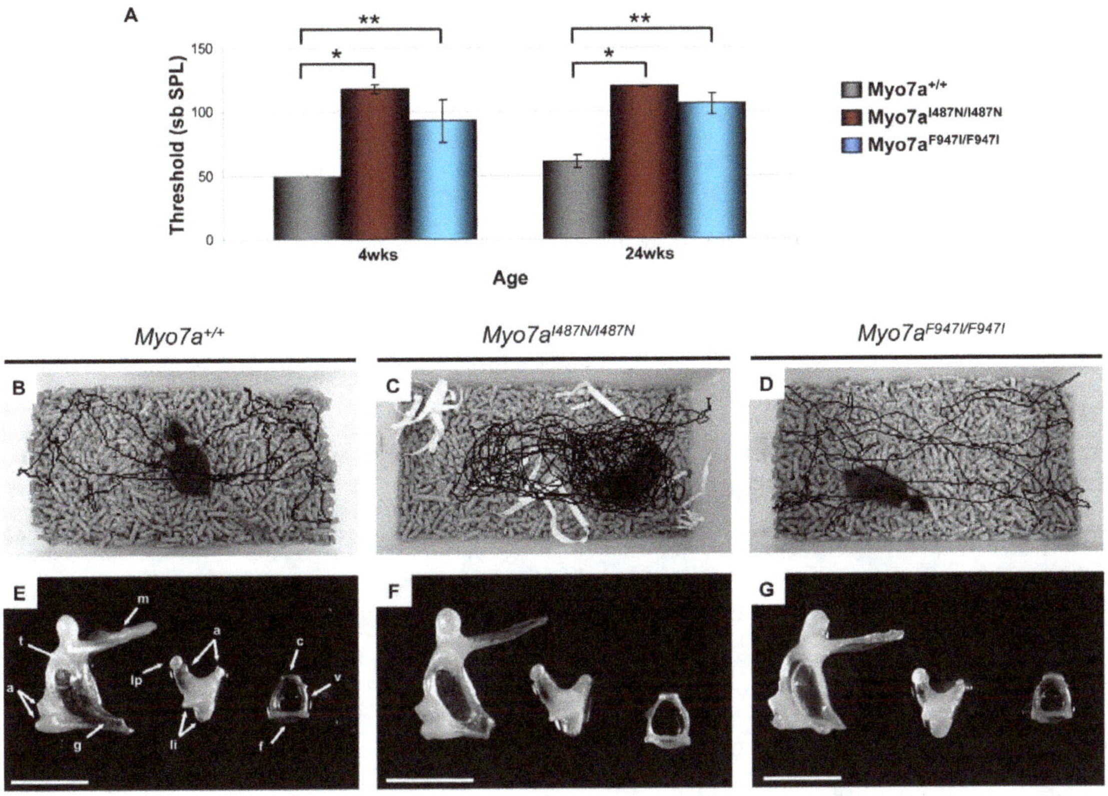

Figure 1. Phenotypic observations of *Myo7a* mutant strains. (**A**) Hearing profile of *Myo7a*$^{+/+}$, *Myo7a*$^{I487N/I487N}$ *ewaso* and *Myo7a*$^{F947I/F947I}$ *dumbo* strains at 4 weeks (*p = 2.2×10^{-25}, **p = 4.5×10^{-10}) and 24 weeks (*p = 3.7×10^{-29}, **p = 7.2×10^{-20}). (**B–G**) Video surveillance and middle ear morphology in *Myo7a* strains. Observations highlighted an increased number of turns in *Myo7a*$^{I487N/I487N}$ *ewaso* mice (**C**), when compared to wild-type (**B**). No such behaviour was seen in *Myo7a*$^{F947I/F947I}$ *dumbo* mutants (**D**). Middle ear bones appear largely normal in *Myo7a*$^{I487N/I487N}$ *ewaso* (**F**) and *Myo7a*$^{F947I/F947I}$ *dumbo* (**G**) mutants, comparable to normal morphology of the malleus, incus and stapes (**E**). M; manubrium of malleus, A; articulation surfaces of malleus and incus joint, T; tubercle, G; gonial angle, LI; attachment points of suspensory ligaments of incus, LP; lenticular process, C; capitulum of stapes, V; arched ventral crus, F; footplate. Scale bar; 1 mm (E–G).

The use of mutant mice generated using the alkylating agent *N*-ethyl-*N*-nitrosourea (ENU) has proven to be highly successful in the discovery and understanding of genes associated with human disease [26–28]. ENU randomly creates point mutations across the genome, meaning the observed phenotypes are likely to be a consequence of a single gene effect [29]. We undertook a comprehensive ENU mouse screen at the Australian Phenomics Facility (APF) to identify and characterise novel mouse models of recessively inherited hearing loss and present data on two novel mouse models of deafness with mutations in the *Myo7a* gene. Understanding the molecular basis of these individual mutations will provide insights into the complex genetic pathways involved in the development and maintenance of hearing.

Materials and Methods

Mice

Mice were screened for hearing loss in two independent screens from a large-scale ENU mutagenesis program at the APF, as described previously [25]. All mouse procedures were approved by the Royal Children's Hospital Animal Ethics Committee, RCH AEEC #A488 and #A585.

Hearing Tests and Phenotypic Observations

Mice were screened for hearing loss initially using a clickbox and subsequently by Auditory Brainstem Response (ABR), as previously described [25]. Specific auditory stimulus in the form of broadband clicks was delivered in a range of decibel sound pressure levels (50–120 dB SPL). Data were analysed using a non-paired T-test and analysis of variance. Behaviour associated with vestibular dysfunction was determined by circling and head tossing/star-gazing observations. Six month old *Myo7a*$^{I487N/I487N}$ *ewaso* and *Myo7a*$^{F947I/F947I}$ *dumbo* mutants were filmed for 1 minute and movements tracked with a computerised image analyzer (Image Pro Plus 6.1; Media Cybernetics Inc).

Mapping and Mutation Analysis

Affected *ewaso* mice were outcrossed to the CBA/H mapping strain and brother-sister progeny crossed to produce affected F2 offspring. Genomic DNA was isolated from tails of hearing and deaf littermates by Proteinase K digestion followed by phenol/chloroform extraction and used for homozygosity mapping and subsequent identification of candidate regions. DNA from 20 affected *ewaso* mice were analysed by genome wide scans using 120 microsatellite markers (AGRF, Australia), and mapping refined using an additional 45 mice with Amplifluor SNP arrays (APF). Deafness loci were mapped using methods described previously [25]. Using the UCSC genome browser [30] linkage intervals were examined for known or putative deafness genes and top candidate genes sequenced.

DNA from affected *dumbo* mice were screened for mutations in the known deafness genes *Tmc1* and *Myo7a*, by sequencing all exons, intron/exon boundaries and most of the 5′ and 3′ untranslated regions of these genes.

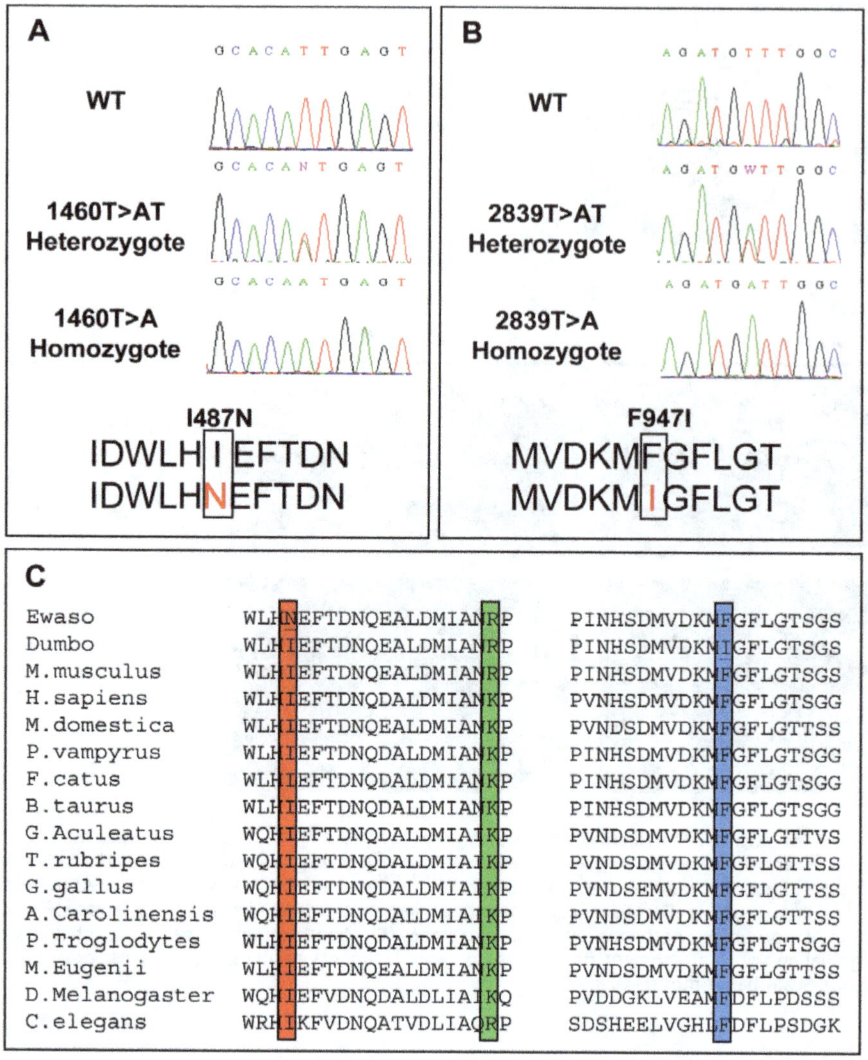

Figure 2. *Myo7a* mutations identified in *Myo7a*$^{I487N/I487N}$ *ewaso* and *Myo7a*$^{F947I/F947I}$ *dumbo* strains. (**A**) Direct sequencing identified a 1460T>A (I487N) missense mutation in *Myo7a*$^{I487N/I487N}$ *ewaso* and a missense mutation 2839T>A (F947I) in the *Myo7a*$^{F947I/F947I}$ *dumbo* mouse strain (**B**). Wildtype and heterozygote sequences are shown for comparison. (**C**) Sequence conservations of *Myo7a*$^{I487N/I487N}$ *ewaso* (red) and *Myo7a*$^{F947I/F947I}$ *dumbo* (blue) mutations, and the closely positioned *Myo7a*$^{sh-1}$ *shaker* mutation (green) showing high evolutionary conservation of our two mutant strains.

PCR, Sequencing and Genotyping

Gene-specific primers were designed for amplification of all 49 exons of the *Myo7a* gene (ENSMUST00000107127) and DNA amplified with HotStar Taq polymerase (Qiagen) or GoTaq® Flexi DNA Polymerase (Promega) using standard PCR cycling conditions with an annealing temperature of 58°C. PCR products were sequenced with a BigDye™ v3.1 Terminator Cycle Sequencing Kit (Applied Biosystems) and products read using an ABI 3130xl capillary genetic analyser (Applied Biosystems). Sequencing chromatograms were compared to the published gDNA sequence using Mutation Surveyor (v2.60) software and any differences identified and determined for potential pathogenicity using Polyphen and SIFT [31,32]. Conservation of Myo7a mutations were analysed using Clustal W [33]. *Myo7a* primer sequences are available on request.

Genomic DNA from all progeny of each strain was amplified as above. PCR primers were designed to disrupt or introduce a restriction enzyme site in the presence of the mutated nucleotide in each strain to produce a different pattern of DNA digestion for each genotype. Primer and enzyme information is detailed in Table S1.

Molecular Modeling of *Myo7a* mutations

To determine whether the *ewaso* p.I487N mutation compromises the structure or function of the Myo7a protein the ATP-bound myosin II structure (pdb entry: 1W9J) was compared to the inactive myosin V structural residues 1 to 780 (pdb entry: 2DFS; http://www.rcsb.org/pdb/home/home.do) to model the structural impact. Models were solvated in 72×96×160A box of water containing ~0.15 M NaCl and simulated for approximately 4 ns at 310K using NAMD molecular dynamics [34]. Molecular modeling images were generated using the VMD software package [35].

As the *dumbo* p.F947I residue is not contained within the 3D protein domain used for analysis of myosin II, and is outside the Myo7a tail crystal structure recently published [36], pathogenicity

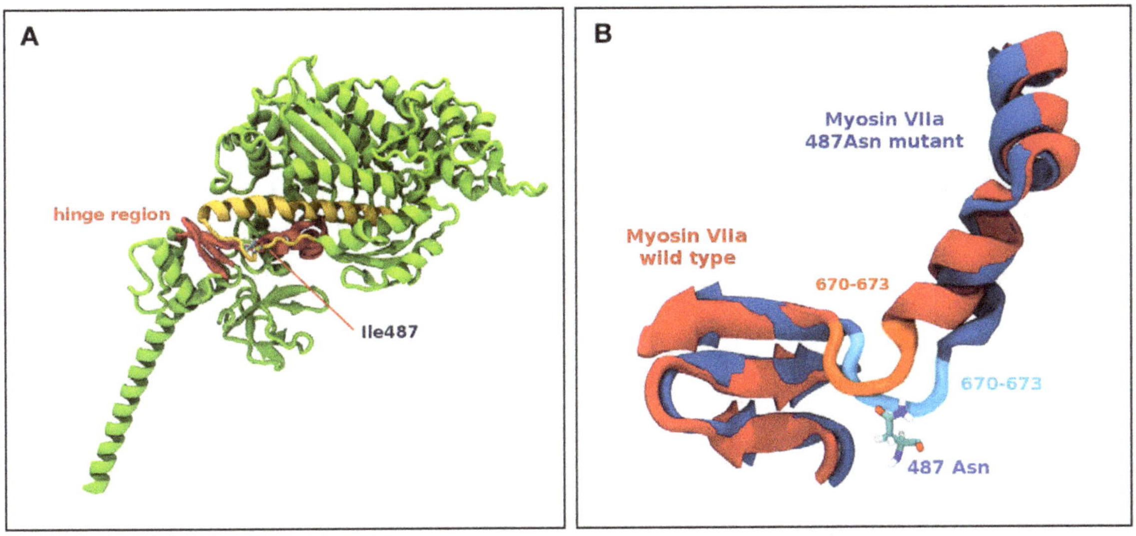

Figure 3. Molecular modelling of the *Myo7a*$^{I487N/I487N}$ *ewaso* mutation. (**A**) Partial ribbon representation of a 3D model of myosin V 2DFS highlighting the Ile^{487} amino acid residue, which is localised to the hinge region between the head and tail domains of the protein. (**B**) Schematic diagram showing superimposed images of the hinge region (*Myo7a*$^{+/+}$ in red and the *Myo7a*$^{I487N/I487N}$ *ewaso* mutation in blue) after 4 ns of molecular dynamics simulation showing a conformational change in the hinge region close to the Ile^{487} mutation site, showing the involvement of residues 670–673 around the hinge region causing the distortion.

of the *dumbo* p.F947I mutation was estimated using Polyphen (http://genetics.bwh.harvard.edu/pph/) where structural query options were set to default. A PSIC score of >2.0 identifies that that particular mutation was never or almost never observed in that protein family and would be classified as 'probably-damaging', scores of 1.5 to 2.0 classified as 'possibly damaging', and scores of <1.5 as 'benign'. A second algorithm, SIFT (http://sift.jcvi.org/) was also used to predict the effect of the *dumbo* p.F947I amino acid substitution on protein function. A SIFT BLink analysis was performed using Myo7a protein ID NP_032689.2.

Tissue Collection

Mice were anaesthetised with isoflurane and culled by cervical dislocation according to the National Health and Medical Research Council Australian code of practice for the care and use of animals for scientific purposes (RCH AEEC approval #A488, #A585). Adult mouse cochleae and postnatal day 5 (P5) cochlear sensory epithelia were dissected and processed as described [24,37,38]. Vestibular sensory epithelia were dissected from the vestibule of P2–P5 mice by removal of the otolithic membrane and otoconia to expose the sensory epithelium of the saccule or utricle maculae.

Ossicles were dissected from half heads of adult (20–28 week old) *Myo7a*$^{+/+}$, *Myo7a*$^{I487N/I487N}$ *ewaso* and *Myo7a*$^{F947I/F947I}$ *dumbo* mice. Briefly, the middle ear was exposed by dissection of the bulla and removal of the tympanic membrane, taking care not to damage the malleus underneath. The malleus, incus and stapes were removed from the middle ear with care, stored in PBS and photographed with a Leica DC200 camera (Leica Microsystems Ltd).

Hematoxylin and Eosin (H&E) Staining

Cochleae were isolated from 4, 8 and 12 week wild-type, heterozygous and homozygous mice for each strain and processed for H&E staining as described previously [25]. A standard H&E protocol was followed with a 4–5 min incubation in hematoxylin and 45 sec staining in eosin, and mounted with Entellan® (Merck) or Pertex (HD Scientific). Images were taken on a Nikon Eclipse 80i microscope (Pathtech).

Immunohistochemistry

P5 cochlear sensory epithelia were processed for immunohistochemistry as previously described [24] using a rabbit polyclonal anti-MyoVIIa primary antibody (1:900; Abcam), an Alexa Fluor® 594-conjugated goat anti rabbit IgG secondary antibody (1:2500; Molecular Probes) and Alexa Fluor® 488 phalloidin (1:250; Molecular Probes). Rabbit IgG (Invitrogen) was used as an isotype control.

Scanning Electron Microscopy (SEM)

Cochleae from P5, 2, 4 and 8 week old wild-type, heterozygous and homozygous mice from each strain were dissected, fixed and processed as previously described [24]. Vestibular sensory epithelia were dissected as above. Tissues were viewed using a Philips XL30 FE scanning electron microscope.

Results

Mice exhibit elevated hearing thresholds with or without vestibular dysfunction

Homozygous *Myo7a*$^{I487N/I487N}$ *ewaso* mice exhibit a profound hearing loss from 4 weeks of age (105–120 dB SPL; Figure 1A). Affected *Myo7a*$^{I487N/I487N}$ *ewaso* mice were identified as having a vestibular dysfunction concomitant with their hearing loss, by exhibiting hyperactivity that manifested as circling/star-gazing behaviour (Figure 1C) and displayed abnormal trunk curling behaviour. An increase in the hearing threshold of *Myo7a*$^{I487N/I487N}$ mice at 24 wks can be attributed to inherent age related hearing loss in the C57BL/6 strain. However, *Myo7a*$^{I487N/I487N}$ heterozygous mice have a statistically significant increase in hearing threshold at 24 wks of age compared to wild-type littermates, indicating semi-dominance in this strain (Figure S1A).

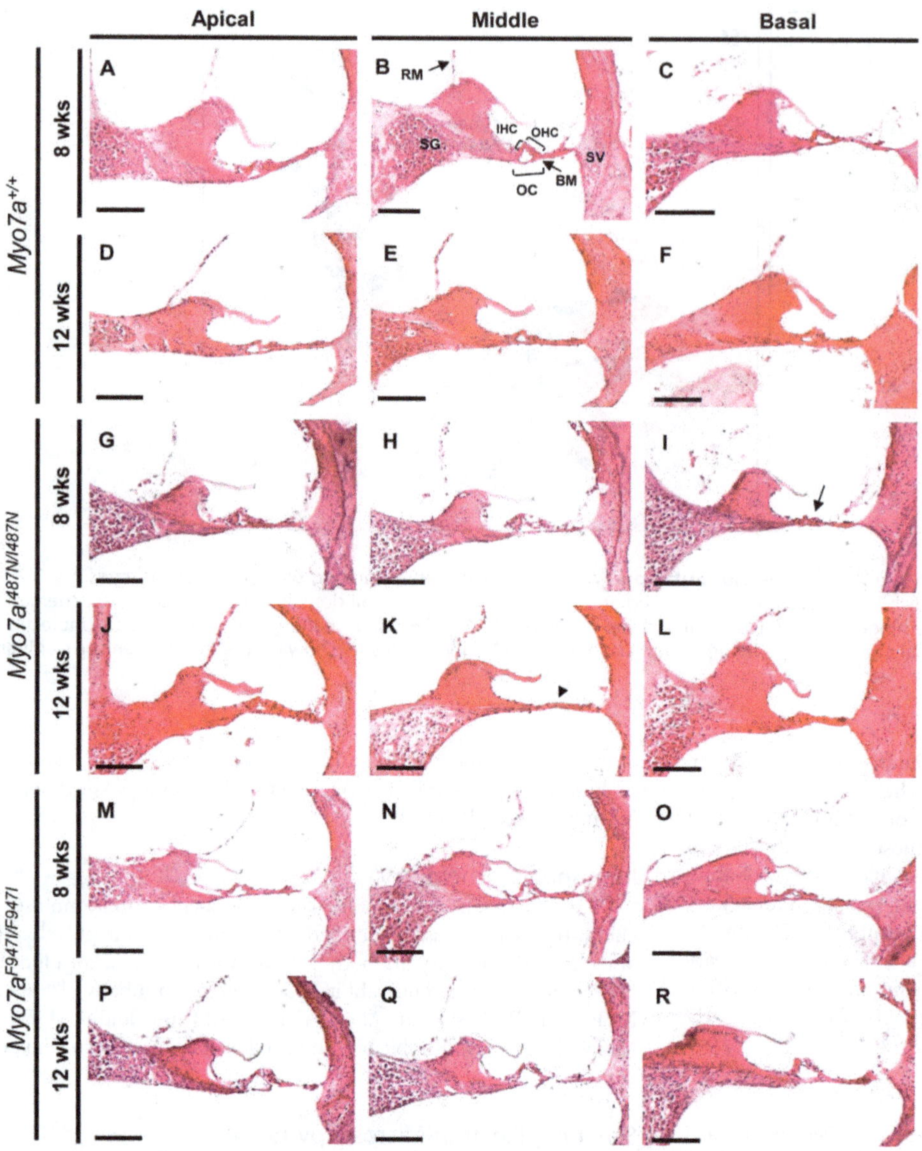

Figure 4. Haematoxylin and Eosin (H&E) staining of cochlear sections from *Myo7a* mutant strains at 8 and 12 weeks old. (**A–F**) $Myo7a^{+/+}$, (**G–L**) $Myo7a^{I487N/I487N}$ *ewaso* and (**M–R**) $Myo7a^{F947I/F947I}$ *dumbo* mice at the apical, middle and basal levels. Normal cochlear morphology shows an intact organ of Corti and the presence of a tunnel containing inner and outer hair cells and intact spiral ganglion and stria vascularis (**B**). Early signs of cochlea degeneration are evident in the basal region of $Myo7a^{I487N/I487N}$ *ewaso* mutant cochleae by 8 weeks of age (**I**), where the OC has collapsed (arrow in I). Complete lack of cellular architecture along the basilar membrane at the mid level is evident in this strain by 12 weeks (arrowhead in K). The cellular architecture in $Myo7a^{F947I/F947I}$ *dumbo* mutants is largely normal at both 8 and 12 weeks. In both mutant strains the the spiral ganglion and the stria vascularis were normal at 8 and 12 weeks of age. RM, Reisner's membrane; SG, spiral ganglion; OHC, outer hair cells; IHC, inner hair cells; OC, organ of Corti; BM, basilar membrane; SV, stria vascularis. Scale bar; 100 µM.

In $Myo7a^{F947I/F947I}$ *dumbo*, homozygote mice have a severe progressive hearing loss, with thresholds of 70–110 dB SPL at 4 weeks of age, reaching 95–110 dB SPL by 12 weeks (Figure 1A and S2), however these mice still retain some residual hearing at 24 weeks (90–110dB SPL; Figure 1A). Consistent with inherent age-related hearing loss in the C57BL/6 strain, wild-type and heterozygote mice also show an elevated hearing threshold by 24 weeks (Figure S1B). The behaviour in homozygous $Myo7a^{F947I/F947I}$ *dumbo* mutants is consistent with a normal vestibular phenotype (Figure 1D).

Middle ear defects can also be associated with elevated ABR thresholds so to determine whether the hearing loss in $Myo7a^{I487N/I487N}$ *ewaso* and $Myo7a^{F947I/F947I}$ *dumbo* mutants was due to a disruption in conductance through the middle ear we examined these structures. In both $Myo7a^{I487N/I487N}$ *ewaso* and $Myo7a^{F947I/F947I}$ *dumbo* mutant mice there was no evidence of infection and the tympanic membrane and bulla were normal. Detailed examination of the ossicles did not highlight any structural differences of the malleus, incus or stapes in $Myo7a^{I487N/I487N}$ *ewaso* (Figure 1F) and $Myo7a^{F947I/F947I}$ *dumbo* (Figure 1G) mutants when compared to wild-type ossicles (Figure 1E). These findings all support a sensoreneural hearing loss in both $Myo7a^{I487N/I487N}$ *ewaso* and $Myo7a^{F947I/F947I}$ *dumbo* mutants.

A *Myo7a* mutation is responsible for hearing loss in *ewaso* and *dumbo* mice

The deafness locus in $Myo7a^{I487N/I487N}$ *ewaso* was localised to a 7Mb region on mouse chromosome 7 by genome-wide homozy-

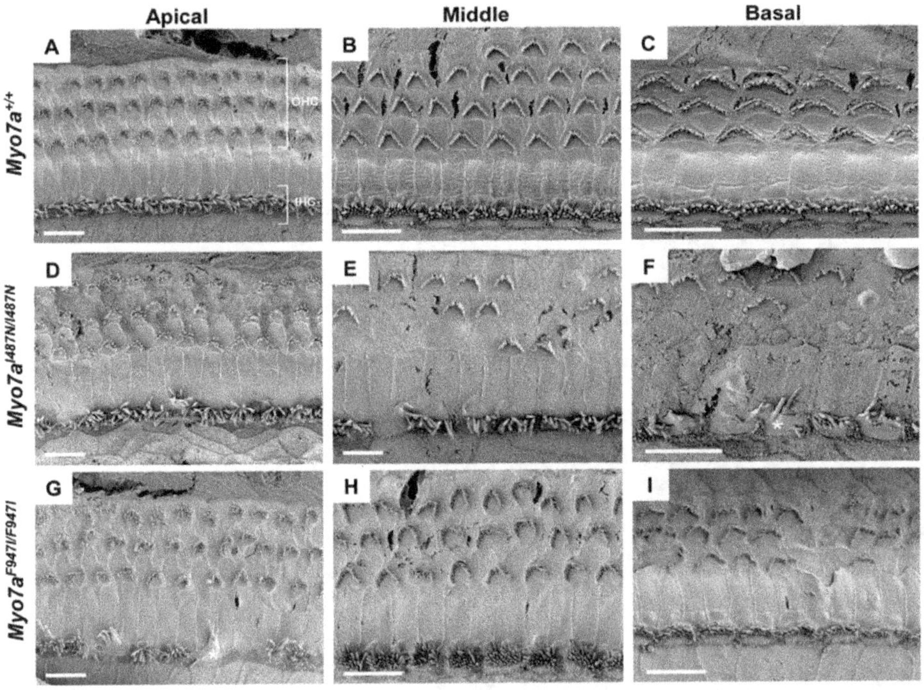

Figure 5. Scanning electron micrographs of cochlear sensory epithelium from *Myo7a* mutant strains at 8 weeks old. (**A–C**) *Myo7a*$^{+/+}$, (**D–F**) *Myo7a*$^{I487N/I487N}$ *ewaso* and (**G–I**) *Myo7a*$^{F947I/F947I}$ *dumbo* mice at the apical, middle and basal cochlear level. Signs of degeneration and/or mis-orientation of OHC bundles is evident in both *Myo7a*$^{I487N/I487N}$ *ewaso* (**D–F**) and *Myo7a*$^{F947I/F947I}$ *dumbo* (**G–I**) mice at all levels of the cochlea. This appears to be more severe in *Myo7a*$^{I487N/I487N}$ *ewaso* mutants, where many bundles are missing in the mid and basal regions (**E and F**). IHC bundles are also affected, appearing disorganised and/or showing signs of fusion in the basal levels of *Myo7a*$^{I487N/I487N}$ *ewaso* cochleae (asterisk in F), and conversely in the apical region of *Myo7a*$^{F947I/F947I}$ *dumbo* mutants (asterisk in G). Scale bar; 10 μM (A–I).

gosity and fine mapping. The critical region was analyzed for known genes using multiple genome browsers (NCBI, http://www.ncbi.nlm.nih.gov; Ensembl, http://www.ensembl.org and UCSC, http://www.genome.ucsc.edu). This region contained the known deafness gene *Myo7a*. Direct sequencing of *Myo7a* revealed a novel T to A transversion at nucleotide position 1460 in exon 13, introducing an Ile to Asn substitution at position 487 in the protein (Figure 2A).

Sequencing of the *Myo7a* gene in *Myo7a*$^{F947I/F947I}$ *dumbo* mice revealed a novel T to A change at nucleotide position 2839 in exon 23 that results in a Phe to Ile amino acid change at position 947 (Figure 2B).

Alignment of Myo7a protein sequences from 14 species identify that the amino acid residues affected by *Myo7a*$^{I487N/I487N}$ *ewaso* and *Myo7a*$^{F947I/F947I}$ *dumbo* mutations are highly conserved across evolution (Figure 2C). The causative mutation identified in these strains segregates with the deafness phenotype in all mice tested (n = 187/187 and 68/68, respectively).

In silico Analysis indicates *Myo7a* mutations impair protein function

The effect of the *ewaso* Myo7a p.I487N mutation on protein structure and function was evaluated using molecular modeling of wild-type and mutant Myo7a head domains, performed based on the 2DFS myosin V structure as a template of amino acid residues 1 to 780 (Figure 3A). A comparative dynamics study between the wild type and mutant form indicates a bulge region between residues 668 and 773 is destabilized by the presence of the Asn^{487} mutation. The mutant Asn^{487} residue is positioned to form hydrogen bonds with the protein backbone and also to Tyr^{477}. Interaction of the mutant Asn^{487} with Tyr^{477} also appears to interfere with salt bridging interactions between Glu^{473}, Arg^{675} and Arg^{668}. Molecular modeling analysis predicts that the *ewaso* Myo7a p.I487N mutation induces a conformational change in the hinge region (amino acids 670–673) of the motor head domain that severely compromises the 'power stroke" action of the protein.

Prediction output from PolyPhen for the *dumbo* Myo7a p.F947I mutation indicates a 'probably damaging' effect of the mutation on protein function, with a PSIC score of 2.001. SIFT prediction output denotes that both *ewaso* Myo7a p.I487N and *dumbo* Myo7a p.947I amino acid changes are 'not tolerated'.

Hair cell structure and stereocilia morphology are abnormal in *Myo7a* mutant strains

No visible structural changes were identified on gross examination of the outer and middle ear structures (Figure 1B–G). Structural integrity of the inner ears was examined in H&E stained cochlear sections from 8 and 12 week old *Myo7a*$^{I487N/I487N}$ *ewaso* and *Myo7a*$^{F947I/F947I}$ *dumbo* revealing morphological differences in *Myo7a*$^{I487N/I487N}$ *ewaso*, but not *Myo7a*$^{F947I/F947I}$ *dumbo* mutants. Hair cell degeneration was observed in *Myo7a*$^{I487N/I487N}$ *ewaso* mice at the basal cochlear region by 8 weeks of age (Figure 4I), evident by collapse of the organ of Corti. This becomes more pronounced by 12 weeks of age, where no cellular architecture is apparent at the mid cochlear level due to a lack of sensory or supporting cells in these mice (Figure 4K). In contrast, the sensory epithelium in *Myo7a*$^{F947I/F947I}$ *dumbo* shows normal morphology (Figure 4M–R). No degeneration of the spiral ganglion or stria vascularis is evident in either strain.

Sensory organs of the cochlear and vestibular system were analysed by SEM. Examination of cochlear sensory epithelium in *Myo7a*$^{I487N/I487N}$ *ewaso* showed mostly normal V-shaped outer hair

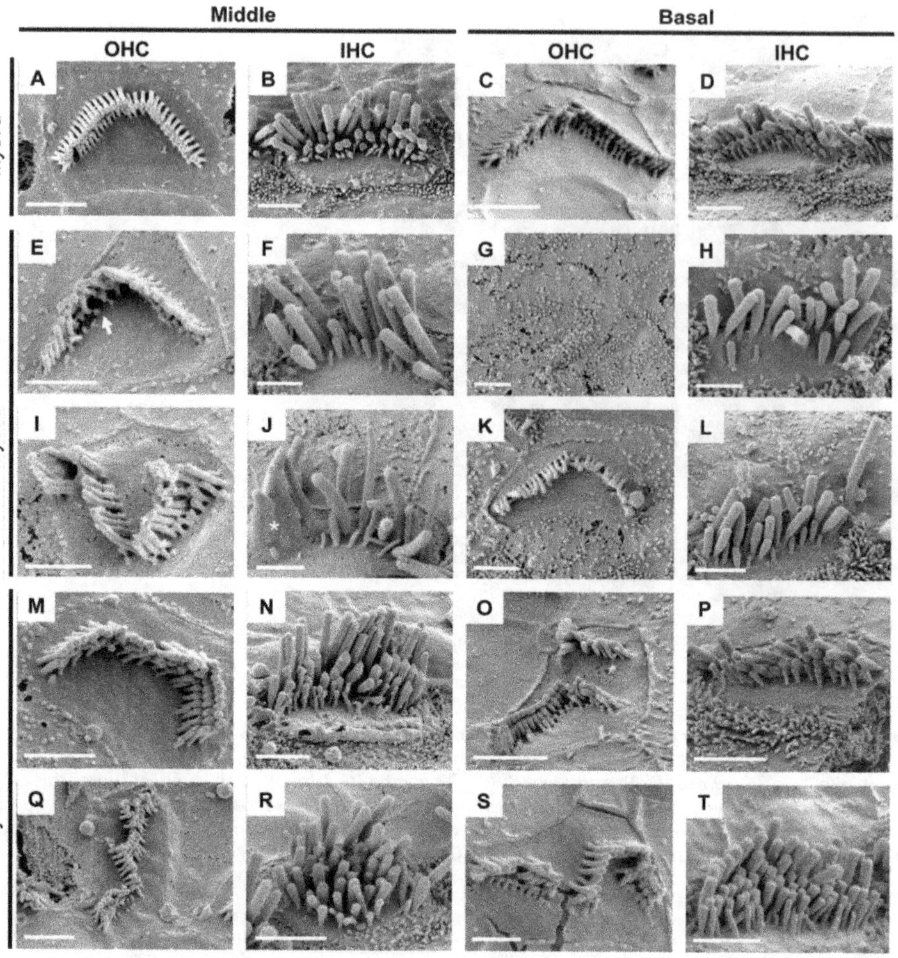

Figure 6. Scanning electron micrographs of inner (IHC) and outer (OHC) hair cells from 8 week old mice. (**A–D**) *Myo7a*$^{+/+}$, (**E–L**) *Myo7a*$^{I487N/I487N}$ *ewaso* and (**M–T**) *Myo7a*$^{F947I/F947I}$ *dumbo* mice at the middle and basal cochlear level. OHC bundles of *Myo7a*$^{I487N/I487N}$ *ewaso* mutants appear to have a regular V shaped array, however are missing the majority of their inner-row stereocilia at the middle level (arrow head in E). This is more severe at the basal level where many OHC bundles are missing (**G**). This phenotype is more severe in *Myo7a*$^{F947I/F947I}$ *dumbo* mutants, where OHC bundles are disoriented, forming an array of OHC-type bundles (**M, Q, O and S**). Many *Myo7a*$^{I487N/I487N}$ *ewaso* IHC bundles are affected at this age, with less numbers of stereocilia within the bundle and those remaining often showing signs of fusion (asterisk in J). The IHC bundles in *Myo7a*$^{F947I/F947I}$ *dumbo* contain additional rows of stereocilia, however do still maintain a staircase-like structure (**N, R, P and T**). Scale bar; 2 µM.

cell (OHC) bundles at P5, although the occasional OHC was misorientated (Figure S3). Some inner hair cell (IHC) bundles showed abnormal morphology at the basal level at this age. At 2wks of age, IHC bundles at the mid and basal levels of the cochlea begin to show signs of disorganisation and/or fusion, and a few OHC bundles are misorientated, predominantly at the basal level (Figure S4). As this strain ages, the progression of abnormal stereocilia bundle morphology becomes evident. From 4 to 8 weeks increasingly more OHC bundles are affected, showing signs of degeneration of whole OHC bundles, as well as within bundles (Figures 5D–F, 6G, I and Figure S5). By 8 weeks large numbers of OHC bundles are missing at the basal and mid levels of the cochlea (Figure 5E and F). IHC bundles also show a progressive degeneration, with many appearing disorganised, comprising fused and often elongated stereocilia (Figure 5F and 6J).

In contrast to that seen in the *Myo7a*$^{I487N/I487N}$ *ewaso* strain, *Myo7a*$^{F947I/F947I}$ *dumbo* hair bundles appear to be more affected at the apical level of the cochlea. As early as P5, a number of OHC bundles are misorientated, however a few bundles also appear to be affected at the mid and basal levels (Figure S3). IHC begin to show abnormal structure by 2 weeks of age at the apical level and more OHC are misorientated at all levels of the cochlea (Figure S4). In addition to the progressive degeneration of IHC bundles, closer inspection of these bundles revealed the presence of additional rows of stereocilia (Figure 6N, R and T). OHC bundles become more severely misorientated with advancing age and some appear disintegrated in parts, forming individual 'bundles' (Figure 6O and S), At 8 weeks of age, the sensory epithelium of *Myo7a*$^{F947I/F947I}$ *dumbo* mice shows minimal degeneration as a whole, as large numbers of OHC bundles are still present (Figure 5G–I).

Vestibular sensory epithelia were examined by SEM in *Myo7a*$^{I487N/I487N}$ *ewaso* mice to determine the sensory organ morphology/defect underlying the circling/star-gazing behaviour in these mice. Normal saccular maculae consist of hair cells arranged in a particular orientation, such that on either side of the midline (striola) of the saccule, the hair cells (and stereocilia bundle) show opposite polarity (Figure 7A). These vestibular hair bundles contain several rows of stereocilia, arranged in a staircase orientation, with the longer stereocilia situated on the kinocilium side (Figure 7B and C). In *Myo7a*$^{I487N/I487N}$ *ewaso* mutant mice, hair bundles are highly irregular, with rows of stereocilia missing

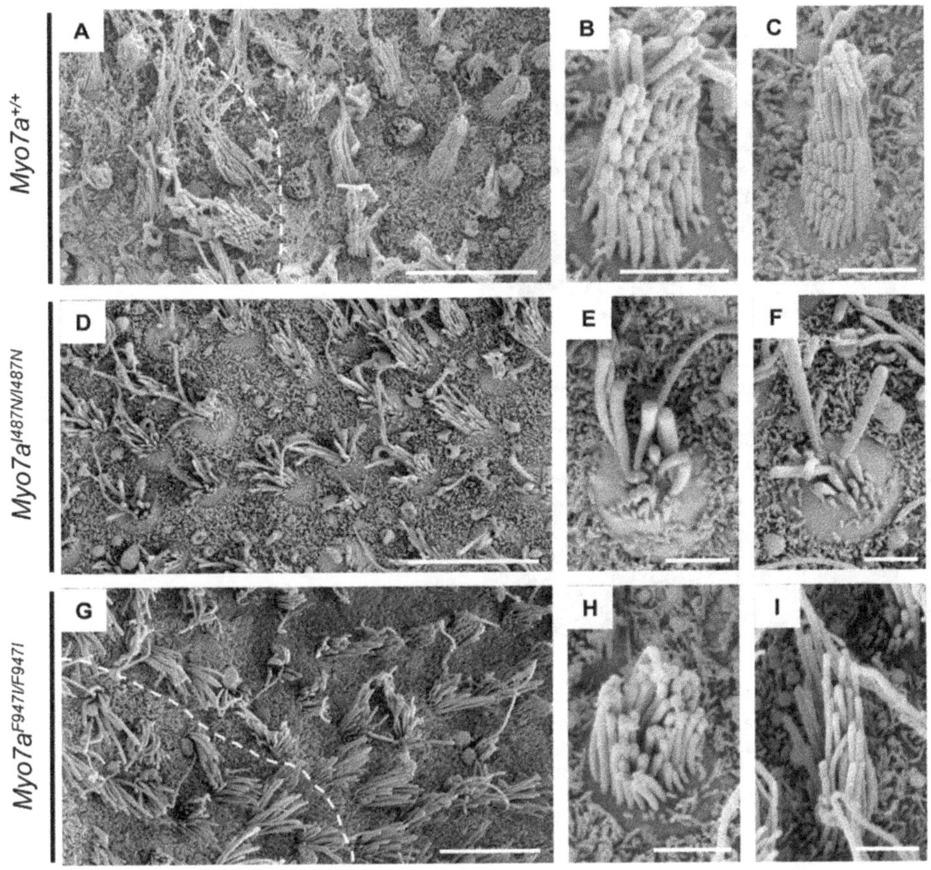

Figure 7. Scanning electron micrographs of P2–5 vestibular epithelia. (**A–C and J**) *Myo7a*$^{+/+}$, (**D–F and K**) *Myo7a*$^{I487N/I487N}$ *ewaso* and (**G–I and L**) *Myo7a*$^{F947I/F947I}$ *dumbo*. A clear line of polarity reversal can be identified in *Myo7a*$^{+/+}$ saccular maculae (**A; dashed line**), and normal hair bundle morphology is apparent, with a staircase arrangement of stereocilia and kinocilium located with the tallest stereocilia (**B and C**). Hair cell bundles are affected in *Myo7a*$^{I487N/I487N}$ *ewaso* saccules, and no clear zone of polarity is evident (**D**). These bundles do contain stereocilia of various lengths, however are generally disorientated and unstructured (**E and F**). A zone of polarity can be identified in *Myo7a*$^{F947I/F947I}$ *dumbo* saccules (**G**), however hair bundles do appear to have a mild phenotype, with bundles missing some of the tallest (**H**) and/or shortest stereocilia (**I**). Scale bar; 10 µM (A, D and G), 2 µM (B, C, E, F, H and I).

and the staircase morphology disrupted (Figure 7E and F). The distorted hair bundles make identification of the zone of polarity reversal difficult in these mice (Figure 7D).

Vestibular sensory epithelia were also examined in *Myo7a*$^{F947I/F947I}$ *dumbo* mutants, despite there being no overt vestibular phenotype evident in these mice. Saccular hair bundles in these mice appear largely normal, with an obvious staircase arrangement, however some of the tallest or shortest stereocilia are missing in some bundles (Figure 7H and I). The zone of polarity reversal however, is evident in *Myo7a*$^{F947I/F947I}$ *dumbo* mutants (Figure 7G).

Myo7a protein expression in *Myo7a* mutant strains

The effect of *Myo7a*$^{I487N/I487N}$ *ewaso* and *Myo7a*$^{F947I/F947I}$ *dumbo* mutations on Myo7a protein expression was examined by immunofluorescence in P5 cochlear sensory epithelium. Myo7a protein localization was confirmed by confocal microscopy in the cytoplasm of inner and outer hair cells (Figure 8B). Reduced levels of Myo7a protein were observed in *Myo7a*$^{F947I/F947I}$ *dumbo* sensory epithelium (Figure 8F), but levels of expression in *Myo7a*$^{I487N/I487N}$ *ewaso* tissue appear to be undetectable, comparable to that seen in tissue incubated with an isotype control (Figure 8D and H).

Discussion

It is well understood that mutations in the *MYO7A* gene can underlie certain forms of syndromic and non-syndromic deafness in the human population, specifically non-syndromic dominant (DFNA11) and recessive (DFNB2) deafness and Usher Syndrome type 1B (USH1B). Myosin VIIA was the first gene identified as a contributing factor to hearing loss in a genetic screen of mutations that lead to inner ear defects in the mouse [39], and until now 9 mouse models with mutations in the *Myo7a* gene have been published [19,39–41]. We report two additional mouse models of deafness with novel mutations in the *Myo7a* gene, identified through an ENU mutagenesis screen. *Myo7a*$^{I487N/I487N}$ *ewaso* mutant mice have a profound hearing loss with vestibular dysfunction due to a missense mutation affecting Ile residue 487, located in the motor head domain of the protein. The mutation identified in *Myo7a*$^{F947I/F947I}$ *dumbo* results in a severe and progressive hearing loss but mice do not exhibit behaviour associated with a vestibular defect. This mutation lies in a linker region between the CC1 (coiled-coil) and first MyTH4 domains of the protein, the first reported in mice outside a functional/structural domain of the Myo7a protein.

The mouse Myo7a protein consists of a 729 aa N-terminal head domain, followed by a tail domain containing five light-chain

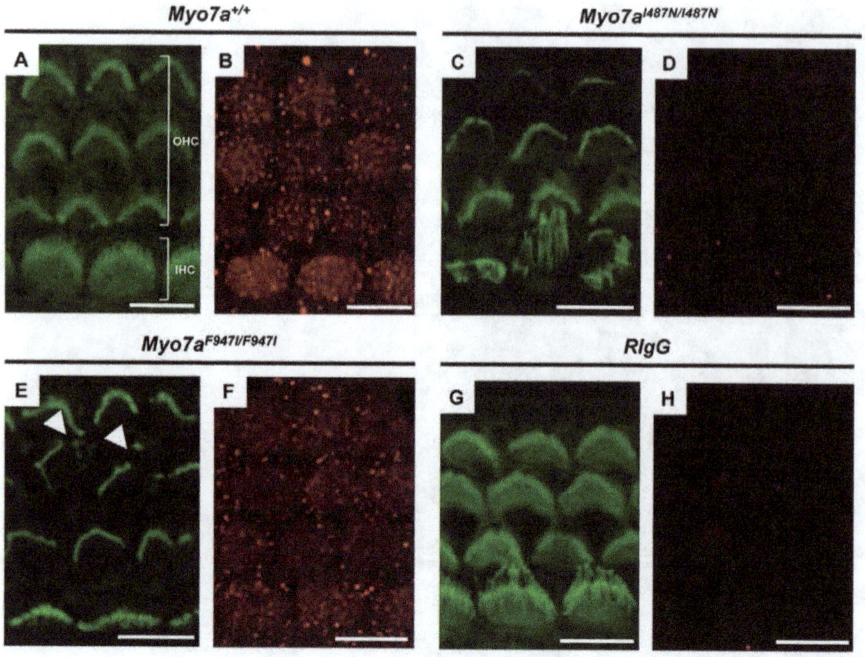

Figure 8. Immunohistochemistry of P5 sensory epithelia. Images of phalloidin (green) and Myo7a (red) stained cochlear sensory epithelium from P5 *Myo7a*$^{+/+}$ (**A and B**), *Myo7a*$^{I487N/I487N}$ *ewaso* (**C and D**) and *Myo7a*$^{F947I/F947I}$ *dumbo* (**E and F**) mice at the basal cochlear level. No Myo7a expression is evident in *Myo7a*$^{I487N/I487N}$ *ewaso* mutant tissue (**D**), and may be slightly reduced in *Myo7a*$^{F947I/F947I}$ *dumbo* mutants (**F**). No difference in protein localisation was observed between wilt-type and *Myo7a*$^{F947I/F947I}$ *dumbo* tissue. Phalloidin staining highlights abnormal IHC structure in *Myo7a*$^{I487N/I487N}$ *ewaso* mutants (**C**) and OHC hair bundles appear misorientated and/or fragmented in *Myo7a*$^{F947I/F947I}$ *dumbo* (arrowheads in E). Scale bar; 8 μM (A–H).

binding IQ (isoleucine-glutamine) motifs, a predicted coiled-coil region (CC1) and two MyTH4-FERM repeats separated by an Src homology 3 domain (SH3; Figure 9, [42]). The head domain binds filamentous actin and undergoes a conformational change upon the hydrolysis of ATP, allowing it to "walk" along the actin structure and provide intracellular forces [43]. Previously reported *Myo7a* mouse models show a spectrum of phenotypes and mutations have been located across the protein (Figure 9, Table 1). The location and severity of these mutations correlate to the particular phenotype in each strain.

Our mouse models, *Myo7a*$^{I487N/I487N}$ *ewaso* and *Myo7a*$^{F947I/F947I}$ *dumbo*, show a variety of features identified in previously reported *Myo7a* strains. The phenotype observed in *Myo7a*$^{I487N/I487N}$ *ewaso* reflects the severity of the highly conserved motor head domain mutation. Degeneration of OHC stereocilia in *Myo7a*$^{I487N/I487N}$ *ewaso* at the mid to basal level of the cochlea is likely to be a consequence of the non-functional Myo7a protein. Molecular modeling data predicts that the *Myo7a*$^{I487N/I487N}$ *ewaso* mutation affects the structure of the hinge region in the motor head domain in such a way that it severely compromises the 'power stroke' action of the protein. These mice also exhibit a severe vestibular phenotype supporting a major role of the motor head domain in Myo7a protein function. Hair cells of the vestibular sensory epithelium are severely disrupted, showing highly irregular

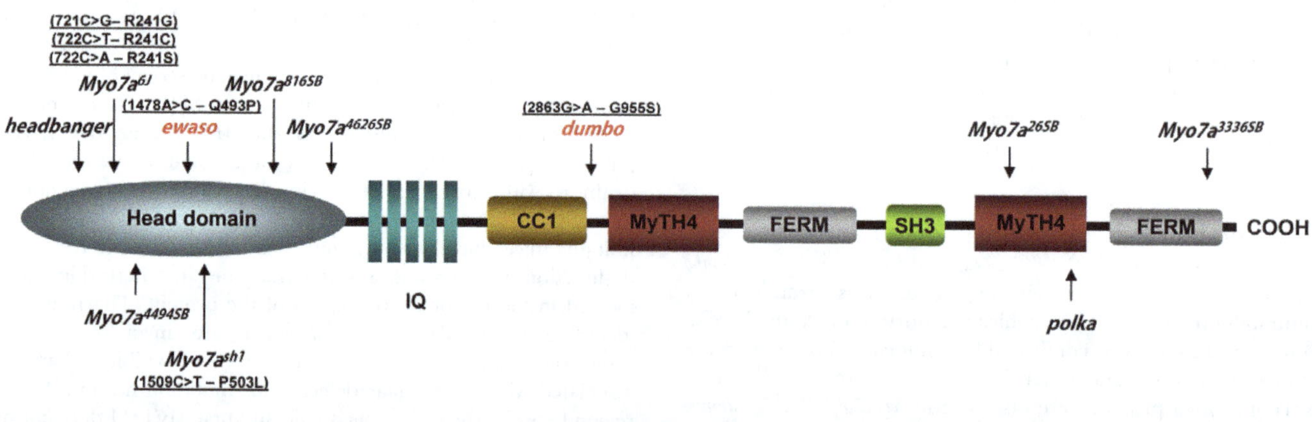

Figure 9. Schematic diagram of Myo7a protein structure showing the location of *Myo7a*$^{I487N/I487N}$ *ewaso* and *Myo7a*$^{F947I/F947I}$ *dumbo* mutations (in red) in relation to reported *shaker* mutations. DFNA11/DFNB2/USH1B human mutations within close proximity to a reported *shaker* mutation are shown in parentheses [14,56,57]. Details of these mouse mutations are included in Table 1. IQ, isoleucine-glutamine motif; CC1, Coiled Coil domain; MyTH4, Myosin Tail Homology 4; SH3, SRC Homology 3 domain.

Table 1. Reported *Myo7a* mouse models.

Mouse Model	*Nucleotide change*	*Protein change*	*Exon*	*Phenotype*	*Affected domain*	*Reference*
ewaso	c.1460T>A	p.I487N	13	USB1B	head domain	This study
dumbo	c.2839T>A	p.F947I	23	DFNB2	linker region	This study
headbanger	c.531A>T	p.I178F	6	USB1B	head domain	[41]
$Myo7a^{4494SB}$	c.592+2T>A	Truncation	In 6–7	USB1B	head domain	[40]
$Myo7a^{6J}$	c.722G>C	p.R241P	7	USB1B	head domain	[39]
$Myo7a^{sh1}$	c.1505G>C	p.R502P	13	USB1B	head domain	[39]
$Myo7a^{816SB}$	c.1934-2A>G	Deletion of α-helix	In 16–17	USB1B	head domain	[39]
$Myo7a^{4626SB}$	c.2158C>T	p.Q720X	18	USB1B	head domain	[40]
$Myo7a^{26SB}$	c.5284T>A	p.F1762I	39	USB1B	MyTH4 2 domain	[40]
polka	c.5472+5G>A	Truncation	In 42–43	USB1B	MyTH4 2 domain	[19]
$Myo7a^{3336SB}$	c.6432T>A	p.C2144X	48	USB1B	FERM domain	[40]

staircase morphology and disruption of polarity, thereby disturbing normal linear and angular acceleration and affecting responses required for balance. This would indicate that stability and function of the mutant protein in the inner ear is severely affected in this strain.

$Myo7a^{F947I/F947I}$ *dumbo* mutants have a less severe phenotype than seen in previously reported tail mutation strains $Myo7a^{26SB}$, $Myo7a^{3336SB}$ and *polka* [19,40]. These mice exhibit similarly disrupted morphology of the cochlear hair cells, although to a lesser degree. In the cochlea, the vibration of the basilar membrane in response to transmitted sound peaks at a location dependent on the sound frequency [42]. The apical to basal severity in $Myo7a^{F947I/F947I}$ *dumbo* cochlea is most similar to that seen in *headbanger* homozygotes, and suggests residual hearing is maintained at higher frequencies (detected in the basal cochlear region) [41]. The mildly affected structure of vestibular hair bundles does not appear to influence balance in $Myo7a^{F947I/F947I}$ *dumbo* mutants as no vestibular behaviour was observed using the methods described. This is the first such *Myo7a* mouse mutant not to exhibit such behaviour and may indicate the existence of an undetected or subtle vestibular phenotype in human patients with hearing loss that do not exhibit an obvious balance defect. It is also worth noting however, that some DFNB2 patients do exhibit some vestibular dysfunction [44]. The $Myo7a^{F947I/F947I}$ *dumbo* mutation affects a highly conserved amino acid, and analysis by Polyphen and SIFT indicates a severe effect. This suggests that Myo7a may be compromised in its motor function due to disruption of the interactions that the Ile residue normally forms. Located several amino acids upstream of the MFS domain (MyTH4-FERM-SH3) it is likely to cause misfolding of the protein, therefore disrupting the Y-shaped architecture of this domain that in turn will disrupt the ability of Myo7a to interact with its scaffold protein sans [36], or in homodimer assembly [1]. It has been observed that in a sans mouse model of hearing loss stereocilia bundles also show a disrupted morphology, suggesting an interaction with Myo7a [45–47]. Data from $Myo7a^{F947I/F947I}$ *dumbo* mice may also indicate that a direct interaction with an unknown protein found only in the auditory system is disrupted in these mice.

Myo7a is evidently required, either directly or indirectly, for maintaining the normal arrangement of stereocilia, and for hair bundle positioning at the top of the hair cell. In all *Myo7a* mouse models an abnormal array is seen across all levels of the cochlea and hair cell polarity defects are observed in many. In the inner ear, Myo7a is involved in transduction and adaption processes in the hair cells [48], controlling hair bundle organization, morphogenesis and polarity [49,50], as well as in the elongation of stereocilia [51]. Our mouse models support this evidence as both $Myo7a^{I487N/I487N}$ *ewaso* and $Myo7a^{F947I/F947I}$ *dumbo* mutants exhibit defects that can be attributed to each of these processes. Protein function and/or interactions appear to be disrupted, thereby affecting signal transduction processes. This may be due to limitations in the physical positioning of hair bundles, or restricted bundle movement in response to external signals. Abnormal development of the hair cell bundle is possibly due to aberrant interactions with harmonin b and cadherin 23, required for development of a coherent structure [49]. Stereocilia reabsorption and abnormal array pattern is likely related to the detachment of individual stereocilia from the bundle via abnormal cross- or tip-links, where Myo7a is thought to play a role [48].

Human Usher syndrome is a dual sensory deficit disorder involving both the audiovestibular and visual systems [52] and in many cases a mutation in *MYO7A* will result in an Usher phenotype: congenital sensorineural hearing loss and retinitis pigmentosa identified by progressive loss of vision [52]. Many of these disease-causing mutations are located within the motor head domain of the protein, and the $Myo7a^{I487N/I487N}$ *ewaso* mutant represents a model for this condition. Analysis of visual acuity and retinal histology in $Myo7a^{I487N/I487N}$ *ewaso* and $Myo7a^{F947I/F947I}$ *dumbo* mutant mice did not indicate any retinal phenotype (Miller et al, unpublished data). The lack of an eye phenotype is consistent with that seen in previously reported *Myo7a* mouse models, and several theories have been proposed to explain this observation such as alternative splicing and functional redundancy [53,54]. However, a 9bp deletion in the coiled-coil domain in humans results in a moderate, progressive, non-syndromic hearing loss, a phenotype reflected in our $Myo7a^{F947I/F947I}$ *dumbo* mutants that carry a mutation located just downstream of this domain [55].

The relationship between a particular mutation and its resulting phenotype is particularly important for improving our understanding of the molecular mechanisms involved in normal hearing, and is a pre-requisite for identifying possible therapeutic targets for sufferers of hearing loss. This requires the availability of mouse models with a range of mutations in a particular gene that recapitulate characteristics seen in humans. These two novel mouse models will facilitate the process of delineating the interactions, molecules and pathways involved in hearing loss. Our $Myo7a^{F947I/F947I}$ *dumbo* strain is of particular interest, as it is the first characterised *Myo7a* mouse model without a vestibular dysfunction, and therefore the first for DFNB2.

Supporting Information

Figure S1 Hearing profile of 4 and 24 wk (**A**) *Myo7a*$^{+/+}$ (n = 16, n = 13), *Myo7a*$^{I487N/+}$ *ewaso* (n = 16, n = 22), *Myo7a*$^{I487N/I487N}$ *ewaso* (n = 13, n = 18) and (**B**) *Myo7a*$^{+/+}$, *Myo7a*$^{F947I/+}$ *dumbo* (n = 13, n = 14) and *Myo7a*$^{F947I/F947I}$ *dumbo* (n = 12, n = 25) mice at 24 weeks of age.*p = 9.8×10^{-12}.

Figure S2 Hearing profile of *Myo7a*$^{F947I/F947I}$ *dumbo* strain from 4 to 24 weeks of age. 4wk (n = 12), 8wk (n = 17), 12wk (n = 24), 24wk (n = 25). *p = 7.2×10^{-20}.

Figure S3 SEM analysis of P5 cochlear sensory epithelium from Myo7a mutant strains. Apical, middle and basal cochlear turns were examined in Myo7a$^{+/+}$ (A, B and C), Myo7a$^{I487N/I487N}$ (D, E and F) and Myo7a$^{F947I/F947I}$ (G, H and I) mice at P5. OHC, outer hair cells; IHC, inner hair cells. Stereocilia on the occasional OHC appear to be misorientated in *Myo7a*$^{I487N/I487N}$ *ewaso* mice at this age (asterix in D), and more commonly in *Myo7a*$^{F947I/F947I}$ *dumbo* mutants. Scale bar; 5 μM.

Figure S4 SEM analysis of 2 week old cochlear sensory epithelium from Myo7a mutant strains. Apical, middle and basal cochlear turns were examined in *Myo7a*$^{+/+}$ (A, B and C), *Myo7a*$^{I487N/I487N}$ *ewaso* (D, E and F) and *Myo7a*$^{F947I/F947I}$ *dumbo* (G, H and I) mice at 2 weeks. Misorientation of stereocilia bundles can be seen in both strains, particularly at the basal level in *Myo7a*$^{I487N/I487N}$ *ewaso* mice (asterisk in F) and at all levels in *Myo7a*$^{F947I/F947I}$ *dumbo* mutants. Fusion of stereocilia of IHC is also evident in *Myo7aI487N/I487N ewaso* at this age (arrowhead in F), and show abnormal structure in *Myo7a*$^{F947I/F947I}$ *dumbo (asterisk in* G). OHC, outer hair cells; IHC, inner hair cells. Scale bar; 5 μM

Figure S5 SEM analysis of 4 week old cochlear sensory epithelium from Myo7a mutant strains. Apical, middle and basal cochlear turns were examined in Myo7a$^{+/+}$ (A, B and C), Myo7a$^{I487N/I487N}$ (D, E and F) and Myo7a$^{F947I/F947I}$ (G, H and I) mice at 4 weeks. OHC, outer hair cells; IHC, inner hair cells. Scale bar; 10 μM.

Table S1 Primer and enzymes used in genotyping assays.

Acknowledgments

We thank Wendy Hutchison, Melissa Arnold, Jessica Cardwell, Thomas Dantoft, Cynthia Luk and Melanie Bahlo for technical assistance and advice, and acknowledge the contribution of the Australian Phenomics Facility (APF). We also thank Matthew Burton for help with the behaviour video traces.

Author Contributions

Conceived and designed the experiments: KM LW ER MK SM HD. Performed the experiments: KM LW MK SM. Analyzed the data: KM LW. Contributed reagents/materials/analysis tools: MK HD. Wrote the paper: KM. Substantial contributions to conception and design, interpretation of data, and critical revision of the manuscript: ER.

References

1. Hilgert N, Smith RJ, Van Camp G (2009) Function and expression pattern of nonsyndromic deafness genes. Curr Mol Med 9: 546–564.
2. Mohr PE, Feldman JJ, Dunbar JL, McConkey-Robbins A, Niparko JK, et al. (2000) The societal costs of severe to profound hearing loss in the United States. Int J Technol Assess Health Care 16: 1120–1135.
3. Friedman TB, Griffith AJ (2003) Human nonsyndromic sensorineural deafness. Annu Rev Genomics Hum Genet 4: 341–402.
4. Keats BJ, Corey DP (1999) The usher syndromes. Am J Med Genet 89: 158–166.
5. Reardon W, Trembath RC (1996) Pendred syndrome. J Med Genet 33: 1037–1040.
6. Morton NE (1991) Genetic epidemiology of hearing impairment. Ann N Y Acad Sci 630: 16–31.
7. Petit C (1996) Genes responsible for human hereditary deafness: symphony of a thousand. Nat Genet 14: 385–391.
8. Liu XZ, Walsh J, Tamagawa Y, Kitamura K, Nishizawa M, et al. (1997) Autosomal dominant non-syndromic deafness caused by a mutation in the myosin VIIA gene. Nat Genet 17: 268–269.
9. Luijendijk MW, Van Wijk E, Bischoff AM, Krieger E, Huygen PL, et al. (2004) Identification and molecular modelling of a mutation in the motor head domain of myosin VIIA in a family with autosomal dominant hearing impairment (DFNA11). Hum Genet 115: 149–156.
10. Liu XZ, Walsh J, Mburu P, Kendrick-Jones J, Cope MJ, et al. (1997) Mutations in the myosin VIIA gene cause non-syndromic recessive deafness. Nat Genet 16: 188–190.
11. Riazuddin S, Nazli S, Ahmed ZM, Yang Y, Zulfiqar F, et al. (2008) Mutation spectrum of MYO7A and evaluation of a novel nonsyndromic deafness DFNB2 allele with residual function. Hum Mutat 29: 502–511.
12. Levy G, Levi-Acobas F, Blanchard S, Gerber S, Larget-Piet D, et al. (1997) Myosin VIIA gene: heterogeneity of the mutations responsible for Usher syndrome type IB. Hum Mol Genet 6: 111–116.
13. Weil D, Blanchard S, Kaplan J, Guilford P, Gibson F, et al. (1995) Defective myosin VIIA gene responsible for Usher syndrome type 1B. Nature 374: 60–61.
14. Weston MD, Kelley PM, Overbeck LD, Wagenaar M, Orten DJ, et al. (1996) Myosin VIIA mutation screening in 189 Usher syndrome type 1 patients. Am J Hum Genet 59: 1074–1083.
15. Hartman MA, Finan D, Sivaramakrishnan S, Spudich JA (2011) Principles of unconventional Myosin function and targeting. Annu Rev Cell Dev Biol 27: 133–155.
16. Sakai T, Umeki N, Ikebe R, Ikebe M (2011) Cargo binding activates myosin VIIA motor function in cells. Proc Natl Acad Sci U S A 108: 7028–7033.
17. Chen ZY, Hasson T, Kelley PM, Schwender BJ, Schwartz MF, et al. (1996) Molecular cloning and domain structure of human myosin-VIIa, the gene product defective in Usher syndrome 1B. Genomics 36: 440–448.
18. Hasson T, Heintzelman MB, Santos-Sacchi J, Corey DP, Mooseker MS (1995) Expression in cochlea and retina of myosin VIIa, the gene product defective in Usher syndrome type 1B. Proc Natl Acad Sci U S A 92: 9815–9819.
19. Schwander M, Lopes V, Sczaniecka A, Gibbs D, Lillo C, et al. (2009) A novel allele of myosin VIIa reveals a critical function for the C-terminal FERM domain for melanosome transport in retinal pigment epithelial cells. J Neurosci 29: 15810–15818.
20. Piatto VB, Nascimento EC, Alexandrino F, Oliveira CA, Lopes AC, et al. (2005) Molecular genetics of non-syndromic deafness. Braz J Otorhinolaryngol 71: 216–223.
21. Bedell MA, Jenkins NA, Copeland NG (1997) Mouse models of human disease. Part I: techniques and resources for genetic analysis in mice. Genes Dev 11: 1–10.
22. Ahituv N, Avraham KB (2002) Mouse models for human deafness: current tools for new fashions. Trends Mol Med 8: 447–451.
23. Avraham KB (2003) Mouse models for deafness: lessons for the human inner ear and hearing loss. Ear Hear 24: 332–341.
24. Manji SS, Miller KA, Williams LH, Andreasen L, Siboe M, et al. (2011) An ENU-induced mutation of Cdh23 causes congenital hearing loss, but no vestibular dysfunction, in mice. Am J Pathol 179: 903–914.
25. Manji SS, Williams LH, Miller KA, Ooms LM, Bahlo M, et al. (2011) A mutation in synaptojanin 2 causes progressive hearing loss in the ENU-mutagenised mouse strain Mozart. PLoS One 6: e17607.
26. Acevedo-Arozena A, Wells S, Potter P, Kelly M, Cox RD, et al. (2008) ENU mutagenesis, a way forward to understand gene function. Annu Rev Genomics Hum Genet 9: 49–69.
27. Caspary T (2010) Phenotype-driven mouse ENU mutagenesis screens. Methods Enzymol 477: 313–327.
28. Hoyne GF, Goodnow CC (2006) The use of genomewide ENU mutagenesis screens to unravel complex mammalian traits: identifying genes that regulate organ-specific and systemic autoimmunity. Immunol Rev 210: 27–39.
29. Nolan PM, Hugill A, Cox RD (2002) ENU mutagenesis in the mouse: application to human genetic disease. Brief Funct Genomic Proteomic 1: 278–289.

30. Kent WJ, Sugnet CW, Furey TS, Roskin KM, Pringle TH, et al. (2002) The human genome browser at UCSC. Genome Res 12: 996–1006.
31. Ng PC, Henikoff S (2002) Accounting for human polymorphisms predicted to affect protein function. Genome Res 12: 436–446.
32. Ramensky V, Bork P, Sunyaev S (2002) Human non-synonymous SNPs: server and survey. Nucleic Acids Res 30: 3894–3900.
33. Borodovsky M, McIninch J (1993) Recognition of genes in DNA sequence with ambiguities. Biosystems 30: 161–171.
34. Phillips JC, Braun R, Wang W, Gumbart J, Tajkhorshid E, et al. (2005) Scalable molecular dynamics with NAMD. J Comput Chem 26: 1781–1802.
35. Humphrey W, Dalke A, Schulten K (1996) VMD: visual molecular dynamics. J Mol Graph 14: 33–38, 27–38.
36. Wu L, Pan L, Wei Z, Zhang M (2011) Structure of MyTH4-FERM domains in myosin VIIa tail bound to cargo. Science 331: 757–760.
37. Manji SS, Sorensen BS, Klockars T, Lam T, Hutchison W, et al. (2006) Molecular characterization and expression of maternally expressed gene 3 (Meg3/Gtl2) RNA in the mouse inner ear. J Neurosci Res 83: 181–190.
38. Whitlon DS, Szakaly R, Greiner MA (2001) Cryoembedding and sectioning of cochleas for immunocytochemistry and in situ hybridization. Brain Res Brain Res Protoc 6: 159–166.
39. Gibson F, Walsh J, Mburu P, Varela A, Brown KA, et al. (1995) A type VII myosin encoded by the mouse deafness gene shaker-1. Nature 374: 62–64.
40. Mburu P, Liu XZ, Walsh J, Saw D Jr, Cope MJ, et al. (1997) Mutation analysis of the mouse myosin VIIA deafness gene. Genes Funct 1: 191–203.
41. Rhodes CR, Hertzano R, Fuchs H, Bell RE, de Angelis MH, et al. (2004) A Myo7a mutation cosegregates with stereocilia defects and low-frequency hearing impairment. Mamm Genome 15: 686–697.
42. Petit C, Levilliers J, Hardelin JP (2001) Molecular genetics of hearing loss. Annu Rev Genet 35: 589–646.
43. Tyska MJ, Warshaw DM (2002) The myosin power stroke. Cell Motil Cytoskeleton 51: 1–15.
44. Weil D, Kussel P, Blanchard S, Levy G, Levi-Acobas F, et al. (1997) The autosomal recessive isolated deafness, DFNB2, and the Usher 1B syndrome are allelic defects of the myosin-VIIA gene. Nat Genet 16: 191–193.
45. Kikkawa Y, Shitara H, Wakana S, Kohara Y, Takada T, et al. (2003) Mutations in a new scaffold protein Sans cause deafness in Jackson shaker mice. Hum Mol Genet 12: 453–461.
46. Kitamura K, Kakoi H, Yoshikawa Y, Ochikubo F (1992) Ultrastructural findings in the inner ear of Jackson shaker mice. Acta Otolaryngol 112: 622–627.
47. Kitamura K, Nomura Y, Yagi M, Yoshikawa Y, Ochikubo F (1991) Morphological changes of cochlea in a strain of new-mutant mice. Acta Otolaryngol 111: 61–69.
48. Kros CJ, Marcotti W, van Netten SM, Self TJ, Libby RT, et al. (2002) Reduced climbing and increased slipping adaptation in cochlear hair cells of mice with Myo7a mutations. Nat Neurosci 5: 41–47.
49. Boeda B, El-Amraoui A, Bahloul A, Goodyear R, Daviet L, et al. (2002) Myosin VIIa, harmonin and cadherin 23, three Usher I gene products that cooperate to shape the sensory hair cell bundle. Embo J 21: 6689–6699.
50. Senften M, Schwander M, Kazmierczak P, Lillo C, Shin JB, et al. (2006) Physical and functional interaction between protocadherin 15 and myosin VIIa in mechanosensory hair cells. J Neurosci 26: 2060–2071.
51. Prosser HM, Rzadzinska AK, Steel KP, Bradley A (2008) Mosaic complementation demonstrates a regulatory role for myosin VIIa in actin dynamics of stereocilia. Mol Cell Biol 28: 1702–1712.
52. Saihan Z, Webster AR, Luxon L, Bitner-Glindzicz M (2009) Update on Usher syndrome. Curr Opin Neurol 22: 19–27.
53. Ahmed ZM, Riazuddin S, Riazuddin S, Wilcox ER (2003) The molecular genetics of Usher syndrome. Clin Genet 63: 431–444.
54. Liu X, Bulgakov OV, Darrow KN, Pawlyk B, Adamian M, et al. (2007) Usherin is required for maintenance of retinal photoreceptors and normal development of cochlear hair cells. Proc Natl Acad Sci U S A 104: 4413–4418.
55. Tamagawa Y, Ishikawa K, Ishikawa K, Ishida T, Kitamura K, et al. (2002) Phenotype of DFNA11: a nonsyndromic hearing loss caused by a myosin VIIA mutation. Laryngoscope 112: 292–297.
56. Bharadwaj AK, Kasztejna JP, Huq S, Berson EL, Dryja TP (2000) Evaluation of the myosin VIIA gene and visual function in patients with Usher syndrome type I. Exp Eye Res 71: 173–181.
57. Jaijo T, Aller E, Beneyto M, Najera C, Graziano C, et al. (2007) MYO7A mutation screening in Usher syndrome type I patients from diverse origins. J Med Genet 44: e71.

13

Changes in Early Cortical Visual Processing Predict Enhanced Reactivity in Deaf Individuals

Davide Bottari[1,2*], Anne Caclin[3,4], Marie-Hélène Giard[3,4], Francesco Pavani[1,2]

1 Department of Cognitive Sciences and Education, University of Trento, Trento, Italy, **2** Center for Mind/Brain Sciences, University of Trento, Trento, Italy, **3** INSERM, U1028; CNRS, UMR5292; Lyon Neuroscience Research Center, Brain Dynamics and Cognition Team, Lyon, France, **4** University Lyon 1, Lyon, France

Abstract

Individuals with profound deafness rely critically on vision to interact with their environment. Improvement of visual performance as a consequence of auditory deprivation is assumed to result from cross-modal changes occurring in late stages of visual processing. Here we measured reaction times and event-related potentials (ERPs) in profoundly deaf adults and hearing controls during a speeded visual detection task, to assess to what extent the enhanced reactivity of deaf individuals could reflect plastic changes in the early cortical processing of the stimulus. We found that deaf subjects were faster than hearing controls at detecting the visual targets, regardless of their location in the visual field (peripheral or peri-foveal). This behavioural facilitation was associated with ERP changes starting from the first detectable response in the striate cortex (C1 component) at about 80 ms after stimulus onset, and in the P1 complex (100–150 ms). In addition, we found that P1 peak amplitudes predicted the response times in deaf subjects, whereas in hearing individuals visual reactivity and ERP amplitudes correlated only at later stages of processing. These findings show that long-term auditory deprivation can profoundly alter visual processing from the earliest cortical stages. Furthermore, our results provide the first evidence of a co-variation between modified brain activity (cortical plasticity) and behavioural enhancement in this sensory-deprived population.

Editor: Angela Sirigu, French National Centre for Scientific Research, France

Funding: This work was supported by a PRIN 2006 grant (Prot. 2006118540_004) from MIUR (Italy), a Galileo grant from Italian and French Universities, and a PAT-CRS grant from University of Trento (Italy). The funders had no role in study design, data collection and analysis, decision to publish, or preparation of the manuscript.

Competing Interests: The authors have declared that no competing interests exist.

* E-mail: davidebottari@gmail.com

Introduction

When coping with profound sensory deprivation, processing of inputs from the intact modalities is critical. In profound deafness, detection of changes in the environment and orienting of attention occurs primarily through vision. Deaf individuals are faster at detecting abrupt visual onsets [1,2,3,4], faster and more accurate at discriminating motion direction of visual stimuli [5], and more efficient in re-orienting attentional resources in visual space [6,7,8]. These abilities have mainly, though not exclusively, been documented for events occurring towards the periphery of the visual field [9].

For profound deafness, it has been proposed that crossmodal changes involving the visual modality occur beyond the early processing stages, through the recruitment of higher-order visual areas as well as the de-afferented auditory cortices [10]. Differences in brain activation between deaf and hearing individuals have been found in the dorsal processing pathway (e.g., MT, MST) in response to motion stimuli [11,12]. In addition, responses to visual stimuli have been recorded outside visually responsive brain regions, in the primary and secondary auditory cortices of deaf individuals [13,14]. Recently Lomber and colleagues [15] showed in deaf cats a causal relationship between the reorganization of portions of the auditory cortex and specific enhancements of visual functions. Finally, two event-related potential (ERP) studies in humans [5,16] found that the visual cortical responses elicited by deaf and hearing individuals started to differ from 180–200 ms latency, in the N1 component known to be generated in extra-striate cortex [17] and sensitive to high-order cognitive processes such as attentional orienting [18].

While ERPs are ideally suited to address the question of when changes in sensory processing occur, the possibility to reveal effects of crossmodal plasticity in early visual processing likely depends upon the specific task demands. The observation of modulations starting from the N1 component, for instance, could result from the use of visual discrimination tasks [5]. Indeed, target identification requires stimulus-feature binding before the response choice: this in turn necessitates orienting of attention towards the stimulus, which is known to modulate the N1 component of visual ERPs [18]. A simple detection task would not imply such processes and could reveal deafness-induced changes in earlier visual processing stages. In the present study, we tested this hypothesis by measuring reaction times and ERPs while deaf and hearing adults performed a simple speeded detection task. We focused our analyses on early (C1, P1) and later (N1) ERP components. In addition, we analysed the relationship between response times and visual ERP components, to highlight possible correlations between behavioural changes and brain responses in the deaf. As a large body of literature suggests that the deaf display enhanced visual performance particularly when the task involves the peripheral portion of the visual field [3,5], we asked our participants to detect targets presented at either peri-foveal or peripheral eccentricities.

Methods

Participants

Ten profoundly deaf individuals (mean age = 33 years, SD = 4, range 18–50 year-old; mean years of education = 14, SD = 2.6; 6 female) were recruited at the National Association for Deaf (Ente Nazionale per la protezione e assistenza dei Sordi, Trento, Italy) and gave their informed consent to participate in the study. All deaf participants had uncorrected bilateral profound hearing loss (>90 dB), and acquired deafness within the first 3 years of age (8 had congenital deafness). All deaf participants were proficient sign-language users (6 learned sign language as first language, the other four had first a training based on Italian lip reading). Ten hearing matched controls (mean age = 29 years, SD = 2.5, range 23–50 years old; mean years of education = 16, SD = 2.6; 5 females) were also recruited to take part in the study. All participants had normal or corrected-to-normal vision and were right-handed by self-report.

The study was approved by the ethical committee at the University of Trento (Italy), and written informed consent was obtained from all participants prior to testing.

Stimuli and apparatus

Visual fixation was a white cross, presented at the centre of the screen throughout the experimental session. The target was a circle opened on left or right side that could be presented at eight possible locations arranged on two invisible concentric circles centred on visual fixation. The radius of the inner circle was 3 degrees of visual angle, and the radius of the outer circle was 8 degrees. Four possible target locations were on the inner circle and four were on the outer (see Fig. 1a). Each location was placed along the two diagonals of the screen, thus resulting in 4 possible stimulus locations in the upper portion of the visual field, and 4 in the lower. From now on we will refer to locations on the inner circle as peri-foveal, and locations on the outer circle as peripheral. Targets appearing at peripheral locations were corrected for the cortical magnification factor [19]. Peri-foveal targets covered a visual angle of 1.5° and peripheral targets of 2.6°. The widths of the lines of the open circles were 1.5 mm and 2.4 mm for the peri-phoveal and peripheral targets, respectively. All stimuli were clearly presented suprathreshold. The luminance of the background was Y = 23, x = .278, y = .301, that of the target stimulus was Y = 83.3, x = .277, y = .297, and that of the cue was Y = 24.2,

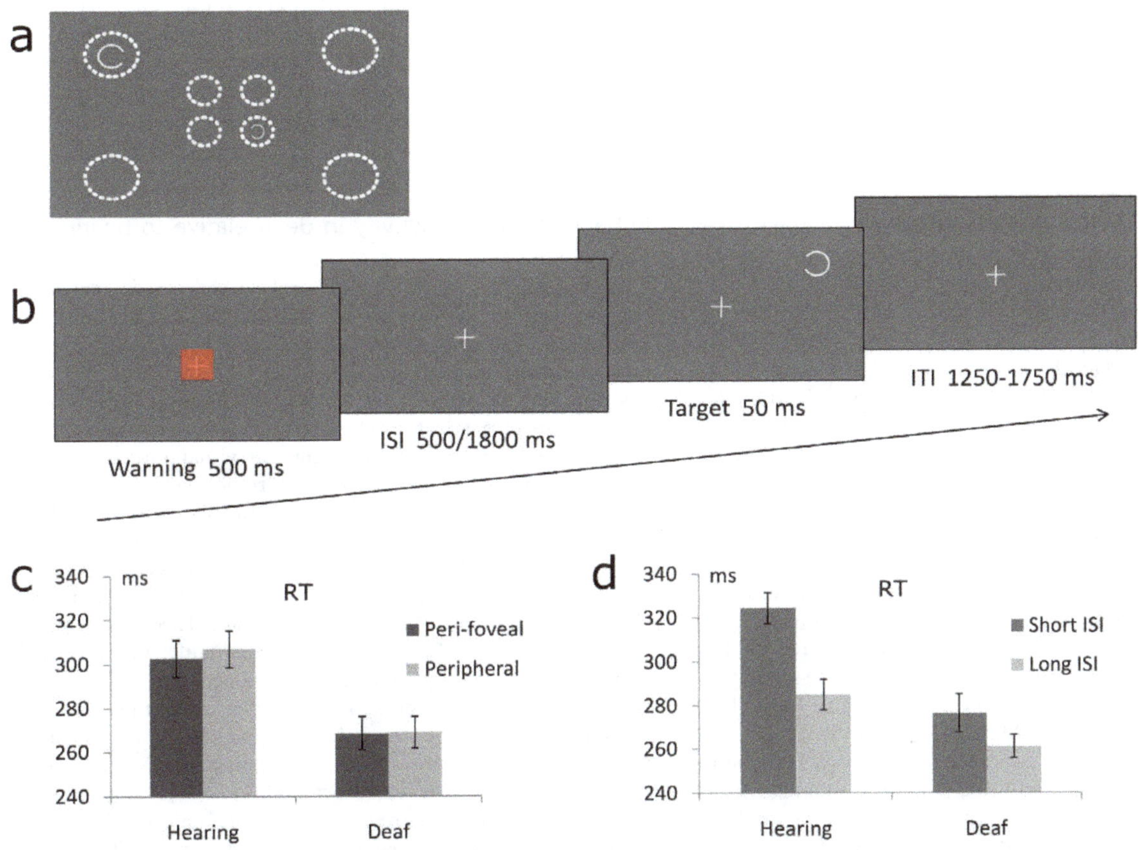

Figure 1. Experimental protocol and behavioural results. (**a**) The target was a single circle opened on the left or right side, presented at one of 8 possible locations. Peri-foveal targets were centred at 3° from fixation and covered a visual angle of 1.5°; peripheral targets were centred at 8° from fixation and covered a visual angle of 2.6° (i.e., targets were corrected for the cortical magnification factor). Dotted place-holders and examples of targets are shown in (a) for illustrative purposes only. (**b**) Each trial began with a warning signal (a red square covering 1.5° of visual angle, presented for 500 ms). The inter-stimulus intervals (ISIs) between the warning signal and the target were, equiprobably, either 500 ms (short ISI) or 1800 ms (long ISI). The target appeared for 50 ms, at any of the 8 possible locations randomly. Participants were instructed to press the response button as soon as possible. The inter-trial interval (ITI) ranged randomly between 1250 and 1750 ms. (**c, d**) Mean (of individual subjects medians) response times (RTs) for deaf and hearing participants as a function of (**c**) target eccentricity (perifoveal or peripheral) and (**d**) ISI (short or long) between the warning and the target. Deaf were overall faster than hearing controls. In addition, they showed no RT cost when reacting to peripheral vs. perifoveal targets, unlike hearing controls (**c**). Finally, the ISI modulated the reactivity performance in the two groups (**d**).

x = .510, y = .301 (measured with Chroma Meter CS-100A, http://www.konicaminolta.com/). All stimuli were presented on a standard 17 inches monitor, with 1024×768 pixels resolution, and 60 Hz refresh rate. The experiment was programmed with E-Studio 1.1.4.1, and run using E-Prime 1.1.4.1 (http://www.pstnet.com).

Procedure

Participants sat at approximately 60 cm from the computer monitor inside a sound-attenuated chamber and were instructed to keep their head and eyes oriented towards fixation throughout testing. The experimental session lasted approximately 60 min. All hearing participants wore ear-plugs.

Each trial began with a warning stimulus consisting of a red square covering 1.5° of visual angle and presented for 500 ms (the visual fixation cross was superimposed on the red square, see Fig. 1b). The warning stimulus was presented for several reasons: first to give an attentional cue to the participants, second to analyze the ERPs to an event placed at fixation, and third to replicate our previous behavioural findings using the same paradigm [3]. The inter-stimulus intervals (ISIs) between the warning stimulus (offset) and the target (onset) were, randomly and equiprobably, either 500 ms (short ISI) or 1800 ms (long ISI). The visual target was presented randomly at any of the 8 possible locations (i.e., 4 central and 4 peripheral) for 50 ms. Participants were required to press as fast as possible the space bar of a computer keyboard upon detection of the target. The inter-trial interval (target offset to warning onset) ranged randomly from 1250 to 1750 ms. This task was designed on the basis of the paradigm used by Bottari and colleagues [3], which showed RT differences between deaf and hearing participants.

In case of anticipated responses (in the first 100 ms after stimulus onset), the sentence "do not anticipate!" appeared on the screen. Before data recording, participants completed a practice block of 24 trials. The experimental session was divided into 10 blocks comprising 96 trials each and lasting approximately 5 minutes. Between blocks, participants were invited to take short breaks. The experiment was a 2 by 2 by 2 factorial design, with target eccentricity (peri-foveal or peripheral) and ISI (short or long) as within-participant factors, and group (deaf individuals or hearing controls) as between-participants factor.

Event-related potentials

The EEG was recorded (analog bandwidth: 0.1–200 Hz, sampling rate: 1 kHz) from 34 scalp sites using the International 10–20 System extended montage (documentation in http://www.easycap.de). Standard 10–20 sites were Fp1, Fp2, F7, F3, Fz, F4, F8, T7, C3, Cz, C4, T8, T5 (P7), P3, Pz, P4, T6 (P8), O1, and O2. Additional intermediate sites were FC5, FC1, FC2, FC6, TP9 (M1), CP5, CP1, CP2, TP10 (M2), PO3, PO4, PO9, Iz, and PO10. All scalp channels were referenced to the nose. Horizontal eye-movements were monitored with a bipolar montage from electrodes at left and right outer canthi. To eliminate the artefacts due to blinks, we performed an Independent Component Analysis (ICA; [20,21]; runica version, implemented on EEGLAB running in MATLAB, http://www.mathworks.com/). The ICA was conducted on EEG epochs running from 1250 ms before the warning signal onset to 2200 ms after (for short-ISI trials), or 3500 ms after (for long-ISI trials). After removal of blink effects, trials including incorrect responses (anticipations, i.e. responses before the target or in the 100 ms following it) or with signals exceeding 100 µV at any electrode were excluded from averaging.

ERPs to the warning signal were averaged over a period of 2700 ms including 500 ms pre-stimulus (on average, 680 trials after artefact rejection). ERPs to the targets were averaged separately for each ISI and target location over a period of 1000 ms including 500 ms pre-stimulus (on average, 188 trials per condition). The responses were corrected relative to a [−100, 0 ms] pre-stimulus baseline with respect to both warning signal and target onsets. In addition, the ERPs to targets were also corrected relative to a [−300, −200 ms] baseline to assess possible group differences in anticipatory activities occurring before the target onset and their potential effects on the subsequent brain responses. Finally, the ERPs were digitally filtered (low-pass filter with a 30-Hz cut-off, slope 24db/octave). Scalp potential maps were generated using spherical spline interpolation [22,23]. All EEG data were analysed with the ELAN-pack software developed at the Brain Dynamics and Cognition team in Lyon [24].

Statistical approach

Before comparing the cortical activity between groups, we evaluated the emergence of visual evoked responses within each group. To this purpose, we run a series of Wilcoxon tests across all participants, comparing to zero the activity recorded at each time sample. We performed this exploratory analysis for the ERPs to the warning signal and to the targets, to select the time windows and electrodes for the main analyses. The selected time windows were thus: C1 [40–95 ms], P1 [80–150 ms] and N1 [150–220 ms]. Main analyses were conducted on peak amplitude and peak latency for the C1, P1 and N1 components, adopting mixed ANOVAs and between-group t-tests. When necessary the Tukey test was used for post-hoc comparisons.

Results

Enhanced visual reactivity in deaf relative to hearing individuals

Response times (RTs) in deaf and hearing participants were computed as the medians for each participant in each condition, and analyzed using an ANOVA with Target Eccentricity (3° or 8°) and Inter-stimulus interval (ISI) between warning signal and target (short or long) as within-subject factors, and Group (deaf, hearing) as between-subject factor. Deaf participants were overall faster than hearing controls at detecting the visual targets (269±10 (SEM) ms vs. 305±10 (SEM) ms, respectively; $F(1,18) = 6.7$, $p<0.02$). In addition, while hearing controls showed a small but consistent RT cost (4 ms; $t(9) = 2.6$, $p<0.03$) when responding to peripheral relative to peri-foveal targets, this cost was negligible in deaf participants (0.4 ms; $t<1$). This resulted in a marginally significant interaction between Group and Target Eccentricity ($F(1,18) = 3.3$, $p<0.08$; see Fig. 1c). Importantly, the faster RTs found in the deaf group compared to hearing controls was not due to a larger number of anticipation responses, as the amount of trials in which the RTs were below 100 ms was comparable in the two groups (proportion of anticipation trials: Hearing = 0.0004±0.0002; Deaf = 0.0009±0.0004; $t(18) = 1.2$, $p = 0.2$). Overall, these findings replicate previous reports [1,2,3] and indicate that profound deafness can enhance reactivity to visual events, particularly towards the periphery of the visual field. An additional behavioural finding was the significant interaction between the warning-to-target ISI and Group factors ($F(1,18) = 8.8$, $p<0.01$; see Fig. 1d). Hearing controls were faster at detecting targets at long than short ISI (285±10 ms vs. 324±10 ms, respectively; $p<0.0002$, Tukey HSD post-hoc test), as predicted by the increased posterior probability for the long ISI targets [25]. This ISI-related difference did not significantly emerge in deaf individuals (261±8 ms vs. 276±12 ms). As a result, reactivity difference between groups was substantial at the short

ISI ($p = 0.02$), and not significant at the long ISI ($p = 0.4$, Tukey HSD tests). Note however that a ceiling effect in deaf individuals might explain this last result.

Brain responses to the central warning signal

The warning signal elicited "classical" visual ERP components on posterior scalp areas in both groups, with however differences between deaf and hearing participants in the latency, amplitude, and morphology of the early visual responses (C1, P1, N1 components).

Both deaf and hearing participants exhibited a significant C1 component of negative polarity [26] within the 40–95 ms time interval, with a maximum amplitude around Iz electrode (see Fig. 2a). Its peak latency was significantly shorter in deaf individuals (80±2 ms) than in hearing participants (87±2 ms; $t(18) = 2.3$, $p<0.04$). There was no significant group difference in peak amplitudes ($t(18)<1.4$). This difference in the C1 peak latency between groups would indicate that the cortical processing between deaf and hearing subjects already differs at the level of the striate cortex [17]. An increasing number of evidence suggests that visual attention might modulate the C1 component [27,28,29,30]. Nonetheless all the observed C1 modulations as a function of attentional and/or perceptual load manipulations emerged as amplitude changes. The present latency difference might reflect changes in striate cortex activity or even in earlier processing stages of deaf individuals' visual pathway. In any case, this result shows that differences in visual processing between deaf individuals and hearing controls can emerge for a central visual event, presented directly at fixation.

Following the C1 deflection, a prominent P1 component was recorded over the posterior electrodes between 80 and 150 ms, with a substantially different morphology between the two groups. As shown in Fig. 2b, the two groups present a similar P1 profile until about 125 ms, with a positive peak around 105 ms. Then, unlike hearing controls, deaf displayed a second positive deflection around 145 ms. This double deflection was observed in 7 out of 10 deaf participants (but only in 2 out of 10 hearing controls). To assess the consistency of these different P1 profiles, we compared between the two groups the mean amplitude of the P1 response in two different latency ranges: 105 ms±10 ms (first P1 peak), and 145 ms±10 ms (second P1 deflection), over the subset of posterior electrodes that better captured this activity (T5-T6-PO9-PO10-TP9-TP10). As expected from the ERP waves in Fig. 2b, the mean amplitude around the first P1 peak did not differ between the two subjects' groups ($t(18)<0.4$), whereas around the second P1 peak deaf individuals displayed a greater positive activity (0.9±0.6 μV)

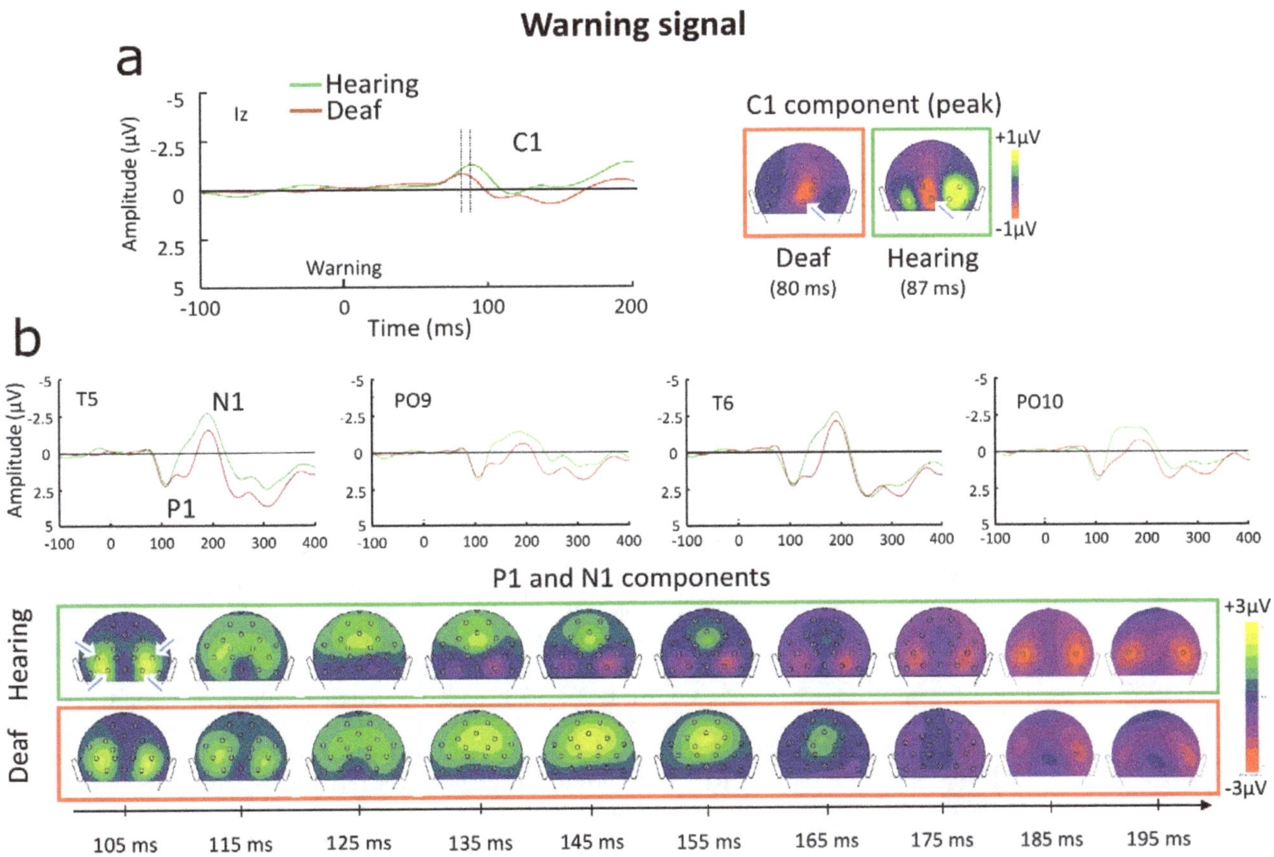

Figure 2. Brain responses to the central warning signal in deaf subjects and in hearing controls. (**a**) Visual ERPs and topography of the C1 component around its peak latency for each group. Arrows indicate the electrode (Iz) at which the ERP curves are shown. (Note that because the C1 peak latency is later in hearing controls than in deaf participants, the emerging P1 can be seen for the controls on each side of the C1 in this figure.) (**b**) P1 and N1 responses at 4 posterior electrodes (T5, PO9, T6, PO10, identified by arrows in the first potential map). The P1 components have a similar profile in the two subjects groups until about 125 ms, then deaf subjects present a second positive deflection (145 ms) compared to hearing controls. The prolonged positivity in deaf subjects (145–165 ms) is clearly seen in the spatiotemporal distribution of the responses (back view of the head). By contrast, although the negative N1 component emerged earlier in control than in deaf subjects, there was no difference in morphology or topography between the two subjects groups.

compared to hearing controls ($-1.2\pm0.8\ \mu V$, $t(18)=4.1$, $p<0.05$). The different morphology of the P1 complex between groups is also evident in the spatiotemporal distribution of the responses between 105 and 195 ms (see lower panel in Fig. 2b). From about 135 to 165 ms, while hearing controls present negative potential fields at the most occipital electrodes (emerging N1 component), deaf individuals still show an enduring positive activity centred over parietal electrodes. This corroborates further our findings that cortical changes in deaf compared to hearing individuals can be detected in early processing and for a centrally displayed stimulus (see also [31] for a result in this direction, showing ERP differences at the P2 level, between cochlear implanted patients and hearing controls for visual stimuli presented at fixation).

Although visual inspection of the topographies (see Fig. 2b) suggests that the N1 component emerged earlier in controls than in deaf individuals around the occipital electrodes (e.g. PO9 and PO10), its morphology was similar between the two groups, and there was no significant difference in the peak amplitude (5.3 vs. 5.0 µV) or peak latency (177 vs. 180 ms, hearing controls vs. deaf individuals respectively, both $ts<1$).

Brain responses to peri-foveal and peripheral targets

In paradigms using a warning signal prior to the occurrence of a visual target, subjects may generate anticipatory activities in sensory cortices before target appearance. To test for this possibility, we measured in each subject the mean ERP amplitude over the 200 ms preceding the target (relative to a baseline taken over the [−300, −200 ms] pre-stimulus period), averaged across parieto-occipital electrodes (PO3-PO4-O1-O2-PO9-PO10-Iz). This mean pre-stimulus activity did not differ from the baseline for either (short or long) ISI condition in the control group. It was however significantly different from the baseline in the deaf group for the targets presented at short (but not at long) ISI ($t(9)=4.5$, $p<0.005$). This result was further confirmed when comparing the mean pre-stimulus amplitudes of the two groups in a two-way ANOVA with the factors ISI and Group, with a significant interaction between the two factors ($F(1,18)=4.6$, $p<0.05$): this was caused by greater mean amplitude (sustained anticipatory activity) in deaf than hearing participants when the target was presented at short ISI ($p=0.05$, Tukey HSD post-hoc test; Fig. 3).

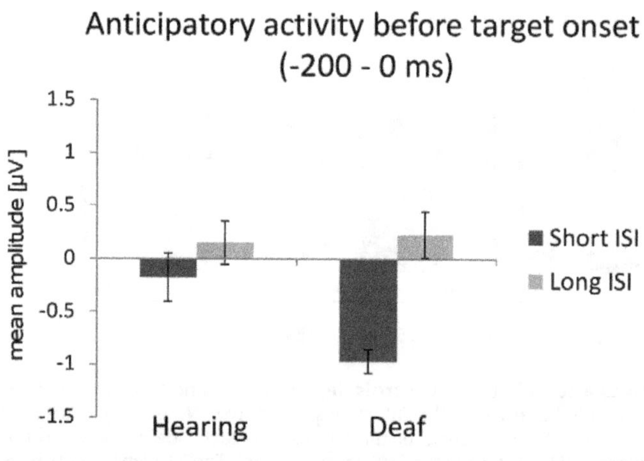

Figure 3. Anticipatory activity recorded before target onset. Deaf individuals show enhanced anticipatory activity (mean amplitude over the 200 ms preceding target onset, with a −300 to −200 ms baseline) compared to hearing controls for target presented at short ISI.

Because the different anticipatory activities in deaf and hearing subjects (over the 200 ms preceding the target presentation) could impact differently on subsequent brain responses, we kept the same [−300, −200 ms] pre-stimulus baseline for ERP component analyses. For completeness, however, we also report the results of the analyses when adopting a [−100, 0 ms] baseline, as for the warning signal, in Table 1. The results remain globally unchanged irrespective of the adopted baseline.

The C1 component elicited by the targets was observable in the grand average responses, with the typical inversion of polarity for upper vs. lower visual field stimulation [26]. However, it could not be further analyzed because it was not well defined in every participant.

Visual inspection of the P1 component to targets did not reveal the clear biphasic morphology seen in the response to the warning signal (see ERP waves in Fig. 4). This can be due to the fact that P1 is usually sensitive to the visual contrast of the stimulus: this contrast was much lower for the targets than for the warning signal (red square). In addition, ERPs to the targets (peri-foveal or peripheral) are averaged responses to stimuli presented at four distinct locations (upper and lower, right and left positions, see Fig. 1a) while the warning signal was always delivered at fixation. Nevertheless, the spatiotemporal distribution of the responses to targets (see topographies in Fig. 4a and Fig. 4b) shows that the development of the P1 and N1 components in the two subjects' groups is similar to that observed in response to the warning signal: deaf display a prolonged P1 relative to hearing controls, with a prominent late phase distributed over parietal scalp sites.

The peak latencies and amplitudes of P1 (determined within the 80–150 ms time window across the posterior electrodes T5-T6-PO3-PO4-P3-P4-Pz-O1-O2-TP9-TP10-PO9-PO10-Iz) were compared between the two groups using ANOVAs with Target Eccentricity (peri-foveal or peripheral) and ISI (short or long) as within-participant factors and Group as between-participant factor. Analysis on P1 peak latency revealed a significant effect of ISI ($F(1,18)=8.4$, $p<0.01$) due to a delayed P1 peak for targets presented at long compared to short ISI, and a marginally significant effect of Target Eccentricity ($F(1,18)=4.2$, $p<0.06$), showing a tendency for delayed P1 peak for peripheral relative to central targets. Most importantly, deaf participants showed a significant peak latency delay (130 ± 5 ms) compared to hearing controls (115 ± 5 ms, $F(1,18)=4.8$, $p<0.05$). There were no other significant interactions involving the Group factor ($Fs<1.5$). In particular, the absence of an ISI-by-Group interaction ($F<1$ with both baseline corrections) suggested that the difference between the two groups in anticipatory activities as a function of ISI reported above had no effect on the P1 peak latency. ANOVA on the P1 peak amplitude showed again a significant effect of ISI ($F(1,18)=13.3$, $p<0.01$), indicating that participants generated larger P1 amplitudes to targets presented at long compared to short ISIs. The interaction between the ISI and Group factors tended towards significance ($F(1,18)=4.2$, $p<0.06$). In particular, deaf tended to show a larger difference between the P1 peak amplitude in the long- compared to the short-ISI condition than hearing controls. (Note that this interaction may have contributed to the main effect of ISI reported above). Lastly, although it did not reach statistical significance, there was a trend for a larger P1 amplitude in deaf ($4.6\pm0.6\ \mu V$) than in hearing subjects ($3.2\pm0.6\ \mu V$, $F(1,18)=2.5$, $p=1.3$).

Analysis of the N1 component (assessed over the 150–220 ms time window) using the same procedure as for the P1 response did not reveal any significant effect of ISI or Group, nor interaction involving the Group factor (all $Fs<3.5$).

Table 1. Analyses (ANOVAs) of the ERPs to targets and their relationships with behavioural responses relative to a baseline taken over the 100 ms preceding the target onset.

Brain responses to peri-foveal and peripheral targets			
P1 component	Factors	- 2 within-subjects: Target Eccentricity (peri-foveal, peripheral), ISI (short, long) - 1 between-subjects: Group	
	Peak latency	*Main effects*	ISI: $F(1,18)=8.7$, $p<0.01$ Target Eccentricity: $F(1,18)=6.5$, $p<0.02$ **Group**: $F(1,18)=5.7$, $p<0.03$
		No interactions involving Group	All $Fs<1$
	Peak Amplitude	*Main effects*	ISI: $F(1,18)=5.7$, $p<0.03$
		Interactions involving Group	**ISI×Group**: $F(1,18)=13.4$, $p<0.01$
N1 component	Factors	- 2 within-subjects: Target Eccentricity (peri-foveal, peripheral), ISI (short, long) - 1 between-subjects: Group	
	Peak latency	*No main effects or interactions involving Group*	Target eccentricity: $F(1,18)=3.7$, $p<0.08$
	Peak Amplitude	*No main effects or interactions involving Group*	All $Fs<2.8$
Changes in early visual ERPs of the profoundly deaf predict enhanced reactivity			
P1 component	Factors	- 2 within-subjects: ISI (short, long), Quartile (1,2,3,4) - 1 between-subjects: Group	
	Peak latency	*No main effects or interactions involving Group*	All $Fs<1.8$, n.s.
	Peak Amplitude	*Main effects*	ISI: $F(1,18)=8.01$, $p<0.02$ Quartile: $F(3,54)=6.3$, $p<0.001$
		Interactions involving Group	ISI×Group: $F(1,18)<1$, n.s. **Quartile×Group**: $F(3,54)=3.5$, $p<0.02$
		Post-hoc* ANOVAs *for each group with ISI and Quartile as factors	**Deaf: Quartile** $F(3,27)=8.3$, $p<0.001$ (linear contrast $F(1,9)=15.7$, $p<0.003$) Hearing: Quartile $F<1.5$, n.s. (linear contrast: $F<1$, n.s.)
N1 component	Factors	- 2 within-subjects: ISI (short, long), Quartile (1,2,3,4) - 1 between-subjects: Group	
	Peak latency	*No main effects or interactions involving Group*	All $Fs<2.4$, n.s.
	Peak Amplitude	*Main effects*	Quartile: $F(3,54)=14.7$, $p<0.0001$ (linear contrast $F(1,18)=22.1$, $p<0.0001$)
		No Interactions involving Group	All $Fs<1$

Significant effects involving the group factor are highlighted with a grey background. Note that the results are similar to those obtained with a [−300, −200 ms] baseline reported in the main text.

Changes in early visual ERPs of the profoundly deaf predict enhanced reactivity

Having demonstrated substantial early visual ERPs differences between deaf and hearing subjects in particular in the P1 latency range, we turned to investigate whether these different ERP profiles could predict the observed behavioural differences in terms of reactivity to the visual targets. To this aim, we separated the RT distribution for each condition (target eccentricity and ISI) and in each participant into four quartiles (Fig. 5b). Trials belonging to each quartile were used to calculate four ERPs for each participant. We could thus re-analyze the main responses to the targets (anticipatory activities, P1, and N1 components) as a function of the RT quartiles. The overall outcome of these analyses is illustrated in Fig. 5.

As we reported above, deaf individuals showed enhanced sustained activity prior to the appearance of the target in the short ISI condition. Because we observed the larger behavioural advantage for deaf compared to hearing subjects precisely for the short ISI, we examined whether enhanced pre-stimulus activity (within the 200 ms prior to target presentation, relative to a [−300, −200 ms] baseline; see Figure 3) could be related to the RTs. A mixed ANOVA with ISI (short or long), Quartile (1, 2, 3, 4) and Group as factors did not reveal significant main effects of Group or Quartile ($F(1,18)=3$, $p<0.1$ and $F<1$, respectively) on pre-stimulus activity, nor significant interactions between Quartile and Group, or between ISI, Quartile and Group ($Fs<1$; as expected from the previous analysis on the anticipatory activity, the ISI×Group interaction was significant $F(1,18)=4.4$, $p=0.05$). These results thus indicate that, whatever the ISI the RTs did not – at least directly – depend on anticipatory activities in visual areas before target appearance (Fig. 5c).

A very different pattern of results emerges when considering the peak amplitude of the P1 component as a function of ISI, Quartile, and Group (note that for this analysis data were pooled across target locations as this factor did not affect P1 or N1 latencies or amplitudes in previous analysis). An ANOVA with ISI, Quartile, and Group as factors revealed a significant main effect of ISI ($F(1,18)=13.7$, $p<0.01$) and an interaction between ISI and Group ($F(1,18)=4.9$, $p<0.04$) showing that deaf individuals displayed an enhanced P1 peak amplitude for targets presented at long than at short ISI ($p<0.01$, Tukey HSD post-hoc test). Most importantly, the analysis revealed a significant main effect of

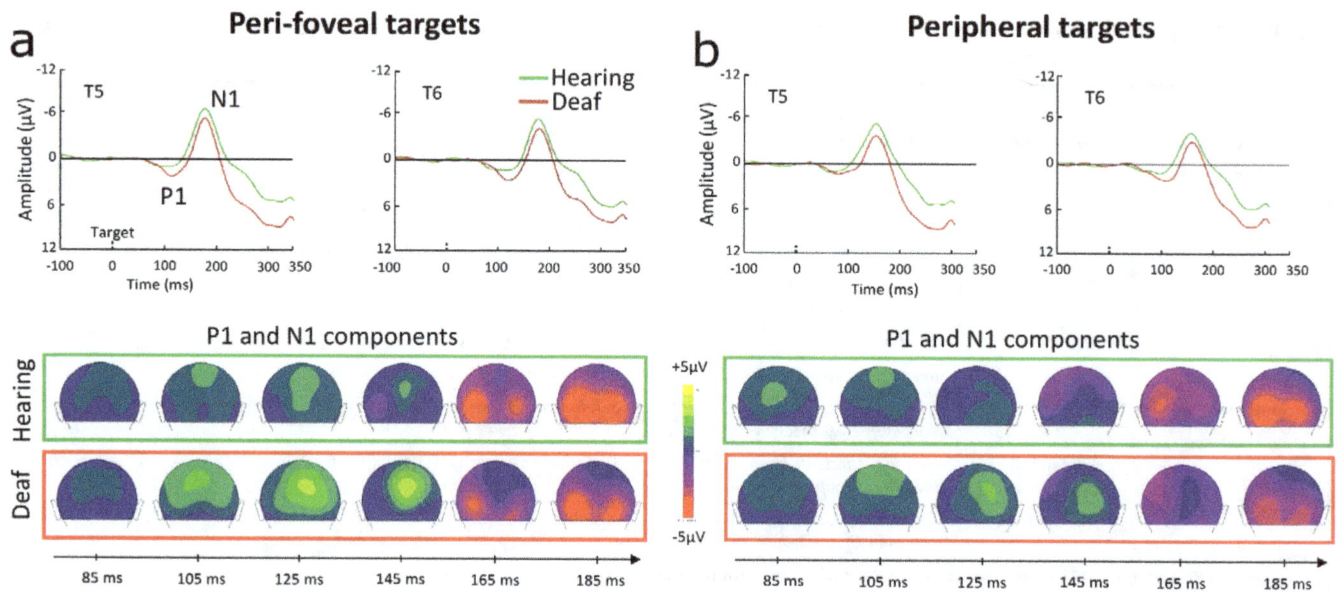

Figure 4. Brain responses to (a) peri-foveal and (b) peripheral targets. Upper panels show ERPs at T5 and T6 electrodes for the targets. Lower panels show spatiotemporal distribution of the responses between 85 and 185 ms in each group. Like in the responses to the warning signal, the P1 component is prolonged in deaf compared to hearing subjects, whereas the N1 is similar.

Quartile ($F(3,54)=5.1$, $p<0.01$) and a significant interaction between Quartile and Group ($F(3,54)=3.7$, $p<0.02$). A separate ANOVA on the deaf data showed a significant effect of Quartile ($F(3,27)=7.9$, $p<0.001$), and a significant linear contrast ($F(1,9)=19.5$, $p<0.003$; see Fig. 5d). Conversely, this relationship between ERP and behaviour was entirely absent in hearing controls (for both baseline corrections, main effect of Quartile: $F<1.5$; linear contrast: $F<1$).

In sum, RTs of deaf individuals slow down as P1 peak amplitude decreases, with a clear linear relationship, whereas no such relationship emerged in hearing controls. Figure 5f illustrates these effects in the topography of the P1 component (around its peak latency) as a function of quartiles. The same analysis on peak latency did not show any significant effect of Quartile ($F<1$ for both baseline corrections) nor any interaction involving the Group factor ($F<1.8$, n.s. for both baseline corrections).

Finally, in both deaf and hearing participants the amplitude of the N1 component predicted RTs. A similar relationship between ERPs and behaviour emerged in the two groups (Fig. 5e; see also Fig. 5g for the topography of the N1 peak as a function of quartiles). ANOVA on the N1 peak amplitude showed a significant main effect of Quartile ($F(3,54)=10.7$, $p<0.0001$) and a linear pattern for this factor (linear contrast: $F(1,18)=17.5$, $p<0.001$). However, no significant interaction involving the Group factor was found ($F<1$ for both baseline corrections). Thus, for both groups faster RTs were associated with an increase in N1 peak amplitude. Similar to the P1 component, there was no effect of the Quartile or Group factors on the N1 peak latency ($F<2.4$, n.s. for both baseline corrections).

Discussion

The current view on visual changes in profound deafness is that they entail crossmodal plasticity resulting in modifications in late visual processing [9,10]. Using a simple speeded detection task, our study challenges this dominant view by providing evidence for modulations of the brain responses in deaf individuals at very early visual processing stages. Neural responses to visual events differed between deaf and hearing participants already in the C1 ERP component (50–95 ms) associated with striate cortex activity. Furthermore, substantial differences between the two subjects' groups emerged in the latency range of the P1 component (80–150 ms) for both warning and target stimuli. The P1 complex was prolonged in deaf relative to hearing participants, with a biphasic morphology in 7 out of 10 deaf participants at least in the responses to the (salient) warning signal. This finding thus sets the initial hallmark for a divergence in visual processing between deaf and hearing individuals at the first cortical stages, about 100 ms before that documented in previous reports [5,16].

Our findings also provide the first evidence that this altered dynamics of early visual ERPs may play a functional role in the changes observed at the behavioural level in the deaf. In both subjects' groups, the speed of the upcoming response was linearly related to the N1 peak amplitude. This finding corroborates previous evidence in hearing individuals [32] showing a linear relationship between RTs and N1 amplitude. Strikingly, our results also revealed that the relationship between the electrical brain response and reaction time dissociates between the two groups, precisely in the early ERP component that differs the most substantially between deaf and hearing individuals (i.e., the P1 complex). In the deaf group only, RTs decreased linearly with P1 peak amplitude . This calls for two remarks. First, it may seem paradoxical that RTs in the Deaf were not related to P1 latency (rather than amplitude) as this component was prolonged in this group, resulting in a change in its peak latency. As noted above however, this prolonged P1 complex stems more from a change in P1 morphology rather than an actual delay of the response. Second, the important point is that the ERP component that predicts the behavioural measures is anticipated in deaf (P1) compared to hearing subjects (N1) by a time globally corresponding to the anticipation of the behavioural responses (it is remarkable to note that the difference between the P1 and N1 peak latencies is around 50 ms, roughly the amount of difference between the RTs of deaf and hearing subjects).

To sum up, changes in initial stages of visual processing predict enhanced visual reactivity in deaf individuals. Thus, the reactivity

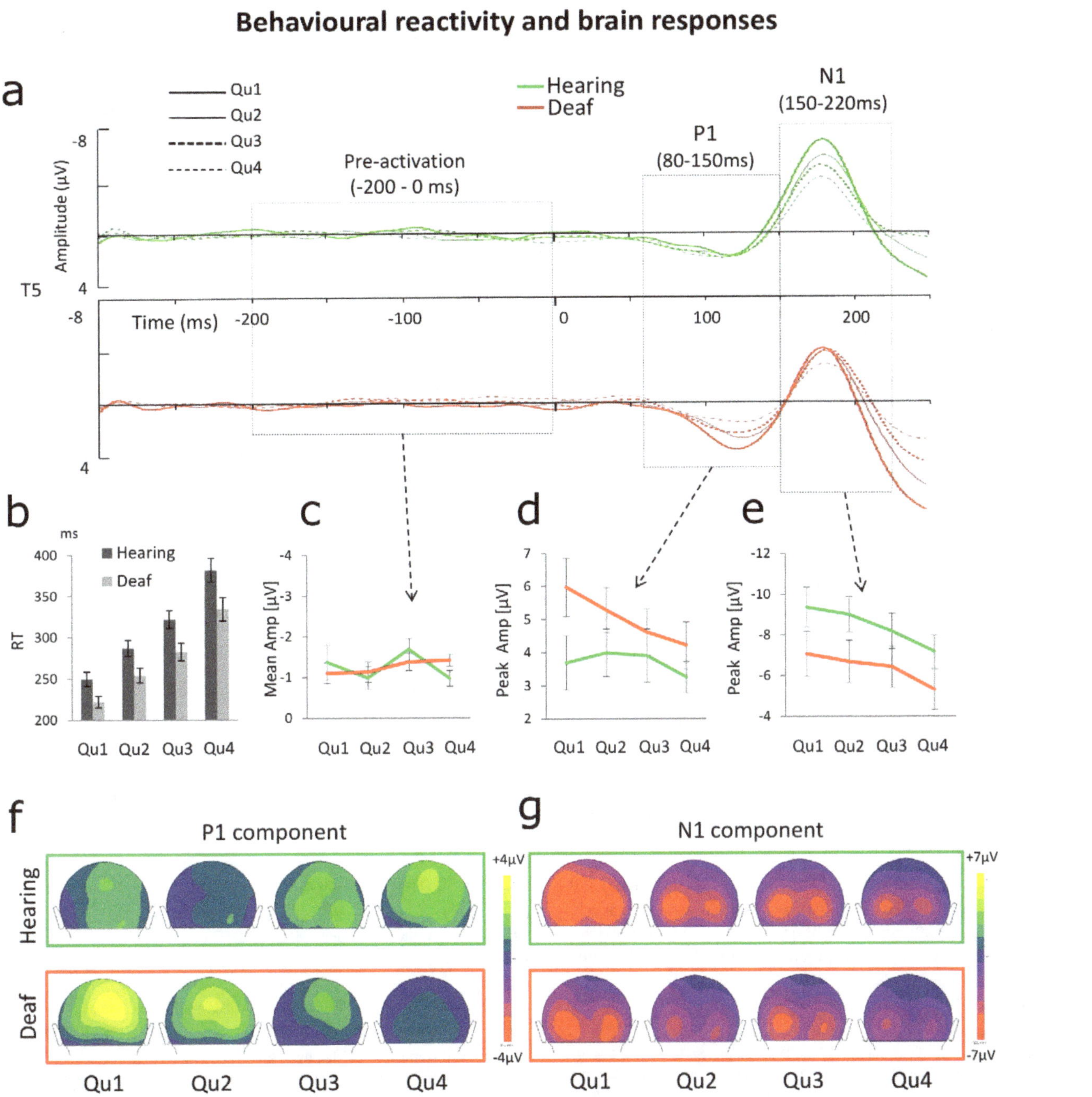

Figure 5. Correlation between behavioural reactivity and brain responses. The figure depicts the main ERP components as a function of RTs in deaf individuals and in hearing controls. (**a**, **b**) For each participant trials were sorted into 4 quartiles as a function of the response speed, from the fastest (Qu1) to the slowest (Qu4), and ERPs were averaged within each quartile. (**c**) In both groups the mean amplitude of the pre-stimulus activity (leftmost dashed area in (**a**) see text) was unrelated to the RTs. (**d**) By contrast, the peak amplitude of the P1 component (central dashed area in (**a**)) decreases linearly as a function of RTs in deaf participants, but not in hearing controls. (**e**) Finally, in both groups the peak amplitude of the N1 component (rightmost dashed area in (**a**) decreased monotonically as a function of RTs. The lower panel illustrates these results by showing the topographies of the P1 (**f**) and N1 (**g**) components around their respective peak latencies in both subjects' groups as a function of the four quartiles: the potential fields related to P1 peak decrease with increasing RTs only for the deaf group, whereas N1 potentials decrease similarly in the two groups with increasing RTs.

advantage in this sensory deprived population cannot be ascribed to response preparation alone, but emerge also within the visual system before response release. This is also corroborated by two observations: (i) in behavioural measurements, the occasional anticipatory responses were comparable between groups, and (ii) in ERPs, the amplitude of preparatory activities did not predict RT advantages (Fig. 5c).

One possible account for the early visual changes we observed in deaf adults is linked to selective attention. Behavioural and neural changes in the visual processing of the profoundly deaf have been linked to changes in selective visual attention [5,6,9]. Although in our task orienting of attentional resources to the target was not a mandatory stage before the response (unlike in visual discrimination tasks), the visual onsets of the salient warning signal and the targets surely captured the participant's exogenous attention. The changes in the P1 dynamics in the deaf may thus reflect stronger exogenous attention capture in deaf compared to hearing subjects. This is compatible with recent data showing that exogenous attention can indeed affect the P1 ERP complex [33], and that specifically the second phase of the P1 component could be modulated by attentional capture [34].

Nonetheless, this attentional account cannot easily explain the latency difference observed in the C1 component. Although an increasing number of evidences suggests that attention and perceptual load can modulate the C1 component [27,28,29,30], all the effects reported were expressed by C1 amplitude changes. As the C1 component reflects the initial stage of striate cortex activity, the observed latency difference could represent a plastic change in V1 or in an earlier visual stage in deaf individuals. As a general remark, it should be noted that morphological changes at various stages of the central nervous system as a consequence of profound deafness could indeed have contributed to the early changes we observed in visual ERPs. Recently Codina and colleagues (2011) [35] found evidence for cross-modal plasticity effects as early as at the retinal level (larger neural rim areas within the neural optic nerve head, suggesting a greater number of retinal ganglion cells in deaf individuals compared to hearing controls). In addition, at the subcortical level, aberrant retinal projections to the auditory thalamus and to the intermediate layers of the superior colliculus have been described in deaf mice [36]. Although to our knowledge, gray matter changes have not been documented in the visual cortex of deaf humans [14], the existence of atypical white matter fibers has been reported in deaf animals and deaf humans. At the cortical level, recent studies using DTI (diffusion tensor imaging) have reported increased anisotropy in the forceps major of the corpus callosum in early deaf adults, suggesting increased connectivity between visual cortices in these individuals [37,38]. These morphological changes, observed at several stages of the visual pathway could be responsible for the modified dynamics of the C1 (striate cortex) and P1 (extra-striate cortices) ERP components in deaf compared to hearing subjects, without claiming an attentional explanation.

A final important aspect of our findings is that the ERP differences between deaf and hearing subjects were largely comparable for visual events at 3 or 8 degrees of eccentricity (targets) and, perhaps more surprisingly, even for visual events delivered at fixation (warning signal). This result is compatible with the observation of enhanced visual reactivity regardless of stimulus eccentricity in deaf compared to hearing subjects [4], but it contrasts with the widespread assumption that compensatory changes of visual processing in the deaf should emerge selectively for events appearing towards the periphery of the visual field. While a special role of the visual periphery in profound deafness is undisputed, and documented also by some aspects of the present findings (see behavioural results in Fig. 1c), our results clearly indicate that early changes in visual processing occur for events at both central and peripheral portions of the visual field.

In conclusion, the present findings extend previous views on the cross-modal effects of deafness on visual processing in various ways. First, they show that auditory deprivation can alter visual processing from the earliest cortical stages. Second, they reveal a link between reactivity to visual events in profound deafness and changes occuring at early stages of visual processing, thus providing the first evidence of co-variation between modified brain activity (cortical plasticity) and behavioural enhancement in this sensory deprived population. This suggests that the stage of visual processing which accumulates the critical perceptual evidence to trigger the simple detection response may be anticipated in deaf compared to hearing individuals. While speculative this interpretation of the relation between brain response and behavioural reactivity suggests that profound deafness may not just re-structure the spatial processing of the visual scene (with enhanced abilities for the periphery of the visual field), but may also modify the timing of visual functions.

Acknowledgments

We wish to thank the Ente Nazionale Sordi (Trento), and particularly Brunella Grigolli for coordinating the recruitment of the deaf participants. We are grateful to Pierre-Emmanuel Aguera, Emmanuel Maby and Massimo Vescovi for the technical support, Veronica Mazza for the help during the EEG recordings, and David Melcher for comments on an earlier version of this manuscript.

Author Contributions

Conceived and designed the experiments: DB FP. Analyzed the data: DB AC M-HG. Wrote the paper: DB AC M-HG FP. Acquired the ERP data: DB.

References

1. Loke WH, Song S (1991) Central and peripheral visual processing in hearing and nonhearing individuals. Bulletin of the Psychonomic Society 29: 437–440.
2. Reynolds HN (1993) Effects of foveal stimulation on peripheral visual processing and laterality in deaf and hearing subjects. The American Journal of Psychology 106: 523–540.
3. Bottari D, Nava E, Ley P, Pavani F (2010) Enhanced reactivity to visual stimuli in deaf individuals. Restorative Neurology and Neuroscience 28: 167–179.
4. Pavani F, Bottari D (in press) Visual abilities in individuals with profound deafness: a critical review. In: Murray MM, Wallace M, eds. Frontiers in the Neural Bases of Multisensory Processes. Boca Raton, FL: CRC Press.
5. Neville HJ, Lawson D (1987) Attention to central and peripheral visual space in a movement detection task: an event-related potential and behavioral study. II. Congenitally deaf adults. Brain Research 405: 268–283.
6. Parasnis I, Samar VJ (1985) Parafoveal attention in congenitally deaf and hearing young adults. Brain and Cognition 4: 313–327.
7. Stivalet P, Moreno Y, Richard J, Barraud PA, Raphel C (1998) Differences in visual search tasks between congenitally deaf and normally hearing adults. Cognitive Brain Research 6: 227–232.
8. Colmenero JM, Catena A, Fuentes LJ, Ramos MM (2004) Mechanisms of visuo-spatial orienting in deafness. European Journal of Cognitive Psychology 16: 791–805.
9. Bavelier D, Dye MW, Hauser PC (2006) Do deaf individuals see better? Trends in Cognitive Sciences 10: 512–518.
10. Merabet LB, Pascual-Leone A (2010) Neural reorganization following sensory loss: the opportunity of change. Nature Reviews Neuroscience 11: 44–52.
11. Bavelier D, Deruelle C, Proksch J (2000) Positive and negative compatibility effects. Perception & Psychophysics 62: 100–112.
12. Bavelier D, Brozinsky C, Tomann A, Mitchell T, Neville H, et al. (2001) Impact of early deafness and early exposure to sign language on the cerebral organization for motion processing. Journal of Neuroscience 21: 8931–8942.
13. Finney EM, Fine I, Dobkins KR (2001) Visual stimuli activate auditory cortex in the deaf. Nature Neuroscience 4: 1171–1173.
14. Fine I, Finney EM, Boynton GM, Dobkins KR (2005) Comparing the effects of auditory deprivation and sign language within the auditory and visual cortex. Journal of Cognitive Neuroscience 17: 1621–1637.
15. Lomber SG, Meredith MA, Kral A (2010) Cross-modal plasticity in specific auditory cortices underlies visual compensations in the deaf. Nature Neuroscience 13: 1421–1427.
16. Armstrong BA, Neville HJ, Hillyard SA, Mitchell TV (2002) Auditory deprivation affects processing of motion, but not color. Cognitive Brain Research 14: 422–434.
17. Di Russo F, Martinez A, Sereno MI, Pitzalis S, Hillyard SA (2002) Cortical sources of the early components of the visual evoked potential. Human Brain Mapping 15: 95–111.
18. Luck SJ, Heinze HJ, Mangun GR, Hillyard SA (1990) Visual event-related potentials index focused attention within bilateral stimulus arrays. II. Functional dissociation of P1 and N1 components. Electroencephalography and Clinical Neurophysiology 75: 528–542.
19. Saarinen J, Rovamo J, Virsu V (1989) Analysis of spatial structure in eccentric vision. Investigative Ophthalmology & Visual Science 30: 293–296.

20. Comon P (1994) Independent Component Analysis, a new concept? Signal Processing 36: 287–314.
21. Mennes M, Wouters H, Vanrumste B, Lagae L, Stiers P (2010) Validation of ICA as a tool to remove eye movement artifacts from EEG/ERP. Psychophysiology 47: 1142–50.
22. Perrin F, Pernier J, Bertrand O, Echallier JF (1989) Spherical splines for scalp potential and current density mapping. Electroencephalography and Clinical Neurophysiology 72: 184–187.
23. Perrin F, Pernier J, Bertrand O, Giard MH, Echallier JF (1987) Mapping of scalp potentials by surface spline interpolation. Electroencephalography and Clinical Neurophysiology 66: 75–81.
24. Aguera PE, Jerbi K, Caclin A, Bertrand O (2011) ELAN: A software package for analysis and visualization of MEG, EEG, and LFP signals. Computational Intelligence and Neuroscience, vol. 2011, Article ID 158970, 11 p. doi: 10.1155/2011/158970.
25. Trillenberg P, Verleger R, Wascher E, Wauschkuhn B, Wessel K (2000) CNV and temporal uncertainty with 'ageing' and 'non-ageing' S1–S2 intervals. Clinical Neurophysiology 111: 1216–1226.
26. Foxe JJ, Strugstad EC, Sehatpour P, Molholm S, Pasieka W, et al. (2008) Parvocellular and magnocellular contributions to the initial generators of the visual evoked potential: high-density electrical mapping of the "C1" component. Brain Topography 21: 11–21.
27. Proverbio AM, Del Zotto M, Zani A (2010) Electrical neuroimaging evidence that spatial frequency-based selective attention affects V1 activity as early as 40–60 ms in humans. BMC Neuroscience 11: 59.
28. Rauss KS, Pourtois G, Vuilleumier P, Schwartz S (2009) Attentional load modifies early activity in human primary visual cortex. Human Brain Mapping 30: 1723–33.
29. Fu S, Fedota JR, Greenwood PM, Parasuraman R (2010) Dissociation of visual C1 and P1 components as a function of attentional load: an event-related potential study. Biological Psychology 85: 171–8.
30. Karns CM, Knight RT (2009) Intermodal auditory, visual, and tactile attention modulates early stages of neural processing. Journal of Cognitive Neuroscience 21: 669–83.
31. Doucet ME, Bergeron F, Lassonde M, Ferron P, Lepore F (2006) Cross-modal reorganization and speech perception in cochlear implant users. Brain 129: 3376–83.
32. Talsma D, Mulckhuyse M, Slagter HA, Theeuwes J (2007) Faster, more intense! The relation between electrophysiological reflections of attentional orienting, sensory gain control, and speed of responding. Brain Research 1178: 92–105.
33. Chica AB, Lupianez J (2009) Effects of endogenous and exogenous attention on visual processing: an Inhibition of Return study. Brain Research 1278: 75–85.
34. Hopfinger JB, West VM (2006) Interactions between endogenous and exogenous attention on cortical visual processing. NeuroImage 31: 774–789.
35. Codina C, Pascalis O, Mody C, Toomey P, Rose J, et al. (2011) Visual advantage in deaf adults linked to retinal changes. PLoS One 6: e20417.
36. Hunt DL, King B, Kahn DM, Yamoah EN, Shull GE, et al. (2005) Aberrant retinal projections in congenitally deaf mice: how are phenotypic characteristics specified in development and evolution? Anat Rec A Discov Mol Cell Evol Biol 287: 1051–1066.
37. Kim DJ, Park SY, Kim J, Lee DH, Park HJ (2009) Alterations of white matter diffusion anisotropy in early deafness. NeuroReport 20: 1032–1036.
38. Emmorey K, Allen JS, Bruss J, Schenker N, Damasio H (2003) A morphometric analysis of auditory brain regions in congenitally deaf adults. Proceedings of National Academy of Science USA 100: 10049–54.

14

Genetic Inactivation of *Trpml3* does not Lead to Hearing and Vestibular Impairment in Mice

Simone Jörs[◔], **Christian Grimm**[◔], **Lars Becker, Stefan Heller***

Departments of Otolaryngology – Head and Neck Surgery and Molecular and Cellular Physiology, Stanford University School of Medicine, Stanford, California, United States of America

Abstract

TRPML3, a member of the transient receptor potential (TRP) family, is an inwardly rectifying, non-selective Ca^{2+}-permeable cation channel that is regulated by extracytosolic Na^+ and H^+ and can be activated by a variety of small molecules. The severe auditory and vestibular phenotype of the TRPML3(A419P) varitint-waddler mutation made this protein particularly interesting for inner ear biology. To elucidate the physiological role of murine TRPML3, we conditionally inactivated *Trpml3* in mice. Surprisingly, lack of functional TRPML3 did not lead to circling behavior, balance impairment or hearing loss.

Editor: Hiroaki Matsunami, Duke University, United States of America

Funding: This work was supported by National Institutes of Health grants DC004563 and P30 DC010363. The funders had no role in study design, data collection and analysis, decision to publish, or preparation of the manuscript.

Competing Interests: The authors have declared that no competing interests exist.

* E-mail: hellers@stanford.edu

◔ These authors contributed equally to this work.

Introduction

The mammalian TRPML gene family consists of TRPML1, TRPML2, and TRPML3. Mutations in human TRPML1 cause the lysosomal storage disease Mucolipidosis Type IV [1–3]. The murine *Trpml2* and *Trpml3* genes were identified in a positional cloning approach to find the gene responsible for the varitint-waddler (*Va*) phenotype [4]. Heterozygote *Va* mice have pigmentation defects, hearing loss, and circling behavior, whereas homozygotes display perinatal lethality [4–6]. The *Va* phenotype is caused by a single mutation (A419P) in the predicted fifth transmembrane-spanning domain (TM5) of TRPML3, which leads to a constitutively open channel, resulting in elevated $[Ca^{2+}]_i$ causing apoptosis [7–11]. Heterologously expressed TRPML3 is regulated by extracytosolic Na^+ and H^+ [8,12,13] and can be activated by a variety of small molecules [13]. Subcellular localization studies of heterologously expressed TRPML channels revealed that TRPML1 and TRPML2 are expressed in late endosomes and lysosomes, whereas TRPML3 presumably shuttles between multiple intracellular compartments and the plasma membrane [14]. The localization to intracellular vesicles and the interaction with a variety of vesicular proteins suggest that all three members may play a role in endocytic and exocytic signalling pathways [15]. In addition, heterologously expressed TRPML protein subunits are able to heteromerize with each other [13,16], and it has been hypothesized that plasma membrane-localized TRPML3 in epidermal melanocytes occurs exclusively as a subunit of uncharacterized heteromeric channels [13].

TRPML3 expression has been detected in inner ear sensory hair cells [4,17], and the *Va* mutation of the channel leads to hair cell degeneration and deafness [4,5]. On the other hand, hair cell death-mediated deafness (due to a constitutive active ion channel) is not sufficient to justify a function in the hearing process itself. To elucidate a relevant function for TRPML3 in hair cells, we generated and examined a mouse model that allows conditional *Trpml3* inactivation. Here we show that ubiquitous as well as hair cell-specific postnatal inactivation of *Trpml3* does not result in hearing and balance impairment when compared with control littermates.

Results and Discussion

Generation of a floxed Trpml3 allele (*Trpml3^{lox}*)

TRP channel knockouts have successfully been generated through targeted deletion of a genomic region encoding the presumptive pore-loop domain of the ion channel [18–20]. Therefore, we decided to target exon 11 of *Trpml3*, which encodes the pore-loop and the pore lining TM6 (Fig. 1A). We generated a targeting vector that, after homologous recombination, resulted in a modified *Trpml3* allele carrying two *loxP* sites flanking exon 11 (Fig. 1B). A *neo^R* cassette, which was used for G418/geneticin selection, was removed with Flp recombinase before the ES cells were injected into host blastocysts to generate chimeric mice (Fig. 1C). After germline transmission and continued breeding, PCR with genomic DNA from progeny of wild-type, heterozygous and homozygous animals showed proper recombination and inheritance of the *Trpml3^{lox}* allele (Fig. 2A,B). Exon 11 of the *Trpml3^{lox}* allele and the genomic sequences surrounding the recombination site were verified by sequencing.

Excision of *Trpml3* exon 11

To investigate whether TRPML3 plays a role in development, we used the X-linked *Hprt$^{Cre/+}$* driver, which mediates ubiquitous and highly efficient excision that is complete at the first stages of development [21]. *Hprt$^{Cre/+}$*;*Trpml3$^{lox/+}$* females were mated with *Trpml3$^{lox/+}$* males. The floxed exon 11 was always excised

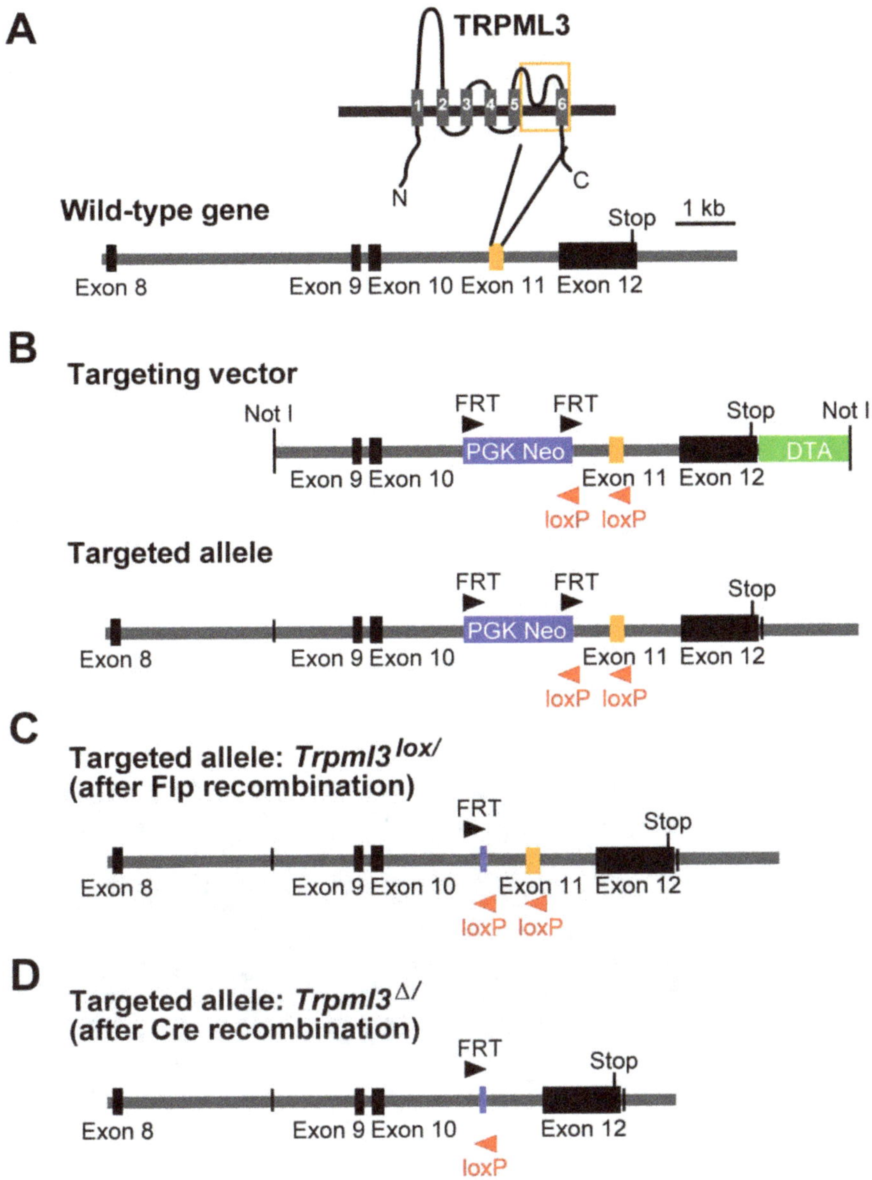

Figure 1. Targeting strategy for disruption of the *Trpml3* gene. A, Transmembrane-spanning domains are depicted as grey bars and numbered from 1–6. The orange frame indicates the part of the TRPML3 protein that is encoded by exon 11, which will be deleted (pore loop and TM6). Exons are shown as black and orange bars on the schematic genomic map below. B, Shown are the targeting vector and the targeted allele after homologous recombination. The blue bar represents the PGK promoter-driven neo^R expression cassette, which was used for positive selection. The DTA cassette, used for negative selection, is shown in green. The black and red arrowheads symbolize position and orientation of *FRT* and *loxP* sites. C, Targeted allele after Flp site-specific recombination in ES cells, resulting in excision of neo^R cassette, and leaving one FRT site behind. D, Excision of exon 11 using Cre site-specific recombinase, resulting in disruption of *Trpml3* gene.

regardless of $Hprt^{Cre}$ inheritance. Oocytes of $Hprt^{Cre}$ females have sufficiently stored Cre recombinase to excise floxed DNA segments already at the zygote or early stages [21], which most likely resulted in *Trpml3* inactivation already in the fertilized egg. The resulting $Trpml3^{\Delta}$ mutation was stably inherited (Fig 2C–E).

To examine whether the $Trpml3^{\Delta}$ allele is being transcribed, RT-PCRs were conducted (Fig. 2D,E). mRNA from kidney and inner ear was purified from dissected organs of mice of each genotype. RT-PCR amplification of specific cDNA sequences before and after the site of deletion indicated that wild-type and $Trpml3^{\Delta}$ mRNA was expressed in kidney and the inner ear of all animals (Fig. 2D,E; RT-2 and 3). Amplification of cDNA encoding exon 11 (RT-1), however, was only possible from mRNA of wild-type ($Trpml3^{+/+}$) and heterozygous animals ($Trpml3^{\Delta/+}$), but not from mRNA of $Trpml3^{\Delta/\Delta}$ mice.

An additional oligonucleotide pair was used (RT-4) to amplify the coding region comprising exons 10, 11, and 12. Sequence analysis revealed that in mutated animals, splicing occurred between exon 10 and exon 12, resulting in a 207 bp shorter message encoding a protein lacking 69 amino acids of the pore loop and TM6, but without frame shift. To demonstrate that a pore-less TRPML3 protein does not function as an ion channel, we generated cDNA encoding a fusion protein of TRPML3(Δ exon11) with yellow fluorescent protein and expressed the mutant channel protein in HEK293 cells. The subcellular distribution of the mutant channel TRPML3(Δ exon11), analyzed by confocal

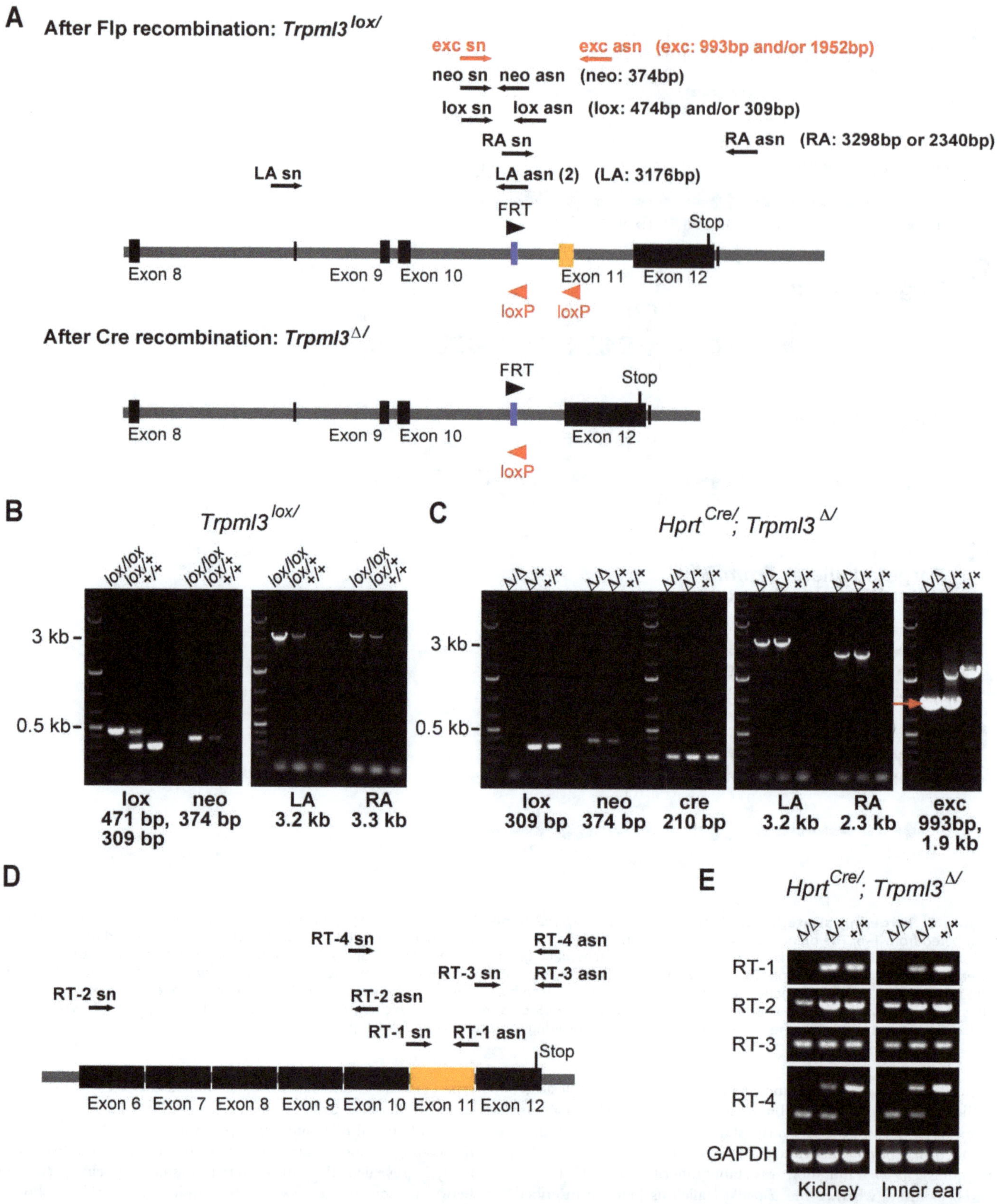

Figure 2. Genotyping analysis. A, Schematic drawing of the *Trpml3* targeted allele before ($Trpml3^{lox/}$) and after Cre recombination ($Trpml3^{\Delta/}$). The positions of sense (sn) and antisense (asn) oligonucleotides are indicated with arrows. The names of PCR products and the corresponding lengths are parenthesized. B, PCR amplification products of *Trpml3* locus of homozygous (lox/lox), heterozygous (lox/+), and wild-type (+/+) $Trpml3^{lox/}$ mice are shown: lox: 309 bp and/or 471 bp, neo: 374 bp, and left arm (LA): 3176 bp and right arm (RA): 3298 bp. C, Genotyping after Cre recombination of representative $Hprt^{Cre/}$;$Trpml3^{\Delta/}$ mice. All mice are heterozygous for *cre* (210 bp). The same sets of oligonucleotides were used as in (B), however lox-PCR only displayed the wild-type 309 bp PCR fragment, since the lox asn-oligonucleotides cannot hybridize after the targeted exon 11 was excised; and RA: 2340 bp, since exon 11 was excised by Cre. The last panel on the right shows the shortened fragment (indicated with a red arrow): 1952 bp

for *Trpml3*$^{lox/}$ and 993 bp for *Trpml3* $^{\Delta/}$. D and E, RT-PCR analysis of TRPML3 mRNA expression in kidney and inner ear from 3-week-old *Hprt*$^{Cre/}$;*Trpml3* $^{\Delta/}$ *mice.* D, Schematic illustration is showing exon 6–12. The sense (sn) and antisense (asn) oligonucleotides are indicated with black arrows. E, Amplification products RT-1 (200 bp), RT-2 (512 bp), RT-3 (181 bp), and RT-4 (473 bp for wild-type cDNA, and 266 bp for Cre targeted *Trpml3* cDNA). Oligonucleotides for GAPDH (442 bp) were used to control for RNA preparation quality. The symbol Δindicates the deleted exon 11 in the *Trpml3* allele generated by recombination of the floxed (*loxP*) locus; +, represents the wild-type locus.

microscopy, was different from wild-type TRPML3-YFP fusion protein. Mutant channel protein appeared to be absent from the plasma membrane and was mainly located intracellularly (Fig. 3A). When we used the TRPML3 agonist SN-2 to activate TRPML3(*Δ* exon11) [13], we detected no change of $[Ca^{2+}]_i$, whereas wild-type TRPML3-expressing cells responded with a robust increase in $[Ca^{2+}]_i$ (Fig. 3B). The average maximum $[Ca^{2+}]_i$ levels were 0.81±0.073 (Δratio 340nm/380nm, n = 10) for wild-type TRPML3 and −0.016±0.009 (Δratio 340nm/380nm, n = 6) for TRPML3(Δ exon11); the latter measurements did not differ significantly from the baseline average ratio of 0.319±0.038 (n = 6), indicating that TRPML3(*Δ* exon11) is an inactive ion channel when expressed in HEK293 cells. Based on these experiments, we presume that *Trpml3* $^{\Delta/\Delta}$ mice lack functional TRPML3 protein.

Evaluation of Balance and Auditory Function

Based on the *Va* phenotype, TRPML3 has been proposed to play a role in hearing and balance and the channel has been put forward as potential candidate for the hair cell mechanoelectrical transduction channel [22]. Consequently, we were curious to find out whether *Trpml3* inactivation would result in hearing and balance defects. Three-week-old *Hprt*$^{Cre/+}$;*Trpml3*$^{+/+}$, *Hprt*$^{Cre/+}$; *Trpml3* $^{\Delta/+}$, and *Hprt*$^{Cre/+}$;*Trpml3* $^{\Delta/\Delta}$ mice had normal Preyer's reflexes, characterized by a distinct movement of the pinna in response to a loud sound [23].

Auditory-evoked brainstem response (ABR) measurements were used to evaluate hearing thresholds of three-week-old mice (Fig. 3). Because the Preyer's reflex and other subjective measures to assess hearing are only effective for identification of profound hearing loss, more objective electroacoustical tests were conducted: Click, 8-, 16-, and 32 kHz tone burst measurements revealed no significant differences in ABR thresholds and interwave latencies among all three groups: *Hprt*$^{Cre/+}$;*Trpml3*$^{+/+}$, *Hprt*$^{Cre/+}$;*Trpml3* $^{\Delta/+}$, and *Hprt*$^{Cre/+}$;*Trpml3* $^{\Delta/\Delta}$ (Fig. 3A,B). Interwave latencies between wave I and wave III at 70 dB, which are indicative of the afferent auditory nerve conductance were 1.9±0.026 msec in *Hprt*$^{Cre/+}$; *Trpml3*$^{+/+}$ animals (n = 6), compared to 1.87±0.026 msec in *Hprt*$^{Cre/+}$;*Trpml3* $^{\Delta/+}$ (n = 6), and 1.86±0.019 msec in *Hprt*$^{Cre/+}$; *Trpml3* $^{\Delta/\Delta}$ littermates (n = 6). These results suggested that TRPML3 is not essential for hair cell function, synaptic signal transmission, performance of spiral ganglion neurons, and auditory nerve function. Nevertheless, because the inactivation of *Trpml3* using *Hprt*^{Cre}–mediated recombination was introduced very early in development, compensation effects cannot be excluded with this approach.

With the goal to circumvent potential compensatory mechanisms, we used tamoxifen-inducible *Math1-Cre*ER^{TM} mice [24] to inactivate TRPML3 in cochlear hair cells between P0–P3. ABR measurements of these mice at three weeks of age revealed no differences (Fig. 3C), suggesting that compensatory mechanisms most likely do not explain the lack of a TRPML3 hearing phenotype. Mice were also analyzed at 3 months of age to determine possible enhancement or early onset of age-related hearing loss. But reviewing audiograms revealed no ABR threshold difference between mutant mice and control mice (data not shown). These experiments have two important limitations. First, the tamoxifen-inducible recombination in cochlear hair cells is not complete, as revealed by analysis of crosses of *Math1-Cre*ER^{TM} mice with *Rosa26-lacZ* reporter mice [24]. Therefore, a substantial number of cochlear hair cells might have been unaffected by Cre-mediated recombination. The fact that mutant TRPML3 protein is being expressed (Fig. 3A) complicates the analysis of Cre-mediated recombination because the mutant pore-less TRPML3 protein is likely to be detectable by immunohistochemistry. Second, three weeks of loss of TRPML3 function might be enough for potential compensatory mechanisms to become effective. Nevertheless, as long as there are no clear candidates or

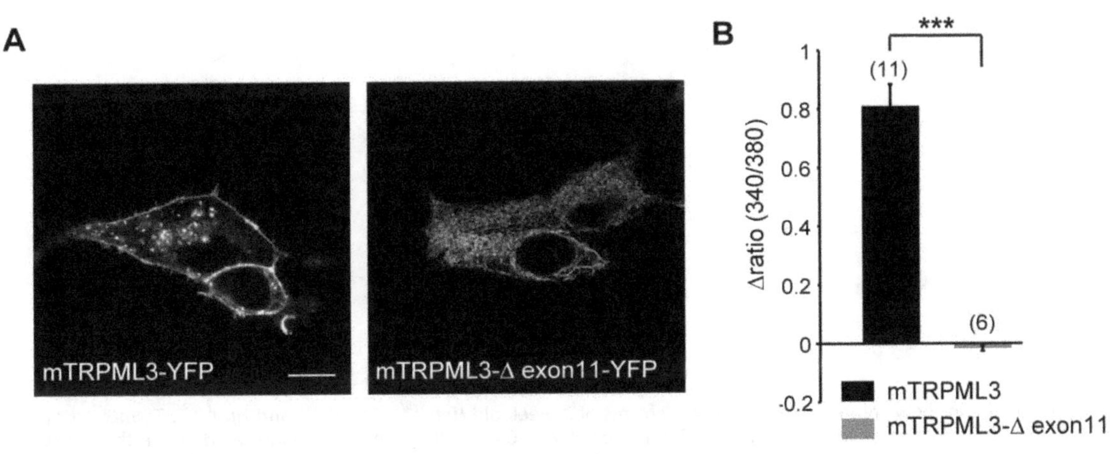

Figure 3. Molecular and functional assessment of mutant TRPML3(Δ exon11) channels. A, Shown are representative cells expressing the respective murine (m) constructs of wild-type TRPML3 or mutant TRPML3(Δ exon11), C-terminally fused to yellow fluorescent protein, 24 h after transfection. Scale bar = 10 μm. B, Ca^{2+} imaging results showing relative $[Ca^{2+}]_i$ increases after application of TRPML3 activator SN-2 in HEK293 cells expressing wild-type TRPML3 or mutant TRPML3(Δ exon11). Shown are mean values ± SEM (numbers in parentheses are the numbers of independent experiments with 10–20 cells each). Statistical comparisons of means were made using Student's *t* test (unpaired); ***p<0.0001.

mechanisms known that could provide compensation for inactivation of *Trpml3*, it is difficult to speculate about the timing of compensatory mechanisms. In summary, the use of *Math1-Cre*ER^{TM} mice did not reveal potential compensatory mechanisms of *Trpml3* inactivation, but because of the limitations of this experiment, we cannot exclude that loss of TRPML3 function is being compensated by an unknown mechanism.

To investigate whether acoustic challenge of the auditory system would reveal a more subtle role of TRPML3, we exposed $Hprt^{Cre/+}$; $Trpml3^{+/+}$ and $Hprt^{Cre/+}$;$Trpml3^{\Delta/\Delta}$ mice for 4 hr to 4 kHz pure tone at 125 dB SPL [25,26]. We compared ABR thresholds of littermates of both genotypes before and one week after the noise exposure, and we detected no difference in noise susceptibility between the two groups (Fig. 4D). Unlike knockout of TRPV4, an ion channel expressed by cochlear hair cells, spiral ganglion neurons, and stria vascularis marginal cells [27], which displays increased susceptibility to acoustic injury [25], mice carrying two inactive *Trpml3* alleles did not show increased acoustic vulnerability.

Besides evaluating the auditory system, we also assessed vestibular function in $Hprt^{Cre/+}$;$Trpml3^{+/+}$ and $Hprt^{Cre/+}$;$Trpml3^{\Delta/\Delta}$

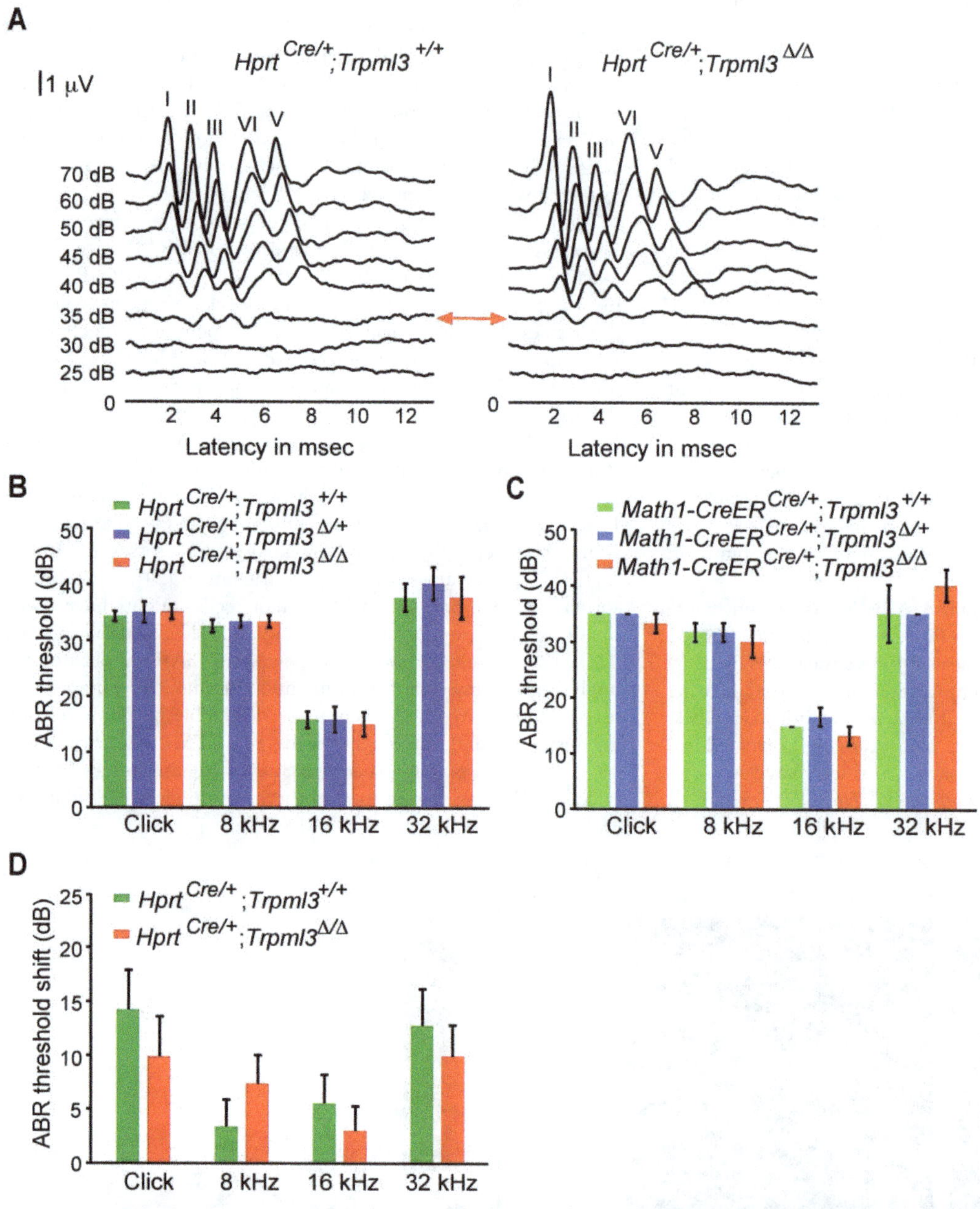

Figure 4. ABR measurements. A, Graph shows representative ABR waveforms of 3-week-old $Hprt^{Cre/+}$; $Trpml3^{+/+}$ and $Hprt^{Cre/+}$; $Trpml3^{\Delta/\Delta}$ mice in response to a click stimulus. ABRs were recorded at sound stimulation intensities of 25–70 dB. ABR waves I–V are indicated above the peaks. Red arrow highlights the hearing threshold, which is at 35 dB in this representative example pair. B, Shown are ABR thresholds (mean values ± SEM) to click, 8-, 16-, and 32 kHz stimuli of $Hprt^{Cre/+}$;$Trpml3^{+/+}$ (n = 6), $Hprt^{Cre/+}$;$Trpml3^{\Delta/+}$ (n = 6), and $Hprt^{Cre/+}$;$Trpml3^{\Delta/\Delta}$ (n = 6) and C, of $Math1\text{-}CreER^{Cre/+}$; $Trpml3^{+/+}$ (n = 3), $Math1\text{-}CreER^{Cre/+}$;$Trpml3^{\Delta/+}$ (n = 3), and $Math1\text{-}CreER^{Cre/+}$;$Trpml3^{\Delta/\Delta}$ (n = 3), respectively. Statistical comparisons of means of different genotypes were made using one-way ANOVA followed by Tukey's post test; $p>0.05$. D, ABR threshold shifts of 3-month-old $Hprt^{Cre/+}$;$Trpml3^{+/+}$ (n = 7) and $Hprt^{Cre/+}$;$Trpml3^{\Delta/\Delta}$ (n = 7) 1 week after the acoustic overexposure of 125 dB SPL at 4 kHz for 4 hr. Shown are mean values ± SEM. No significant differences were observed between genotypes ($p>0.05$, one-way ANOVA, followed by Tukey's post test).

mice. We did not notice circling behavior, head-bobbing, waddling, or imbalance when walking or when walking along the top of the 3 mm thin cage wall, suggesting normal vestibular function (data not shown). To obtain more objective and quantitative data on potential balance deficits, we performed Rotarod tests [28]. We did not measure a significant difference between *Hprt*$^{Cre/+}$;*Trpml3*$^{+/+}$ and *Hprt*$^{Cre/+}$;*Trpml3* $^{\Delta/\Delta}$ mice for the 6-day-period tested (Fig. 5), indicating that inactivation of *Trpml3* does not lead to balance defects in this test.

Despite the strong *Va* phenotype, which is caused by constitutively active TRPML3, no overt inner ear phenotype was detectable in mice with ubiquitous *Trpml3* inactivation or when the gene was inactivated from P0–P3 onwards. This finding supports the previous conclusion that the TRPML3(A419P) mutation of *Va* mice is a gain-of-function mutation, which has been hypothesized to cause Ca^{2+}-loading of cells and subsequently apoptotic cell death [7–11]. Loss of functional *Trpml3*, on the other hand, is not causing a detectable phenotype in the inner ear. Moreover, *Hprt*$^{Cre/+}$;*Trpml3* $^{\Delta/\Delta}$ mice were indistinguishable from their wild-type littermates in size and weight. *Trpml3* $^{\Delta/\Delta}$ mice inherited the mutation stably and homozygous mutant animals displayed normal breeding performance.

We suggest several possible explanations for the lack of a phenotype in *Trpml3* $^{\Delta/\Delta}$ mice. The first possibility is that *Trpml3* is not essential for inner ear function and that in *Va* mice, the channel protein is turned into a constitutively active and cytotoxic channel. This would mean, however, that the native TRPML3 channel does not fulfill essential detectable functions in the inner ear *in vivo*. Another possibility is that our tests were not sufficient to reveal more subtle roles of TRPML3 such as potential modulatory roles in hair cells or other parts of the auditory and vestibular system.

Finally, it is a distinct possibility that native TRPML3 proteins are dispensable subunits of heteromeric channels. A different TRP channel, such as the related TRPML2 might compensate for loss of TRPML3. Heteromerisation of TRPML channels has been shown previously [12,15]. This hypothesis is supported by the observation that a dominant negative isoform of TRPML3, when transfected into epidermal melanocytes, is able to inhibit activation of a presumptively heteromeric channel consisting of TRPML3 and other unknown subunits [13]. Such a mechanism is potentially testable by generation of mice with inactivating mutations in *Trpml3* and one or more additional genes that encode potential heteromeric subunits. This strategy might ultimately reveal the physiological function of TRPML3-containing channels in sensory hair cells and other cell types of the body.

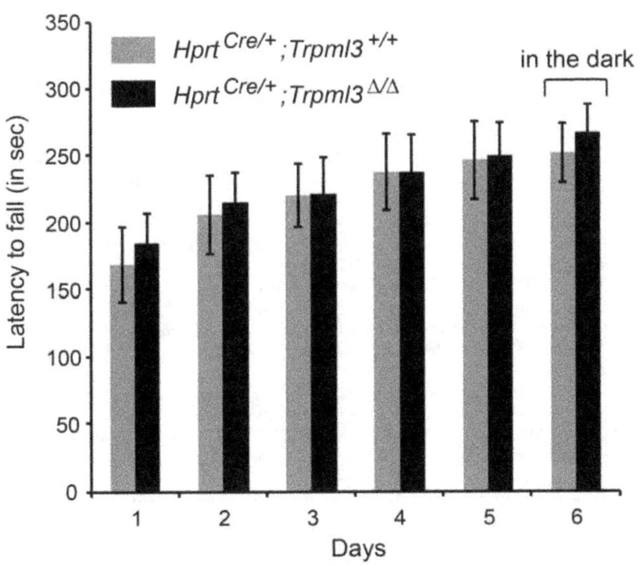

Figure 5. Rotarod experiments. The average latencies to fall ± SEM (in sec) are shown for 3-month-old *Hprt*$^{Cre/+}$;*Trpml3*$^{+/+}$ (n = 8) and *Hprt*$^{Cre/+}$;*Trpml3* $^{\Delta/\Delta}$ (n = 8) mice. The experiment was executed over a time range of 6 days. The day 6 experiment was performed in the dark to exclude compensation via visual cues. The difference between genotypes was not statistically significant at any given time point ($p>0.05$, one-way ANOVA, followed by Tukey's post test).

Materials and Methods

Targeting construct

Genomic 129sv/svj mouse DNA was used for PCR-amplification of DNA sequences flanking exon 11 of *Trpml3* (Fig. 1). pBluescript II SK(+) vector (Stratagene): Left arm (*Sal*I), FRT-flanked neomycin resistance marker (*neo*^{R}) (*Hind*III), *loxP*-flanked Intron-Exon11-Intron (*Eco*RI), right arm (*Sma*I), and Diphteria toxin A (DTA) cassette (*Spe*I and *Sac*I). The sequence-verified and linearized targeting vector DNA was electroporated into 129sv/svj ES cells (Stanford transgenic research center (http://med.stanford.edu/transgenic)) and two independent clones with proper homologous recombination were selected by PCR amplification and sequencing of the integration sites. The *neo*^{R}-cassette was excised with Flp recombinase and the ES cells carrying the targeted *Trpml3* allele were injected into blastocysts to generate chimeras. Mating of male chimeras with C57BL/6J females produced heterozygous transgenic founders that were crossed and maintained in FVB/NJ background, which was selected for analysis because this strain does not exhibit early onset age-related hearing loss [29].

Mice and Genotyping

FVB/NJ mice (Jackson Laboratory stock number 001800), *Math1-Cre*ER^{TM} mice (provided by Dr. S.J. Baker, St. Jude, Memphis, TN), and *Hprt*^{Cre} mice (provided by Dr. M. Krasnow, Stanford University) were used. Both driver strains were crossed for at least ten generations into FVB/NJ background before crossing them with mice carrying the *Trpml3*^{lox} allele. *Trpml3*^{lox} mice had been crossed into FVB/NJ background for at least three generations. Genomic DNA was isolated from mouse tails (DNEasy, Qiagen, Valencia, CA). Animal studies were conducted in accordance with protocols approved by the Administrative Panel on Laboratory Animal Care at Stanford University. The protocol number is #11961.

Induction of Cre activity

Tamoxifen (Sigma) was dissolved in prewarmed sterile corn oil (Sigma) at a concentration of 3 mg/ml. A 26-gauge needle insulin syringe was used for intraperitoneal injections between P0 and P3 at 3–4 mg/40 g body weight. Three injections were separated by 24 hours.

Heterologous expression of TRPML3 isoforms and calcium imaging

HEK293 cells were grown and maintained in a standard humidified 37°C incubator, with 95% air and 5% CO_2. The cells were maintained in DMEM (Cellgro), supplemented with 10% fetal bovine serum (Omega scientific), and 100 µg/ml penicillin and streptomycin (Cellgro). For calcium imaging experiments and localization studies all plasmid constructs were transiently expressed in HEK293 cells with the use of Genejammer (Stratagene), and analyzed 24 hr after transfection. Expression vectors were based on pcDNA3.1 (Invitrogen). For calcium imaging experiments, the cells were loaded with 4 μM fura-2-AM (Invitrogen) in a solution containing 138 mM NaCl, 6 mM KCl, 2 mM $MgCl_2$, 2 mM $CaCl_2$, 10 mM HEPES, and 5.5 mM D-glucose (300 mOsmol/kg and adjusted to pH 7.4 with NaOH). Measurements of $[Ca^{2+}]_i$ with the fluorescent indicator were performed using a monochromatic-based imaging system (iMIC platform and Polychrome V monochromator, TILL Photonics). TRPML3 activator SN-2 (5-mesityl-3-oxa-4-azatricyclo[5.2.1.02,6]dec-4-ene) (Specs) was used at a final concentration of 10 μM [13].

Auditory brainstem response (ABR) measurements and noise exposure

The ABR procedure was done as previously described [11]. The absolute threshold was obtained for each animal by reducing the stimulus intensity in 5 dB steps to identify the lowest intensity at which the first ABR wave was detectable. The latency (time delay from when the stimulus is presented (0 msec) until its peak occurs) was determined after detecting all peaks in click ABR waveforms I–V at 70 dB. Interwave latencies between the peaks of ABR waves I and III were calculated. Three months old $Hprt^{Cre/+}$; $Trpml3^{+/+}$ and $Hprt^{Cre/+}$;$Trpml3^{\Delta/\Delta}$ mice were exposed 4 hr to 4 kHz pure tone at 125 dB SPL (sound pressure level) in a truncated pyramid-shaped exposure box [26] to examine the effects of TRPML3 inactivation on acoustic injury of the cochlea. Shifts in the ABR thresholds were determined after 1 week.

Motor coordination tests

A four track Rotarod (Columbus Instruments) was used to test for a balance or motoric impairment in 3 months old $Hprt^{Cre/+}$; $Trpml3^{+/+}$ and $Hprt^{Cre/+}$;$Trpml3^{\Delta/\Delta}$. The mice were acquainted with the instrument (without rotating) daily for five days, and one day before the first trial, the mice were placed on the Rotarod for 90 sec at a constant speed of 3 rpm to familiarize them with the procedure. For testing, the mice were placed onto the rod for a 330 sec trial with constant acceleration from 3 rpm to 40 rpm. Four trials with 45 min inter-trial periods were performed each day. The trials on day 6 were performed in the dark. The time until fall was automatically recorded, while the maximal time was noted for mice staying until 40 rpm.

Statistical analysis

Data are presented as mean ± SEM with the number of independent experiments indicated (n). Statistical comparisons were made using either one-way ANOVA followed by Tukey's post test or Student's *t* test (unpaired) and KaleidaGraph Synergy software. Differences were considered significant when $p<0.01$ (*), and highly significant when $p<0.0001$ (***).

Acknowledgments

We thank Dr. H. Zeng (Stanford Transgenic Research Facility) for assistance with generating the floxed allele, Dr. G. Popelka (Stanford) for technical support with ABR measurements, and Dr. D. Salih (Stanford) for help with Rotarod tests.

Author Contributions

Conceived and designed the experiments: SJ CG SH. Performed the experiments: SJ CG LB. Analyzed the data: SJ CG LB SH. Wrote the paper: SJ CG SH.

References

1. Bargal R, Avidan N, Ben-Asher E, Olender Z, Zeigler M, et al. (2000) Identification of the gene causing mucolipidosis type IV. Nat Genet 26: 118–123.
2. Sun M, Goldin E, Stahl S, Falardeau JL, Kennedy JC, et al. (2000) Mucolipidosis type IV is caused by mutations in a gene encoding a novel transient receptor potential channel. Hum Mol Genet 9: 2471–2478.
3. Bach G (2001) Minireview Mucolipidosis Type IV. Mol Genet Metab 73: 197–203.
4. Di Palma F, Belyantseva IA, Kim HJ, Vogt TF, Kachar B, et al. (2002) Mutations in Mcoln3 associated with deafness and pigmentation defects in varitint-waddler (Va) mice. Proc Natl Acad Sci U S A 99: 14994–14999.
5. Cable J, Steel KP (1998) Combined cochleo-saccular and neuroepithelial abnormalities in the Varitint-waddler-J (Va^J) mouse. Hear Res 123: 125–136.
6. Kim HJ, Jackson T, Noben-Trauth K (2003) Genetic analyses of mouse deafness mutation Varitint-waddler (Va) and Jerker ($Espn^{je}$). J Assoc Res Otolaryngol 4: 83–90.
7. Grimm C, Cuajungco MP, van Aken AF, Schnee M, Jörs S, et al. (2007) A helix-breaking mutation in TRPML3 leads to constitutive activity underlying deafness in the varitint-waddler mouse. Proc Natl Acad Sci U S A 104: 19583–19588.
8. Kim HJ, Li Q, Tjon-Kon-Sang S, So I, Kiselyov K, et al. (2007) Gain-of-function mutation in TRPML3 causes the mouse Varitint-Waddler phenotype. J Biol Chem 282: 36138–36142.
9. Nagata K, Zheng L, Madathany T, Castiglioni AJ, Bartles JR, et al. (2008) The varitint-waddler (Va) deafness mutation in TRPML3 generates constitutive, inward rectifying currents and causes cell degeneration. Proc Natl Acad Sci U S A 105: 353–358.
10. Xu H, Delling M, Li L, Dong X, Clapham DE (2007) Activating mutation in a mucolipin transient receptor potential channel leads to melanocyte loss in varitint-waddler mice. Proc Natl Acad Sci U S A 104: 18321–18326.
11. Grimm C, Jörs S, Heller S (2009) Life and death of sensory hair cells expressing constitutively active TRPML3. J Biol Chem 284: 13823–13831.
12. Kim HJ, Li Q, Tjon-Kon-Sang S, So I, Kiselyov K, et al. (2008) A novel mode of TRPML3 regulation by extracytosolic pH absent in the varitint-waddler phenotype. EMBO J 27: 1197–1205.
13. Grimm C, Jörs S, Saldana A, Obukov AG, Pan B, et al. (2010) Small molecule activators of TRPML3. Chemistry & Biology 17: 135–148.
14. Kim HJ, Soyombo AA, Tjon-Kon-Sang S, So I, Muallem S (2009) The Ca^{2+} channel TRPML3 regulates membrane trafficking and autophagy. Traffic 10: 1157–1167.
15. Cheng X, Shen D, Samie M, Xu H (2010) Mucolipins: Intracellular TRPML1–3 channels. FEBS Letters 584: 2013–2021.
16. Venkatachalam K, Hofmann T, Montell C (2006) Lysosomal localization of TRPML3 depends on TRPML2 and the mucolipidosis-associated protein TRPML1. J Biol Chem 281: 17517–17527.
17. van Aken AF, Atiba-Davies M, Marcotti W, Goodyear RJ, Bryant JE, et al. (2008) TRPML3 mutations cause impaired mechano-electrical transduction and depolarization by an inward-rectifier cation current in auditory hair cells of varitint-waddler mice. J Physiol 586: 5403–5418.
18. Kwan KY, Allchorne AJ, Vollrath MA, Christensen AP, Zhang D, et al. (2006) TRPA1 contributes to cold, mechanical and chemical nociception but is not essential for hair-cell transduction. Neuron 59: 277–289.
19. Bautista DM, Jordt SE, Nikai T, Tsuruda PR, Read AJ, et al. (2006) TRPA1 mediates the inflammatory action of environmental irritants and proalgesic agents. Cell 124: 1269–1282.
20. Moqrich A, Wook Hwang S, Earley TJ, Petrus MJ, Murray AN, et al. (2005) Impaired thermosensation in mice lacking TRPV3, a heat and camphor sensor in the skin. Science 307: 1468–1472.
21. Tang SHE, Silva FJ, Tsark WMK, Mann JR (2002) A Cre/loxP-deleter transgenic line in mouse strain 129S1/SvImJ. Genesis 32: 199–202.
22. Cuajungco MP, Grimm C, Heller S (2007) TRP channels as candidates for hearing and balance abnormalities in vertebrates. Biochimica et Biophysica Acta 1772: 1022–1027.
23. Jero J, Coling DE, Lalwani AK (2001) The use of Preyer's reflex in evaluation of hearing in mice. Acta Oto-Laryngologica 121: 585–589.
24. Chow LML, Tian Y, Weber T, Corbett M, Zuo J, et al. (2006) Inducible Cre recombinase activity in mouse cerebellar granule cell precursors and inner ear hair cells. Dev Dyn 235: 2991–2998.
25. Tabuchi K, Suzuki M, Mizuno A, Hara A (2005) Hearing impairment in TRPV4 knockout mice. Neurosci Lett 382: 304–308.
26. Liberman MC, Gao WY (1995) Chronic chochlear de-efferentation and susceptibility to permanent acoustic injury. Hearing Research 90: 158–168.
27. Liedtke W, Choe Y, Martí-Renom MA, Bell AM, Denis CS, et al. (2000) Vanilloid receptor-related osmotically activated channel (VR-OAC), a candidate vertebrate osmoreceptor. Cell 103: 525–535.
28. Jones BJ, Roberts DJ (1968) The quantitative measurement of motor inco-ordination in naive mice using an accelerating rotarod. J Pharm Pharmac 20: 302–304.
29. Zheng QY, Johnson KR, Erway LC (1999) Assessment of hearing in 80 inbred strains of mice by ABR threshold analyses. Hear Res 130: 94–107.

Tracking the Expression of Excitatory and Inhibitory Neurotransmission-Related Proteins and Neuroplasticity Markers after Noise Induced Hearing Loss

Cherylea J. Browne, John W. Morley, Carl H. Parsons*

Department of Anatomy and Cell Biology, School of Medicine, The University of Western Sydney, Sydney, New South Wales, Australia

Abstract

Excessive exposure to loud noise can damage the cochlea and create a hearing loss. These pathologies coincide with a range of CNS changes including reorganisation of frequency representation, alterations in the pattern of spontaneous activity and changed expression of excitatory and inhibitory neurotransmitters. Moreover, damage to the cochlea is often accompanied by acoustic disorders such as hyperacusis and tinnitus, suggesting that one or more of these neuronal changes may be involved in these disorders, although the mechanisms remain unknown. We tested the hypothesis that excessive noise exposure increases expression of markers of excitation and plasticity, and decreases expression of inhibitory markers over a 32-day recovery period. Adult rats (n = 25) were monaurally exposed to a loud noise (16 kHz, 1/10th octave band pass (115 dB SPL)) for 1-hour, or left as non-exposed controls (n = 5). Animals were euthanased at either 0, 4, 8, 16 or 32 days following acoustic trauma. We used Western Blots to quantify protein levels of $GABA_A$ receptor subunit $\alpha 1$ ($GABA_A\alpha 1$), Glutamic-Acid Decarboxylase-67 (GAD-67), N-Methyl-D-Aspartate receptor subunit 2A (NR2A), Calbindin (Calb1) and Growth Associated Protein 43 (GAP-43) in the Auditory Cortex (AC), Inferior Colliculus (IC) and Dorsal Cochlear Nucleus (DCN). Compared to sham-exposed controls, noise-exposed animals had significantly ($p<0.05$): lower levels of $GABA_A\alpha 1$ in the contralateral AC at day-16 and day-32, lower levels of GAD-67 in the ipsilateral DCN at day-4, lower levels of Calb1 in the ipsilateral DCN at day-0, lower levels of $GABA_A\alpha 1$ in the ipsilateral AC at day-4 and day-32. GAP-43 was reduced in the ipsilateral AC for the duration of the experiment. These complex fluctuations in protein expression suggests that for at least a month following acoustic trauma the auditory system is adapting to a new pattern of sensory input.

Editor: Giorgio F. Gilestro, Imperial College London, United Kingdom

Funding: This work was supported by a University of Western Sydney project grant pg82909. C.J. Browne is the recipient of a UWS post-graduate research award. The funders had no role in study design, data collection and analysis, decision to publish, or preparation of the manuscript.

Competing Interests: The authors have declared that no competing interests exist.

* E-mail: c.parsons@uws.edu.au

Introduction

Noise-induced hearing loss (NIHL) is a major and growing problem in the world today. At present, more people are exposed to damaging levels of noise in the workplace, at entertainment venues and the increasing use of personal listening devices (PLD) such as iPods, radios, CD players and mp3 players, is becoming a major concern [1,2,3]. It is known that intense noise exposure leads to temporary threshold shifts in hearing, but also that in some instances permanent loss occurs and this may be accompanied by auditory disorders such as tinnitus and hyperacusis in humans [4]. Noise exposure causes a range of changes throughout the auditory pathway including an imbalance of excitatory and inhibitory transmitter systems [5,6,7,8,9,10]. This suggests that these molecular changes may be involved in causing auditory disorders, although the mechanisms and site/s of generation have yet to be identified.

This study focuses on the excitatory and inhibitory neurotransmission-related proteins and changes in neuroplasticity-related proteins in the auditory pathway up to one month following acoustic trauma. The central nervous system relies on a fine balance of excitatory and inhibitory inputs [11], and an imbalance may have significant physiological implications in the auditory system. An imbalance may influence the reorganization of tonotopy and could lead to changes in spontaneous activity, which has been previously reported after acoustic trauma [12,13,14,15,16,17,18,19]. Many studies have reported changes in expression of excitatory and inhibitory neurotransmission-related proteins and the level of neuroplasticity-related proteins in the auditory pathway after acoustic trauma. Changes have been observed in the NMDA receptor subunit 2A (NR2A) mRNA [5], Gamma-Amino-Butyric-Acid (GABA) [7,8], $GABA_A$ receptor alpha 1 subunit ($GABA_A\alpha 1$) [6], Glutamic-Acid Decarboxylase (GAD-67) [6,8], Calbindin (Calb1) [20] and GAP-43 [21]. However, the findings of these studies vary significantly from one another, due to the species used, the age of the animals, method of acoustic trauma, method of quantification and assessing protein changes at differing time points.

As mentioned above, many investigations have centered on changes in the central auditory pathway following acoustic exposure. Clearly partial or total hearing loss results in significant changes throughout the auditory pathway that cannot be explained by peripheral loss alone. This statement is supported by the fact that tinnitus persists in patients with acoustic neuroma after transection of the auditory nerve [22,23]. The Auditory Cortex (AC), Inferior Colliculus (IC) and the Dorsal Cochlear

Nucleus (DCN) have each been investigated as sites where hearing related disorders may be generated after acoustic exposure. The AC has been shown to be vulnerable to acoustic exposure through the development of tonotopic reorganisation [15,16,18,24,25]. The IC has been reported to be functionally and neurochemically altered after acoustic trauma [8,10,25]. The DCN has also been implicated as a possible site for the generation of tinnitus-producing signals owing to its tendency to become hyperactive following exposure to tinnitus inducing agents such as intense sound and cisplatin [26].

We have attempted to find the possible site of generation of acoustic disorders. Our investigations centre on the protein changes in the contralateral and ipsilateral AC, IC and DCN within the same animals following acoustic trauma, with the aim of determining which brain regions may be involved in the generation of auditory disorders by assessing the relative changes in protein expression over time. There are also limited investigations into the development of these changes over time, the majority of studies sample time points before and immediately after acoustic exposure, with limited investigations systematically sampling time points after acoustic exposure. Understanding the development of changes that occur after acoustic trauma is of utmost importance for the development of treatments for auditory disorders. Accordingly, we tracked the expression of excitatory and inhibitory neurotransmission-related proteins and the expression of neuroplasticity-related proteins in the contralateral and ipsilateral AC, IC and DCN over 32 days after acoustic trauma. We hypothesized that acoustic trauma would lead to an increase in excitatory and neuroplasticity marker expression and a decrease in inhibitory marker expression in the AC, IC and DCN over time.

Materials and Methods

Animals

Ethics statement. The experimental procedures were approved by the University of Western Sydney Animal Care and Ethics Committee (ACEC A6670) and conformed to the Australian code of practice for the care and use of animals for scientific purposes – 7th edition. Thirty Long Evans rats aged between 11–14weeks (250 g–350 g) were randomly assigned to 6 groups used to assess the effect of acoustic trauma on the expression of excitatory and inhibitory neurotransmission-related proteins and of neuroplasticity-related proteins in the contralateral and ipsilateral AC, IC and DCN. These groups were a control group (n = 5), day 0 (n = 5), day 4 (n = 5), day 8 (n = 5), day 16 (n = 5) and day 32 (n = 5) post-acoustic trauma group.

Acoustic Trauma

Each rat was anaesthetised via an intraperitoneal (i.p.) injection of ketamine/medetomidine (75 mg/kg;0.5 mg/kg). The animal was placed on a feedback-controlled heating pad with a rectal probe to maintain a constant body temperature of 37°C (Physitemp, Clifton, NJ; Cat #TCAT 2LV Controller). A small tube, 3 mm inner diameter and originating from a speaker (CTS Powerline, Piezo Electric, Woburn, MA) was tightly and securely placed in the animals left ear canal. Rats were unilaterally exposed to a 16 kHz band pass (1/10th octave noise (115 dB SPL)) for 1 hour. The right ear canal remained unblocked during the acoustic trauma. The power spectrum of this stimulus is presented in Figure 1. Control animals were not exposed to the acoustic trauma, but were exposed to a sham acoustic trauma procedure: they underwent the same protocol as the exposed rats, in regards to anaesthesia, ABR testing and were placed in a sound proof room for 1 hour next to the acoustic

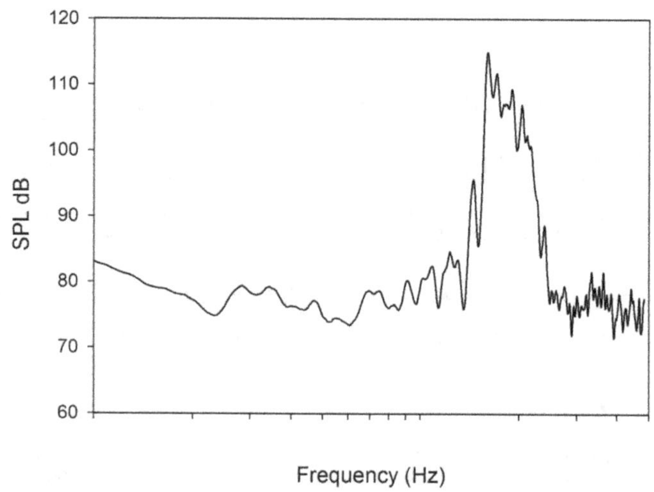

Figure 1. Energy distribution of the noise used in the experiment.

trauma speaker. The speaker was not turned on during this period. To reverse the effects of the anaesthesia following both procedures, a subcutaneous injection of atipamezole (1 mg/kg) was administered.

Auditory Brainstem Response Audiograms

Auditory brainstem response (ABR) audiograms were performed before and after acoustic trauma and at 4, 8, 16 and 32 days post acoustic trauma, on both ipsilateral and contralateral ears. The ABR was performed within a sound attenuated room. The animal was anaesthetised as previously described and placed on a heating pad with a rectal probe to maintain a constant body temperature of 37°C. Tucker Davis Technologies (TDT) system 3 Software (OpenEx) and hardware were used to generate stimuli and to acquire data. Stimuli were generated using an RX6 multifunction processor with a sampling rate of 100 kHz. Stimuli were attenuated using TDT PA5 attenuators, and transduced using TDT EC1 electrostatic speakers. The sound was presented to the animal via a small tube, 3.5 mm in diameter, originating from a speaker (TDT EC1), placed gently in the ear canal. Animals were presented with tones at 1, 2, 4, 8, 16 and 32 kHz at a range of 0 dB–85 dB SPL (90 dB was the maximum that the software could deliver). Tone bursts were 3 ms in duration, presented every 17 ms. Each frequency/SPL combination was presented 500 times sequentially from lowest to highest. The resulting evoked potentials were measured using stainless steel electrodes placed subdermally; behind left ear (active), behind right ear (active), in the midline 2.5 cm anterior to the intra-aural axis (reference) and in the rear leg (ground). At the conclusion of the experiment, the electrodes were removed and animals were given a sub-cutaneous (s.c.) injection of atipamezole (1 mg/kg).

Western Blotting for NR2A, Calb1, GABA$_A$Rα1, GAD-67 and GAP-43 protein

Five animals from each of the six exposure groups and their respective controls (30 in total) were decapitated at 0, 4, 8, 16 or 32 days post acoustic trauma and their brains snap frozen in liquid nitrogen and stored at −80°C until processed. At the time of the experiment, the brains were semi-thawed in 3 ml of protease inhibitor cocktail (Sigma-Aldrich Inc. Cat #8340) and the contralateral and ipsilateral AC, IC and DCN were removed. Regions were identified in accordance with a rat atlas [27]. Each tissue sample was placed in 500 µl of protease inhibitor cocktail. All tissue samples were kept on ice (4°C) throughout the experiment unless otherwise specified. Tissues were homogenised with protease inhibitor cocktail with a hand held tissue grinder (Pellet Pestle Motor, Kontes, Vineland, NJ). The homogenate was passed through a 27G syringe needle to further shear the tissue, then was centrifuged for 10 minutes at 1000 rpm and the supernatant was collected. The supernatant was then centrifuged for 20 minutes at 12000 rpm and the pellet was collected. The pellet was resuspended in protease inhibitor cocktail; 100 µL (AC and IC) and 50 µL (DCN), and passed through a 30G syringe needle. Five µl was removed from each sample for a protein assay (Bio-Rad, Hercules, CA). Each sample received 2× sample buffer; 100 µL (AC and IC) and 50 µL (DCN). Forty µg of protein was loaded in each well and samples were run for 30 minutes at 60 volts and 90 minutes at 120 volts on 10% SDS-PAGE gel. The gel was transferred overnight at 30 mA for a minimum of 17 hours. The gel was transferred onto 0.2 µm pore size nitrocellulose membrane (Sigma-Aldrich, St Louis, MO). The resulting membranes were blocked with 5% skim milk on a rotator for 1 hour. The membrane was probed with a primary antibody multiplex diluted in 3% skim milk for 2 hours, which consisted of $GABA_AR\alpha1$ (Chemicon, Temecula, CA; Cat #06-868) at a concentration of 1:4000, GAD-67 (Santa Cruz Biotechnologies; Cat #28376) at a concentration of 1:400, NR2A (Abcam, Cambridge, MA; Cat #14596-50) at a concentration of 1:3000, Calb1 (Abcam, Cambridge, MA; Cat #9481-500) at a concentration of 1:150 and GAP-43 (Abcam, Cambridge, MA; Cat #50608) at a concentration of 1:400. The membrane was washed repeatedly and probed with secondary antibodies, goat anti rabbit (Sigma-Aldrich, St Louis, MO; Cat #4914) at a concentration of 1:1000 and goat anti mouse (Sigma-Aldrich, St Louis, MO; Cat #4416) at a concentration of 1:750 for 1 hour. The membrane was incubated for 5 minutes with chemiluminescent substrate, Supersignal West Pico (Pierce, Rockford, IL; Cat #34087) and Supersignal West Femto (Pierce, Rockford, IL; Cat #34094) when the signal was low. The membranes were placed on CL exposure films (Pierce, Rockford, IL; Cat #34090) for varying times depending on the signal. The films were processed in an x-ray film processor (Agfa CP-1000). The films were scanned in a LAS-4000 imaging system (Fujifilm Life Science, USA) and images were digitised. The images were analysed using Multi-Gauge Analysis Software Version 2.0 (Fujifilm Life Science, USA), which quantifies the level of density in each band selected compared to the background. Deep Purple Total Protein Stain (GE Healthcare Life Sciences; Cat #RPN6305) was used to standardise results.

Statistical analysis

Statistical analyses were performed using SPSS (IBM Corporation, Somers, NY). The pre and post ABR audiograms (specifically the SPLs) of the groups were compared at individual frequencies, but not across frequencies, using a two tailed student's t-test with a P value of <0.05 considered significant. Control and post acoustic trauma ABR threshold shifts were compared at individual frequencies, but not across frequencies, using a one-way ANOVA and Tukey's post-hoc multiple comparison test with a P value of <0.05 considered significant. If no response was evoked at a SPL of 85 dB, we assigned a SPL threshold of 90 dB. For multiple comparisons of the western blot data, a one-way ANOVA and Tukey's post-hoc multiple comparison test were used with a P value of <0.05 considered significant.

Results

Auditory Brainstem Response Audiograms

ABR audiograms indicate significant threshold shifts following acoustic trauma. Figure 2A–F presents the mean ABR audiograms of all animals obtained prior to the acoustic trauma and at 0 (Fig. 2B), 4 (Fig. 2C), 8 (Fig. 2D), 16 (Fig. 2E) and 32 (Fig. 2F) days post acoustic trauma. All values in the figures are expressed as mean ± SEM. The control sham trauma group showed no significant difference across all frequencies (Fig. 2A), which was expected as the animals received no acoustic trauma. The 0 (Fig. 2B), 4 (Fig. 2C), 8 (Fig. 2D), 16 (Fig. 2E) and 32 (Fig. 2F) day groups showed a significant threshold increase across most frequencies. The lesioned (ipsilateral) ear indicated significant threshold shifts after acoustic trauma. These increases were sustained up to 4 days. At day 8, the high frequencies remained elevated (16 kHz and 32 kHz), whilst the lower frequencies returned to normal levels. At 16 days, these threshold shifts increased again, except for 1 kHz which remained at normal. At 32 days, threshold shifts across all frequencies were significantly increased. Table 1 presents the threshold shifts in dB SPL/frequency/group with p values. The ABR audiograms of the contralateral ear are presented in Table 2 and indicate no significant changes in threshold shifts.

Protein Expression in dominant Auditory Pathway (Contralateral AC, Contralateral IC and Ipsilateral DCN)

Figure 3 shows the pattern of protein expression in contralateral AC, contralateral IC and ipsilateral DCN, which is the dominant auditory pathway with respect to the exposed ear. Tukey's post-hoc analysis showed statistically significant changes in the dominant auditory pathway compared with the control animals and between groups, and these are summarized in the following sections. GAP-43 protein did not show any significant changes in any of the groups over time.

Excitatory neurotransmission related proteins

In the contralateral IC, NR2A showed a 44% decrease when comparing day 0 to day 32 ($p<0.01$) (Fig. 3B). In the ipsilateral DCN, Calb1 showed a 50% decrease at day 0 ($p<0.05$), compared to controls, and showed a 118% increase when comparing day 0 to day 32 ($p<0.05$) (Fig. 3C).

Inhibitory neurotransmission related proteins

In the contralateral AC, $GABA_A\alpha1$ showed a 44% decrease at day 16 ($p<0.05$) and a 51% decrease at day 32 ($p<0.01$), compared to controls (Fig. 3A). In the contralateral IC, GAD-67 showed a 45% decrease when comparing day 0 to day 16 ($p<0.05$) (Fig. 3B). In the ipsilateral DCN, GAD-67 showed a 49% decrease at day 4 ($p<0.05$), compared to controls (Fig. 3C).

Protein Expression in non-dominant Auditory Pathway (Ipsilateral AC, Ipsilateral IC and Contralateral DCN)

Figure 4 shows the pattern of protein expression in ipsilateral AC, ipsilateral IC and contralateral DCN, which is the non-dominant auditory pathway with respect to the exposed ear. Tukey's post-hoc analysis showed statistically significant changes in the dominant auditory pathway compared to the control animals and between groups, and these are summarized as follows.

Excitatory neurotransmission related proteins

In the ipsilateral AC, Calb1 showed a 117% increase when comparing day 0 to day 16 ($p<0.05$) (Fig. 4A). In the contralateral

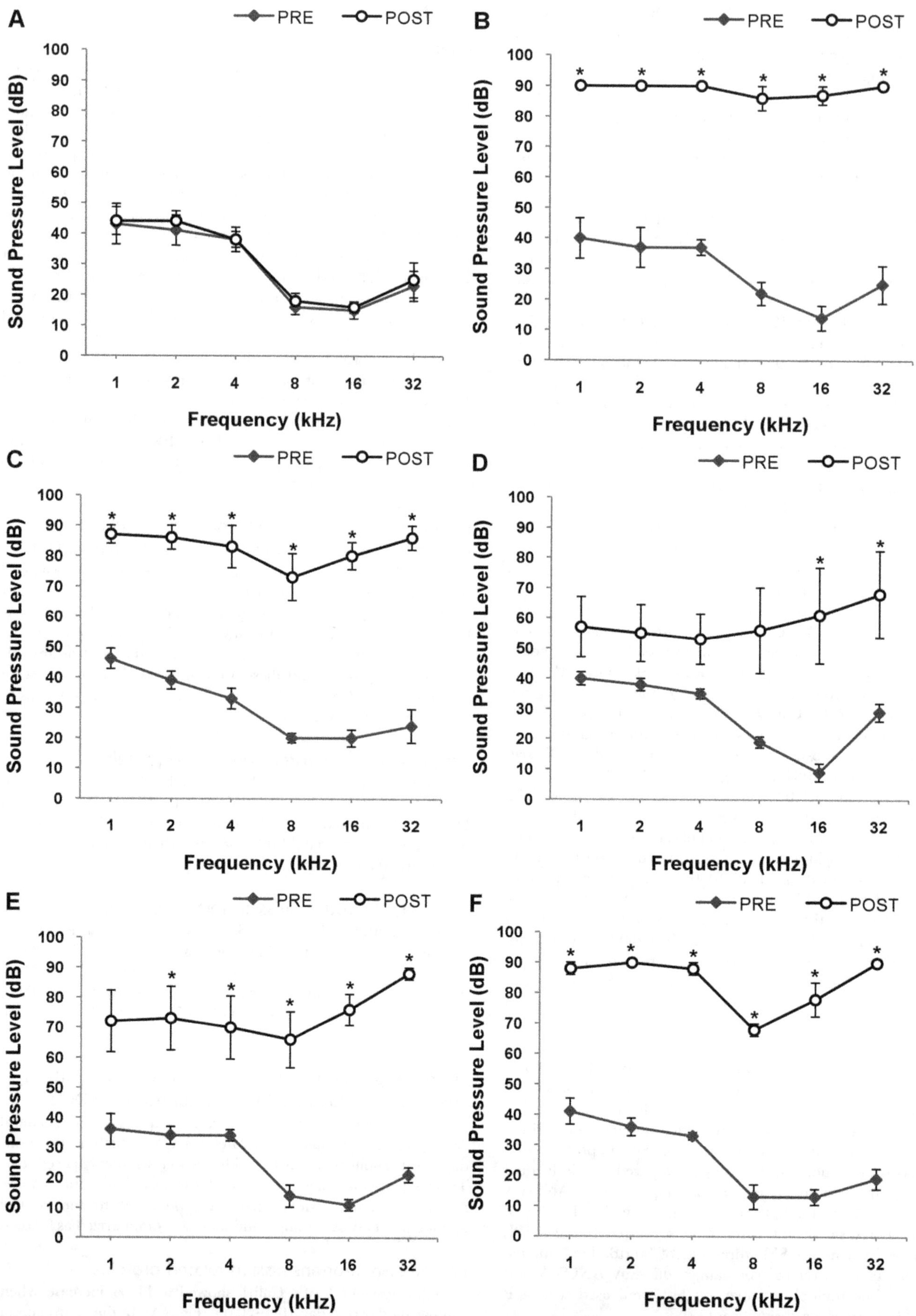
A
PRE
POST
Sound Pressure Level (dB)
Frequency (kHz)
B
PRE
POST
Sound Pressure Level (dB)
Frequency (kHz)
C
PRE
POST
Sound Pressure Level (dB)
Frequency (kHz)
D
PRE
POST
Sound Pressure Level (dB)
Frequency (kHz)
E
PRE
POST
Sound Pressure Level (dB)
Frequency (kHz)
F
PRE
POST
Sound Pressure Level (dB)
Frequency (kHz)

Figure 2. ABR Audiograms of absolute thresholds. Pre-lesion recordings are compared to (A) post-lesion (SHAM); (B) 0 days post-lesion; (C) 4 days post-lesion; (D) 8 days post-lesion; (E) 16 days post-lesion and (F) 32 days post-lesion recordings. Results are presented as the mean ± SEM of SPL (dB). *p<0.05.

DCN, Calb1 showed a 45% decrease when comparing day 0 to day 8 ($p<0.05$) (Fig. 4C). NR2A protein did not show any significant changes in any of the groups.

Inhibitory neurotransmission related proteins

In the ipsilateral AC, $GABA_A\alpha 1$ showed a 19% decrease at day 4 ($p<0.05$) and a 35% decrease at day 32 ($p<0.05$) compared to controls, GAD-67 showed a 39% decrease at day 0 ($p<0.05$) compared to controls (Fig. 4A). In the ipsilateral IC, GAD-67 showed a 48% decrease at day 4 ($p<0.05$) compared to controls and an 86% increase when comparing day 4 to day 32 ($p<0.05$) (Fig. 4B). In the contralateral DCN, GAD-67 showed a 50% decrease when comparing day 0 to day 8 ($p<0.05$) and a 53% decrease when comparing day 0 to day 32 ($p<0.05$) (Fig. 4C).

Neuroplasticity related proteins

In the ipsilateral AC, GAP-43 showed a 58–68% decrease when comparing day 0 ($p<0.05$), day 4 ($p<0.01$), day 8 ($p<0.01$) and day 16 ($p<0.05$) to controls (Fig. 4A).

Discussion

We have quantified the protein expression of $GABA_AR\alpha 1$, GAD-67, NR2A, Calb1 and GAP-43 in the ipsilateral and contralateral AC, IC and DCN of the young adult rat up to 32 days following acoustic trauma. We have demonstrated that acoustic trauma significantly alters the normal levels of excitatory and inhibitory neurotransmission-related proteins and neuroplasticity-related proteins in the auditory pathway of the rat over time. Our findings suggest that these changes in protein expression may serve as part of the molecular mechanism underlying significant physiological changes which lead to acoustic disorders following acoustic trauma.

The Effect of Acoustic Trauma on Hearing Thresholds

The degree of hearing loss produced by exposure to a sound is dependent on the loudness of the sound and the duration of the exposure. Temporary Threshold Shifts (TTS), which are temporary shifts in hearing thresholds, may be observed immediately following exposure [28,29,30], and if the sound is loud enough it may produce permanent elevations in thresholds resulting in permanent threshold shifts (PTS) [31].

The hearing loss produced by our stimulus can be characterized by significant threshold shifts across all frequencies and all time points. The threshold shifts ranged from 49–74 dB at Day 0, 46–67 dB at Day 4, 18–48 dB at Day 8, 31–65 dB at Day 16 and 47–67 dB at Day 32. It is interesting to note the gradual reduction of hearing thresholds over the first eight days. Day 8 suggests that some hearing function has recovered after the acoustic trauma. However, this recovery is not sustained and hearing thresholds begin to increase.

The acoustic trauma we used caused a significant increase in hearing thresholds for the duration of our study. Others who have used a similar acoustic trauma treatment have shown mixed results. Turner [32], using the same strain of rats reported that after 4 months recovery thresholds remained elevated for all frequencies tested (except 10 kHz and 32 kHz). Additionally, Bauer [29] reported that threshold shifts remained elevated 7 months after being exposed to a 16 kHz octave band noise at 105 dB for 1 hour. In contrast, Wang and Caspary [33] using Fisher Brown Norway rats showed full recovery by 16 weeks post-exposure. It should be noted that the maximum hearing loss in the present study occurred at 16 kHz and 32 kHz and at those frequencies the losses were greater than those of comparable studies [29,32,33].

The initial threshold shifts may be a result of peripheral damage to the auditory system. The immediate changes that occur in inner hair cells (IHC) and outer hair cells (OHC) of the cochlea are quite variable (see [34] for extensive review). It is known that IHC and OHC cannot regenerate in humans and most mammals [35], The observation of the Day 8 recovery may suggest a combination of central and peripheral events playing a role in the temporary recovery of hearing function after acoustic trauma. It is not in disagreement with findings which suggest that peripheral recovery can occur, followed by central degenerative changes [36,37] or changes in excitatory transmission [38].

Protein Expression

Western blot data demonstrated that all proteins of interest were expressed in the contralateral and ipsilateral AC, IC and DCN of the adult Long Evans rat. Fluctuations in the expression of excitatory and inhibitory neurotransmission-related proteins may play a role in excitotoxicity, decreased neuronal survival and the

Table 1. Post Acoustic Trauma Threshold shifts in all exposure groups (Ipsilateral Ear).

	Frequency					
Group	**1 kHz**	**2 kHz**	**4 kHz**	**8 kHz**	**16 kHz**	**24 kHz**
Control (SHAM)	1 dB (p = 0.9)	3 dB (p = 0.6)	0 dB (p = 1.0)	2 dB (p = 0.6)	1 dB (p = 0.8)	2 dB (p = 0.8)
Day 0	50 dB **(p = 0.003)**	53 dB **(p = 0.002)**	53 dB **(p<0.001)**	64 dB **(p<0.001)**	73 dB **(p<0.001)**	65 dB **(p<0.001)**
Day 4	41 dB **(p = 0.019)**	47 dB **(p = 0.007)**	50 dB **(p = 0.001)**	53 dB **(p = 0.004)**	60 dB **(p = 0.001)**	62 dB **(p<0.001)**
Day 8	17 dB (p = 0.723)	17 dB (p = 0.807)	18 dB (p = 0.491)	37 dB (p = 0.076)	52 dB **(p = 0.003)**	39 dB **(p = 0.018)**
Day 16	36 dB (p = 052)	39 dB **(p = 0.038)**	36 dB **(p = 0.017)**	52 dB **(p = 0.005)**	65 dB **(p<0.001)**	67 dB **(p<0.001)**
Day 32	47 dB **(p = 0.006)**	54 dB **(p = 0.002)**	55 dB **(p<0.001)**	55 dB **(p = 0.002)**	65 dB **(p<0.001)**	71 dB **(p<0.001)**

Significant p values in bold.

Table 2. Post Acoustic Trauma Threshold shifts in all exposure groups (Contralateral Ear).

	Frequency					
Group	**1 kHz**	**2 kHz**	**4 kHz**	**8 kHz**	**16 kHz**	**24 kHz**
Control (SHAM)	5 dB (p = 0.8)	2 dB (p = 0.6)	2 dB (p = 1.0)	2 dB (p = 0.6)	6 dB (p = 0.8)	1 dB (p = 1.0)
Day 0	−3 dB (p = 0.8)	−1 dB (p = 1.0)	3 dB (p = 1.0)	3 dB (p = 1.0)	2 dB (p = 0.9)	0 dB (p = 1.0)
Day 4	−4 dB (p = 0.7)	−3 dB (p = 0.9)	−7 dB (p = 0.5)	−5 dB (p = 0.6)	−3 dB (p = 0.3)	−3 dB (p = 1.0)
Day 8	−13 dB (p = 0.8)	9 dB (p = 0.8)	3 dB (p = 1.0)	1 dB (p = 1.0)	7 dB (p = 1.0)	−2 dB (p = 1.0)
Day 16	−1 dB (p = 1.0)	0 dB (p = 1.0)	1 dB (p = 1.0)	1 dB (p = 1.0)	2 dB (p = 0.9)	−1 dB (p = 1.0)
Day 32	−4 dB (p = 0.7)	−4 dB (p = 0.9)	0 dB (p = 1.0)	−2 dB (p = 0.9)	−1 dB (p = 0.5)	−3 dB (p = 1.0)

Significant p values in bold.

overall decrease of inhibitory neurotransmission. A significant decrease in neuroplasticity-related proteins may play a role in reorganization of tonotopic maps, which has been shown to occur after acoustic trauma [16,18,19,25]. These changes could ultimately lead to the development of acoustic disorders, such as tinnitus and hyperacusis.

The Effect of Acoustic Trauma on Excitatory Neurotransmission-Related Proteins

We found that the expression of the calcium binding protein (CBP) Calb1 decreased immediately after acoustic trauma in the ipsilateral DCN, followed by a recovery to normal level over the 32 days. Calb1 decreased slightly in the contralateral AC followed by recovery at Day 16. It has been postulated that Calb1 has a neuroprotective effect against excitotoxic damage caused by disruption of intracellular calcium homeostasis [39]. A possible reason for the decrease in Calb1 could be that the production of Calb1 is disrupted and therefore could be responsible for excitotoxic damage that may occur in the auditory system after acoustic trauma. Excitotoxicity in the cochlea and central auditory pathway has been researched extensively and is postulated to be a major contributor to the development of acoustic disorders [38,40]. Indeed, Muly and colleagues have reported evidence of excitotoxic damage following unilateral acoustic trauma in the chinchilla [38]. In excitotoxicity, elevations of Ca^{2+} progress to an irreversible loss of Ca^{2+} homeostasis and neuronal death. In this study, a reduction of Calb1 in the ipsilateral AC and DCN could suggest that a dysfunction has occurred in the production of Calb1 which would affect its function as a cytoplasmic calcium buffer, thereby no longer being able to protect cells against excitotoxic damage. However, it is known that there are other CBPs such as Calretinin and Parvalbumin, which carry out similar functions to Calb1 [41]. Thus it would be important to investigate the changes of other CBP after acoustic trauma as Calb1 levels were not increased. It has been shown that Calretinin and Parvalbumin protein levels increase in mice that were exposed to repeated noise trauma [42]. The immediate decrease of Calb1 in the ipsilateral DCN and the contralateral AC that we observed has not been shown in other studies. The expression of Calb1 in the contralateral DCN slightly increased immediately but returned to normal levels over time. These contralateral DCN findings support previous studies which have found that Calb1 increases in the DCN immediately after acoustic trauma [43,44].

The other excitatory neurotransmission-related protein that we investigated was NR2A. The expression of NR2A protein had a tendency to decrease over the month following the trauma in the contralateral IC. NMDA receptors containing the NR2A subunit display fast kinetics and NR2A is the most widespread NMDA receptor subunit in the mature brain [45]. This decrease could suggest that the auditory system attempts to compensate for increased excitation; the down regulation of the receptors may serve to reduce increased levels of excitation. Kim and colleagues showed an increase in glutamate release after acoustic trauma, followed by a decrease and a subsequent increase [37]. Our results support previous research by Marionowski et al, which found a decrease in the expression of NR2A mRNA after ototoxic exposure in IC and CN of young rats [5].

A decrease in the expression of NR2A in the contralateral IC could also suggest a reduction in neuronal survival and subsequently neuronal death, because injury induced activation of NR2A containing NMDARs functions as a pro-survival signal [46]. A decrease in neuronal survival after acoustic trauma has been shown in numerous studies. An increase of apoptotic markers was observed in the CN after severe acoustic trauma [47]. Other studies have observed an increased in cell death and degeneration after acoustic trauma in the CN [48,49], IC [49] MGB and AC [49,50].

The fluctuations we observed in the protein levels of the CBP, Calb1, suggest that there may be fluctuations of excitation in central auditory structures after acoustic trauma. The slight decreases we observed in the protein levels of the NMDA receptor subunit NR2A suggests that they may not have a direct effect on excitation changes, but may have an effect on neuronal survival of auditory neurons.

The Effect of Acoustic Trauma on *Inhibitory Neurotransmission-Related Proteins*

This is the first study that has investigated the effect of acoustic trauma on the expression of $GABA_A\alpha1$ in the ipsilateral and contralateral AC. After acoustic trauma, the expression of $GABA_A\alpha1$ decreased over time firstly in the ipsilateral AC and followed by the contralateral AC. Previous studies have shown that the expression of $GABA_A\alpha1$ also decreases in other regions of the auditory pathway, such as the IC and DCN [6,14]. This down-regulation could result in a significant decrease in inhibition in these auditory areas on both ipsilateral and contralateral sides. A consequence of the reduction of inhibitory processes is that increased excitation may occur in the AC after acoustic trauma, resulting in an altered pattern of spontaneous activity in the AC. Indeed, changes in spontaneous activity and neuronal excitability has been observed across the auditory pathway after acoustic trauma, specifically in DCN [26], the IC [6,14,17] and the AC [12,19].

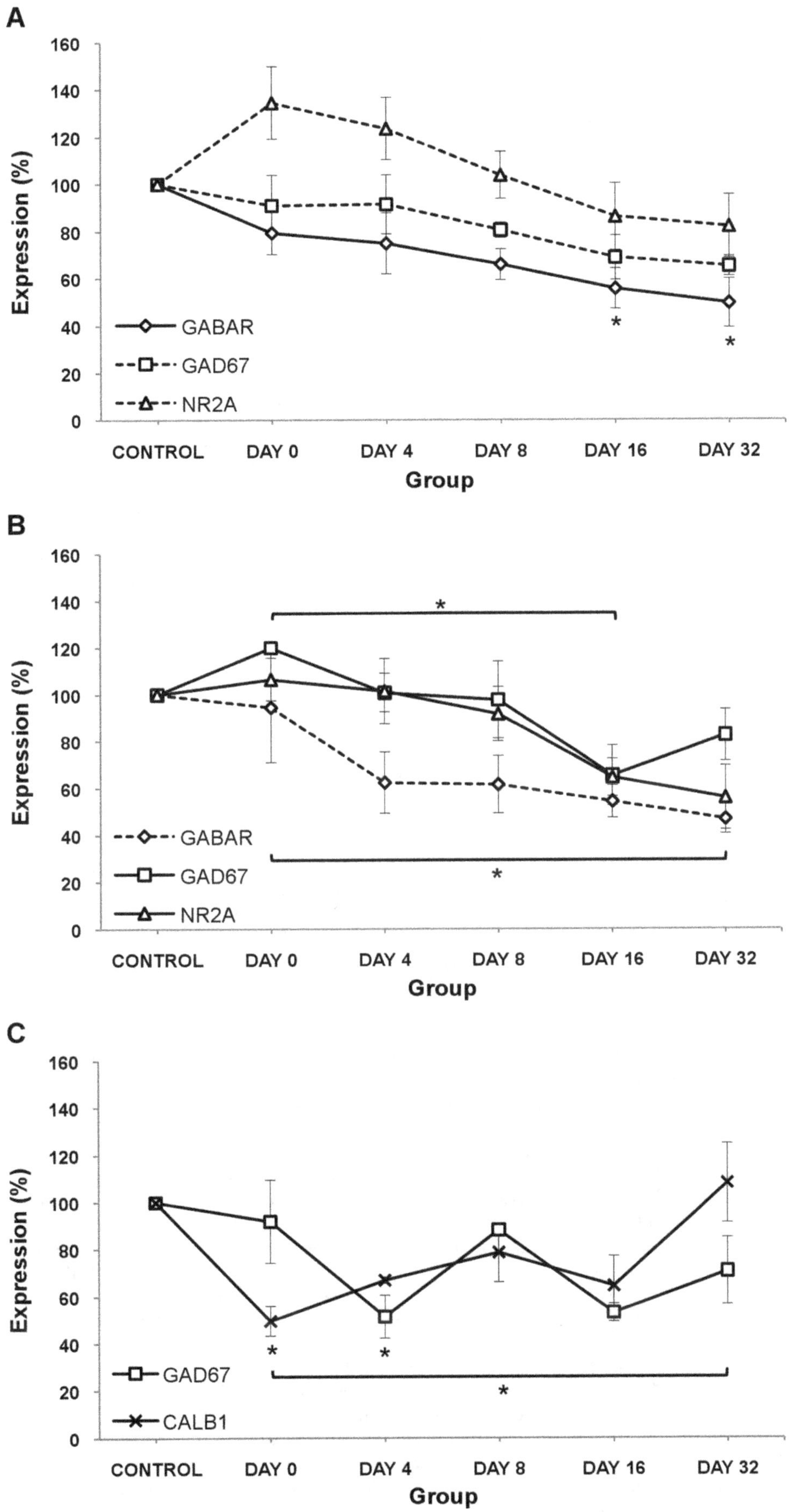
A
Expression (%)
GABAR
GAD67
NR2A
CONTROL
DAY 0
DAY 4
DAY 8
DAY 16
DAY 32
Group
B
Expression (%)
GABAR
GAD67
NR2A
CONTROL
DAY 0
DAY 4
DAY 8
DAY 16
DAY 32
Group
C
Expression (%)
GAD67
CALB1
CONTROL
DAY 0
DAY 4
DAY 8
DAY 16
DAY 32
Group

Figure 3. Expression of proteins of interest after acoustic trauma in Dominant Auditory Pathway. (A) Contralateral AC; (B) Contralateral IC and (C) Ipsilateral DCN. Results presented are the mean ± SEM of density units expressed as a % compared to controls. NOTE: only protein expression that reached statistical significance (full lines) or indicates trends (dotted lines) are plotted on the graphs. * $p<0.05$.

After unilateral acoustic trauma, the expression of GAD-67 increased slightly in the contralateral IC and DCN, followed by a recovery to normal levels over time. A decrease was observed immediately in the ipsilateral AC, within the first week in the ipsilateral IC but the levels of GAD-67 in both regions returned to normal over time. Slight fluctuations were observed in the contralateral DCN followed by a recovery to normal levels over time. GAD-67 is an enzyme that converts intracellular glutamate into the neurotransmitter GABA [51]. A decreased expression of GAD-67 will lead to reduced levels of GABA, which has been previously observed after acoustic trauma [8,52], and can ultimately lead to an overall decrease in inhibition. The changes of GAD-67 were the most widespread finding in this study and suggest that a disruption in inhibitory transmission plays an important role in the development of acoustic disorders.

The decreases we observed in the protein levels of the $GABA_A\alpha1$ receptor subunit and the GABA synthesis enzyme GAD-67 supports the theory of Dong et al., implying that both pre- and post-synaptic mechanisms contribute to deafness- related loss of inhibition [53]. The possibility that presynaptic GABA synthesis may diminish in the auditory pathway after ipsilateral partial deafness is supported by a study showing a loss of GABA positive neurons in the CN of aged rats with hearing loss [52] and decreased GABA release in the IC [8]. It has been demonstrated that GABA release and binding, as well as GAD-67 expression are down-regulated in the IC after hearing loss [54,55,56]. The down-regulation of $GABA_A\alpha1$ and GAD-67 would most likely result in an overall decrease in neuronal inhibition in the auditory pathway. This could lead to increases in spontaneous activity, neuronal synchrony and excitability, which has been observed across the auditory pathway after acoustic trauma [13,17,19,57]. Prolonged synchronous firing has been observed in the AC after acoustic trauma [12,19], which can lead to use-dependent synaptic modifications, Long Term Potentiation (LTP). LTP is thought to promote the increase of synaptic strength and this may lead to the development of auditory disorders such as tinnitus [58].

Neuroplasticity-related proteins

The expression of GAP-43 has been shown to increase during heightened levels of neuroplasticity, as it is located in the growth cones of neurons [59]. Previous research indicates that GAP-43 also plays a key role in axonal guidance [60,61], GAP-43 (−/−) mice show defects in path finding of retinal ganglion cell axons across the optic chiasm [62]. Over expression of GAP-43 leads to formation of new synapses and enhanced sprouting after injury whereas reduced sprouting is found with a mutant GAP-43 that cannot be phosphorylated by Protein Kinase C. This control of sprouting implies that GAP-43 is an intrinsic determinant of the neurons growth state. We observed a significant decrease in the overall expression of GAP-43 in the ipsilateral AC. This may have an impact on anatomical reorganization of tonotopic maps after NIHL, as previous studies suggest that reduced GAP-43 expression may alter the fine tuning of a cortical map through a combination of path finding and synaptic plasticity mechanisms [63].

Significance of Time-Course Changes

To date, there are limited investigations into the time-course of changes that occur in the auditory pathway after acoustic trauma. This is the first study that has investigated changes in the ipsilateral and contralateral AC, IC and DCN in the same animals over time.

Samples were taken as early as 30 minutes after noise trauma (day 0 time point). At this time point we observed significant changes in the expression of Calb1; in the ipsilateral DCN, GAD-67 and GAP-43; in the ipsilateral AC. This observation indicates that these proteins act immediately after the acoustic trauma and may suggest a role in an immediate active fine-tuning process.

Significant changes in both contralateral and ipsilateral DCN involved GAD-67 and Calb1. Over the time-course, GAD-67 and Calb1 were very closely related, both experiencing fluctuations at similar time points. As Calb1 is an indicator of excitation and GAD-67 is involved in synthesizing GABA, it may suggest that there is a connection between these proteins that acts to balance excitatory and inhibitory actions in the DCN normally and after an acoustic insult. These fluctuations over time may indicate that the nervous system continually attempts to rebalance the changes that are occurring in response to altered input. For example when the Calb1 increased, GAD-67 increased in order to produce more GABA, and when Calb1 decreased, GAD-67 also decreases due to the decreased demand for GABA. A previous study has shown that neurons in the olfactory bulbs of mice co-express Calb1 and GAD-67 [64], however there is no study that has looked at the co-expression of these two proteins over time. It is not known the extent to which the levels of Calb1 and GAD-67 relative to each other over time.

The contralateral AC and IC show similar significant decreases and near-significant trends in the levels of NR2A, GAD-67 and $GABA_A\alpha1$. This may indicate the AC and IC contralateral to the lesioned ear respond in a similar fashion. The overall potential of the cells would be excitatory which as previously discussed can lead to LTP and may facilitate synaptic plasticity. It would be beneficial to research into the tonotopic changes of the AC and IC to identify whether these protein changes correlate to cortical reorganization and increases of spontaneous activity over time.

The ipsilateral IC experienced a decrease in the expression of GAD-67 within the first week after acoustic trauma. The decrease in the GAD-67 may indicate a malfunction, which would lead to decreased levels of GABA which would result in increased excitation. However, there were no significant changes in the expression of excitatory neurotransmission related proteins in the ipsilateral IC across the time-course. There have been no other reports of the ipsilateral IC changing significantly after acoustic trauma.

Many significant changes were observed in the ipsilateral AC. GAD-67 and $GABA_AR\alpha1$ protein levels were observed to be closely related over the time-course. This was expected as both of these proteins work together in maintaining the balance of excitation and inhibition. We observed fluctuations of Calb1 over the time-course which may indicate that excitation fluctuations were. The decrease GAP-43 may suggest that the ipsilateral AC experiences maladaptive plastic changes, due to the neuronal path finding properties of GAP-43.

In summary, we provide the first 32 day time-course investigation of protein expression of NR2A, Calb1, $GABA_AR\alpha1$, GAD-67 and GAP-43 in the contralateral and ipsilateral AC, IC and DCN utilizing a rat model of unilateral NIHL. We have investigated the development of these protein changes, in order to gain a deeper understanding of the underlying mechanisms of

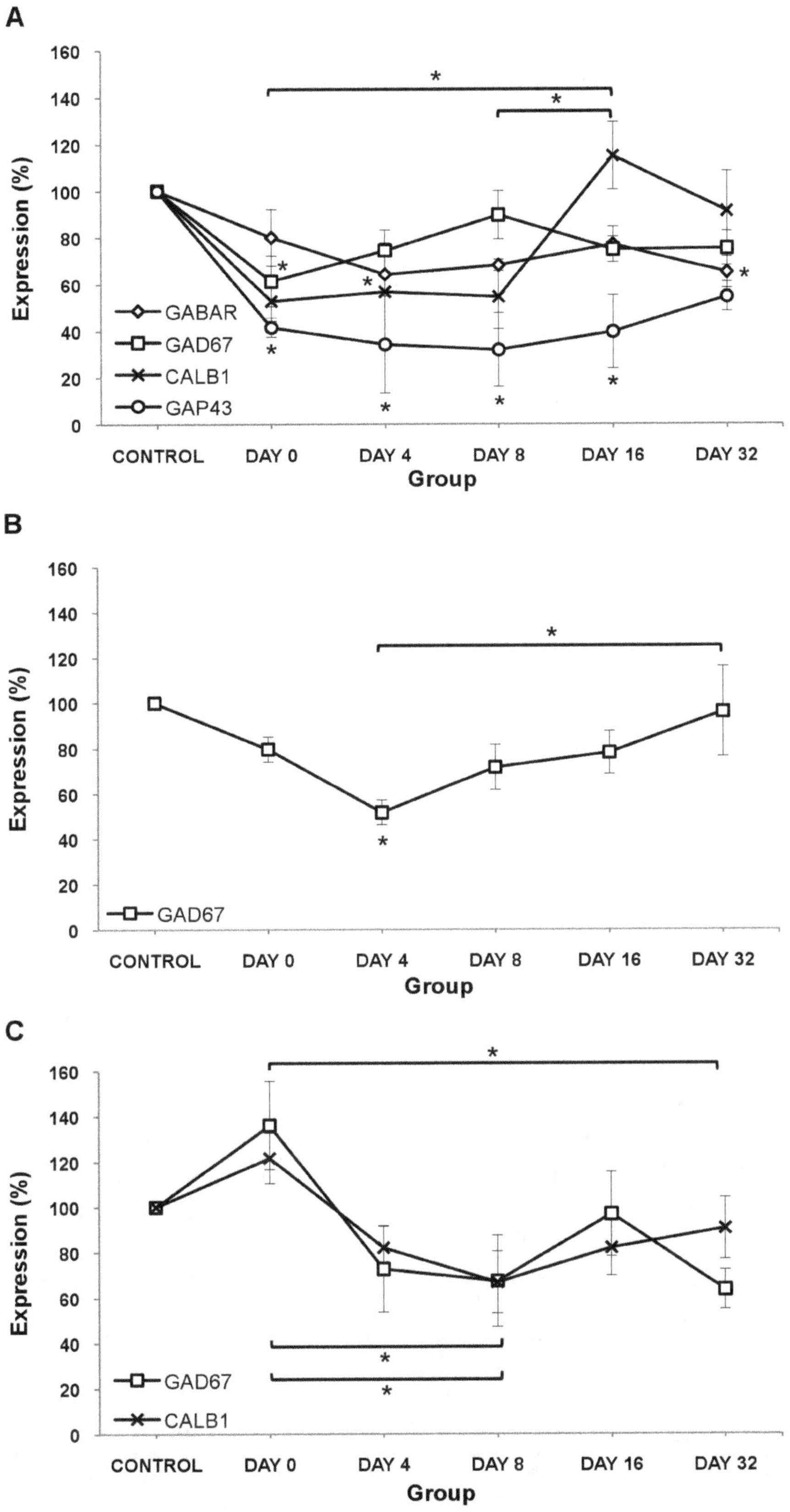

Figure 4. Expression of proteins of interest after acoustic trauma in Non-dominant Auditory Pathway. (A) Ipsilateral AC; (B) Ipsilateral IC and (C) Contralateral DCN. Results presented are the mean ± SEM of density units expressed as a % compared to controls. NOTE: only protein expression that reached statistical significance are plotted on the graphs. * $p<0.05$.

NIHL. Gaining more knowledge about the underlying mechanisms of NIHL is crucial for the development of therapeutic intervention.

Our findings provide evidence that acoustic trauma significantly affects the balance of excitatory and inhibitory neurotransmission-related proteins and neuroplasticity-related proteins in the rat auditory pathway. Our results suggest that the characteristic decrease of inhibition that previous researchers have observed after acoustic trauma, may not necessarily be due to significant increases of excitatory neurotransmission-related proteins; rather a significant *decrease* of inhibitory-neurotransmission related proteins which leads to an overall increase in excitation. This does not support our original hypothesis.

In addition to confirming changes in excitatory and inhibitory-neurotransmission related protein expression, we have shown for the first time that mechanisms from the contralateral auditory pathway may play a role in functional compensation after NIHL. Changes in the ipsilateral and contralateral AC, IC and DCN, may reflect an attempt to balance excitatory and inhibitory transmission following noise-induced hearing loss. The resulting imbalances may contribute to the generation of acoustic disorders.

Acknowledgments

We would like to thank Sindy Kueh for her assistance with the Western Blots.

Author Contributions

Conceived and designed the experiments: CHP CJB JWM. Performed the experiments: CJB. Analyzed the data: CJB CHP JWM. Contributed reagents/materials/analysis tools: CHP JWM. Wrote the paper: CJB CHP JWM.

References

1. Kumar A, Mathew K, Alexander S, Kiran C (2009) Output sound pressure levels of personal music systems and their effect on hearing.(Article)(Report). Noise and Health 11: 132.
2. Peng JH, Tao ZZ, Huang ZW (2007) Risk of damage to hearing from personal listening devices in young adults. J Otolaryngol 36: 181–185.
3. Kurmis AP, Apps SA (2007) Occupationally-acquired noise-induced hearing loss: a senseless workplace hazard. Int J Occup Med Environ Health 20: 127–136.
4. Axelsson A, Sandh A (1985) Tinnitus in noise-induced hearing loss. Br J Audiol 19: 271–276.
5. Marianowski R, Liao WH, Van Den Abbeele T, Fillit P, Herman P, et al. (2000) Expression of NMDA, AMPA and GABA(A) receptor subunit mRNAs in the rat auditory brainstem. I. Influence of early auditory deprivation. Hear Res 150: 1–11.
6. Dong S, Mulders WH, Rodger J, Robertson D (2009) Changes in neuronal activity and gene expression in guinea-pig auditory brainstem after unilateral partial hearing loss. Neuroscience 159: 1164–1174.
7. Tan J, Ruttiger L, Panford-Walsh R, Singer W, Schulze H, et al. (2007) Tinnitus behavior and hearing function correlate with the reciprocal expression patterns of BDNF and Arg3.1/arc in auditory neurons following acoustic trauma. Neuroscience 145: 715–726.
8. Milbrandt JC, Holder TM, Wilson MC, Salvi RJ, Caspary DM (2000) GAD levels and muscimol binding in rat inferior colliculus following acoustic trauma. Hear Res 147: 251–260.
9. Zettel ML, O'Neill WE, Trang TT, Frisina RD (2003) The effects of early bilateral deafening on calretinin expression in the dorsal cochlear nucleus of aged CBA/CaJ mice. Hear Res 183: 57–66.
10. Alvarado JC, Fuentes-Santamaria V, Franklin SR, Brunso-Bechtold JK, Henkel CK (2005) Unilateral cochlear ablation in adult ferrets results in upregulation in calretinin immunostaining in the central nucleus of the inferior colliculus. Neuroscience 136: 957–969.
11. Sun YJ, Wu GK, Liu B-h, Li P, Zhou M, et al. (2010) Fine-tuning of pre-balanced excitation and inhibition during auditory cortical development. Nature 465: 927–931.
12. Noreña AJ, Eggermont JJ (2003) Changes in spontaneous neural activity immediately after an acoustic trauma: implications for neural correlates of tinnitus. Hearing Research 183: 137–153.
13. Chang H, Chen K, Kaltenbach JA, Zhang J, Godfrey DA (2002) Effects of acoustic trauma on dorsal cochlear nucleus neuron activity in slices. Hear Res 164: 59–68.
14. Dong S, Mulders WH, Rodger J, Woo S, Robertson D (2010) Acoustic trauma evokes hyperactivity and changes in gene expression in guinea-pig auditory brainstem. Eur J Neurosci 31: 1616–1628.
15. Harrison RV, Ibrahim D, Mount RJ (1998) Plasticity of tonotopic maps in auditory midbrain following partial cochlear damage in the developing chinchilla. Exp Brain Res 123: 449–460.
16. Kaltenbach JA, Czaja JM, Kaplan CR (1992) Changes in the tonotopic map of the dorsal cochlear nucleus following induction of cochlear lesions by exposure to intense sound. Hear Res 59: 213–223.
17. Mulders WH, Robertson D (2009) Hyperactivity in the auditory midbrain after acoustic trauma: dependence on cochlear activity. Neuroscience 164: 733–746.
18. Robertson D, Irvine DR (1989) Plasticity of frequency organization in auditory cortex of guinea pigs with partial unilateral deafness. J Comp Neurol 282: 456–471.
19. Seki S, Eggermont JJ (2003) Changes in spontaneous firing rate and neural synchrony in cat primary auditory cortex after localized tone-induced hearing loss. Hear Res 180: 28–38.
20. Idrizbegovic E, Bogdanovic N, Canlon B (1999) Sound stimulation increases calcium-binding protein immunoreactivity in the inferior colliculus in mice. Neurosci Lett 259: 49–52.
21. Illing RB, Horvath M, Laszig R (1997) Plasticity of the auditory brainstem: effects of cochlear ablation on GAP-43 immunoreactivity in the rat. J Comp Neurol 382: 116–138.
22. House JW, Brackmann DE (1981) Tinnitus: surgical treatment. Ciba Found Symp 85: 204–216.
23. Matthies C, Samii M (1997) Management of vestibular schwannomas (acoustic neuromas): the value of neurophysiology for evaluation and prediction of auditory function in 420 cases. Neurosurgery 40: 919–929; discussion 929–930.
24. Irvine DR, Wright BA (2005) Plasticity of spectral processing. Int Rev Neurobiol 70: 435–472.
25. Izquierdo MA, Gutierrez-Conde PM, Merchan MA, Malmierca MS (2008) Non-plastic reorganization of frequency coding in the inferior colliculus of the rat following noise-induced hearing loss. Neuroscience 154: 355–369.
26. Kaltenbach JA, Zhang J, Finlayson P (2005) Tinnitus as a plastic phenomenon and its possible neural underpinnings in the dorsal cochlear nucleus. Hear Res 206: 200–226.
27. Paxinos G, Watson C (2007) The rat brain in stereotaxic coordinates Academic Press.
28. Syka J, Rybalko N (2000) Threshold shifts and enhancement of cortical evoked responses after noise exposure in rats. Hearing Research 139: 59–68.
29. Bauer CA (2003) Animal models of tinnitus. Otolaryngol Clin North Am 36: 267–285, vi.
30. Puel JL, Ruel J, Gervais d'Aldin C, Pujol R (1998) Excitotoxicity and repair of cochlear synapses after noise-trauma induced hearing loss. Neuroreport 9: 2109–2114.
31. Clark WW (1991) Recent studies of temporary threshold shift (TTS) and permanent threshold shift (PTS) in animals. J Acoust Soc Am 90: 155–163.
32. Turner JG, Brozoski TJ, Bauer CA, Parrish JL, Myers K, et al. (2006) Gap detection deficits in rats with tinnitus: a potential novel screening tool. Behav Neurosci 120: 188–195.
33. Wang H, Brozoski TJ, Turner JG, Ling L, Parrish JL, et al. (2009) Plasticity at glycinergic synapses in dorsal cochlear nucleus of rats with behavioral evidence of tinnitus. Neuroscience 164: 747–759.
34. Nordmann AS, Bohne BA, Harding GW (2000) Histopathological differences between temporary and permanent threshold shift. Hear Res 139: 13–30.
35. Edge ASB, Chen Z-Y (2008) Hair cell regeneration. Current Opinion in Neurobiology 18: 377–382.
36. Lin HW, Furman AC, Kujawa SG, Liberman MC (2011) Primary neural degeneration in the Guinea pig cochlea after reversible noise-induced threshold shift. J Assoc Res Otolaryngol 12: 605–616.
37. Kim JJ, Gross J, Morest DK, Potashner SJ (2004) Quantitative study of degeneration and new growth of axons and synaptic endings in the chinchilla cochlear nucleus after acoustic overstimulation. J Neurosci Res 77: 829–842.
38. Muly SM, Gross JS, Potashner SJ (2004) Noise trauma alters D-[3H]aspartate release and AMPA binding in chinchilla cochlear nucleus. J Neurosci Res 75: 585–596.
39. Mattson MP, Rychlik B, Chu C, Christakos S (1991) Evidence for calcium-reducing and excito-protective roles for the calcium-binding protein calbindin-D28k in cultured hippocampal neurons. Neuron 6: 41–51.
40. Pujol R, Puel JL (1999) Excitotoxicity, synaptic repair, and functional recovery in the mammalian cochlea: a review of recent findings. Ann N Y Acad Sci 884: 249–254.
41. Heizmann CW (1992) Calcium-binding proteins: basic concepts and clinical implications. Gen Physiol Biophys 11: 411–425.
42. Arun P, Wang Y, Wei Y, Oguntayo S, Biggemann L, et al. (2007) Repeated Blast Exposures Lead to Changes in Hearing Related Gene Expression in Mice Brain. In: Branch B-IN, ed. Silver Spring, MD 20910, .
43. Idrizbegovic E, Bogdanovic N, Canlon B (1998) Modulating calbindin and parvalbumin immunoreactivity in the cochlear nucleus by moderate noise

exposure in mice. A quantitative study on the dorsal and posteroventral cochlear nucleus. Brain Res 800: 86–96.

44. Forster CR, Illing RB (2000) Plasticity of the auditory brainstem: cochleotomy-induced changes of calbindin-D28k expression in the rat. J Comp Neurol 416: 173–187.

45. Monyer H, Burnashev N, Laurie DJ, Sakmann B, Seeburg PH (1994) Developmental and regional expression in the rat brain and functional properties of four NMDA receptors. Neuron 12: 529–540.

46. DeRidder MN, Simon MJ, Siman R, Auberson YP, Raghupathi R, et al. (2006) Traumatic mechanical injury to the hippocampus in vitro causes regional caspase-3 and calpain activation that is influenced by NMDA receptor subunit composition. Neurobiol Dis 22: 165–176.

47. Coordes A, Groschel M, Ernst A, Basta D (2011) Apoptotic Cascades in the Central Auditory Pathway after Noise Exposure. J Neurotrauma.

48. Watanabe M, Inoue Y, Sakimura K, Mishina M (1992) Developmental changes in distribution of NMDA receptor channel subunit mRNAs. Neuroreport 3: 1138–1140.

49. Groschel M, Gotze R, Ernst A, Basta D (2010) Differential impact of temporary and permanent noise-induced hearing loss on neuronal cell density in the mouse central auditory pathway. J Neurotrauma 27: 1499–1507.

50. Basta D, Tzschentke B, Ernst A (2005) Noise-induced cell death in the mouse medial geniculate body and primary auditory cortex. Neurosci Lett 381: 199–204.

51. Erlander MG, Tillakaratne NJK, Feldblum S, Patel N, Tobin AJ (1991) Two genes encode distinct glutamate decarboxylases. Neuron 7: 91–100.

52. Yang W, Wu W, Fang Y (1998) [Changes of GABA immunoreactivity in aged rat cochlear nucleus]. Zhonghua Yi Xue Za Zhi 78: 30–32.

53. Dong S, Rodger J, Mulders WHAM, Robertson D (2010) Tonotopic changes in GABA receptor expression in guinea pig inferior colliculus after partial unilateral hearing loss. Brain Research 1342: 24–32.

54. Suneja SK, Potashner SJ, Benson CG (1998) Plastic changes in glycine and GABA release and uptake in adult brain stem auditory nuclei after unilateral middle ear ossicle removal and cochlear ablation. Exp Neurol 151: 273–288.

55. Caspary DM, Holder TM, Hughes LF, Milbrandt JC, McKernan RM, et al. (1999) Age-related changes in GABA(A) receptor subunit composition and function in rat auditory system. Neuroscience 93: 307–312.

56. Mossop JE, Wilson MJ, Caspary DM, Moore DR (2000) Down-regulation of inhibition following unilateral deafening. Hear Res 147: 183–187.

57. Bauer CA, Turner JG, Caspary DM, Myers KS, Brozoski TJ (2008) Tinnitus and inferior colliculus activity in chinchillas related to three distinct patterns of cochlear trauma. J Neurosci Res 86: 2564–2578.

58. Weisz N, Dohrmann K, Elbert T (2007) The relevance of spontaneous activity for the coding of the tinnitus sensation. In: B. Langguth GHTKAC, Møller AR, eds. Progress in Brain Research Elsevier. pp 61–70.

59. Meiri KF, Pfenninger KH, Willard MB (1986) Growth-associated protein, GAP-43, a polypeptide that is induced when neurons extend axons, is a component of growth cones and corresponds to pp46, a major polypeptide of a subcellular fraction enriched in growth cones. Proc Natl Acad Sci U S A 83: 3537–3541.

60. Benowitz LI, Routtenberg A (1997) GAP-43: an intrinsic determinant of neuronal development and plasticity. Trends Neurosci 20: 84–91.

61. Benowitz LI, Perrone-Bizzozero NI (1991) The expression of GAP-43 in relation to neuronal growth and plasticity: when, where, how, and why? Prog Brain Res 89: 69–87.

62. Strittmatter SM, Fankhauser C, Huang PL, Mashimo H, Fishman MC (1995) Neuronal pathfinding is abnormal in mice lacking the neuronal growth cone protein GAP-43. Cell 80: 445–452.

63. McIlvain VA, Robertson DR, Maimone MM, McCasland JS (2003) Abnormal thalamocortical pathfinding and terminal arbors lead to enlarged barrels in neonatal GAP-43 heterozygous mice. J Comp Neurol 462: 252–264.

64. Parrish-Aungst S, Shipley MT, Erdelyi F, Szabo G, Puche AC (2007) Quantitative analysis of neuronal diversity in the mouse olfactory bulb. The Journal of Comparative Neurology 501: 825–836.

16

Epithelial Cell Stretching and Luminal Acidification Lead to a Retarded Development of Stria Vascularis and Deafness in Mice Lacking Pendrin

Hyoung-Mi Kim¤**, Philine Wangemann***

Anatomy and Physiology Department, Kansas State University, Manhattan, Kansas, United States of America

Abstract

Loss-of-function mutations of *SLC26A4*/pendrin are among the most prevalent causes of deafness. Deafness and vestibular dysfunction in the corresponding mouse model, *Slc26a4*$^{-/-}$, are associated with an enlargement and acidification of the membranous labyrinth. Here we relate the onset of expression of the HCO_3^- transporter pendrin to the luminal pH and to enlargement-associated epithelial cell stretching. We determined expression with immunocytochemistry, cell stretching by digital morphometry and pH with double-barreled ion-selective electrodes. Pendrin was first expressed in the endolymphatic sac at embryonic day (E) 11.5, in the cochlear hook-region at E13.5, in the utricle and saccule at E14.5, in ampullae at E16.5, and in the upper turn of the cochlea at E17.5. Epithelial cell stretching in *Slc26a4*$^{-/-}$ mice began at E14.5. pH changes occurred first in the cochlea at E15.5 and in the endolymphatic sac at E17.5. At postnatal day 2, stria vascularis, outer sulcus and Reissner's membrane epithelial cells, and utricular and saccular transitional cells were stretched, whereas sensory cells in the cochlea, utricle and saccule did not differ between *Slc26a4*$^{+/-}$ and *Slc26a4*$^{-/-}$ mice. Structural development of stria vascularis, including vascularization, was retarded in *Slc26a4*$^{-/-}$ mice. In conclusion, the data demonstrate that the enlargement and stretching of non-sensory epithelial cells precedes luminal acidification in the cochlea and the endolymphatic sac. Stretching and luminal acidification may alter cell-to-cell communication and lead to the observed retarded development of stria vascularis, which may be an important step on the path to deafness in *Slc26a4*$^{-/-}$ mice, and possibly in humans, lacking functional pendrin expression.

Editor: Eliana Abdelhay, Instituto Nacional de Câncer, Brazil

Funding: This work was supported by the following grants: KSU-SMILE, NIH-R01-DC00212, and NIH-P20-RR017686. The funders had no role in study design, data collection and analysis, decision to publish, or preparation of the manuscript.

Competing Interests: The authors have declared that no competing interests exist.

* E-mail: wange@vet.ksu.edu

¤ Current address: Department of Otolaryngology, Pochon-CHA University College of Medicine, Seoul, Korea

Introduction

Mutations of *SLC26A4* are found in some populations in as many as 13.7% of deaf subjects and are thereby among the most prevalent causes of deafness [1,2,3,4,5]. Phenotypes associated with mutations of *SLC26A4* include deafness at birth and fluctuating hearing loss that progresses toward deafness during childhood [6,7,8]. Deafness is associated with balance dysfunction in a subset of patients [9]. The high incidence of this disorder provides a strong imperative to investigate the etiology of the disease with the ultimate goal to develop strategies to preserve hearing in afflicted individuals.

The gene *SLC26A4* codes for the protein pendrin, which is an anion-exchanger that is expressed in apical membranes of inner ear epithelial cells and transports HCO_3^- into the luminal fluid [10,11]. Pendrin-mediated HCO_3^- secretion is responsible for the pH of cochlear endolymph to be higher than the pH of perilymph, which is the fluid surrounding the cochlear duct.

Work toward an understanding of the role of pendrin in hearing and balance has been accelerated by a conventional knock out mouse model, *Slc26a4*$^{-/-}$, formerly called *Pds*$^{-/-}$ [12]. Studies using this mouse model have revealed that key events in the etiology of deafness are an acidification and enlargement of the membranous labyrinth that includes a ~10-fold enlargement of the cochlear lumen [12,13,14,10]. The enlargement of the cochlea lumen begins at embryonic day (E) 14.5, which is ~19 days before the onset of hearing at postnatal day (P) 12 [12,13,14]. The enlargement is the result of fluid secretion in the vestibular labyrinth that 'pumps up' the cochlea and a failure of fluid absorption in the endolymphatic sac that 'drains' the cochlea at this age [14]. The enlargement and the acidification spread the effect of lacking pendrin-expression from affecting solely pendrin-expressing cells themselves to affecting a multitude of other cells in the cochlea and vestibular labyrinth, thereby ultimately leading to a failure to develop proper hearing and vestibular function.

The question how lack of pendrin affects fluid transport in the embryonic inner ear is complicated by the fact that pendrin is expressed in multiple epithelial cell types that are located in small domains throughout the inner ear. Based on studies in adult mice, pendrin is expressed in the cochlea in outer sulcus and spiral prominence epithelial cells and in spindle cells of stria vascularis [15,16]. Further, pendrin is expressed in the vestibular labyrinth in transitional cells of the saccule, utricle, and ampullae and in the mitochondria-rich cells of the endolymphatic sac [15,16,17]. The onset of pendrin expression and the onset of pH changes associated with a lack of functional pendrin are important toward an understanding of the role of pendrin in fluid transport. Thus, the first goal of the present study was to determine the onset of pendrin expression in different parts of the inner ear, including the cochlea, saccule, utricle, ampullae, and endolymphatic sac and to determine the onset of pH changes that occur in the cochlea and endolymphatic sac when functional pendrin expression is present or lacking.

Loss of functional pendrin expression leads to an enlargement of the membranous labyrinth that displaces mesenchymal cells that normally surround the epithelial duct. This displacement impairs mesenchymal-epithelial cell communication including cochlear thyroid hormone signaling, which is important for the early postnatal development of the cochlea. Disruption of cochlear thyroid hormone signaling in *Slc26a4*$^{-/-}$ mice leads to cochlear hypothyroidism in the early postnatal phase of development [13]. The enlargement of the cochlea lumen may not only disrupt communication between mesenchymal and epithelial cells but may also disrupt cell signaling between adjacent epithelial cells. Stretching of epithelial cells can be expected to lengthen diffusional distances, which would dampen or delay the arrival of diffusional signals. Normal cochlear development depends on cell-to-cell communication. Loss of cell-to-cell communication, i.e. due to lack of connexin 26 expression, leads to retarded development and failure to acquire hearing [18,19,20]. Impairment of cell signaling and disruption of proper orchestration of development may also be a cause for the failure to develop hearing and balance in mice and possibly in humans lacking pendrin expression. Thus, the second goal of this study was to determine the onset of epithelial cell stretching in the cochlea and the endolymphatic sac and to determine which epithelial cell types are stretched in the cochlea and the vestibular labyrinth of mice lacking functional pendrin expression.

Methods

Animals

A colony of *Slc26a4*$^{-/-}$ and *Slc26a4*$^{+/-}$ mice was maintained at Kansas State University. Pairs of *Slc26a4*$^{+/-}$ dams and *Slc26a4*$^{-/-}$ sires were housed together. Litters sizes averaged 5.1 pups with *Slc26a4*$^{+/-}$ and *Slc26a4*$^{-/-}$ offspring in the Mendelian ratio of 50.1 to 49.9. The gestational period was 21 days. Genetic drift was limited by occasional back-crossing to the original strain, 129SvEvTac, maintained by Taconic, Germantown, NY. The colony was maintained free of known and suspected murine pathogens. Serologic tests (Radil, Columbia, MO), that were consistently and repeatedly negative, included the following antibodies: EDIM (Epizootic diarrhea of infant mice virus - a mouse rotavirus), TMEV (Theiler's murine encephalomyelitis virus - mouse poliovirus, strain GDVII), MHV (Mouse hepatitis virus - a mouse coronavirus), MVM (Minute virus of mice - a mouse parvovirus), MNV (Murine norovirus - a mouse calicivirus), M. pulmonis (Mycoplasma pulmonis – the agent of murine mycoplasmosis), MPV (a mouse parvovirus), Parvo NS-1 (a conserved recombinant parvoviral protein, rNS1) and Sendai (Sendai virus – a type 1 paramyxovirus).

Slc26a4$^{+/-}$ and *Slc26a4*$^{-/-}$ mice ranging in age from embryonic (E) day 11.5 to postnatal (P) day 7 were used in the present study. Time-pregnant dams were deeply anesthetized with 4% tri-bromo-ethanol and sacrificed by decapitation after harvesting embryos by sterile laparotomy. Gestational age was counted from the day, when a vaginal plug was detected. This day was set to E0.5. Gestational age, however, was verified, and in rare cases corrected, by evaluating gross morphological features including limbs, digits, and appearance of the pinna and auditory meatus [21,22]. Neonatal mice (P2–P3) were anesthetized by a combination of i.p. injection of 0.013 ml/g body weight of 4% tri-bromo-ethanol and rapid cooling on an ice-water slush. Older mice (P7) were anesthetized solely by i.p. injection of 0.013 ml/g body weight of 4% tri-bromo-ethanol. Embryos and postnatal mice were sacrificed by decapitation.

Ethics Statement

All procedures involving animals were approved by the Institutional Animal Care and Use Committee of Kansas State University (IACUC#: 2613 and 2961).

Immunocytochemistry

For whole-mounts, tissues were isolated by microdissection and fixed at 4°C for 2 hrs in a PBS-solution containing (in mM) 150 NaCl, 3.6 KCl, 5 HEPES, 1 $CaCl_2$, 1 $MgCl_2$ and 5 glucose, pH 7.4 and 4% paraformaldehyde. Whole-mounts were blocked for 1 hr with 5% bovine serum albumin (BSA) in PBS-TX solution containing (in mM) 137 NaCl, 2.7 KCl, 10.1 Na_2HPO_4, 1.8 KH_2PO_4, pH 7.4, and 0.2% Triton-X-100.

For cryo-sections, isolated otocysts from embryos and isolated inner ear from postnatal mice were fixed at 4°C for 2 hrs in a PBS-solution containing 4% paraformaldehyde. Fixed tissues were processed through a sucrose gradient (10% and 20%, each 20 min, followed by 30% overnight, all at 4°C), infiltrated with polyethylene glycol (Cat# 72592-B, Electron Microscopy Sciences, Hatfield, PA) and cryo-sectioned (12 µm, CM3050S, Leica, Germany). Serial sections throughout the entire cochlea were obtained embryos aged E11.5 and E14.5 and mid-modiolar sections of the cochlea were obtained from embryos between ages E15.5 and E18.5 and from neonates aged P2–P7. Sections were mounted on charged slides (Cat#22-230-900, Fisher) and blocked for 1 hr with 5% bovine serum albumin (BSA) in PBS-TX solution.

For immunocytochemistry, whole-mounts or sections were incubated overnight at 4°C with diluted primary antibody (1:200 rabbit anti-pendrin, a gift from Dr. Søren Nielsen, Aarhus University, Denmark; 1:200 rabbit-anti-Cx26 (Invitrogen, Carlsbad, CA) or 1:200 rabbit anti-Na^+/K^+ ATPase alpha1 subunit (Novus Biologicals, Littleton, CO). Primary antibodies were diluted with PBS-TX containing 1–3% BSA. Whole-mounts or sections were washed three times in PBS-TX and incubated for 1 hr at room temperature with secondary antibody (Alexa594 conjugated goat-anti-rabbit (Invitrogen) diluted 1:1,000 with PBS-TX containing 1–3% BSA. After washing three times in PBS-TX, whole-mounts or sections were incubated at room temperature for 20 min with phalloidin and 5 min with DAPI diluted with PBS-TX at 1:40 and 1:1,000, respectively. After staining, whole-mounts or sections were washed again three times with PBS-TX, cover-slipped with FluorSave (Calbiochem, La Jolla, CA) and observed by confocal laser scanning microscopy (LSM 510 Meta, Carl Zeiss, Göttingen, Germany).

Morphometric measurements including determinations of circumferences and cell surface areas were obtained using software provided with the confocal laser scanning microscope (Aim, LSM 510 Meta, Carl Zeiss). Observations reported are based on at least three independent observations.

Electrophysiological pH measurements

The endolymphatic pH and the transepithelial potential were measured *in vitro* with double-barreled microelectrodes. Procedures were developed by modifying previously described protocols [23,11]. Otocysts were isolated from embryonic mice aged E14.5–E17.5 in cold (4°C) dissection solution containing (mM):

150 NaCl, 4 KCl, 10 HEPES, 1.5 $CaCl_2$, 1 $MgCl_2$, and 5 glucose, pH 7.4. For pH measurements, otocysts were transferred into a bath chamber, stabilized with a suction pipette and superfused with warm (37°C) bicarbonate-solution containing (mM): 135 NaCl, 25 $NaHCO_3^-$, 4 KCl, 1.5 $CaCl_2$, 1 $MgCl_2$ and 5 glucose, bubbled with 5% CO_2 95% O_2 to assume pH 7.3–7.4. Measurements in the cochlea were made via a round-window approach, which yields data from the hook-region of the cochlea. Measurements in the endolymphatic sac were made in the intermediate portion. Data were recorded digitally (DIGIDATA 1322A and AxoScope 9, Axon Instruments) and analyzed using custom software written by P.W. in LabTalk (Origin 6.0, The Origin Company, Northhampton, MA).

Calibration consisted of taking a reference value in the superfused bath solution and then obtaining the slope of the electrode in a perfused agar cup placed into the bath chamber. Agar cups holding ~100 µl were prepared with warm (37°C) weakly-buffered Ringer solution. This method was devised to minimize the contribution of electrode drift and differences between reference electrodes. pH sensitive electrodes had a slope of 58±3 mV/pH unit (n = 40). Three calibration solutions with different pH values were used. Calibration solution contained (in mM): pH 6: 130 NaCl, 20 MES; pH 7: 130 NaCl, 20 HEPES; and pH 8: 130 NaCl, 20 tricine.

Double-barreled glass microelectrodes were manufactured from filament-containing glass tubing (World Precision Instruments 1B100F-4, Sarasota, FL) using a micropipette puller (Narishige PD-5, Tokyo, Japan). Prior to silanization, microelectrodes were baked at 180°C for 2 hrs to ensure dryness. The longer ion-selective barrel was mounted in the lid of a beaker. The beaker was heated to 210°C and silanized by a 90 s exposure to 0.02 ml dimethyldichlorosilane (Fluka 40136) at RT. The shorter reference barrel was protected from silanization by sealing the open end with Parafilm (Alcan Packaging, Chicago, IL). After silanization, microelectrodes were baked at 180°C for 3 hrs and tips were broken to a final O.D. of ~3 µm. The reference barrel was filled with 1 M KCl and the ionselective barrel was filled at the tip with liquid ion exchanger (Hydrogen ionophore II - Cocktail A, Fluka 95297) and back-filled with buffer solution (500 mM KCl, 20 mM HEPES, pH 7.4).

Statistics

Data are generally presented as average ± sem with N being the number of animals. In some instances averages are presented with SD, as indicated. Data acquired in paired experiments using littermates were evaluated by paired t-test. Significance was assumed when $p<0.05$.

Results

Onset of pendrin expression

In a first series of experiments, we determined the onset of pendrin expression in the embryonic cochlea, the vestibular labyrinth and the endolymphatic sac and duct. In the cochlea, pendrin expression was found in the outer sulcus region of the lateral wall. The onset of expression progressed from the hook region to the basal turn and then to the upper turn of the cochlea. The first expression was found at E13.5–E14.5 in the hook region of the cochlea (Fig. 1A–C). At this age, there was yet no expression in the basal turn. At E16.5, expression was found in the basal turn but not yet in the upper turn (Fig. 1D and E) and at E17.5 pendrin expression was found throughout the cochlea (Fig. 1F and G).

In the vestibular labyrinth, pendrin expression was found in transitional cells surrounding the sensory cells in the utricle, saccule and semicircular canal ampullae, as well as in epithelial cells that line the saccular duct. The onset of pendrin expression in the anterior semicircular canal ampulla was at E16.5 (Fig. 2A–D), which is two days after the onset of expression in utricular transitional cells, which occurred at E14.5 (Fig. 2E–I). In the saccule, the onset of pendrin expression in transitional cells was at E14.5 (Fig. 3A–C) and in cells lining the saccular duct was at E15.5–E16.5 (Fig. 3D–F).

The endolymphatic sac at E10.5 was identified as a pouch-like structure composed of epithelial cells expressing Na^+/K^+ ATPase that projected from the dorso-medial side of the otocyst opposite to the cochlea duct that emerged at the ventral side (Fig. 4A). A fluid-filled lumen was formed in the endolymphatic sac at E11.5–E12.5 (Fig. 4B and D). The onset of pendrin expression was at E11.5 (Fig. 4B). The number of cells expressing pendrin increased with development (Fig. 4B–J). The overall organ size grew notably from E13.5 to E14.5 (Fig. 4E and G). From E14.5 onward, almost 30% of cells in the distal portion of endolymphatic sac expressed pendrin (Fig. 4G and H). At E17.5 and P2, the endolymphatic sac epithelium became increasingly rugous with infoldings and tubular protrusions (Fig. 4I and J).

Onset of pendrin-dependent pH changes

In a second series of experiments, we measured in isolated *in vitro* superfused otocysts the transepithelial potential and the pH of endolymph and perilymph in the hook region of the cochlea. Further, we measured the transepithelial potential and the pH of endolymph in the endolymphatic sac. Measurements were made in *Slc26a4*$^{+/-}$ and *Slc26a4*$^{-/-}$ littermates ranging from age E14.5 to E17.5. The transepithelial potential in the cochlea and the endolymphatic sac was near zero at all ages and genotypes (*data not shown*). The perilymphatic pH in the cochlea was 7.32±0.05 (SD; n = 15) and did not vary with development or genotype (Fig. 5A). The endolymphatic pH was dependent on the age and genotype of the embryo. At E14.5, the pH of cochlear endolymph was by ~0.1 pH-units larger than the pH of perilymph with no difference between *Slc26a4*$^{+/-}$ and *Slc26a4*$^{-/-}$ mice. At E15.5 and E17.5 the pH of cochlear endolymph in *Slc26a4*$^{+/-}$ mice remained by ~0.1-pH-units more alkaline than the pH of perilymph but the endolymphatic pH in *Slc26a4*$^{-/-}$ became ~0.3 pH-units more acid than the endolymphatic pH in *Slc26a4*$^{+/-}$ mice.

The pH of the bath fluid surrounding the endolymphatic sac was 7.35±0.04 (SD; n = 25). At E14.5 the pH in the endolymphatic sac of *Slc26a4*$^{+/-}$ and *Slc26a4*$^{-/-}$ mice was ~0.1 pH-units lower than the pH of the bath solution (Fig. 5B). At E15.5 and E17.5 the endolymphatic pH in *Slc26a4*$^{+/-}$ mice dropped to ~0.3 and ~0.5 pH-units below the pH of the bath fluid, respectively. No differences were observed between *Slc26a4*$^{+/-}$ and *Slc26a4*$^{-/-}$ mice at E14.5 and E15.5, however, at E17.5 the endolymphatic pH in *Slc26a4*$^{-/-}$ mice was ~0.8 pH-units more acidic than the pH of the bath solution and ~0.2 pH-units more acid than endolymphatic pH in *Slc26a4*$^{+/-}$ mice.

Pendrin-dependent luminal enlargement and epithelial cell stretching

In a third series of experiments, we evaluated epithelial cell stretching by measuring the circumference of the cochlear lumen and by measuring the apical surface areas of individual epithelial cells. Measurements of the circumference of the cochlea lumen were made in matched cross-sections of the basal turn of *Slc26a4*$^{+/-}$and *Slc26a4*$^{-/-}$ littermates (Fig. 6A–B). At E14.5 the length of the circumference of the cochlear lumen was larger in *Slc26a4*$^{-/-}$ mice compared to *Slc26a4*$^{+/-}$ mice, although the increase in length was not substantial, factor 1.1. With further development the difference in length of the circumference between *Slc26a4*$^{+/-}$ and *Slc26a4*$^{-/-}$

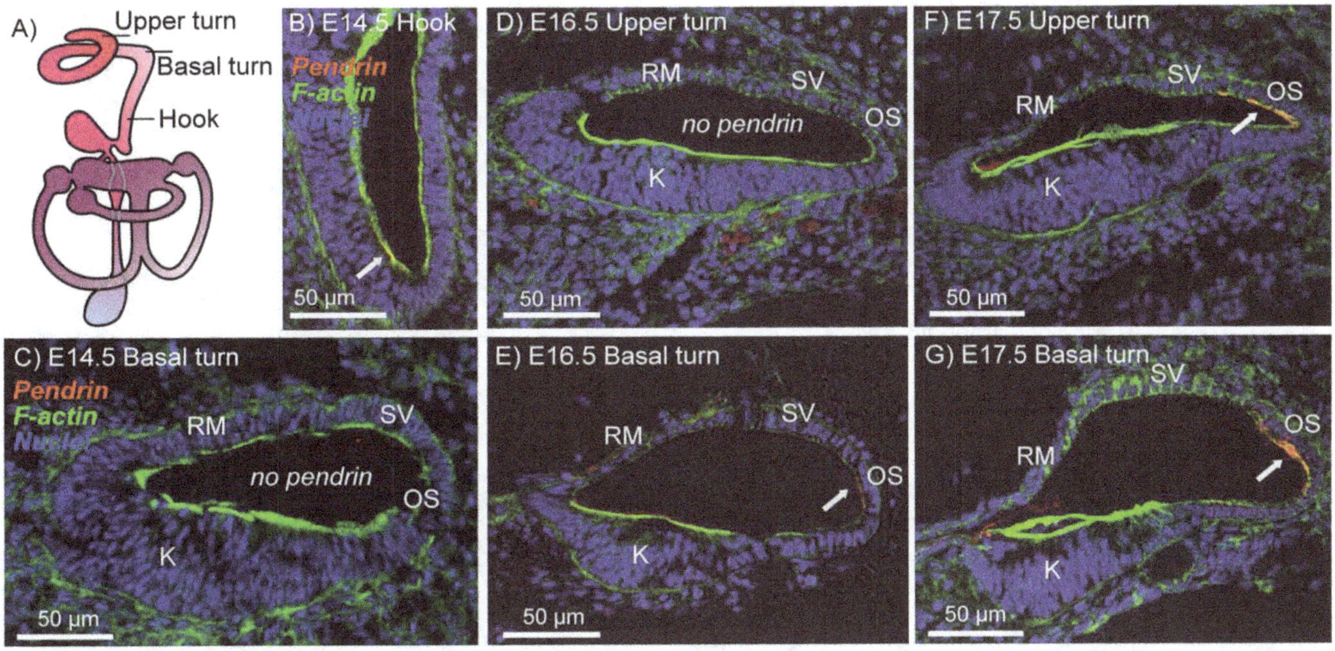

Figure 1. Onset of pendrin expression in the cochlea. Pendrin (*red*) was visualized by immunocytochemistry. F-actin (*green*) and nuclei (*blue*) were labeled. A: Diagram of the inner ear. B–G: Cross-sections of the cochlear duct in the hook region (B), basal turn (C, E and G) and upper turn (D and F) of *Slc26a4*$^{+/-}$ mice at age E14.5 (B and C), E16.5 (D and E) and E17.5 (F and G). Abbreviations: K, Kölliker's organ; RM, Reissner's membrane; SV, stria vascularis; OS, outer sulcus. Pendrin expression is marked by arrows.

mice grew from a factor of 1.1 to a factor of 2.3 at E16.5 and 2.7 at E18.5 (Fig. 6B).

The overall organ size of the endolymphatic sac at E13.5 was similar between *Slc26a4*$^{+/-}$ and *Slc26a4*$^{-/-}$ mice, however, one day later, at E14.5, the endolymphatic sac was notably enlarged in *Slc26a4*$^{-/-}$ mice (Fig. 6C–D). Consistently, apical cell surface areas in the endolymphatic sac were similar at E13.5 but enlarged at E14.5 (Fig. 6E), however, apical cells surface areas in the

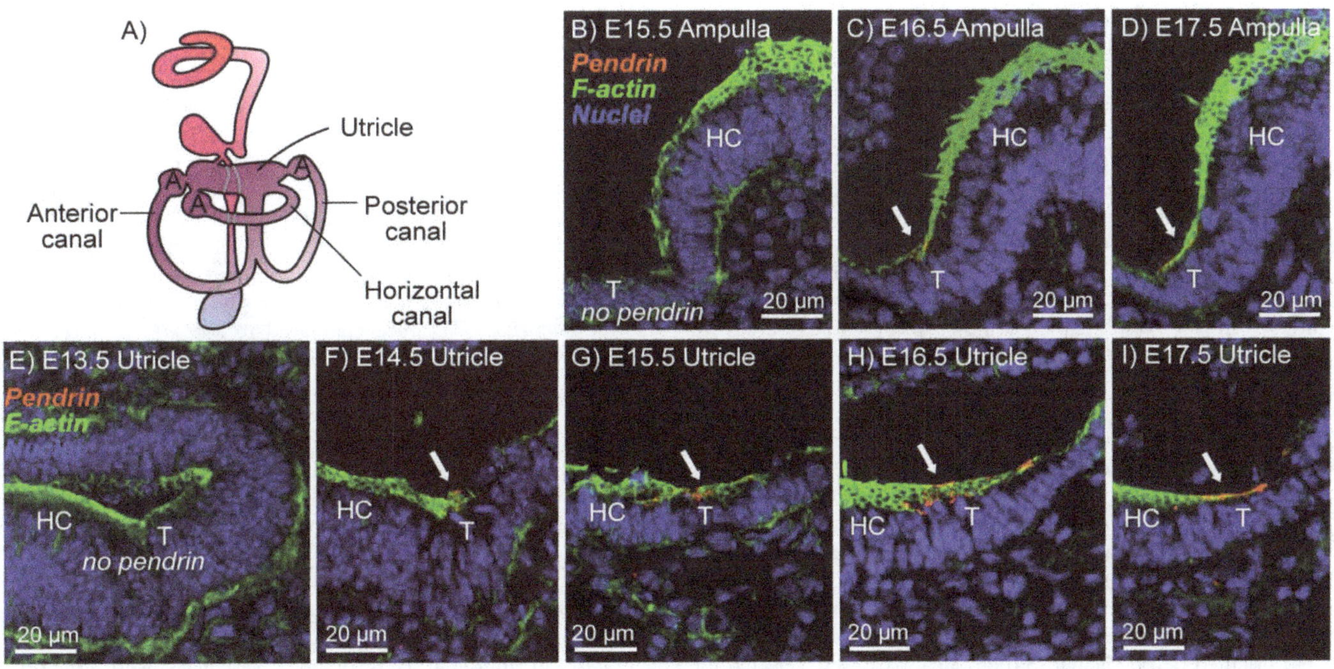

Figure 2. Onset of pendrin expression in the ampullae and utricle of the vestibular labyrinth. Pendrin (*red*) was visualized by immunocytochemistry. F-actin (*green*) and nuclei (*blue*) were labeled. A: Diagram of the inner ear. B–D: Cross-sections of the anterior canal ampulla of *Slc26a4*$^{+/-}$ mice at age E15.5–E17.5. E–I: Cross-sections of utricle of *Slc26a4*$^{+/-}$ mice at age E13.5–E17.5. Abbreviations: A, Ampulla; T, transitional cells; HC, hair cells. Pendrin expression is marked by arrows.

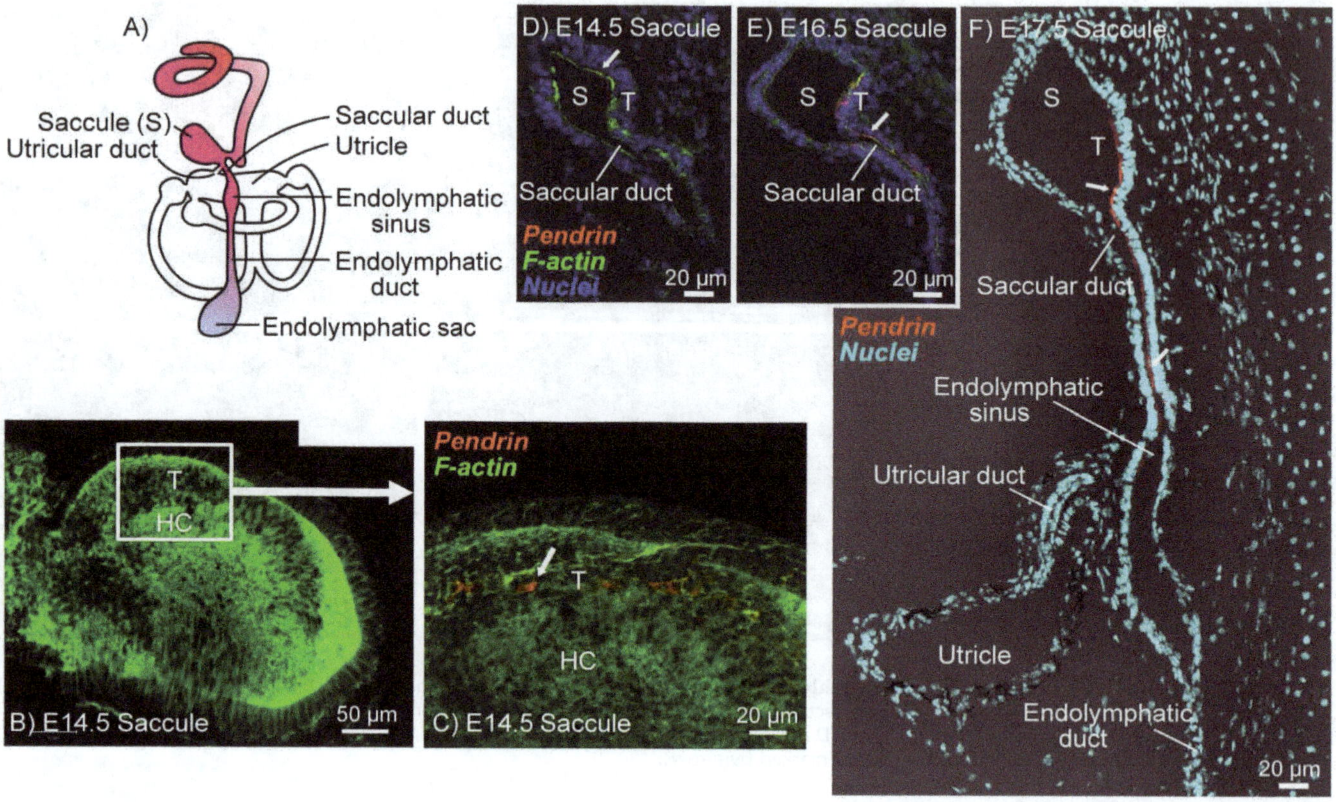

Figure 3. Onset of pendrin expression in the saccule of the vestibular labyrinth. Pendrin (*red*) was visualized by immunocytochemistry. F-actin (*green*) and nuclei (*blue*) were labeled. A: Diagram of the inner ear. B–C: Whole-mount of the saccule from a *Slc26a4*$^{+/-}$ mice at age E14.5. D–F: Cross-sections of the saccule from *Slc26a4*$^{+/-}$ mice at age E14.5–E17.5. Abbreviations: S, Saccule; T, transitional cells; HC, hair cells. Pendrin expression is marked by arrows.

endolymphatic duct remained similar between *Slc26a4*$^{+/-}$ and *Slc26a4*$^{-/-}$ mice at E13.5 and at E14.5 (Fig. 6F).

Stretching of epithelial cells in the cochlea, the vestibular labyrinth and the endolymphatic sac and duct was evaluated in greater detail by measuring apical surface areas in *Slc26a4*$^{+/-}$ and *Slc26a4*$^{-/-}$ mice at age P2 (Fig. 7). In the cochlea, apical surface areas of strial marginal cells, outer sulcus epithelial cells, and Reissner's membrane epithelial cells were enlarged in *Slc26a4*$^{-/-}$ mice compared to *Slc26a4*$^{+/-}$ mice (Fig. 7A–C and I). In contrast, apical surface areas of inner and outer hair cells were similar and not different between *Slc26a4*$^{+/-}$ and *Slc26a4*$^{-/-}$ mice (Fig. 7D and I). In the vestibular labyrinth, apical surface areas of transitional cells in the utricle and saccule were enlarged in *Slc26a4*$^{-/-}$ mice compared to *Slc26a4*$^{+/-}$ mice, however, similar to the cochlea, apical surface areas of hair cells did not differ between *Slc26a4*$^{+/-}$ and *Slc26a4*$^{-/-}$ mice (Fig. 7E–F and J). The epithelium of the endolymphatic sac in *Slc26a4*$^{+/-}$ was heavily folded and included tubular protrusions, as shown in Fig. 4J. In contrast, the epithelium in *Slc26a4*$^{-/-}$ mice was planar due to cell stretching caused by the enlargement. Mitochondria-rich cells that expressed pendrin in *Slc26a4*$^{+/-}$ mice were distinguished from ribosome-rich cells in *Slc26a4*$^{+/-}$ and *Slc26a4*$^{-/-}$ mice by their dense actin expression near the apical membrane (Fig. 7G). Cells oriented perpendicular to the optical path were selected for apical surface area measurements in *Slc26a4*$^{+/-}$ and *Slc26a4*$^{-/-}$ mice. Apical surface areas of mitochondria-rich and ribosome-rich cells were found to be enlarged in *Slc26a4*$^{-/-}$ mice compared to *Slc26a4*$^{+/-}$ mice (Fig. 7J). Further, apical surface areas of epithelial cells lining the endolymphatic duct were found to be enlarged in *Slc26a4*$^{-/-}$ mice compared to *Slc26a4*$^{+/-}$ mice (Fig. 7H and J).

In a fourth series of experiments, we evaluated expression patterns of connexin 26 and Na^+/K^+ ATPase in the cochlea of *Slc26a4*$^{+/-}$ and *Slc26a4*$^{-/-}$ mice. At E14.5, connexin 26 was expressed in gap junction plaques in Kölliker's organ and in outer sulcus epithelial cells. The expression pattern at this age was similar in *Slc26a4*$^{+/-}$ and *Slc26a4*$^{-/-}$ mice (Fig. 8A and B). At E16.5, the region of connexin 26 expression in Kölliker's organ became distinct from the region of in outer sulcus epithelial cells (Fig. 8C and D). Cell height of outer sulcus epithelial cells was lower in *Slc26a4*$^{-/-}$ mice compared to *Slc26a4*$^{+/-}$ mice. This thinning of the epithelium is most likely due to stretching. The stretch-related reduction in the area of lateral approximation between epithelial cells was reflected in the staining pattern of connexin 26 that appeared concentrated toward the tight-junction complexes. At E18.5, connexin 26 expression was found in *Slc26a4*$^{+/-}$ and *Slc26a4*$^{-/-}$ mice in Kölliker's organ, in outer sulcus epithelial cells and in fibrocytes of the suprastrial region (Fig. 9A and C). Expression of Na^+/K^+ ATPase was found in all epithelial lining the cochlea lumen (Fig. 9B). The highest intensity of Na^+/K^+ ATPase expression was found in stria vascularis. At P3, intense expressions of connexin 26 in basal cells and of Na^+/K^+ ATPase in marginal cells of stria vascularis were found in *Slc26a4*$^{+/-}$ and *Slc26a4*$^{-/-}$ mice (Fig. 10A–D).

Tissue height of stria vascularis was much lower in *Slc26a4*$^{-/-}$ mice compared to *Slc26a4*$^{+/-}$ mice. This thinning of the tissue is most likely due to stretching. Interestingly, the onset of connexin 26 expression in basal cell of stria vascularis appeared earlier in

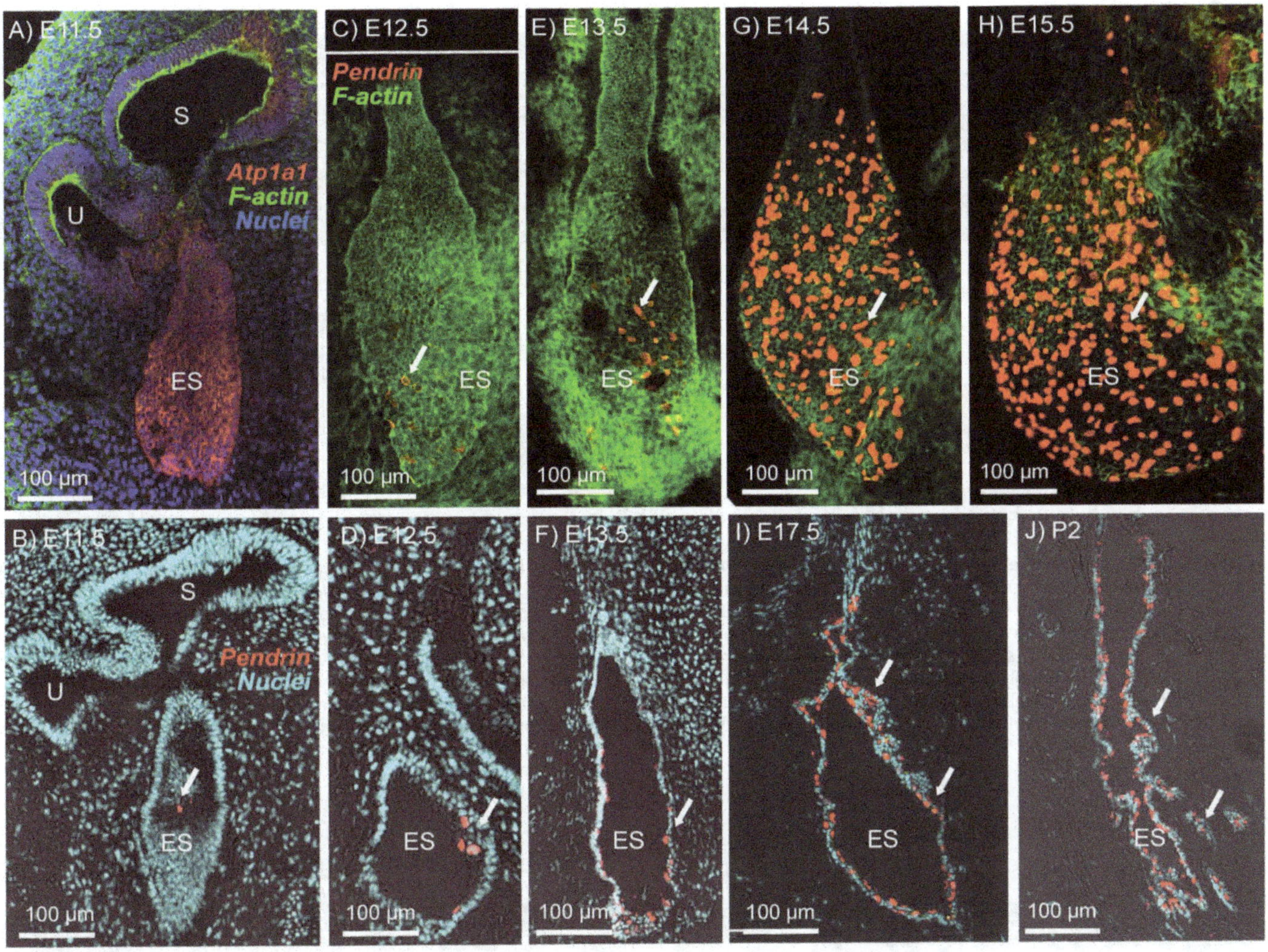

Figure 4. Onset of pendrin expression in the endolymphatic sac. Na^+/K^+ ATPase or pendrin (*red*) were visualized by immunocytochemistry. F-actin (*green*) and nuclei (*blue*) were labeled. A, B, D, F, I and J: Cross-sections of the endolymphatic sac from *Slc26a4*$^{+/-}$ mice at ages E11.5-P2. C, E, G and H: Whole-mounts of the endolymphatic sac from *Slc26a4*$^{+/-}$ mice at age E12.5–E15.5. Abbreviations: U, utricle; S, saccule; ES, endolymphatic sac. Pendrin expression is marked by arrows.

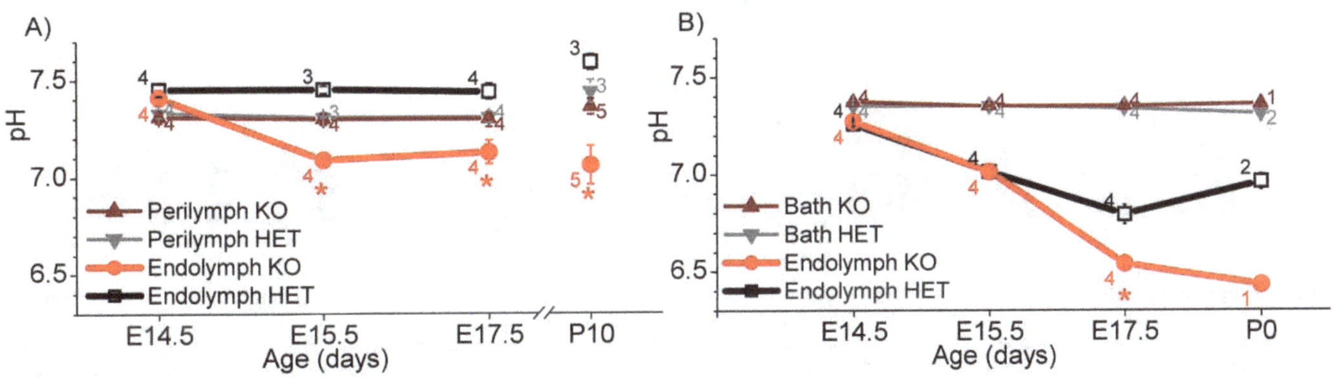

Figure 5. pH measurements in the embryonic inner ear. A: Measurements of the endolymphatic and perilymphatic pH in the cochlea of isolated *in vitro* superfused otocysts from *Slc26a4*$^{+/-}$ (HET) and *Slc26a4*$^{-/-}$ (KO) mice aged E14.5–E17.5. Data from P10 *Slc26a4*$^{+/-}$ mice, obtained by *in situ* measurements and reported earlier [11], are shown here for comparison. B: Measurements of the endolymphatic pH in the endolymphatic sac of isolated otocysts from *Slc26a4*$^{+/-}$ (HET) and *Slc26a4*$^{-/-}$ (KO) mice aged E14.5–E17.5. Numbers next to the bars represent the N number of otocysts. Significant differences between endolymph from *Slc26a4*$^{+/-}$ (*black*) and *Slc26a4*$^{-/-}$ (*red*) mice are marked with a star.

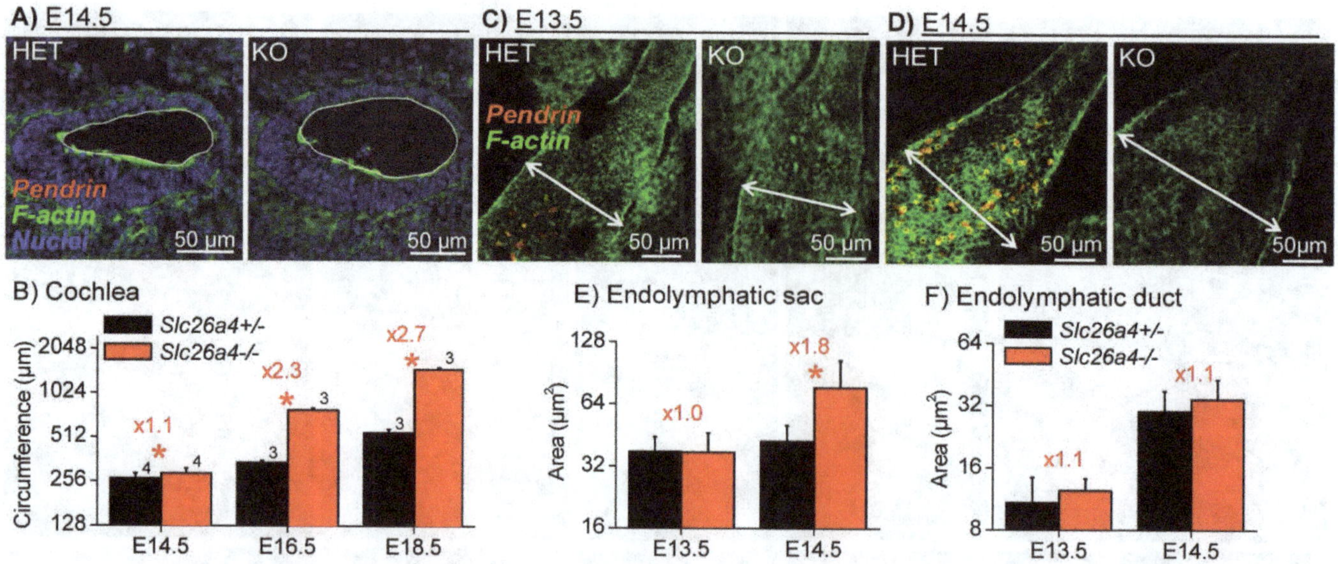

Figure 6. Onset of cell stretching in cochlea and endolymphatic sac. Pendrin (*red*) was visualized by immunocytochemistry. F-actin (*green*) and nuclei (*blue*) were labeled. A: Cross-sections of the basal turn of the cochlea from $Slc26a4^{+/-}$ (HET) and $Slc26a4^{-/-}$ (KO) mice at age E14.5. The circumference of the cochlear lumen is marked by a white line. B: Summarized measurements (avg±sem) of the luminal circumference of the cochlea at ages E14.5–E18.5. Numbers next to the bars represent the N number of otocysts. Significant differences between $Slc26a4^{+/-}$ (*black*) and $Slc26a4^{-/-}$ (*red*) mice are marked with a star. C–D: Whole-mounts of the endolymphatic sac from $Slc26a4^{+/-}$ (HET) and $Slc26a4^{-/-}$ (KO) mice at ages E13.5 and E14.5. The width of the endolymphatic sac is marked by a double-arrow. E–F: Summarized measurements (avg±SD, each bar N = 15) of the apical surface area of epithelial cells in the endolymphatic sac and duct at ages E13.5–E14.5. Significant differences between $Slc26a4^{+/-}$ (*black*) and $Slc26a4^{-/-}$ (*red*) mice are marked with a star. Figures preceded by 'x' indicate the factor between measurements in $Slc26a4^{+/-}$ and $Slc26a4^{-/-}$ mice.

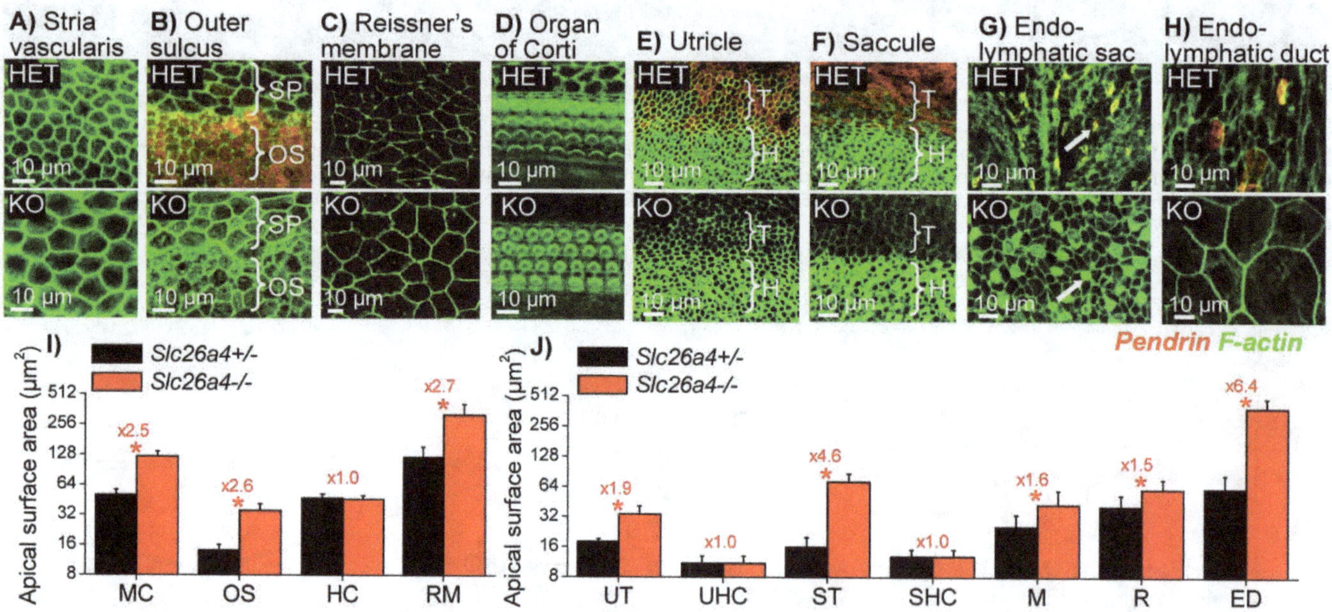

Figure 7. Epithelial cell stretching in the cochlea and the vestibular labyrinth at P2. Pendrin (*red*) was visualized by immunocytochemistry and F-actin (*green*) was labeled in $Slc26a4^{+/-}$ (HET) mice and $Slc26a4^{-/-}$ (KO) mice. A–D: Whole-mounts of epithelial cells from the cochlea. Abbreviations: SP, spiral prominence epithelial cells; OS, outer sulcus epithelial cells. E–H) Whole-mounts of epithelial cells from the vestibular labyrinth and endolymphatic sac. Mitochondria-rich cells in endolymphatic sac from $Slc26a4^{+/-}$ and $Slc26a4^{-/-}$ mice are marked by arrows. Abbreviations: T, transitional cells; H, hair cells. I: Summary of apical cell surface area measurements (avg±SD, N = 15) made on cochlea epithelial cells. Abbreviations: MC, marginal cells of stria vascularis; OS, outer sulcus epithelial cells; HC, hair cells; RM, Reissner's membrane epithelial cells. J: Summary of apical cell surface area measurements (avg±SD, N = 15) made on vestibular epithelial cells. Abbreviations: UT, utricular transitional cells; UHC, utricular hair cells; ST, saccular transitional cells; SHC, saccular hair cells; M, mitochondria-rich cells; R, ribosome-rich cells; ED, endolymphatic duct epithelial cells. Significant differences between $Slc26a4^{+/-}$ (*black*) and $Slc26a4^{-/-}$ (*red*) mice are marked with a star. Figures preceded by 'x' indicate the factor between measurements in $Slc26a4^{+/-}$ and $Slc26a4^{-/-}$ mice.

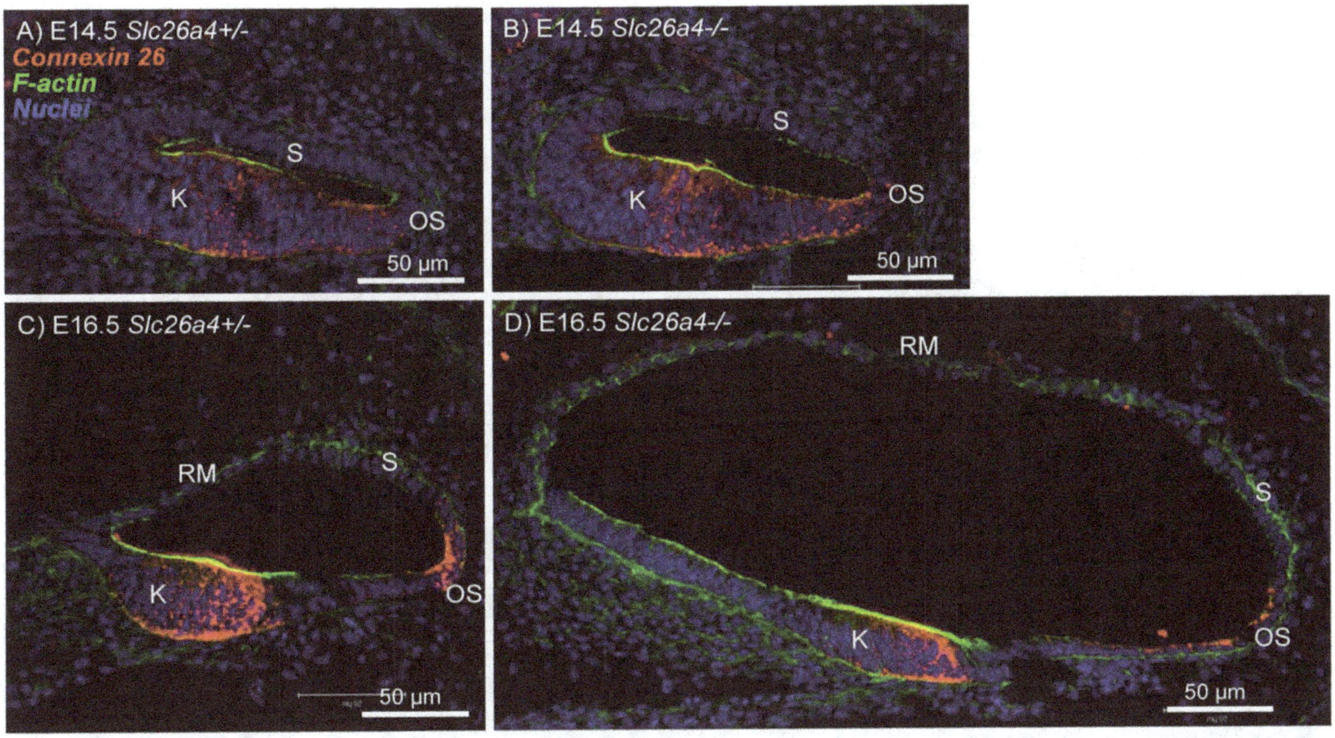

Figure 8. Connexin 26 expression in the cochlea of *Slc26a4*$^{+/-}$ and *Slc26a4*$^{-/-}$ mice at E14.5 and E16.5. Connexin 26 (*red*) was visualized by immunocytochemistry. F-actin (*green*) and nuclei (*blue*) were labeled. A–B: Cross-sections of the basal turn of the cochlea from *Slc26a4*$^{+/-}$ and *Slc26a4*$^{-/-}$ mice at age E14.5. C–D: Cross-sections of the basal turn of the cochlea from *Slc26a4*$^{+/-}$ and *Slc26a4*$^{-/-}$ mice at age E16.5. Abbreviations: K, Kölliker's organ; RM, Reissner's membrane; S, stria vascularis; OS, outer sulcus.

Slc26a4$^{-/-}$ mice compared to *Slc26a4*$^{+/-}$ mice: Expression was found at E18.5 in *Slc26a4*$^{-/-}$ mice but not yet in *Slc26a4*$^{+/-}$ mice (Fig. 9A and C). At P3, the intensity of expression appeared similar in *Slc26a4*$^{+/-}$ and *Slc26a4*$^{-/-}$ mice (Fig. 10A and C).

The development of stria vascularis was evaluated between E14.5 and P7 (Fig. 11). The expression pattern of Na^+/K^+ ATPase was similar between *Slc26a4*$^{+/-}$ and *Slc26a4*$^{-/-}$ mice, however, from E16.5 to P3, tissue height of stria vascularis was lower in *Slc26a4*$^{-/-}$ mice. At P3, stria vascularis became visibly endowed with a network of capillaries (Fig. 11C). The diameter of individual capillaries was smaller in *Slc26a4*$^{-/-}$ mice and the capillary network appeared less dense compared to *Slc26a4*$^{+/-}$ mice. At P7, tissue height of stria vascularis appeared similar in *Slc26a4*$^{+/-}$ and *Slc26a4*$^{-/-}$ mice (Fig. 11D). Diameters of individual capillaries appeared similar at this age, however, the density of the capillary network remained less, which is consistent with tissue stretching.

Discussion

The most salient findings of the present study are: 1) expression of pendrin in the inner ear begins in the endolymphatic sac followed by the onset of expression in the cochlea and vestibular labyrinth. 2) failure to express pendrin causes acidification of the luminal fluid in the cochlea and the endolymphatic sac and that this acidification occurs in the cochlea within 1–2 days of the failed onset of expression and in the endolymphatic sac after more than 4 days after the failed onset. 3) failure to express pendrin causes an enlargement of the endolymphatic sac that develops within 3 days of the failed onset of expression, whereas the enlargement of the cochlea precedes the onset of expression by ~1 day. 4) failure to express pendrin causes stretching of non-sensory epithelial cells and a retarded development of stria vascularis.

Pendrin protein expression

The expression pattern of pendrin in the developing inner ear is consistent with the pattern that had previously been determined in the adult inner ear [15,16]. Accordingly, pendrin expression was found in the developing cochlea in outer sulcus epithelial cells, in transitional cells of the developing semicircular canal ampullae, utricle and saccule as well as in the developing endolymphatic sac (Fig. 1, 2, 3, 4). An additional location of expression was the epithelium that lines the saccular duct (Fig. 3). The role of this epithelium in inner ear fluid homeostasis is unknown.

The observation that pendrin protein expression was found to occur first in the endolymphatic sac is consistent with earlier investigations monitoring the onset of pendrin mRNA expression [24]. Our data document the onset of expression at E11.5, which is 2 days prior to the earlier report that was based on *in situ* hybridization. This difference is important, because the onset of pendrin expression in the endolymphatic sac at E11.5 coincides with the onset of H^+ ATPase expression [25]. H^+ ATPase, like pendrin, is expressed in the apical membrane of mitochondrial-rich cells in the endolymphatic sac. The coincidental onset of expression suggests that both transporters form a functional unit that transports HCO_3^- buffered H^+ across the apical membrane.

Failure to express pendrin causes luminal pH changes

We have previously shown in the adult cochlea that the endolymphatic pH is higher than the perilymphatic pH when pendrin is expressed and lower than the perilymphatic pH when pendrin is absent [11]. Similar observations have now been made

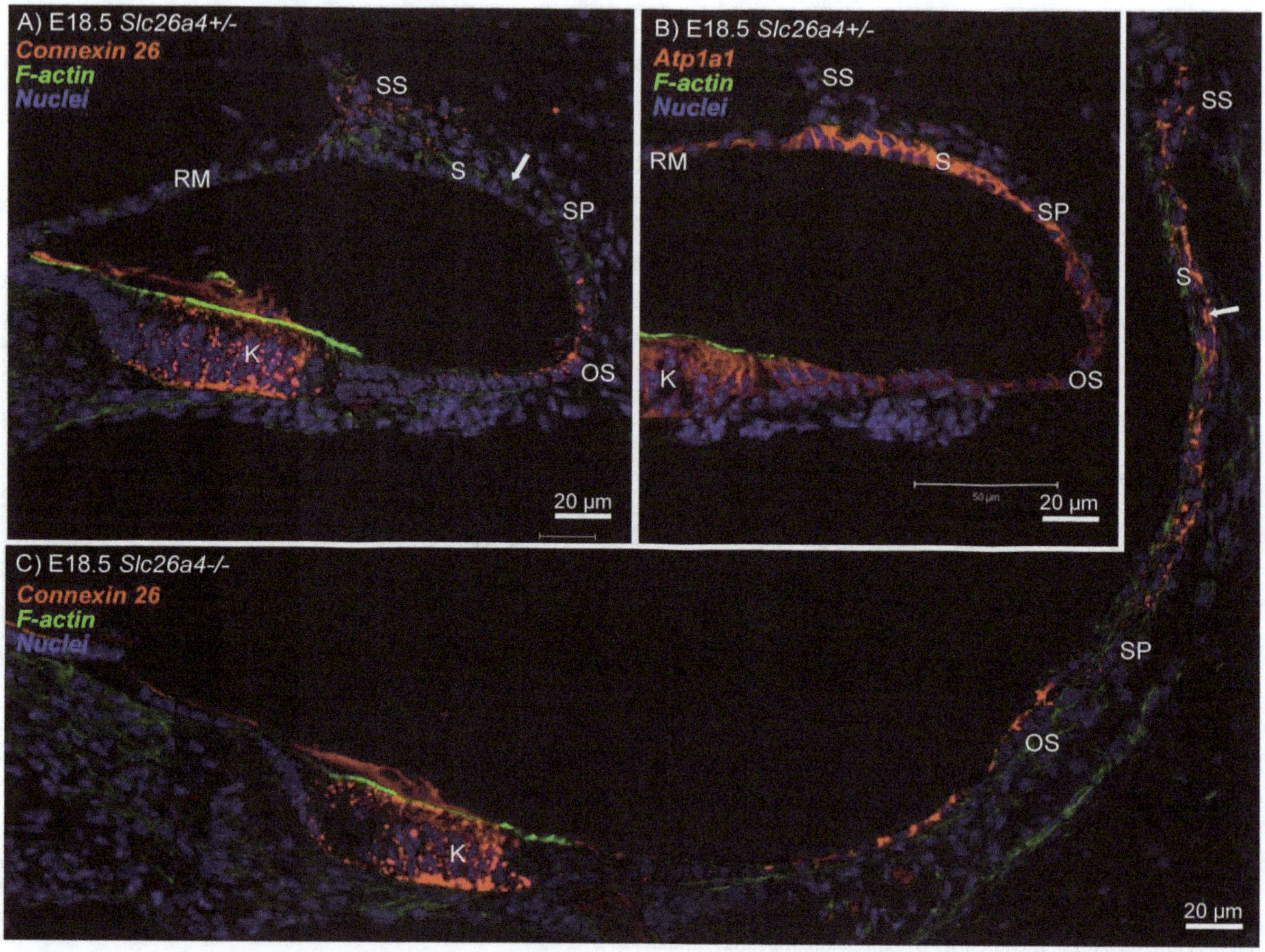

Figure 9. Connexin 26 and Na$^+$/K$^+$ ATPase expression in the cochlea of *Slc26a4*$^{+/-}$ and *Slc26a4*$^{-/-}$ mice at E18.5. Connexin 26 and Na$^+$/K$^+$ ATPase (both *red*) were visualized by immunocytochemistry. F-actin (*green*) and nuclei (*blue*) were labeled. A–B: Cross-sections of the basal turn of the cochlea from *Slc26a4*$^{+/-}$ mice at age E18.5. C: Cross-sections of the basal turn of the cochlea from *Slc26a4*$^{-/-}$ mice at age E18.5. Abbreviations: K, Kölliker's organ; RM, Reissner's membrane; SS, fibrocytes in the suprastrial region; S, stria vascularis; SP, spiral prominence; OS, outer sulcus. The arrows in A and C point to basal cells at E18.5 that lack connexin 26 expression in *Slc26a4*$^{+/-}$ mice but express connexin 26 prematurely in *Slc26a4*$^{-/-}$ mice.

in the developing cochlea as early as E15.5, which is 1–2 days after the onset of pendrin expression in the cochlea (Fig. 5). Interestingly, one day earlier, at E14.5, the endolymphatic pH was by ~0.1 pH-units higher than the perilymphatic pH regardless of the absence of presence of pendrin. This observation suggests the presence of other acid or base transport systems that contribute to the elevated pH of endolymph at least at this stage of development.

In contrast to the endolymphatic pH in the cochlea, the pH of the endolymphatic sac was found to be more acidic than the surrounding fluid. This acidic pH was observed as early as E14.5, which is 3 days after the onset of pendrin and H$^+$ ATPase expression [25] (Fig. 5). The finding of an acidic pH in the developing endolymphatic sac is consistent with measurements in the adult endolymphatic sac [26,27,28]. Interestingly, up to E15.5, which is 4 days after the onset of pendrin expression, no difference in the endolymphatic pH was found between *Slc26a4*$^{+/-}$ and *Slc26a4*$^{-/-}$ mice. It remains undetermined, whether this delay in luminal pH changes is due to compensatory mechanisms possibly consisting of a coupling between the rates of ATPase-mediated H$^+$ secretion and pendrin-mediated HCO_3^- secretion. Alternatively, the delay in the appearance of luminal pH changes could be related to the enlarged luminal volume found in *Slc26a4*$^{-/-}$ mice or simply be a function of luminal pH buffering. Buffering of the luminal pH can be expected to be stronger in the endolymphatic sac compared to the cochlea since the endolymphatic sac, at least in adult animals, contains a higher concentration of proteins [29,30,31].

Failure to express pendrin causes stretching and retarded development of epithelial cells

We have previously reported that lumen formation in the embryonic cochlea is controlled by fluid secretion in the vestibular labyrinth and fluid absorption in the endolymphatic sac and that fluid absorption in the endolymphatic sac depends on pendrin [14]. The observation that the onset of the cochlear enlargement precedes the onset of pendrin expression (Fig. 6) supports the concept that the enlargement is initially driven by fluid secretion in the vestibular labyrinth rather than by defect of local cochlear fluid transport. Nothing is known about ion and fluid transport in the embryonic vestibular labyrinth, although the observation that the endolymphatic sac forms an open lumen at E11.5–E12.5 suggests

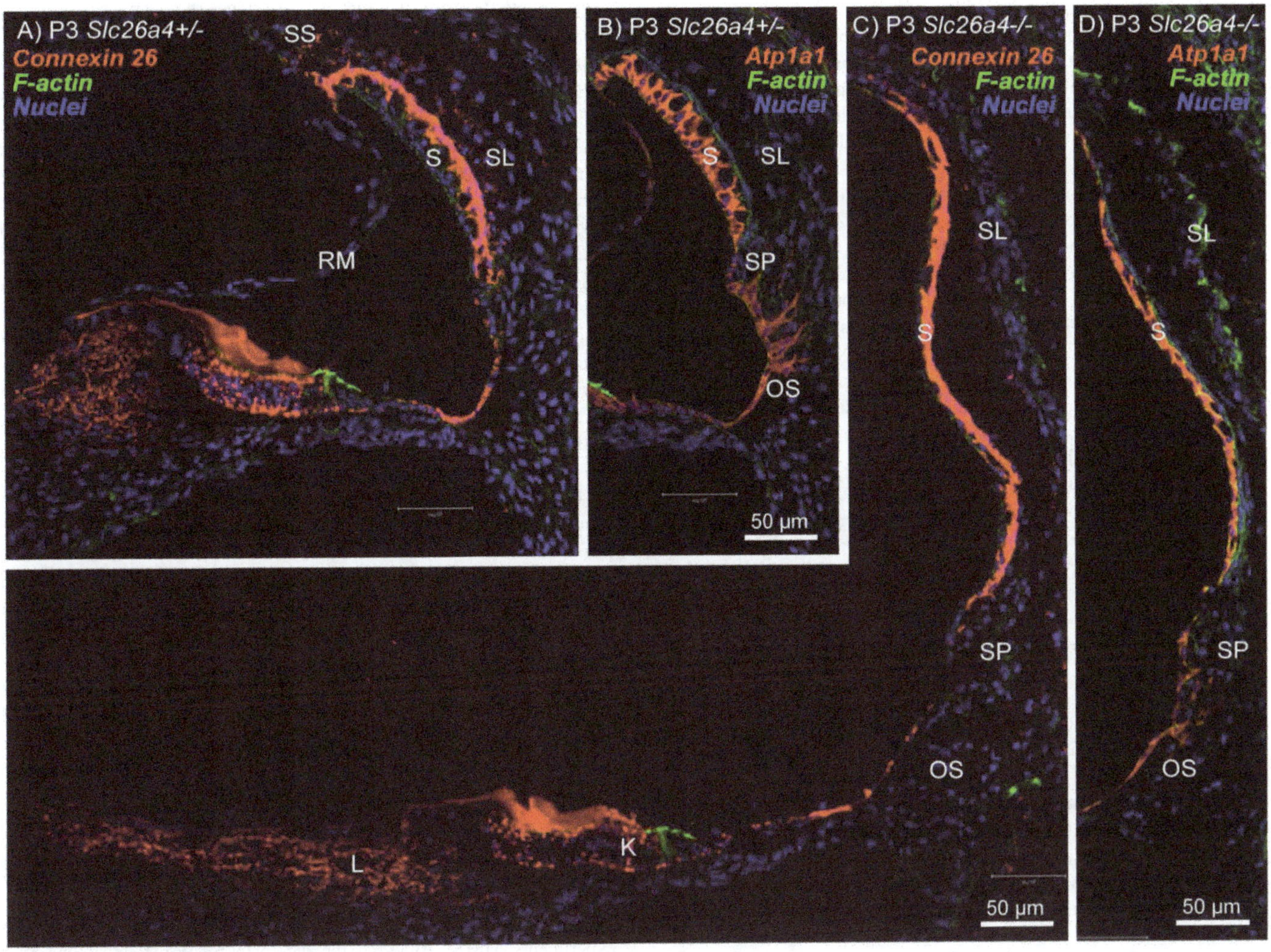

Figure 10. Connexin 26 and Na$^+$/K$^+$ ATPase expression in the cochlea of *Slc26a4*$^{+/-}$ and *Slc26a4*$^{-/-}$ mice at P3. Connexin 26 and Na$^+$/K$^+$ ATPase (both *red*) were visualized by immunocytochemistry. F-actin (*green*) and nuclei (*blue*) were labeled. A–B: Cross-sections of the basal turn of the cochlea from *Slc26a4*$^{+/-}$ mice at age P3. C–D: Cross-sections of the basal turn of the cochlea from *Slc26a4*$^{-/-}$ mice at age P3. Abbreviations: K, Kölliker's organ; L, fibrocytes in the spiral limbus; RM, Reissner's membrane; SS, fibrocytes in the suprastrial region; S, stria vascularis; SL, spiral ligament; SP, spiral prominence; OS, outer sulcus.

that fluid secretion in the vestibular labyrinth is present at this time. It is an attractive hypothesis to assume that the cochlea and the endolymphatic sac, which both form as pouches protruding from the otocyst, are 'pumped up' by fluid secretion in the otocyst that forms the vestibular labyrinth. The observation that the onset of the enlargement of the cochlea and the onset of the enlargement

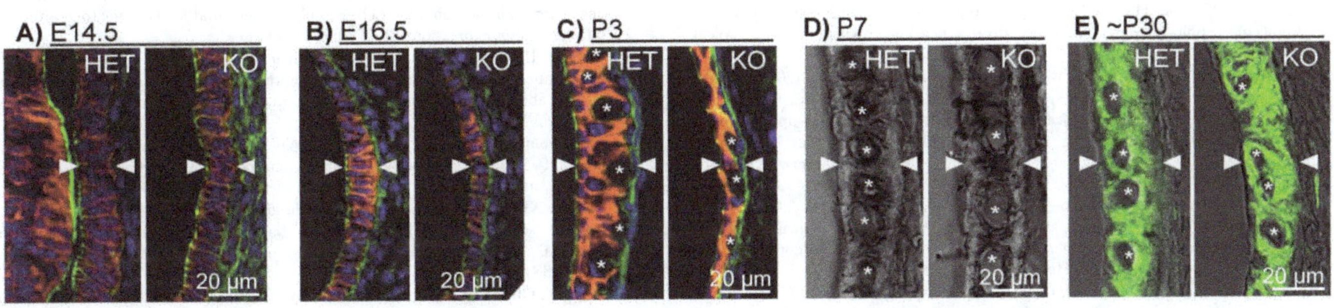

Figure 11. Retarded development of stria vascularis. A–C: Cross-sections of stria vascularis of *Slc26a4*$^{+/-}$ (HET) and *Slc26a4*$^{-/-}$ (KO) mice at E14.5, E16.5 and P3. Na$^+$/K$^+$ ATPase (*red*) was visualized by immunocytochemistry. F-actin (green) and nuclei (*blue*) were labeled. D: Cross-sections of stria vascularis at P7 visualized by laser-scanning microscopy without any stain. E: Cross-sections of stria vascularis at ~P30. The Na$^+$/2Cl$^-$/K$^+$ cotransporter *Slc12a2* was visualized by immunocytochemistry. The ~P30 data, previously reported [16], were added here for comparison. Tissue height of stria vascularis is marked by arrow-heads. Cross-sections of individual capillaries are marked with a star.

of the endolymphatic sac coincide at E14.5 (Fig. 6), is consistent with the hypothesis of a common source of fluid secretion.

The role of the vestibular labyrinth in the control of the cochlear lumen is limited to the phase of development prior to E16.5, since the utricular duct, which connects the utricle to the saccule, is closed after E16.5 [32]. Closing of the utricular duct creates two independent fluid systems. One system consisting of the cochlea, saccule and endolymphatic sac and the other consisting of the utricle, ampullae and semicircular canals [32]. The observation that the cochlear lumen continues to increase after E16.5 suggests the presence of a local defect in fluid homeostasis leading to abnormally high rates of fluid secretion or abnormally low rates of fluid reabsorption [14]. Abnormally low rates of fluid absorption are conceivably due to an impairment of Na^+ reabsorption in Reissner's membrane epithelial cells. Reissner's membrane epithelial cells, analogous to principal cells in the renal cortical collecting duct, are engaged in Na^+ reabsorption via ENaC Na^+ channels and face a fluid compartment that is controlled in its pH and HCO_3^- concentration by pendrin [33,34]. Recent observations in the renal collecting duct suggest that a lower HCO_3^- concentration reduces the abundance of ENaC Na^+ channel subunits [35]. How this mechanism works and whether it is present in the inner ear is unknown.

The enlargement of the cochlear lumen is clearly a key event in the etiology of deafness in mice lacking pendrin [12,14]. The enlargement impairs cell communication between mesenchymal and epithelial cells and causes stretching of epithelial cells. Stretching lengthens diffusional distances and thereby may impair cell-to-cell communication among epithelial cells. Interestingly, non-sensory cells are stretched but sensory cells are not (Fig. 7). This difference is most likely the result of differences in the epithelial rigidity. Sensory cells are endowed with a thick actin-ring near their apical tight junctions, which may provide the sensory epithelia with a greater rigidity which limits cell stretching to the more compliant non-sensory cells.

The enlargement and the acidification spread the effect of lacking pendrin-expression from affecting just pendrin-expressing cells to affecting a multitude of other cells. Expression patterns of connexin 26 and Na^+/K^+ ATPase in Kölliker's organ and the outer sulcus region appeared qualitatively similar in *Slc26a4*$^{+/-}$ and *Slc26a4*$^{-/-}$ mice (Fig. 8, 9, 10). However, the onset of connexin 26 expression in basal cells of stria vascularis occurred in *Slc26a4*$^{-/-}$ prematurely (Fig. 9) and the expression pattern of connexin 26 and Na^+/K^+ ATPase highlighted stretching and thinning of stria vascularis (Fig. 10). The discrepancy in development of stria vascularis between *Slc26a4*$^{+/-}$ and *Slc26a4*$^{-/-}$ mice was most apparent at P3 (Fig. 11). The observation that loss of pendrin leads to a retarded development of stria vascularis including a retarded vascularization is consistent with an impairment of cell-to-cell communication. Structural differences between stria vascularis of *Slc26a4*$^{+/-}$ and *Slc26a4*$^{-/-}$ mice diminished at P7, however, oxidative stress and a reduced endocochlear potential have been found in *Slc26a4*$^{-/-}$ mice at P10 and stria vascularis undergoes degeneration at P30 including an invasion of macrophages [36,37,11]. Taken together, these observations demonstrate that the retarded development of stria vascularis precludes normal function of stria vascularis in the postnatal cochlea.

In summary, the present study documents the onset of pendrin expression and the onset of functional consequence resulting from a failed onset of expression. Lack of pendrin expression leads to epithelial cell stretching and luminal acidification, which may alter cell signaling to result in the observed retarded development of stria vascularis. Retarded development of stria vascularis and possibly of other non-sensory epithelial cells may be an important step on the path to deafness in *Slc26a4*$^{-/-}$ mice, and possibly humans, lacking functional pendrin expression.

Author Contributions

Conceived and designed the experiments: HMK PW. Performed the experiments: HMK. Analyzed the data: HMK. Wrote the manuscript: HMK PW. Designed and wrote software used in analysis: PW.

References

1. Fraser GR (1965) Association of congenital deafness with goitre (Pendred's syndrome) a study of 207 families. Ann Hum Genet 28: 201–249.
2. Reardon W, Coffey R, Phelps PD, Luxon LM, Stephens D, et al. (1997) Pendred syndrome–100 years of underascertainment? QJM 90: 443–447.
3. Park HJ, Shaukat S, Liu XZ, Hahn SH, Naz S, et al. (2003) Origins and frequencies of SLC26A4 (PDS) mutations in east and south Asians: global implications for the epidemiology of deafness. J Med Genet 40: 242–248.
4. Albert S, Blons H, Jonard L, Feldmann D, Chauvin P, et al. (2006) SLC26A4 gene is frequently involved in nonsyndromic hearing impairment with enlarged vestibular aqueduct in Caucasian populations. Eur J Hum Genet 14: 773–779.
5. Yuan Y, You Y, Huang D, Cui J, Wang Y, et al. (2009) Comprehensive molecular etiology analysis of nonsyndromic hearing impairment from typical areas in China. J Transl Med 7: 79–.
6. Luxon LM, Cohen M, Coffey RA, Phelps PD, Britton KE, et al. (2003) Neuro-otological findings in Pendred syndrome. Int J Audiol 42: 82–88.
7. Colvin IB, Beale T, Harrop-Griffiths K (2006) Long-term follow-up of hearing loss in children and young adults with enlarged vestibular aqueducts: relationship to radiologic findings and Pendred syndrome diagnosis. Laryngoscope 116: 2027–2036.
8. Choi BY, Stewart AK, Madeo AC, Pryor SP, Lenhard S, et al. (2009) Hypo-Functional SLC26A4 variants associated with nonsyndromic hearing loss and enlargement of the vestibular aqueduct: Genotype-phenotype correlation or coincidental polymorphisms? Hum Mutat 30: 599–608.
9. Abe S, Usami S, Hoover DM, Cohn E, Shinkawa H, et al. (1999) Fluctuating sensorineural hearing loss associated with enlarged vestibular aqueduct maps to 7q31, the region containing the Pendred gene. Am J Med Genet 82: 322–328.
10. Nakaya K, Harbidge DG, Wangemann P, Schultz BD, Green E, et al. (2007) Lack of pendrin HCO3- transport elevates vestibular endolymphatic [Ca2+] by inhibition of acid-sensitive TRPV5 and TRPV6. Am J Physiol Renal Physiol 292: 1314–1321.
11. Wangemann P, Nakaya K, Wu T, Maganti R, Itza EM, et al. (2007) Loss of cochlear HCO3- secretion causes deafness via endolymphatic acidification and inhibition of Ca2+ reabsorption in a Pendred syndrome mouse model. Am J Physiol Renal Physiol 292: 1345–1353.
12. Everett LA, Belyantseva IA, Noben-Trauth K, Cantos R, Chen A, et al. (2001) Targeted disruption of mouse Pds provides insight about the inner-ear defects encountered in Pendred syndrome. Hum Mol Genet 10: 153–161.
13. Wangemann P, Kim HM, Billings S, Nakaya K, Li X, et al. (2009) Developmental delays consistent with cochlear hypothyroidism contribute to failure to develop hearing in mice lacking Slc26a4/pendrin expression. Am J Physiol Renal Physiol 297: F1435–F1447.
14. Kim HM, Wangemann P (2010) Failure of fluid absorption in the endolymphatic sac initiates cochlear enlargement that leads to deafness in mice lacking *pendrin* expression. PLoS One 5: e14041–.
15. Royaux IE, Belyantseva IA, Wu T, Kachar B, Everett LA, et al. (2003) Localization and functional studies of pendrin in the mouse inner ear provide insight about the etiology of deafness in pendred syndrome. J Assoc Res Otolaryngol 4: 394–404.
16. Wangemann P, Itza EM, Albrecht B, Wu T, Jabba SV, et al. (2004) Loss of KCNJ10 protein expression abolishes endocochlear potential and causes deafness in Pendred syndrome mouse model. BMC Medicine 2: 30.
17. Dou H, Xu J, Wang Z, Smith AN, Soleimani M, et al. (2004) Co-expression of pendrin, vacuolar H^+-ATPase alpha4-subunit and carbonic anhydrase II in epithelial cells of the murine endolymphatic sac. J Histochem Cytochem 52: 1377–1384.
18. Wang Y, Chang Q, Tang W, Sun Y, Zhou B, et al. (2009) Targeted connexin26 ablation arrests postnatal development of the organ of Corti. Biochem Biophys Res Commun 385: 33–37.
19. Inoshita A, Iizuka T, Okamura HO, Minekawa A, Kojima K, et al. (2008) Postnatal development of the organ of Corti in dominant-negative Gjb2 transgenic mice. Neuroscience 156: 1039–1047.
20. Kudo T, Kure S, Ikeda K, Xia AP, Katori Y, et al. (2003) Transgenic expression of a dominant-negative connexin26 causes degeneration of the organ of Corti and non-syndromic deafness. Hum Mol Genet 12: 995–1004.

21. Theiler K (1972) The house mouse Springer Verlag. 168 p.
22. Rugh R (1968) The mouse: Its reproduction and development Burgess Publishing Company. pp 430.
23. Marcus DC, Rokugo M, Thalmann R (1985) Effects of barium and ion substitutions in artificial blood on endocochlear potential. Hear Res 17: 79–86.
24. Everett LA, Morsli H, Wu DK, Green ED (1999) Expression pattern of the mouse ortholog of the Pendred's syndrome gene (Pds) suggests a key role for pendrin in the inner ear. Proc Natl Acad Sci U S A 96: 9727–9732.
25. Dou H, Finberg K, Cardell EL, Lifton R, Choo D (2003) Mice lacking the B1 subunit of H^+ -ATPase have normal hearing. Hear Res 180: 76–84.
26. Couloigner V, Teixeira M, Hulin P, Sterkers O, Bichara M, et al. (2000) Effect of locally applied drugs on the pH of luminal fluid in the endolymphatic sac of guinea pig. Am J Physiol Regul Integr Comp Physiol 279: R1695–R1700.
27. Couloigner V, Teixeira M, Sterkers O, Ferrary E (1999) In vivo study of the electrochemical composition of luminal fluid in the guinea pig endolymphatic sac. Acta Otolaryngol 119: 200–202.
28. Tsujikawa S, Yamashita T, Amano H, Kumazawa T, Vosteen KH (1992) Acidity in the endolymphatic sac fluid of guinea pigs. ORL J Otorhinolaryngol Relat Spec 54: 198–200.
29. Ishida T, Hatae T, Nishi N, Araki N (2006) Soluble megalin is accumulated in the lumen of the rat endolymphatic sac. Cell Struct Funct 31: 77–85.
30. Peters TA, Tonnaer EL, Kuijpers W, Curfs JH (2003) Changes in ultrastructural characteristics of endolymphatic sac ribosome-rich cells of the rat during development. Hear Res 176: 94–104.
31. Thalmann I, Comegys TH, Liu SZ, Ito Z, Thalmann R (1992) Protein profiles of perilymph and endolymph of the guinea pig. Hear Res 63: 37–42.
32. Cantos R, Cole LK, Acampora D, Simeone A, Wu DK (2000) Patterning of the mammalian cochlea. Proc Natl Acad Sci U S A 97: 11707–11713.
33. Kim YH, Pech V, Spencer KB, Beierwaltes WH, Everett LA, et al. (2007) Reduced ENaC protein abundance contributes to the lower blood pressure observed in pendrin-null mice. Am J Physiol Renal Physiol 293: F1314–F1324.
34. Kim SH, Kim KX, Raveendran NN, Wu T, Pondugula SR, et al. (2009) Regulation of ENaC-mediated sodium transport by glucocorticoids in Reissner's membrane epithelium. Am J Physiol Cell Physiol 296: C544–C557.
35. Pech V, Pham TD, Hong S, Weinstein AM, Spencer KB, et al. (2010) Pendrin modulates ENaC function by changing luminal HCO_3^-. J Am Soc Nephrol 21: 1928–1941.
36. Singh R, Wangemann P (2008) Free radical stress mediated loss of Kcnj10 protein expression in stria vascularis contributes to deafness in Pendred syndrome mouse model. Am J Physiol Renal Physiol 294: F139–F148.
37. Jabba SV, Oelke A, Singh R, Maganti RJ, Feming S, et al. (2006) Macrophage invasion contributes to degeneration of stria vascularis in Pendred syndrome mouse model. BMC Med 4: 37–ff.

17

A Rapid Method for Simultaneous Screening of Multi-Gene Mutations Associated with Hearing Loss in the Korean Population

Borum Sagong[1¶], Jeong-In Baek[1¶], Se-Kyung Oh[1], Kyung Jin Na[2], Jae Woong Bae[1], Soo Young Choi[3], Ji Yun Jeong[4], Jae Young Choi[5], Sang-Heun Lee[2], Kyu-Yup Lee[2*], Un-Kyung Kim[1*]

1 Department of Biology, College of Natural Sciences, Kyungpook National University, Daegu, South Korea, **2** Department of Otorhinolaryngology-Head and Neck Surgery, College of Medicine, Kyungpook National University, Daegu, South Korea, **3** Department of Medicine, University of Pennsylvania, Philadelphia, Pennsylvania, United States of America, **4** Department of Endocrinology and Metabolism, Kyungpook National University Hospital, Kyungpook National University School of Medicine, Daegu, South Korea, **5** Department of Otorhinolaryngology, Yonsei University College of Medicine, Seoul, South Korea

Abstract

Hearing loss (HL) is a congenital disease with a high prevalence, and patients with hearing loss need early diagnosis for treatment and prevention. The *GJB2*, *MT-RNR1*, and *SLC26A4* genes have been reported as common causative genes of hearing loss in the Korean population and some mutations of these genes are the most common mutations associated with hearing loss. Accordingly, we developed a method for the simultaneous detection of seven mutations (c.235delC of *GJB2*, c.439A>G, c.919-2A>G, c.1149+3A>G, c.1229C>T, c.2168A>G of *SLC26A4*, and m.1555A>G of the *MT-RNR1* gene) using multiplex SNaPshot minisequencing to enable rapid diagnosis of hereditary hearing loss. This method was confirmed in patients with hearing loss and used for genetic diagnosis of controls with normal hearing and neonates. We found that 4.06% of individuals with normal hearing and 4.32% of neonates were heterozygous carriers. In addition, we detected that an individual is heterozygous for two different mutations of *GJB2* and *SLC26A4* gene, respectively and one normal hearing showing the heteroplasmy of m.1555A>G. These genotypes corresponded to those determined by direct sequencing. Overall, we successfully developed a robust and cost-effective diagnosis method that detects common causative mutations of hearing loss in the Korean population. This method will be possible to detect up to 40% causative mutations associated with prelingual HL in the Korean population and serve as a useful genetic technique for diagnosis of hearing loss for patients, carriers, neonates, and fetuses.

Editor: Gisela Nogales-Gadea, University Hospital Vall d'Hebron, Spain

Funding: This research was supported by the Basic Science Research Program through the National Research Foundation of Korea funded by the Ministry of Education, Science and Technology (2011-0028066) and by a grant from the Korea Health Technology Research & Development Project, Ministry of Health & Welfare, Republic of Korea. (A111345). The funders had no role in study design, data collection and analysis, decision to publish, or preparation of the manuscript.

Competing Interests: The authors have declared that no competing interests exist.

* E-mail: kylee@knu.ac.kr (KYL); kimuk@knu.ac.kr (UKK)

¶ These authors contributed equally to this work.

Introduction

Congenital hearing loss (HL) is a common sensory impairment that occurs in approximately one in 1000 neonates, and more than 50% of cases are hereditary [1]. The occurrence of HL in early childhood could have serious effects on language acquisition, while later onset of severe hearing defect compromises sociality [2]. Currently, the best provision for hereditary HL is prevention of outbreak through early diagnosis and continuous management. Therefore, a precise rapid genetic diagnosis may be the most effective support for treatment and prevention of HL.

More than over 150 loci have been mapped in HL, and 57 genes of them have been shown to cause nonsyndromic HL [3]. Among these, mutations of the *GJB2* gene (OMIM 121011) are the most common cause of hereditary HL in many Caucasian populations [4]. One of them, mutation c.35delG, accounts for up to 70% of the pathologic alleles in European and Caucasian populations [5]. Unlike Caucasian populations, *GJB2* mutations seem to account for a lower percentage of hereditary HL in East Asian populations; however, approximately 43% of the *GJB2* hearing loss are caused by c.235delC mutation in Koreans [6–8]. Moreover, mutations of the *SLC26A4* gene (OMIM 605646), which cause both Pendred syndrome and nonsyndromic HL with enlarged vestibular aqueduct, appear to be common in Asian populations [9]. Especially, five mutations of this gene account for up to 90% of all mutant alleles [8,10]. Mitochondrial DNA mutations have also been reported in both nonsyndromic and syndromic HL. Among these mutations, only the m.1555A>G mutation of the *MT-RNR1* gene (OMIM 561000) has been identified repeatedly in Koreans with HL by our previous studies [11,12]. Based on the prevalence of mutations from the previous studies, we selected 7 mutations which show the high frequencies in Korean hearing loss population and designed the method to detect effectively mutant alleles through rapid screening: c.235delC of *GJB2*, c.919-2A>G and c.2168A>G of *SLC26A4* and m.1555A>G of the *MT-RNR1* gene. All of the 7 mutations selected in this study had been reported that mutations cause abnormal function. The c.235delC mutation of *GJB2* gene caused a loss of targeting activity to the cell membrane and severe deterioration of gap junction activity [13]. The m.1555A>G in *MT-RNR1* gene made the human mitochondrial ribosome more bacteria-like and alter binding sites for aminoglycosides [14]. The p.M147V and p.H723R mutations of *SLC26A4* gene caused loss of Cl^-/HCO_3^- and Cl^-/I^- exchange activity [15–17]. The p.T410M mutation in *SLC26A4* gene caused loss of iodide efflux [17,18]. The c.919-2A>G and c.1149+3A>G mutations of *SLC26A4* gene resulted in premature termination of translation on gene expression, respectively [10,19]. Accordingly, these mutations have been screened by priority during genetic testing of HL. Because all of these mutations are recessive in their effect except the mitochondrial mutation (m.1555A>G), analysis of individual genotype for these mutations can provide crucial genetic information for inheritance of autosomal recessive hearing loss.

In this study, we developed a rapid and low cost multiplex genetic diagnosis of common mutations in Koreans using SNaPshot minisequencing for patients with HL and heterozygous carriers.

Materials and Methods

Subjects and DNA preparation

To set up the SNaPshot minisequencing methods, five patients with mutations in *GJB2*, *MT-RNR1*, and *SLC26A4* and one normal hearing individual without any mutations were used as positive and normal controls, respectively. One hundred ninety-seven unrelated Koreans with normal hearing from Kyungpook National University Hospital were used as controls aged 20 and 64 years. In addition, 139 Korean neonates of unrelated individuals who were born in Kyungpook National University Hospital were recruited for this study with the consent of their parents. Written informed consent was obtained from all participants, and this study was approved by the local ethics committee.

The genomic DNA of normal controls and neonates was extracted from peripheral blood and buccal cells using a FlexiGene DNA kit (Qiagen, Hilden, Germany) or a Gentra Puregene Buccal Cell kit (Qiagen, Hilden, Germany) following the manufacturer's instructions.

PCR multiplex amplification

Fourteen primers were used for amplification of the mutation region, and amplification was conducted in a reaction mixture with a final volume of 25 µl that contained 20 ng of DNA template, 0.2 mM deoxynucleotide, 1 X multiplex polymerase chain reaction (PCR) primer mixture that consisted of seven pairs of primers, 1 X h-Taq reaction buffer, and 0.5 U of h-Taq DNA Polymerase (Solgent, Daejeon, Korea) (Table 1). The PCR conditions were as follows: initial denaturation at 95°C for 15 min, followed by 40 cycles of denaturation at 94°C for 20 sec, annealing at 57°C for 20 sec, and extension at 72°C for 40 sec and then final extension at 72°C for 5 min. Five microliters of the PCR products were separated and visualized following electrophoresis on a 2% agarose gel. Shrimp alkaline phosphatase (SAP) (USB, Cleveland, OH, USA) and exonuclease I (USB, Cleveland, OH, USA) were used for post-PCR purification of the examined PCR products.

SNaPshot minisequencing reaction

The single base extension (SBE) reaction was performed in a reaction mixture with a final volume of 15 µl that contained 2.45 µl of purified multiplex PCR product, 1 X extension primer mixture (Table 2), and 3 µl of SNaPshot Multiplex Ready Reaction Mix (Applied Biosystems, Foster City, CA, USA). The reaction mixture was subjected to 30 SBE cycles of denaturation at 96°C for 10 sec, primer annealing at 50°C for 5 sec, and primer extension at 60°C for 30 sec. SAP (USB, Cleveland, OH, USA) was used for post-SBE purification of the SBE reaction products.

For electrophoresis, 2 µl of purified multiplex SBE reaction products were mixed with 0.3 µl of GeneScan 120 LIZ Size Standard (Applied Biosystems, Foster City, CA, USA) and 7.7 µl of Hi-Di Formamide (Applied Biosystems, Foster City, CA, USA)

Table 1. Multiplex PCR primer sequences.

Gene	Exon		PCR primers (5′→3′)	Concentration* (pmol/µl)	Product size (bp)	Nucleotide change	Protein change
GJB2	2	F	TCTTTTCCAGAGCAAACCGC	0.2	416	c.235delC	p.L79CfsX3
		R	GATGCGGACCTTCTGGGTTT	0.2			
MT-RNR1	-	F	CGTCACCCTCCTCAAGTATACTTC	0.04	137	m.1555A>G	-
		R	GCTTTGTGTTAAGCTACACTCTGG	0.04			
SLC26A4	5	F	TTTTTAAACCCTATGCAGACACA	0.5	175	c.439A>G	p.M147V
		R	TTAATACAGTTCCATTGCTGCTG	0.5			
SLC26A4	7	F	CAAAATCCCAGTCCCTATTCCTA	0.4	363	c.919-2A>G	-
		R	GGTTGTTTCTTCCAGATCACACAC	0.4			
SLC26A4	9	F	GCTTGTTCTCGGAGATGCTG	0.15	301	c.1149+3A>G	-
		R	AGTGATGCAGTGTGTCTATTCC	0.15			
SLC26A4	10	F	GGATCGTTGTCATCCAGTCTC	0.5	488	c.1229C>T	p.T410M
		R	TTACCAGGCCATCTGTCTCC	0.5			
SLC26A4	19	F	CCTGGGCAATAGAATGAGACTC	0.15	227	c.2168A>G	p.H723R
		R	AAATGGAACCTTGACCCTCTTG	0.15			

*Final concentration in the reaction mixture.

Table 2. Extension primer sequences.

Gene	Mutation		Extension primers (5′→3′)	Concentration* (pmol/μl)	Primer size (bp)	WT allele (peak color)	MT allele (peak color)
GJB2	c.235delC	F	ACGATCACTACTTCCCCATCTCCCACATCCGGCTATGGGCC	4	41	C (Black)	T (Red)
MT-RNR1	m.1555A>G	F	TTAACTAAAACCCCTACGCATTTATATAGAGGAG	0.07	34	A (Green)	G (Blue)
SLC26A4	c.439A>G	F	TTAATAACTGATTAATTGTTAGAGACTTTTTTTCCCCAGGA CCTTTTCCAGTGGTGAGTTTA	0.05	62	A (Green)	G (Blue)
SLC26A4	c.919-2A>G	F	AAGTTCAGCATTATTTGGTTGACAAACAAGGAATTATTAAA ACCAATGGAGTTTTTAACATCTTTTGTTTTATTTC	0.03	76	A (Green)	G (Blue)
SLC26A4	c.1149+3A>G	R	TATGTTTTTTTCCTGTTTCCAGCCCTATAAAACCAGTTCAGCA AAAGGGCACCCA	0.07	55	A (Red)	G (Black)
SLC26A4	c.1229C>T	F	CCTTTGGGATCAGCAACATCTTCTCAGGATTCTTCTCTTGTTTT GTGGCCACCACTGCTCTTTCCCGCA	6.67	69	C (Black)	T (Red)
SLC26A4	c.2168A>G	F	GGTTCTTTGACGACAACATTAGAAAGGACACATTCTTTTTGACG GTCC	0.07	48	A (Green)	G (Blue)

*Final concentration in the reaction mixture.

and denatured at 95°C for 2 min. The fluorescently labeled fragments were resolved by capillary electrophoresis on an ABI 3130*xl* Genetic Analyzer (Applied Biosystems, Foster City, CA, USA). The resulting data were analyzed with the GeneMapper v3.7 (Applied Biosystems, Foster City, CA, USA) software.

Sanger sequencing

Specific DNA fragments containing each mutation were amplified by PCR to confirm the genotype. PCR was conducted using a reaction mixture composed of 0.2 mM deoxynucleotide, 10 pmol of each forward and reverse primer, and 0.25 U of h-Taq DNA Polymerase (Solgent, Daejeon, Korea) in a final volume of 25 μl. The PCR conditions were as follows: initial denaturation at 95°C for 15 min, followed by 35 cycles of denaturation at 94°C for 20 sec, annealing at 55°C, depending on the primers for 40 sec, and extension at 72°C for 50 sec followed by final extension at 72°C for 5 min. The quality of the PCR products was examined by electrophoresis on 2% agarose gels. SAP (USB, Cleveland, OH, USA) and exonuclease I (USB, Cleveland, OH, USA) were used for purification of the examined PCR products. The sequences of the purified PCR products were obtained by direct sequencing using a BigDye Terminator v3.1 Cycle Sequencing Kit (Applied Biosystems, Foster City, CA, USA). Extended products were purified by ethanol precipitation. A 3130*xl* Genetic Analyzer (Applied Biosystems, Foster City, CA, USA) was used to resolve the products and the data were analyzed using the Chromas Lite v2.01 (Technelysium Pty Ltd., Tewantin, QLD, Australia) software.

Results

Development of the multiplex amplification and multiplex SNaPshot minisequencing

The seven genomic segments containing each mutation were amplified in a single multiplex PCR reaction, after which the amplified DNA fragments were separated and visualized on agarose gel (Figure 1). We developed a genetic diagnostic technique consisting of SNaPshot multiplex minisequencing of seven mutations in three genes. Five positive controls for the mutant allele of the seven mutations and one normal control with wild-type alleles were analyzed and correctly genotyped in all reactions (Figure 2). Normal controls were genotyped to wild-type in every mutant region (Figure 2, first panel). Positive controls were genotyped mutant types in each mutant region (Figure 2, second to sixth panels). Relative differences in peak heights between each allele were observed because fluorescence emission can be directly influenced by interaction between other fluorophores. In addition, the results of SNaPshot minisequencing were

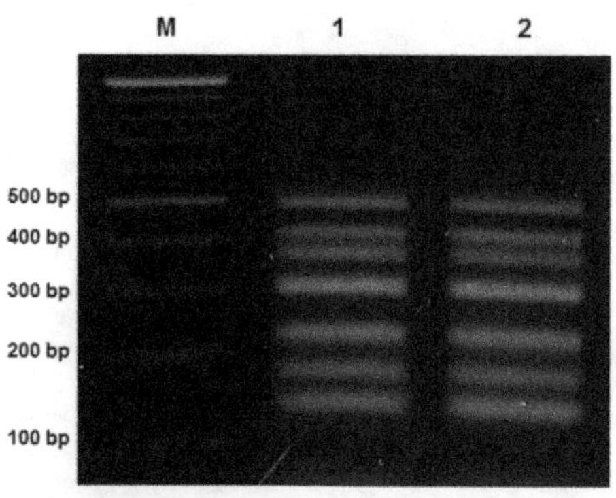

Product size (bp)	Gene	Exon	Nucleotide change
488	*SLC26A4*	10	c.1229C>T
416	*GJB2*	2	c.235delC
363	*SLC26A4*	7	c.919-2A>G
301	*SLC26A4*	9	c.1149+3A>G
227	*SLC26A4*	19	c.2168A>G
175	*SLC26A4*	5	c.439A>G
137	*MT-RNR1*	-	m.1555A>G

Figure 1. The products of multiplex amplification. Agarose gel electrophoresis pattern of digested PCR products stained with ethidium bromide shows the multiplex amplification products of wild type (lane 1), mutant type (lane 2), 100 bp ladder marker (lane M), and corresponding size (bp) for each band of multiplex PCR products (table).

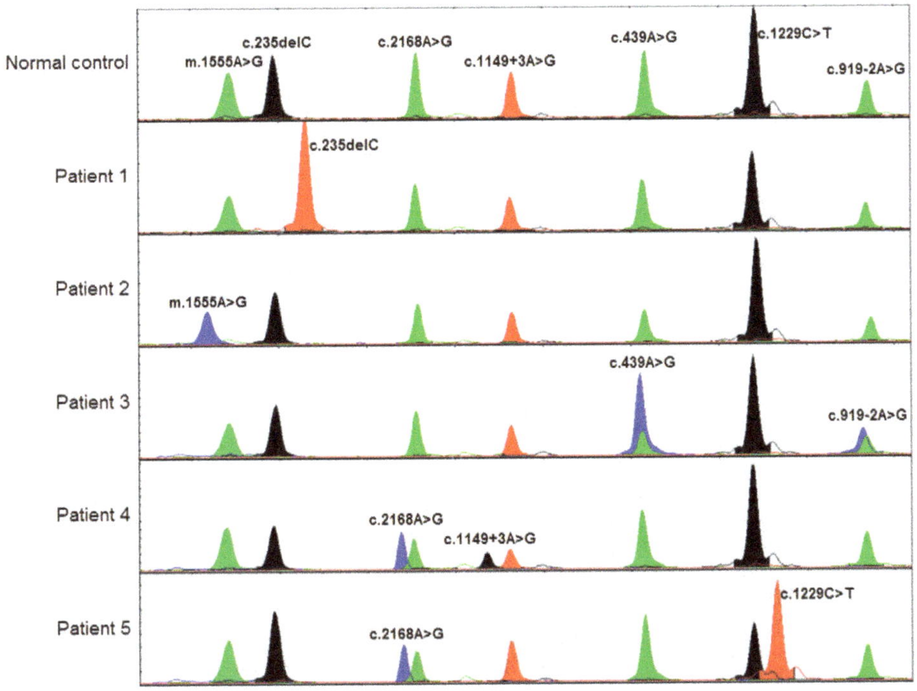

Figure 2. Electropherograms of Genescan Analysis of the SNaPshot multiplex minisequencing. On the top, a control DNA sample with the position and nucleotide of the wild type allele indicated. Following, electropherograms for the most frequent hearing loss mutations in homozygote, compound heterozygote forms on *GJB2*, *SLC26A4* genes, and homoplasmy in the *MT-RNR1* gene.

compared with those of Sanger sequencing of control samples, and these results were matched exactly.

SNaPshot minisequencing in the normal hearing controls and neonates

To investigate the frequency of these common mutations in the Korean normal hearing population, the genotypes of 197 normal hearing controls and 139 neonates were analyzed for the seven mutations using SNaPshot multiplex minisequencing. Analysis revealed a 20-year-old female with normal hearing that had heteroplasmy of m.1555A>G in the *MT-RNR1* gene, which is the most common cause of aminoglycoside-induced HL. In addition, a 35-year-old female with normal hearing was found to have two different heterozygous alleles (c.235delC in *GJB2* and c.2168A>G in *SLC26A4* gene). Moreover, eight normal hearing controls and six neonates were diagnosed as carriers of each mutation. In the normal hearing controls, c.235delC of the *GJB2* gene and c.919-2A>G and c.2168A>G of the *SLC26A4* gene mutations were detected in one, two and four heterozygotes, respectively (Table 3, left panel). In the neonates, three, two and one individuals were found to be heterozygous carriers of the c.235delC *GJB2* gene mutation, c.919-2A>G and c.2168A>G *SLC26A4* mutation, respectively (Table 3, right panel). These genotypes diagnosed by the SNaPshot multiplex minisequencing matched those determined by direct sequencing.

Discussion

The SNaPshot minisequencing technique, which was developed at first by Smith *et al.* [20], has been utilized in various branches of biology, including population genetics and phylogenetics, with a high level of accuracy and effectiveness. Several studies have applied this technique for haplogroup classification of human

Table 3. Frequencies of seven hearing loss mutations in normal controls and neonates.

Gene	Mutation	Normal hearing controls		Neonates	
		No. of alleles (n = 394)	Allele frequency (%)	No. of alleles (n = 278)	Allele frequency (%)
GJB2	c.235delC	2	0.51	3	1.08
MT-RNR1	m.1555A>G heteroplasmy	1	0.51	0	0
SLC26A4	c.439A>G	0	0	0	0
SLC26A4	c.919-2A>G	2	0.51	2	0.72
SLC26A4	c.1149+3A>G	0	0	0	0
SLC26A4	c.1229C>T	0	0	0	0
SLC26A4	c.2168A>G	5	1.27	1	0.36

mitochondrial DNA, which provides crucial information for phylogenetic analysis and forensic identification of individuals [21,22]. Simultaneous identification of several different species using the multiplex SNaPshot reaction has also been attempted in many studies, and their strong possibility of industrial application has been authenticated [23,24].

Recently, SNaPshot minisequencing has been used for effective detection of numerous pathogenic mutations that cause human hereditary disorders such as *CYP21*, *PIK3CA*, *CYP3A5*, *MDR1*, and *BRCA1/2* genes [25–30]. Especially, it is greatly effective at genetic diagnosis of heterogeneous diseases that have a number of causative genes, as well as large single gene diseases because this technique allows simultaneous detection of several variations in a single reaction. Most heterogeneous diseases have several major common causative mutations generated from different genes. Therefore, SNaPshot multiplex minisequencing of selected common mutations provides temporal and economic efficiency rather than direct sequencing of all genes.

Based on previous genetic studies of HL in the Korean population, we selected the seven most common mutations that lead to hereditary HL [8–12,31]. Multiplex genotyping of these seven mutations was successfully performed using SNaPshot minisequencing, which produced accurate data and a detection rate of the mutations that was found to account for up to 40% of the causative mutant alleles associated with prelingual HL in Koreans [8]. These results suggest that this strategy is suitable for use as a precise and rapid genetic diagnosis tool.

To verify the applicability of this technique as a genetic diagnosis tool and a tool for building a population genetic database of type and frequency of mutations in the Korean population, we analyzed genotypes of normal hearing adults and neonates. As a result, we detected heterozygous carriers successfully. Specifically, we found that 4.06% of individuals with normal hearing and 4.32% of neonates were heterozygous carriers. In addition, we identified one carrier having two different heterozygous alleles, and one normal hearing having possibility to cause the HL. The frequencies of two mutations (*GJB2* c.235delC and c.2168A>G of the *SLC26A4* gene) presented that the allele frequency of c.235delC mutation (0.52%) in normal hearing controls by other studies were very similar to the result of this study (0.51%) [10,31–33], and the c.2168A>G mutation presented higher frequency than the other *SLC26A4* mutations in this study and the previous studies in Koreans [9,10,31]. The c.439A>G, c.1149+3A>G, and c.1229C>T mutations of *SLC26A4* were not detected in this study. Likewise, results of this study show similar results of previous studies. These findings suggest that the developed strategy can be highly effective for identification of carriers of mutations associated with HL in the Korean population. Moreover, these results indicate the potential for mitigation and prevention of HL via genetic counseling before the HL begins to possible detection of carriers having each heterozygous allele in different genes and individuals with normal hearing having genes with the potential to cause disease.

This method enables the detection of seven mutations associated with HL at once and costs less than $12 per sample from blood or buccal swab to genotype analysis (based on $1 = 1133.90 KRW), making this method rapid and cost-effective when compared with other diagnostic tools using PCR-RFLP or real-time quantitative PCR [34–37]. Bardien *et al.* elucidated that an estimated cost comparison between the two methods was less than $16 per sample for the SNaPshot method versus less than $30 per sample for the PCR-RFLP method (based on $1 = 10.39 ZAR) [37]. These results verified economical effectiveness of the SNaPshot method compared with other methods. Additionally, the analysis is quick and easy because the results of SNaPshot minisequencing show different colored peaks that reflect single bases of mutations required for analysis. Furthermore, the method can be easily performed in any location equipped with a thermal cycler and DNA sequencer. Because each mutation is simultaneously but independently amplified using specific primers, it is simple and easy to add more mutations by inserting the primers for multiplex PCR and SBE reaction. Thus, if primers are inserted for SBE reaction of other mutations identified in Korean HL, this method will be applicable to identification of genetic diagnosis of more individuals. The present science technology is very advanced, so it is possible to screen large-scale sequences in the short-term using next generation sequencing (NGS). However, the method is still somewhat expensive; therefore, known mutations should be filtered prior to NGS to identify the causative mutations. Nevertheless, our method will be fast and efficient as a method of first-pass screening. To date, this technique has been found to be useful for detection of mutations in fetal DNA from maternal plasma [38,39], as well as both blood DNA from adults and small amounts of DNA from buccal swabs of neonates. Therefore, the developed method will make diagnosis of hereditary HL in fetuses possible as well.

Because hereditary HL is heterogeneous disorder and the major causative gene in Korean population has not been identified, it is almost impossible that all patients with genetic HL are diagnosed by single standardized diagnosis platform, even if it is highly effective techniques to detect a number of mutations. Nevertheless, three genes (*GJB2*, *SLC26A4*, and *MT-RNR1*) are the most common causative genes in Korean population, and their 7 mutations selected in this study account for up to 70% of hearing loss caused by these 3 genes [8]. It obviously suggests that detection of these 7 frequent mutations has the highest diagnosis rate than any other mutations. For this reasons, primary mutation screening of these 3 genes are essentially being required in all genetic studies of hearing loss. It means that analysis of these 7 major mutations using SNaPshot minisequencing tool is very useful for researches of hereditary hearing loss.

In conclusion, we successfully developed a rapid, accurate, robust, and cost-effective genetic tool for diagnosis of HL using SNaPshot minisequencing. It is possible to detect up to 40% causative mutations associated with prelingual HL in the Korean population using this method, and this technique is applicable to other fields including genetic diagnosis of fetuses or first-pass screening prior to NGS screening.

Author Contributions

Conceived and designed the experiments: KYL UKK. Performed the experiments: BS JIB SKO JWB SYC JYJ. Analyzed the data: BS JIB KJN. Contributed reagents/materials/analysis tools: KJN JYC KYL UKK SHL. Wrote the paper: BS JIB UKK.

References

1. Marazita ML, Ploughman LM, Rawlings B, Remington E, Arnos KS, et al. (1993) Genetic epidemiological studies of early-onset deafness in the U.S. school-age population. Am J Med Genet 46: 486–491.

2. Petit C, Levilliers J, Hardelin JP (2001) Molecular genetics of hearing loss. Annu Rev Genet 35: 589–646.

3. Lin X, Tang W, Ahmad S, Lu J, Colby CC, et al. (2012) Applications of targeted gene capture and next-generation sequencing technologies in studies of human deafness and other genetic disabilities. Hear Res 288: 67–76.
4. Cohn ES, Kelley PM (1999) Clinical phenotype and mutations in connexin 26 (DFNB1/GJB2), the most common cause of childhood hearing loss. Am J Med Genet 89: 130–136.
5. Gasparini P, Rabionet R, Barbujani G, Melchionda S, Petersen M, et al. (2000) High carrier frequency of the 35delG deafness mutation in European populations. Genetic Analysis Consortium of GJB2 35delG. Eur J Hum Genet 8: 19–23.
6. Lee KY, Choi SY, Bae JW, Kim S, Chung KW, et al. (2008) Molecular analysis of the GJB2, GJB6 and SLC26A4 genes in Korean deafness patients. Int J Pediatr Otorhinolaryngol 72: 1301–1309.
7. Yan D, Park HJ, Ouyang XM, Pandya A, Doi K, et al. (2003) Evidence of a founder effect for the 235delC mutation of GJB2 (connexin 26) in east Asians. Hum Genet 114: 44–50.
8. Shin J-W, Lee S-C, Lee H-K, Park H-J (2012) Genetic Screening of GJB2 and SLC26A4 in Korean Cochlear Implantees: Experience of Soree Ear Clinic. Clin Exp Otorhinolar 5: S10–S13.
9. Park HJ, Shaukat S, Liu XZ, Hahn SH, Naz S, et al. (2003) Origins and frequencies of SLC26A4 (PDS) mutations in east and south Asians: global implications for the epidemiology of deafness. J Med Genet 40: 242–248.
10. Park HJ, Lee SJ, Jin HS, Lee JO, Go SH, et al. (2005) Genetic basis of hearing loss associated with enlarged vestibular aqueducts in Koreans. Clin Genet 67: 160–165.
11. Bae JW, Lee KY, Choi SY, Lee SH, Park HJ, et al. (2008) Molecular analysis of mitochondrial gene mutations in Korean patients with nonsyndromic hearing loss. Int J Mol Med 22: 175–180.
12. Bae JW, Kim DB, Choi JY, Park HJ, Lee JD, et al. (2012) Molecular and Clinical Characterization of the Variable Phenotype in Korean Families with Hearing Loss Associated with the Mitochondrial A1555G Mutation. PLoS One 7: e42463.
13. Choung YH, Moon SK, Park HJ (2002) Functional study of GJB2 in hereditary hearing loss. Laryngoscope 112: 1667–1671.
14. Guan MX (2011) Mitochondrial 12S rRNA mutations associated with aminoglycoside ototoxicity. Mitochondrion 11: 237–245.
15. Yoon JS, Park HJ, Yoo SY, Namkung W, Jo MJ, et al. (2008) Heterogeneity in the processing defect of SLC26A4 mutants. J Med Genet 45: 411–419.
16. Ishihara K, Okuyama S, Kumano S, Iida K, Hamana H, et al. (2010) Salicylate restores transport function and anion exchanger activity of missense pendrin mutations. Hear Res 270: 110–118.
17. Dossena S, Nofziger C, Tamma G, Bernardinelli E, Vanoni S, et al. (2011) Molecular and functional characterization of human pendrin and its allelic variants. Cell Physiol Biochem 28: 451–466.
18. Taylor JP, Metcalfe RA, Watson PF, Weetman AP, Trembath RC (2002) Mutations of the PDS gene, encoding pendrin, are associated with protein mislocalization and loss of iodide efflux: implications for thyroid dysfunction in Pendred syndrome. J Clin Endocrinol Metab 87: 1778–1784.
19. Yang JJ, Tsai CC, Hsu HM, Shiao JY, Su CC, et al. (2005) Hearing loss associated with enlarged vestibular aqueduct and Mondini dysplasia is caused by splice-site mutation in the PDS gene. Hear Res 199: 22–30.
20. Smith WM, Van Orsouw NJ, Fox EA, Kolodner RD, Vijg J, et al. (1998) Accurate, high-throughput "snapshot" detection of hMLH1 mutations by two-dimensional DNA electrophoresis. Genet Test 2: 43–53.
21. Paneto GG, Kohnemann S, Martins JA, Cicarelli RM, Pfeiffer H (2011) A single multiplex PCR and SNaPshot minisequencing reaction of 42 SNPs to classify admixture populations into mitochondrial DNA haplogroups. Mitochondrion 11: 296–302.
22. Grignani P, Peloso G, Achilli A, Turchi C, Tagliabracci A, et al. (2006) Subtyping mtDNA haplogroup H by SNaPshot minisequencing and its application in forensic individual identification. Int J Legal Med 120: 151–156.
23. La Neve F, Civera T, Mucci N, Bottero MT (2008) Authentication of meat from game and domestic species by SNaPshot minisequencing analysis. Meat Sci 80: 216–224.
24. Huang CH, Chang MT, Huang MC, Lee FL (2011) Application of the SNaPshot minisequencing assay to species identification in the Lactobacillus casei group. Mol Cell Probes 25: 153–157.
25. Fiorentino F, Magli MC, Podini D, Ferraretti AP, Nuccitelli A, et al. (2003) The minisequencing method: an alternative strategy for preimplantation genetic diagnosis of single gene disorders. Mol Hum Reprod 9: 399–410.
26. Speiser PW, White PC (2003) Congenital adrenal hyperplasia. N Engl J Med 349: 776–788.
27. Li SY, Wang W, Li JM, Wang Z, Wen RY, et al. (2011) PIK3CA mutation is an independent indicator of malignant phenotype and prognosis in breast cancer. Zhonghua Zhong Liu Za Zhi 33: 605–608.
28. Dudarewicz M, Baranska M, Rychlik-Sych M, Trzcinski R, Dziki A, et al. (2012) C3435T polymorphism of the ABCB1/MDR1 gene encoding P-glycoprotein in patients with inflammatory bowel disease in a Polish population. Pharmacol Rep 64: 343–350.
29. Garcia-Roca P, Medeiros M, Reyes H, Rodriguez-Espino BA, Alberu J, et al. (2012) CYP3A5 polymorphism in Mexican renal transplant recipients and its association with tacrolimus dosing. Arch Med Res 43: 283–287.
30. Kirchhoff T, Gaudet MM, Antoniou AC, McGuffog L, Humphreys MK, et al. (2012) Breast cancer risk and 6q22.33: combined results from Breast Cancer Association Consortium and Consortium of Investigators on Modifiers of BRCA1/2. PLoS One 7: e35706.
31. Song MJ, Lee ST, Lee MK, Ji Y, Kim JW, et al. (2011) Estimation of carrier frequencies of six autosomal-recessive Mendelian disorders in the Korean population. J Hum Genet 57: 139–144.
32. Han SH, Park HJ, Kang EJ, Ryu JS, Lee A, et al. (2008) Carrier frequency of GJB2 (connexin-26) mutations causing inherited deafness in the Korean population. J Hum Genet 53: 1022–1028.
33. Park HJ, Hahn SH, Chun YM, Park K, Kim HN (2000) Connexin26 mutations associated with nonsyndromic hearing loss. Laryngoscope 110: 1535–1538.
34. Zhao J, Wu LQ, Feng Y, Hu H, Pan Q, et al. (2009) [Rapid detection of the hot spot gene mutations in Chinese patients with nonsyndromic hearing loss by polymerase chain reaction-restrictive fragment length polymorphism]. Zhonghua Yi Xue Yi Chuan Xue Za Zhi 26: 518–520.
35. Kato T, Nishigaki Y, Noguchi Y, Ueno H, Hosoya H, et al. (2010) Extensive and rapid screening for major mitochondrial DNA point mutations in patients with hereditary hearing loss. J Hum Genet 55: 147–154.
36. Kokotas H, Grigoriadou M, Hatzaki A, Antoniadi T, Giannoulia-Karantana A, et al. (2010) Easy, rapid, and cost-effective methods for identifying carriers of recurrent GJB2 mutations causing nonsyndromic hearing impairment in the Greek population. Genet Test Mol Biomarkers 14: 189–192.
37. Bardien S, Human H, Harris T, Hefke G, Veikondis R, et al. (2009) A rapid method for detection of five known mutations associated with aminoglycoside-induced deafness. BMC Med Genet 10: 2.
38. Lo YM, Corbetta N, Chamberlain PF, Rai V, Sargent IL, et al. (1997) Presence of fetal DNA in maternal plasma and serum. Lancet 350: 485–487.
39. Poon LL, Leung TN, Lau TK, Chow KC, Lo YM (2002) Differential DNA methylation between fetus and mother as a strategy for detecting fetal DNA in maternal plasma. Clin Chem 48: 35–41.

18

Platelet Glycoproteins and Fibrinogen in Recovery from Idiopathic Sudden Hearing Loss

Daniel Weiss[1], Bruno Neuner[2], Kerstin Gorzelniak[3], Alexis Bremer[1], Claudia Rudack[1], Michael Walter[4*]

1 Department of Otorhinolaryngology, Head and Neck Surgery, University of Münster, Münster, Germany, 2 Department of Anaesthesiology and Intensive Care Medicine, Campus Virchow-Klinikum and Campus Charité-Mitte, Charité – University Medicine, Berlin, Germany, 3 Institute of Laboratory Medicine, Unfallkrankenhaus Berlin, Berlin, Germany, 4 Institute of Laboratory Medicine, Clinical Chemistry and Pathobiochemistry, Campus Virchow-Klinikum, Charité – University Medicine & Labor Berlin – Charité Vivantes Services GmbH, Berlin, Germany

Abstract

Background: The pathomechanism and location of idiopathic sudden sensorineural hearing loss (ISSHL) is unclear. In a previous case-control study, we found elevated fibrinogen concentrations and a higher prevalence of T allele carriers of the glycoprotein (Gp) Ia C807T polymorphism in ISSHL patients.

Methodology: 127 patients with ISSHL (mean age 53.3 years, 48.8% females), who underwent a standard therapy with high dose steroids, pentoxifyllin and sterofundine over 8 days were included. We examined the influence of GpIa genotype and fibrinogen (BcII-, A312-, HaeIII-) genotype and fibrinogen plasma levels on hearing recovery after 8 weeks (change from baseline: 0 dB = no recovery, >0 to 10 dB = moderate recovery, >10 dB = good recovery). In a subsample of 59 patients with ISSHL, we further studied the association of platelet glycoprotein GpIa, Ib and IIIa densities on hearing recovery as well as the possible effect-modification of platelet glycoproteins on hearing recovery by plasma fibrinogen.

Results: In univariate analysis, neither the GpIa genotype nor fibrinogen genotype (all $p>0.1$) but lower fibrinogen levels ($p=0.029$), less vertigo ($p=0.002$) and lower GpIIIa receptor density ($p=0.037$, $n=59$) were associated with hearing recovery. In multivariate analysis, fibrinogen significantly modified the effect of GPIa receptor density on good hearing recovery (effect-modification on multiplicative scale OR = 0.45 (95% confidence interval (0.21–0.94)), $p=0.03$). GPIb receptor density below the mean was associated with a 2-fold increase in good hearing recovery both in patients with fibrinogen levels above ($p=0.04$) as well as in patients with fibrinogen levels below the mean ($p=0.06$). There was no indication for an effect-modification ($p=0.97$).

Conclusions: The findings suggest a vascular/rheological origin of ISSHL with unique features of thrombosis in the inner ear artery that may include complex interrelationships among platelet glycoproteins and plasma fibrinogen.

Editor: Christian Schulz, King's College London School of Medicine, United Kingdom

Funding: Landesversicherungsanstalt Rheinprovinz (LVA)" (to MW), and the Foundation for Pathobiochemistry and Molecular Diagnostics, German Society for Clinical Chemistry and Laboratory Medicine e.V. (DGKL, Bonn, Germany) (to MW). The funders had no role in study design, data collection and analysis, decision to publish, or preparation of the manuscript.

Competing Interests: The authors have declared that no competing interests exist.

* E-mail: m.walter@charite.de

These authors contributed equally to this work.

Introduction

Sudden sensorineural hearing loss (SSHL) is a dysfunction of the inner ear characterized by sudden onset and rapid progression of hearing impairment within hours or days. It can occur at every age, but mostly affects elderly people and has an estimated incidence of 10-20/100,000/year [1,2]. The true incidence however is likely much higher when taking into account an ageing population in industrialized countries and the fact that hearing impairment is often misdiagnosed or regarded as an age-related, unavoidable fate [2,3]. Hearing impairment is mostly unilateral with varying severity, but can potentially lead to total deafness. It is often accompanied by vertigo, tinnitus and/or ear pressure [4]. At the time of onset, the aetiology of SSHL is usually unknown. In a recent systematic analysis of 23 research papers, Chau et al could demonstrate that 71% of SSHL cases were classified as idiopathic SSHL (ISSHL) because no underlying pathology could be found. In 13% of cases, infection was shown to be the culprit, whereas 5% were attributed to otologic aetiology, 4% to trauma, 3% to hematologic causes, 2% to neoplasia and another 2% to other causes [5].

Hearing recovery in ISSHL varies widely from complete, spontaneous recovery to non-recovery and shows an unpredictable course [6–8]. Reduced blood flow in the inner ear, viral infections and autoimmune processes are hypothetical aetiologies for ISSHL. These possible pathomechanisms have been deduced from animal studies and sporadic histological findings [9], but an allocation of one of these mechanisms to individual cases is difficult. Even the exact location of the disorder (vascular, neuronal, inner ear, cerebral) is not clear. One treatment option involves administration of high-dose steroids intravenously, orally or via intratympanic routes. However, the effectiveness of steroids (oral or systemic) for the treatment of ISSHL remains unproven [10].

One hypothetical scenario in ISSHL is a sudden reduction of the blood flow in the labyrinthic artery, which is a functional end artery. The blood flow in the labyrinthic artery is regulated mainly by adrenergic receptors on smooth muscle cells. It is also influenced by plasma viscosity and local regulatory mechanisms, but not by central regulatory mechanisms as in larger vessels. Due to the possible ischemia-like cause of ISSHL, it was hypothesized that risk factors, comparable to those associated with ischaemic or thromboembolic diseases, such as heart disease, stroke and thrombosis [11–13], may play an underlying role in disease-aetiology. However, these studies were not conclusive and, in part, contradictory [14,15]. The strongest argument for a vascular or haemorheological origin of ISSHL is the observation that outcome is significantly improved in ISSHL patients who underwent combined LDL and fibrinogen apheresis [16]. Because raised fibrinogen and LDL cholesterol-levels are risk factors for such vascular diseases as ischaemic heart disease, stroke and other thromboembolic diseases [17,18], this observation supports the idea that the aetiology of ISSHL is vascular.

We have recently shown that fibrinogen concentrations are significantly elevated in ISSHL patients [19]. We did not, however, find differences in LDL or HDL cholesterol levels between patients and controls, nor could we find a higher incidence of atherothrombotic fibrinogen polymorphisms in ISSHL patients. The only genetic factor that could be allocated to ISSHL was found in the gene encoding glycoprotein Ia (GpIa) [19]. The GpIa-receptor on the surface of thrombocytes is composed of integrin $\alpha_2\beta_1$, which is involved in the early steps of platelet adhesion. Here we extended our previous studies to investigate the influence of fibrinogen and glycoprotein Ia and related glycoproteins Ib and IIIa on hearing recovery. It is well known that platelet glycoproteins and fibrinogen interact on various levels in complex interrelationships [20]. GpIa, GpIb and GpIIIa are involved in adhesion of platelets to the vessel wall, fibrinogen binding and propagation of the activation process, whereas fibrinogen is intimately involved in final clot formation. We therefore wanted to additionally evaluate whether the effect of platelet glycoproteins on hearing recovery was modified by fibrinogen.

Materials and Methods

Patients and Controls

Initially, 142 consecutive German patients with a pantonal, sudden, sensorineural hearing loss (ISSHL) were included in the study: 75 male and 67 female patients aged between 14 and 83 years. Patients have previously been described [16] and were recruited from a cross-sectional study that consecutively selected ISSHL patients of a typical outpatient department. Hearing loss, measured by pure-tone audiometry, was unilateral and did not exceed two weeks of duration in all cases. Patients included had idiopathic hearing loss of at least 60dB in at least 3 frequencies between 125 and 8,000 Hz compared to the healthy ear. A non-idiopathic hearing loss was ruled out by a thorough otorhinolaryngological examination including ear microscopy, magnetic resonance imaging and serological blood investigations for herpes simplex, varizella zoster and borrelia burgdorferi infections. All patients had a negative anamnesis for familial deafness, chronic otological history, trauma, previous ear surgery, or prior sudden deafness. We excluded patients with a medical condition rendering the use of corticosteroids unsafe, such as: pregnancy, poorly controlled diabetes, chronic infections, peptic ulcer, uncompensated heart disease, recent surgery, and psychiatric disease. All patients underwent a standard therapy with high dose steroids (250 mg prednisolone reduced by 25 mg per day), 1000 ml sterofundine and 400 mg pentoxifylline per day over 8 days. Hearing recovery was calculated by comparing the pure-tone thresholds before and 8 weeks after the therapy. We registered hearing recovery [dB] in 4 selected frequencies: 250 Hz, 1,000 Hz, 2,000 Hz and 4,000 Hz. By the 8 week follow-up, 15 patients had dropped out permanently, reducing the final study population to 127 participants. The control group consisted of 81 healthy German subjects (mean age 49.9 +/− 12.6 years) matched for age and sex. The controls were taken from the Prospective Cardiovascular Münster Study (PROCAM). As shown in table 1, the mean age of the ISSHL study participants was 53.3 years, with 48.8% females. Around three-quarters of participants suffered from tinnitus and roughly one-third from vertigo. Compared with age- and sex-matched controls, patients had higher fibrinogen plasma levels (patients: 280.1 +/− 78.9 mg/dl vs. controls: 230.9 mg/dl +/− 107.9; p= 0.001), higher smoking prevalence (patients: 54.8% vs. controls: 17.7%, $p<0.001$) and a higher percentage of T-allele carriers in the GpIa C807T-polymorphism (patients: 77.9% vs. controls 65.0%, p=0.041). A subgroup of 59 patients was used for additional monitoring of platelet glycoprotein (GpIa, GPIb, and GPIIIa) receptor-densities. Except for age (patients with glycoprotein receptor analysis were older than patients without glycoprotein receptor analysis, $p<0.001$) there were no differences regarding basic patients characteristics, laboratory-results, and hearing recovery between groups that underwent receptor-density analysis and those who did not (table 1).

Blood Samples and Routine Measurements

Blood was drawn by venipuncture at the time when hearing recovery was determined, which was at least 8 weeks after ISSHL to avoid acute phase reactions secondary to the acute event. Fibrinogen was measured in citrated plasma after centrifugation for 15 min at 2,500 g. The sample analysis was done within 1 h after venipuncture. DNA was extracted from EDTA-treated blood by a spin column procedure (Quiagen, Germany).

Fibrinogen was determined using the Multifibren U reagent (BCS analyzer; Dade Behring). The coagulation process was initiated by adding a large excess of thrombin to the plasma sample. The time until formation of a fibrin clot was measured. The fibrinogen concentration was then calculated from a standard curve prepared by measuring fibrinogen calibrators of a known concentration. All other routine measurements were performed as previously described [19].

Flow Cytometry Analysis

The platelet-surface GPIa receptor density (integrin $\alpha_2\beta_1$) was determined by flow cytometry analysis using the antibody originally sold by American Diagnostica, which can now be obtained from Biocytex (Marseille, France). Measurements were performed as described by the company (manual reference number 7008). In order to maintain platelet integrity, utmost care was exercised to avoid platelet activation during collection. The anticoagulant used was trisodium citrate 0.129 M (using a ratio 9:1 volumes). Blood samples were treated within 4 hours after collection. Blood was stored at room temperature before testing (18–25°C). The test was performed on platelet rich plasma (PRP). 25 μL of PRP was diluted and then added to 20 μL of anti GpI, GpIb or GpIIIa mouse antibody. Tubes were gently vortexed for 1 to 2 seconds, secondary polyclonal anti-mouse IgG-FITC

Table 1. Comparison of study participants with and without data on glycoprotein receptor density, n = 127.

Variable		All patients; n = 127	Patients stratified for glycoprotein receptor analysis		
			With analysis; n = 59 (46.5%)	Without analysis; n = 68 (53.5%)	p
Basic patients' characteristics	Age in years, mean (sd)	53.3 (17.1)	59.5 (13.6)	48.0 (18.1)	**< 0.001**
	Female gender, n (%)	62 (48.8)	27 (45.8)	35 (51.5)	0.521
	Smoker, n (%)[&]	68 (54.8)	32 (56.1)	36 (53.7)	0.788
	Tinnitus, n (%)[&&]	91 (75.2)	39 (72.2)	52 (77.6)	0.495
	Vertigo, n (%)[&&]	46 (37.7)	18 (32.7)	28 (41.8)	0.304
Laboratory values	GPIa-gene				
	CC (wild type), n (%)	28 (22.1)	9 (15.3)	19 (27.9)	0.085
	TC or TT, n (%)	99 (77.9)	50 (84.7)	49 (72.1)	
	BcLI-gene				
	CC (wild type), n (%)	82 (64.6)	40 (67.8)	42 (61.8)	0.478
	TC or TT, n (%)	45 (35.4)	19 (32.2)	26 (38.2)	
	A312-gene				
	CC, n (%)	77 (60.6)	33 (55.9)	44 (64.7)	0.313
	TC or TT, n (%)	50 (39.4)	26 (44.1)	24 (35.3)	
	HaeIII-gene				
	CC (wild type), n (%)	78 (61.4)	37 (62.7)	41 (60.3)	0.780
	TC or TT, n (%)	49 (58.6)	22 (37.3)	27 (39.7)	
	Fibrinogen in mg/dl, mean (sd)	280.1 (78.9)	277.5 (72.7)	282 (84.5)	0.729
Hearing recovery	None, n (%)	43 (33.9)	18 (30.5)	25 (36.8)	
	1-10 dB, n (%)	46 (36.2)	19 (32.2)	27 (39.7)	0.160[§]
	> 10 dB, n (%)	38 (29.9)	22 (37.3)	16 (23.5)	

& = data missing on 3 patients; && = data missing on 6 patients; CC = wild type, TC = heterozygous; TT = homozygous; § = Mantel-Haenszel Chi-square test.

antibody was added and incubated at room temperature for 10 minutes, and finally diluted with 2 ml of dilution solution (obtained from the test kit) before measurements were performed within 2 hours of obtaining the samples. Before cytometric analysis on a FACS-STAR (Coulter) cytometer the PRP antibody mixture was stored at 2–8°C. For calibration analysis, beads coated with increasing and accurately known quantities of mouse IgG were stained in parallel with the sample using the same secondary IgG-FITC antibody and incubated for the same amount of time as per the manufacturer's recommendations. The bead population was gated using a discriminator on forward scatter to minimize background. Mean fluorescence intensity values were interpolated on the calibration curve and the number of molecules read off directly. The GpIa, GpIb and GpIIIa platelet-surface receptor densities were determined in parallel in the same experimental setting. According to the manufacturer, the values for negative isotypic controls were very low (~300 sites per platelet), so that these controls were not included in the test kit. The number of glycoprotein molecules per platelet, as described by the manufacturer for a normal population, was: 53,000±12,000 for GpIIIa, 38,000±11,000 for GpIb, and 5,000±2,800 for GpIa. In the experiments described here, the number of glycoprotein molecules per platelet was in the same range, except for the case of GPIa, in which 6 participants receptor density markedly exceeded this range (>7,000 molecules per platelet). Therefore, these 6 outliers were removed and data on glycoprotein density analysed for the 53 remaining patients.

Genetic Analysis

Fibrinogen polymorphisms. The fibrinogen polymorphisms BclI, Aα312, HaeIII and Dusart that may influence fibrinogen concentration or function [21] were determined by real time PCR, using assay-by-design kits on the TaqMan-system (Applied Biosystems, Weiterstadt, Germany). Sequence information for primers and minor grove binder probes are as follows:

fibrinogen *BclI:*	Sequence
Forward primer	-ATCCAGCAATCTCACTTTTAGGCATAT-
Reverse primer	-GGGCATCATATAAAGGACCTGAACA -
Probe 1 (labeled with the fluorescent dye VIC)	- CATCTGTGGTCATTGC -
Probe 2 (labeled with the fluorescent dye FAM)	- CATCTGTGATCATTGC -

fibrinogen *Aα312:*	
Forward primer	- GAGGGACTGCAACCTGGAAAC -
Reverse primer	- CAGTTCCAGAGCTCCCAGAGTT -
Probe 1 (labeled with the fluorescent dye VIC)	- TGGAAGTACTGGAAGC -
Probe 2 (labeled with the fluorescent dye FAM)	- TGGAAGTGCTGGAAG -

fibrinogen HaeIII:	
Forward primer	- GAGGGACTGCAACCTGGAAAC -

Reverse primer - CAGTTCCAGAGCTCCCAGAGTT -
Probe 1 (labeled with the fluorescent dye VIC) - CATCTGTGGTCATTGC -
Probe 2 (labeled with the fluorescent dye FAM) - TGGAAGTGCTGGAAG -

fibrinogen Dusart:
Forward primer - CATCACCCTGGGATAGCTGAAT -
Reverse primer - TCGTGCTACTAGTAAATTGTTTGCTGTA-
Probe 1 (labeled with the fluorescent dye VIC) - ACCACGGGAAGGG -
Probe 2 (labeled with the fluorescent dye FAM) - ACCACAGGAAGGGA -

Platelet glycoprotein Ia C807T

Determination of the C or T allele at position 807 of the GPIa gene was performed by mutagenically separated PCR. We determined the C807T genotype indirectly by identifying the linked G873A genotype. The three following primers were used:

Primer 873A in 5′ of exon:
5′-TATTCAGCAGAGTCTGGTGGGCGACGAAGTGCTT-CA-3′;
Primer 873G in 3′of exon:
5′-CTTCTGGTGGGCGACGAAGTGCTATG-3′;
Primer 1 in 5′of exon:
5′-CTCAGTATATTGTCATGGTTGCATTG-3′;

The DNA fragments were visualized on a 3 or 5% agarose gel after staining with ethidium bromide by ultraviolet transillumination.

Ethics

The study protocol was reviewed and approved by the ethics committee of the University of Münster, Germany. Written informed consent was obtained from all patients. If participants were minors, written informed consent was obtained from next of kin, caretakers, or guardians.

Statistical Analysis

Descriptive statistics encompassed the mean (standard deviation) for normally distributed metric variables and the median (range) for not-normally distributed metric variables, respectively. To test for differences between 2 independent subgroups, we used student's t-test for normally distributed metric variables and Mann-Whitney-U-Test for not normally distributed, metric variables. To test for differences between >2 independent ordered groups (of hearing recovery), we used the Mantel-Haenszel Chi-square test in binary and ordinal variables, and ANOVA for normally distributed metric variables respectively Kruskal-Wallis-Test for not-normally distributed metric variables. Binary logistic regression was used to examine the independent association of fibrinogen plasma level, glycoprotein receptor densities and their interaction with hearing recovery >10 dB (averaged over 4 frequencies, 250 Hz, 1,000 Hz, 2,000 HZ, and 4,000 Hz) versus hearing recovery ≤10 dB. We assumed a positive effect of low levels of both fibrinogen and glycoprotein receptors on hearing recovery [22,23]. Therefore, glycoprotein receptor densities and fibrinogen levels were dichotomized using their mean values, and levels above mean were taken as reference categories. Following the recommendations by Knol and VanderWeele [24], we present odds ratios and their 95% confidence intervals with a single reference category (patients with high fibrinogen levels and high glycoprotein receptor levels) for the association of fibrinogen and glycoprotein receptor density with good hearing recovery. Results of glycoprotein receptor densities were displayed stratified for both levels of fibrinogen. Interaction measures were calculated both on additive (relative excess risk due to interaction, RERI) and on multiplicative scale [24]. As the analyses were explorative, no adjustment for multiple testing was done and the statistical significance was accepted at a level of $p<0.05$.

Results

Univariate analysis of platelet integrin $\alpha_2\beta_1$ (GpIa), GpIb and GpIIIa expression in ISSHL patients and controls

The C807T polymorphism in GpIa is a silent polymorphism: it does not alter the deduced amino acid sequence of the translated protein. However, an association between the expression levels of integrin $\alpha_2\beta_1$ on platelets and the C807T polymorphism has been suggested [25], raising the possibility that integrin $\alpha_2\beta_1$ expression may influence ISSHL incidence and/or recovery from ISSHL.

The concentration of platelet integrin $\alpha_2\beta_1$ was measured using a highly sensitive fluorescence-based method (Fig. 1). In healthy age- and sex-matched controls, we could find a significant 1.4-fold higher mean number of integrin $\alpha_2\beta_1$ molecules per platelet in T-allele carriers compared to non-T-allele carriers (TT carriers 5,916 +/− 888; TC carriers 4,844 +/− 715; CC carriers 3,681 +/− 900; p<0.05 for TT vs. TC; p<0.001 for TT vs. CC and for TC vs. CC; Fig. 2a, right panel). In patients, we found a 1.2-fold higher mean number of integrin $\alpha_2\beta_1$ molecules per platelet in T-allele carriers compared to non-T-allele carriers (TT carriers 4,446 +/− 1,188; TC carriers 4,766 +/− 1,166; CC carriers 3,905 +/− 1,012; NS for all comparisons; Fig. 2a, left panel). We found no significant difference in the number of integrin $\alpha_2\beta_1$ molecules per platelet between patients and controls, neither in allele carriers nor in non-allele carriers.

We also measured the platelet expression of the glycoproteins Ib (GpIb), as shown in Fig. 2b, and IIIa (GpIIIa), as shown in Fig. 2c. GpIb, in the form of the platelet glycoprotein Ib/IX/V receptor complex, plays a key role in the platelet binding to von Willebrand Factor and the initial adhesion of platelets to the vessel wall, whereas GpIIIa is, in form of the glycoprotein IIb/IIIa complex, also known as integrin $\alpha_{IIb}\beta_3$, an important receptor for fibrinogen [20]. We did not observe an association of GpIa genotype with GpIb or GpIIIa platelet densities. No significant differences in the levels of GpIb or GpIIIa between patients and controls were observed either.

Univariate analysis of basic patients' characteristics, platelet integrin $\alpha_2\beta_1$ (GpIa), GpIb, GpIIIa expression, GPIa genotype, fibrinogen concentration, and fibrinogen genotype in ISSHL patients with different hearing recovery

As shown in table 2, after averaging hearing recovery over 4 frequencies (250 Hz, 1,000 Hz, 2,000 Hz, and 4,000 Hz) there was no hearing recovery in 43 (33.9%) study participants while 46 (36.2%) showed a mean hearing recovery up to 10 dB (moderate recovery). Another 38 (29.9%) patients showed hearing recovery of >10 dB (good recovery). The 3 groups did not differ in their basic patients' characteristics except for vertigo: patients with good hearing recovery showed the lowest prevalence of vertigo (24.3%), while in patients with no hearing recovery, vertigo prevalence was 58.5% (p for trend = 0.002). Fibrinogen plasma levels differed significantly across groups of hearing recovery (p = 0.029), with the highest fibrinogen levels being found in patients with no hearing recovery. However, 3 fibrinogen polymorphisms: the B2 allele of the BclI restriction fragment length polymorphism of the

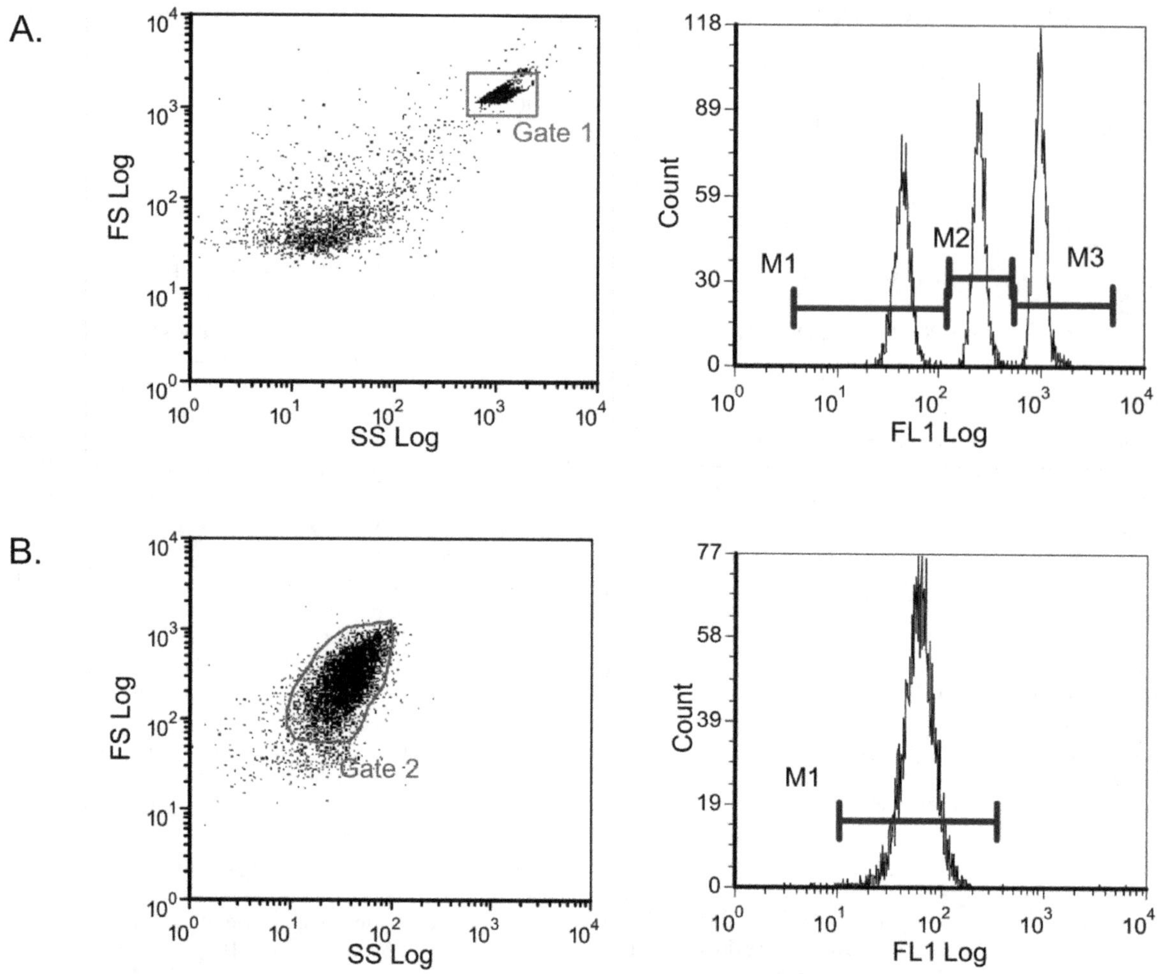

Figure 1. Test calibration cytogram with cursor settings in gated fluorescence histogram (a) and platelet rich plasma cytogram with Gpla immune-labelling cursor settings (b). A single color flow cytometric analysis of the platelet glycoproteins Gpla, Gplb and Gpllla was used (Biocytex, Marseille, France). The number of antigenic sites is determined by converting the fluorescence intensity into the corresponding number of sites per platelet based on calibrated bead standards (a). In all experiments, more than 90% of the platelets of the PRP were gated for the experiment, as shown here for Gpla (b).

fibrinogen β-chain, the 312Ala (GCT) allele of the Aα312 polymorphism of the fibrinogen α-chain [21] and the β-fibrinogen Hae III (-455 G-A) gene variant did not vary between groups. Similarly, a Gpla C807T polymorphism that may influence concentration and function of GPIa, did not vary between groups of hearing recovery. In a subgroup of 59 patients the expression of platelet Gpla, Gplb and GpIIIa receptor was measured. Significant differences between the 3 groups of hearing recovery were found for GPIIIa expression ($p = 0.037$).

Modification of the effect of platelet integrin $\alpha_2\beta_1$ (Gpla), Gplb, Gpllla expression on hearing recovery by fibrinogen in ISSHL patients

As shown in tables 3-5, after adjustment for smoking and vertigo, lower levels of all three platelet glycoproteins (except for Gpla in patients with fibrinogen below mean) were associated with better hearing recovery although this association was significant solely for GPIb in patients with fibrinogen levels above the mean (table 4). As shown in table 3, fibrinogen modified the effect of GPIa receptor density on hearing recovery: in participants with fibrinogen levels below the mean, lower GPIa receptor levels were associated with decreased probability of hearing improvement, while in patients with fibrinogen levels above the mean, the probability of hearing recovery was increased. The modification effect of fibrinogen on the association of GPIa receptor level and hearing recovery was significant on a multiplicative scale (ratio of ORs. 0.47 (95% confidence interval: 0.22 – 0.99; $p = 0.048$). For GPIb, no such effect modification by fibrinogen was observed (table 4): in both strata of fibrinogen levels, the effect of GPIb receptor density on hearing recovery was nearly identical ($OR = 2.00$ versus $OR = 1.98$, ratio of $ORs = 0.99$ (95% confidence interval: 0.52 – 1.86; $p = 0.968$). Fibrinogen did not modify the effect of GPIIIa on hearing recovery either (table 5): the ratio of ORs was 1.16 (95% confidence interval: 0.61 – 2.20; $p = 0.650$). In all three platelet glycoproteins, there was also no indication of a significant positive effect modification of platelet glycoprotein receptor density across strata of fibrinogen on an additive scale.

Discussion

The C807T polymorphism has previously been shown to be a risk factor for incidence of ISSHL [19] and other acute thrombotic events like myocardial infarction, stroke and retinal vein throm-

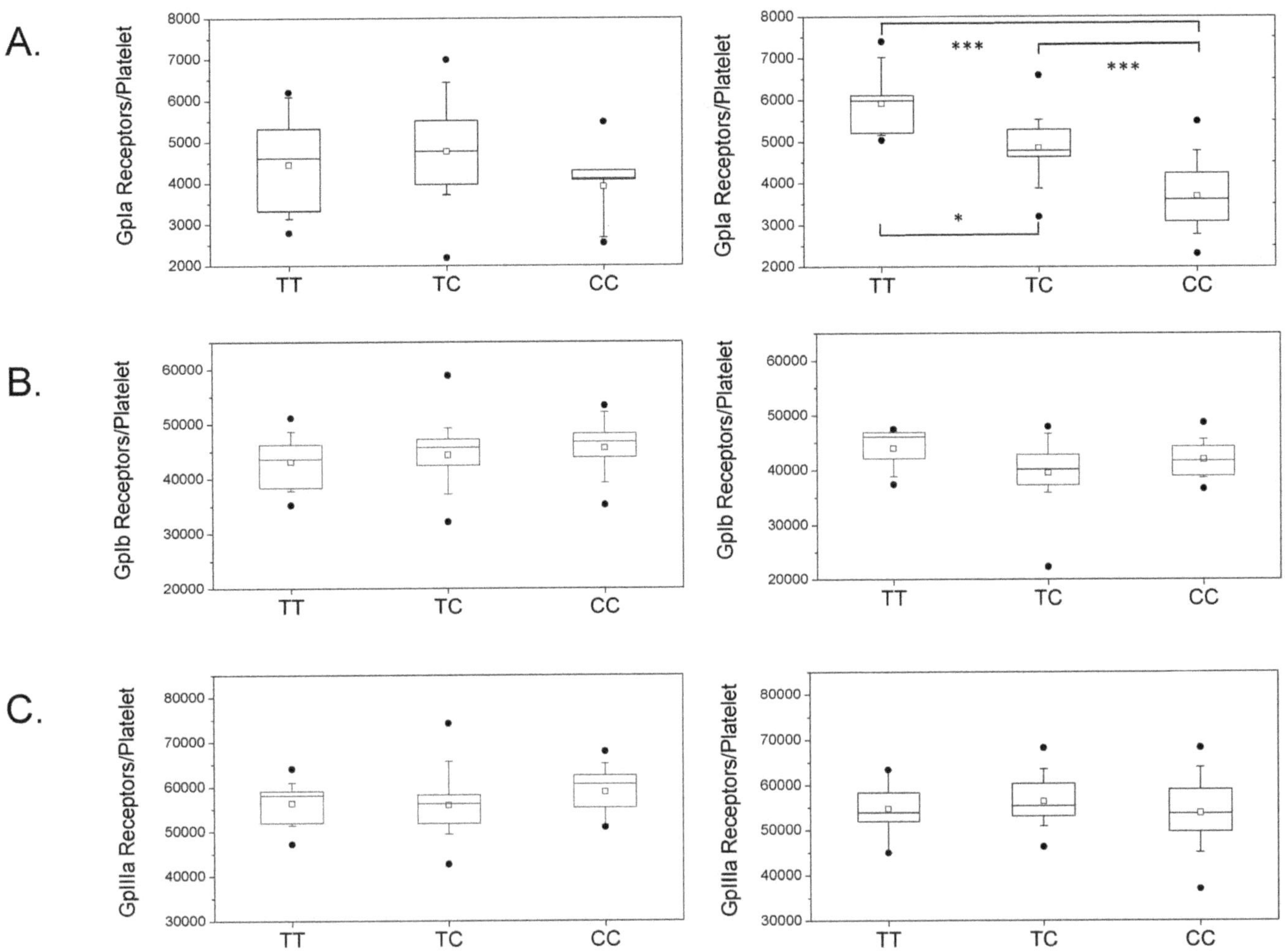

Figure 2. Number of GpIa (a), GpIb (b) and GpIIIa (c) receptor molecules per platelet in patients (left) and controls (right). The values are shown as boxplots, separated for T allele carriers (phenotype TT or CT) and CC allele carriers. The boundary of the box closest to zero indicates the 25th percentile, the line within the box marks the median, the square indicates the mean, and the boundary of the box farthest from zero indicates the 75th percentile. Whiskers above and below the box indicate the 90th and 10th percentiles. The points represent the 1st and 99th percentiles. P indicates the level of significance according to the Mann-Whitney-U-test. *, P<0.05; ***, P<0.001.

bosis, particularly in younger patients [30,31]. In this study, the polymorphism C807T directly correlated with a higher number of $\alpha_2\beta_1$ molecules on the platelet surface of patients and controls, suggesting a direct amplifying influence of the C807T polymorphism on $\alpha_2\beta_1$ integrin expression. These data are in accordance with a previous study [25] and support the model that the 'silent' mutation C807T in GpIa significantly influences platelet expression of $\alpha_2\beta_1$ integrin. However, this effect was moderate (1.2-1.4-fold) and significant only in controls. Moreover, we found no significant difference in the number of integrin $\alpha_2\beta_1$ molecules per platelet between patients and controls, neither in allele carriers nor in non-allele carriers. We had also no indication for any secondary effects of GpIa genotype on concentrations of other platelet glycoproteins, or for aberrant levels of GpIb or GpIIIa in ISSHL patients. These findings suggest that, certainly beyond the critical acute phase, receptor densities are not different between ISSHL patients and healthy controls. A higher GpIa expression in T allele carriers is *per se* apparently not sufficient to trigger an ISSHL.

Fibrinogen level ($p = 0.029$), vertigo ($p = 0.002$) and lower GpIIIa receptor density ($p = 0.037$) varied between groups with different hearing recovery.

We found a significant association between lower plasma fibrinogen levels and good hearing recovery. However, there was no significant association of fibrinogen polymorphisms (that may influence fibrinogen concentration or function) with hearing recovery, suggesting that this effect might have resulted from factors other than genetics. Suckfüll et al showed that fibrinogen apheresis improves the outcome in ISSHL patients [16]. This observation and the current study suggest that higher fibrinogen is not only a surrogate marker of increased ISSHL risk, but a pathogenetic factor in the development of ISSHL itself.

Fibrinogen can be influenced by various non-genetic factors, which include: smoking, obesity, diabetes, hormones, and acute inflammation or trauma [27,28]. It was remarkable that the majority of ISSHL patients in this investigation were smokers. Smoking may have influenced fibrinogen plasma concentration, platelet function [28,29] and hearing recovery. However, in univariate analysis, the percentage of smokers was rather (non significantly) higher in groups with better hearing recovery. We have no explanation for this apparent paradox.

Hearing impairment in ISSHL is often accompanied by vertigo [4], which is caused by a disturbed vestibular system. The blood

Table 2. Basics characteristics in groups with different hearing recovery, n = 127 respectively n = 59.

Variable		All patients stratified for hearing recovery			
		None	1–10 dB	> 10 dB	p
		n = 43 (33.9%)	n = 46 (36.2%)	n = 38 (29.9%)	
Basic patients' characteristics	Age in years, mean (sd)	53.4 (16.8)	52.8 (19.1)	53.8 (15.3)	0.966#
	Female gender, n (%)	25 (58.1)	21 (45.7)	16 (42.1)	0.146§
	Smoker, n (%)&	21 (48.8)	24 (54.6)	23 (62.2)	0.236§
	Tinnitus, n (%)&&	30 (75.0)	32 (72.7)	29 (78.4)	0.741§
	Vertigo, n (%)&&	24 (58.5)	13 (29.6)	9 (24.3)	**0.002**§
Laboratory values	GPIa-gene				
	CC (wild type), n (%)	29 (67.4)	31 (67.4)	30 (79.0)	0.268§
	TC or TT, n (%)	14 (32.6)	15 (23.6)	8 (21.1)	
	BcLI-gene				
	CC (wild type), n (%)	27 (62.8)	29 (63.0)	26 (68.4)	0.606§
	TC or TT, n (%)	16 (37.2)	17 (37.0)	12 (31.6)	
	A312-gene				
	CC (wild type), n (%)	28 (65.1)	27 (58.7)	22 (57.9)	0.501§
	TC or TT, n (%)	15 (34.9)	19 (41.3)	16 (42.1)	
	HaeIII-gene				
	CC (wild type), n (%)	26 (60.5)	26 (56.5)	26 (68.4)	0.485§
	TC or TT, n (%)	17 (39.5)	20 (43.5)	12 (31.6)	
	Fibrinogen in mg/dl, mean (sd)	306.0 (91.5)	266.6 (62.2)	267.2 (76.3)	**0.029**$
Receptor density	GPIa, mean (SD), n = 53$$	4,162.9 (1,398.1)	4,929.9 (1,104.1)	4,590.6 (940.2)	0.169$
(n = 59/53)	GPIb, mean (SD)	43,604.1 (5,099.6)	45,947.0 (5,361.6)	43,300.1 (5,118.5)	0.239$
	GPIIIa, mean (SD)	56,658.1 (5,433.4)	58,976.9 (6,377.1)	54,190.3 (5,516.4)	**0.037**$

Sd = standard deviation; # = Kruskal-Walis-Test; & = data missing on 3 patients; && = data missing on 6 patients; § = Mantel-Haenszel Chi-square test; CC = wild type, TC = heterozygous; TT = homozygous; $ = ANOVA, $$ = 6 outlier removed.

supply to the inner ear originates from the vertebrobasilar system, and vertebrobasilar ischemic stroke can present with vertigo and hearing loss due to infarction of the inner ear [26]. Thus, one possible explanation for vertigo experienced by ISSHL patients with poor prognosis (no or only limited recovery) might be an expression of a more extended degree of thrombotic damage.

The possible positive effect of low platelet concentrations of GPIIIa on hearing recovery in ISSHL patients has been shown for the first time in this study. The Glycoprotein IIb/IIIa complex (also known as integrin $\alpha_{IIb}\beta_3$) is a receptor for fibrinogen and aids in platelet activation. It is a target of several well-established drugs including abciximab, eptifibatide and tirofiban, which are used in treating patients who have unstable angina, certain types of heart

Table 3. Results of binary logistic regression analyses, dependent variable = hearing improvement >10 dB, independent variables = GPIa receptor density and fibrinogen, n = 49#.

	GPIa receptor density above mean		GPIa receptor density below mean		ORs (95%-CI) for GPIa receptor density within different strata of fibrinogen
	N with/without hearing improvement	OR (95% CI)	N with/without hearing improvement	OR (95% CI)	
Fibrinogen above mean	1/9	1.0	5/10	1.24 (0.59 – 2.60); p = 0.568	1.24 (0.59 – 2.60); p = 0.568
Fibrinogen below mean	8/13	1.50 (0.71 – 3.14); p = 0.286	5/17	0.84 (0.29 – 2.42); p = 0.741	0.56 (0.25 – 1.24); p = 0.150

Measure of effect modification on additive scale: relative excess risk due to interaction, RERI (95% CI) = −0.90 (−1.97 – 0.17)
Measure of effect modification on multiplicative scale: ratio of ORs (95% CI) = 0.45 (0.21 – 0.94), p = **0.034**
ORs are adjusted for smoking and vertigo, # = 4 datasets missing due to missing covariates.

Table 4. Results of binary logistic regression analyses, dependent variable = hearing improvement > 10 dB, independent variables = GPIb receptor density and fibrinogen, n = 55#.

	GPIb receptor density above mean		GPIb receptor density below mean		ORs (95%-CI) for GPIb receptor density within different strata of fibrinogen
	N with/without hearing improvement	OR (95% CI)	N with/without hearing improvement	OR (95% CI)	
Fibrinogen above mean	3/14	1.0	4/9	2.00 (1.04 - 3.86); p = **0.038**	2.00 (1.04 - 3.86); p = **0.038**
Fibrinogen below mean	4/15	1.28 (0.68 - 2.41); p = 0.453	10/17	2.52 (0.96 - 6.64); p = 0.061	1.98 (0.88–4.43); p = 0.098

Measure of effect modification on additive scale: relative excess risk due to interaction, RERI (95% CI) = 0.24 (−1.46 - 1.95)
Measure of effect modification on multiplicative scale: ratio of ORs (95% CI) = 0.99 (0.52– 1.86), p = 0.968
ORs are adjusted for smoking and vertigo, # = 4 datasets missing due to missing covariates.

attacks, and are used in combination with angioplasty with or without stent placement. Further studies are recommended to prove possible beneficial effects of these drugs in ISSHL. Additionally, because ADP induces exposure of fibrinogen-binding determinants on GpIIb/IIIa complexes, ADP antagonists such as clopidogrel, ticlopidine or prasugrel may have positive effects in ISSHL.

After adjustment for smoking and vertigo, lower levels of all three platelet glycoproteins were associated with better hearing recovery, although this association was significant solely for GPIb.

GpIb, as component of the GpIb/V/IX complex, binds von Willebrand factor and allows platelet adhesion and plug formation at sites of vascular injury. However, there have been conflicting reports on a possible association of polymorphisms of this glycoprotein with myocardial infarction and coronary artery disease [32–39]. A possible positive effect of low platelet concentrations of GPIb on hearing recovery has not been described before.

Fibrinogen significantly modified the effect of GPIa receptor density on hearing recovery, but in an unexpected manner: a putative protective effect of low GpIa concentrations, after adjustment for vertigo and smoking, was significantly diminished in patients with lower fibrinogen levels. There was a harmful effect modification by fibrinogen on a multiplicative scale. The origin of this effect is unclear. Apart from complex interactions between fibrinogen and GpIa [22], it is possible that pathogenetic factors other than fibrinogen may play a major role in these cases and that protective effects of lower GpIa levels become less significant when plasma fibrinogen is not elevated. A possible interrelationship between GpIa and fibrinogen is of interest insofar as GpIa, as GpIa/IIa complex, functions as receptor engaged in platelet adhesion to collagen and is believed to be associated with the risk of myocardial infarction or ischemic stroke [30,31]. In contrast to GpIa, the protective effect of lower GPIb and GPIIIa receptor density on hearing recovery was not modified by fibrinogen.

Limitations of our study are the relatively small number of patients for whom glycoprotein receptors were measured and the relative high percentage of smokers, both of which may have influenced and biased results. The power of this study was not sufficient to allow for sensitivity analyses in subgroups (e.g. in smokers/non-smokers) or for more complex analyses of interactions between genetics, environmental factors and platelet glycoproteins. Another meaningful supplement to our analysis would have been evaluation of hearing recovery in speech audiometry. Other investigators were able to show that speech audiometry might be more sensitive in detecting differences in hearing recovery [16].

Altogether, data from this study further suggest a vascular/rheological origin of ISSHL with unique features of thrombosis in the inner ear artery that may include a complex interrelationship among platelet glycoproteins and plasma fibrinogen. Further studies with prospective design are necessary to confirm and

Table 5. Results of binary logistic regression analyses, dependent variable = hearing improvement > 10 dB, independent variables = GPIIIa receptor density and fibrinogen, n = 55#.

	GPIIIa receptor density above mean		GPIIIa receptor density below mean		ORs (95%-CI) for GPIIIa receptor density within different strata of fibrinogen
	N with/without hearing improvement	OR (95% CI)	N with/without hearing improvement	OR (95% CI)	
Fibrinogen above mean	2/11	1.0	5/12	1.57 (0.81 - 3.03); p = 0.178	1.57 (0.81 - 3.03); p = 0.178
Fibrinogen below mean	5/17	1.44 (0.76 - 2.70); p = 0.260	9/15	2.62 (0.96 - 7.15); p = 0.060	1.82 (0.83 - 4.01); p = 0.135

Measure of effect modification on additive scale: relative excess risk due to interaction, RERI (95% CI) = 0.61 (−1.11 - 2.34)
Measure of effect modification on multiplicative scale: ratio of ORs (95% CI) = 1.16 (0.61– 2.20), p = 0.650
ORs are adjusted for smoking and vertigo, # = 4 datasets missing due to missing covariates.

deepen the findings described here and to prove the proposed therapeutic options, particularly glycoprotein blockade.

Acknowledgments

The expert technical assistance of Margit Käse is gratefully acknowledged. We thank Dr. Helmut Schulte (PROCAM) for his help with the manuscript preparation and Dr. Sabine Ziemer for critical reading of the manuscript.

Author Contributions

Conceived and designed the experiments: CR MW. Performed the experiments: DW AB CR MW. Analyzed the data: DW KG AB MW BN. Contributed reagents/materials/analysis tools: CR MW. Wrote the paper: MW KG BN.

References

1. Nakashima T, Itoh A, Misawa H, Ohno Y (2000). Clinicoepidemiological features of sudden deafness diagnosed and treated at university hospitals in Japan. Otolaryngol Head Neck Surg 123: 593–597.
2. Klemm E, Schaarschmidt W (1989) Epidemiological survey on sudden deafness, vestibular dysfunction and Meniere's Disease [Article in German]. HNO-Praxis 14: 295–299.
3. Klemm E, Deutscher A, Mösges R (2009). A present investigation of the epidemiology in idiopathic sudden sensorineural hearing loss. Laryngorhinootologie 88: 524–527.
4. Koc A, Sanisoglu O (2003) Sudden sensorineural hearing loss: Literature review on recent studies. J Otolaryngol 32: 308–313.
5. Chau JK, Cho JJ, Fritz DK (2012) Evidence-based practice: management of adult sensorineural hearing loss. Otolaryngol Clin North Am 45: 941–958.
6. Heiden C, Porzsolt F, Biesinger E, Hoing R (2000) Spontaneous remission of sudden deafness. HNO 48: 621–623.
7. Fuse T, Aoyagi M, Funakubo T, Sakakibara A, Yoshida S (2002) Short-term outcome and prognosis of acute low-tone sensorineural hearing loss by administration of steroid. ORL J Otorhinolaryngol Relat Spec 64: 6–10.
8. Tamhankar M, Solomon D (2004) Acute Hearing Loss. Curr Treat Options Neurol 6: 55–65.
9. Tran Ba HP (2002) Endolymphatic deafness: a particular variety of cochlear disorder. ORL J Otorhinolaryngol Relat Spec 64:120–124.
10. Conlin AE, Parnes LS (2007) Treatment of sudden sensorineural hearing loss: a systematic review. Arch Otolaryngol Head Neck Surg 133:573–581. Review
11. Selmani Z, Pyykko I, Ishizaki H, Marttila TI (2001) Cochlear blood flow measurement in patients with Meniere's Disease and other inner ear disorders. Acta Otolaryngol Suppl 545: 10–13.
12. Hirano K, Ikeda K, Kawase T, Oshima T, Kekehata S, et al. (1999) Prognosis of sudden deafness with special reference to risk factors of microvascular pathology. Auris Nasus Larynx 26: 111–115.
13. Valbonesi M, Mora F, Mora R, Carlier P (2004) Rheopheresis for sudden hearing loss (SHL). Int J Artif Organs 27: 806–809.
14. Marcucci R, Alessandrello Liotta A, Cellai AP, Rogolino A, Berloco P, et al. (2005) Cardiovascular and thrombophilic risk factors for idiopathic sudden sensorineural hearing loss. J Thromb Haemost 3: 929–934.
15. Cadoni G, Scipione S, Rocca B, Agostino S, La Greca C, et al. (2006). Lack of association between inherited thrombophilic risk factors and idiopathic sudden sensorineural hearing loss in Italian patients. Ann Otol Rhinol Laryngol 115: 195–200.
16. Suckfüll M, et al. (2002) Fibrinogen and LDL apheresis in treatment of sudden hearing loss: a randomised multicentre trial. The Lancet 360:1811–1817.
17. Ernst E, Resch KL (1993). Fibrinogen as a cardiovascular risk factor: A meta-analysis and review of the literature. Ann Int Med 118: 956–963.
18. Balleisen L, Assmann JB, Epping P-H, Schulte H, Van de Loo JCW (1985) Epidemiological Study on Factor VII and fibrinogen in an industrial population-II. Baseline data on the relation to blood pressure, blood glucose, uric acid and lipid fractions. Thromb Haemost 54: 721–723.
19. Rudack C, Langer C, Stoll W, Rust S, Walter M (2006) Vascular risk factors in sudden hearing loss. Thromb Haemost 95: 454–461.
20. Rivera JR, Lozano ML, Navarro-Nunez L, Vicente V (2009) Platelet receptors and signalling in the dynamics of thrombus formation. Hematologica 94: 700–711.
21. Hamsten A, Iselius L, De Faire U, Blomback M (1987) Genetic and cultural inheritance of plasma fibrinogen concentration. Lancet 2: 988–991.
22. Reiner AP, Siscovick DS, Rosendaal FR (2001). Platelet glycoprotein gene polymorphisms and risk of thrombosis: facts and fancies. Rev Clin Exp Hematol 5: 262–287.
23. Kannel WB (2005). Overview of hemostatic factors involved in atherosclerotic cardiovascular disease. Lipids 40: 1215–1520.
24. Knol MJ, VanderWeele TJ (2012) Recommendations for presenting analyses of effect modification and interaction. Int J Epidemiol 41:514–520.
25. Kritzik M, Savage B, Nugent DJ, Santoso S, Ruggeri ZM, et al. (1998) Nucleotid polymorphisms in the α_2 gene define multiple alleles that are associated with differences in platelet $\alpha_2\beta_1$ density. Blood 92: 2382–2388.
26. Kim HJ, Lee SH, Park JH, Choi JY, Kim JS (2013) Isolated vestibular nuclear infarction: report of two cases and review of the literature. J Neurol [Epub ahead of print].
27. De Maat MP, Pietersma A, Kofflard M, Sluiter W, Kluft C (1996) Association of plasma fibrinogen levels with coronary artery disease, smoking and 7. inflammatory markers. Atherosclerosis 121: 185–191.
28. Lu JT, Creager MA (2004) The relationship of cigarette smoking to peripheral arterial disease. Rev Cardiovasc Med 5: 189–193.
29. Nascetti S, Elosua R, Pena A, Covas MI, Senti M, et al. (2001) Variables associated with fibrinogen in a population-based study: interaction between smoking and age on fibrinogen concentration. Eur J Epidemiol 7:953–958.
30. Carlsson LE, Santoso S, Spitzer C, Kessler C, Greinacher A (1993) The alpha2 gene coding sequence T807/A873 of the platelet collagen receptor integrin alpha2beta1 might be a genetic risk factor for the development of stroke in younger patients. Blood 93: 3583–3586.
31. Santoso S, Kunicki TJ, Kroll H, Haberbosch W, Gardemann A (1999) Association of the platelet glycoprotein Ia C807T gene polymorphism with nonfatal myocardial infarction in younger patients. Blood 93: 2449–2453.
32. Pellikka M, Narhi L, Perola M, Penttila A, Karhunen PJ, et al. (2008) Platelet GPIb alpha, GPIV and vWF polymorphisms and fatal pre-hospital MI among middle-aged men. J Thromb Thrombolysis 26:91–96.
33. Ishida F, Ito T, Takei M, Shimodaira S, Kitano K, et al. (2000) Genetic linkage of Kozak sequence polymorphism of the platelet glycoprotein Ib alpha with human platelet antigen-2 and variable number of tandem repeats polymorphism, and its relationship with coronary artery disease. Br J Haematol. 111:1247–1249.
34. Cadroy Y, Sakariassen KS, Charlet JP, Thalamas C, Boneu B, et al. (2001) Role of 4 platelet membrane glycoprotein polymorphisms on experimental arterial thrombus formation in men. Blood 98:3159–3161.
35. Meisel C, Afshar-Kharghan V, Cascorbi I, Laule M, Stangl V, et al. (2001) Role of Kozak sequence polymorphism of platelet glycoprotein Ibalpha as a risk factor for coronary artery disease and catheter interventions. J Am Coll Cardiol 38:1023–1027.
36. Kenny D, Muckian C, Fitzgerald DJ, Cannon CP, Shields DC (2002) Platelet glycoprotein Ib alpha receptor polymorphisms and recurrent ischaemic events in acute coronary syndrome patients. J Thromb Thrombolysis 13:13–19.
37. Croft SA, Hampton KK, Daly ME, Steeds RP, Channer KS, et al. (2000) Kozak sequence polymorphism in the platelet GPIbalpha gene is not associated with risk of myocardial infarction. Blood 95:2183–2184.
38. Frank MB, Reiner AP, Schwartz SM, Kumar PN, Pearce RM, et al. (2001) The Kozak sequence polymorphism of platelet glycoprotein Ibalpha and risk of nonfatal myocardial infarction and nonfatal stroke in young women. Blood 97:875–879.
39. Douglas H, Michaelides K, Gorog DA, Durante-Mangoni E, Ahmed N, et al. (2002) Platelet membrane glycoprotein Ibalpha gene -5T/C Kozak sequence polymorphism as an independent risk factor for the occurrence of coronary thrombosis. Heart 87:70–74.

Identifying MicroRNAs Involved in Degeneration of the Organ of Corti during Age-Related Hearing Loss

Qian Zhang[1], Huizhan Liu[1], JoAnn McGee[2], Edward J. Walsh[2], Garrett A. Soukup[1]*, David Z. Z. He[1]*

1 From the Department of Biomedical Sciences, Creighton University School of Medicine, Omaha, Nebraska, United States of America, **2** Boys Town National Research Hospital, Omaha, Nebraska, United States of America

Abstract

MicroRNAs (miRNAs), a class of short non-coding RNAs that regulate the expression of mRNA targets, are important regulators of cellular senescence and aging. We questioned which miRNAs are involved in age-related degeneration of the organ of Corti (OC), the auditory sensory epithelium that transduces mechanical stimuli to electrical activity in the inner ear. Degeneration of the OC is generally accepted as the main cause of age-related hearing loss (ARHL), a progressive loss of hearing in individuals as they grow older. To determine which miRNAs are involved in the onset and progression of ARHL, miRNA gene expression in the OC of two mouse strains, C57BL/6J and CBA/J, was compared at three different ages using GeneChip miRNA microarray and was validated by real-time PCR. We showed that 111 and 71 miRNAs exhibited differential expression in the C57 and CBA mice, respectively, and that downregulated miRNAs substantially outnumbered upregulated miRNAs during aging. miRNAs that had approximately 2-fold upregulation included members of miR-29 family and miR-34 family, which are known regulators of pro-apoptotic pathways. In contrast, miRNAs that were downregulated by about 2-fold were members of the miR-181 family and miR-183 family, which are known to be important for proliferation and differentiation, respectively. The shift of miRNA expression favoring apoptosis occurred earlier than detectable hearing threshold elevation and hair cell loss. Our study suggests that changes in miRNA expression precede morphological and functional changes, and that upregulation of pro-apoptotic miRNAs and downregulation of miRNAs promoting proliferation and differentiation are both involved in age-related degeneration of the OC.

Editor: Arun Rishi, Wayne State University, United States of America

Funding: This work has been supported by the National Institutes of Health (NIH) grant R01 DC004696 to DH from the NIDCD. QZ has been supported by a graduate student fellowship from Creighton University School of Medicine. GS is supported by NIH grant R01 DC 009025 from the NIDCD. We acknowledge the use of the Integrated Biological Imaging Facility (supported by the Creighton University School of Medicine and C06 Grant RR17417-01 from the NCRR, NIH) and the University of Nebraska Microarray Facility (supported by P20 Grant RR 018788 from the NCRR, NIH). The funders had no role in study design, data collection and analysis, decision to publish, or preparation of the manuscript.

Competing Interests: The authors have declared that no competing interests exist.

* E-mail: GarrettSoukup@creighton.edu (GS); hed@creighton.edu (DH)

Introduction

Age-related hearing loss (ARHL), also known as presbycusis, is a progressive sensorineural hearing loss that occurs as people get older. It has been reported that as many as 35% to 50% of the population aged between 65 and 75 have ARHL [1,2]. Although gradual morphological and physiological changes in the central auditory system can also contribute to hearing impairment and difficulty understanding spoken language, it is generally accepted that degeneration of the organ of Corti (OC) is the primary cause of ARHL. The OC contains mechanosensitive hair cells, which convert mechanical stimuli into electrical activity.

miRNAs are endogenous, small (20–23 nt), non-coding RNAs that bind to complementary sequences within target messenger RNA (mRNA) transcripts and typically result in translational repression or target degradation and gene silencing [3]. miRNAs are collectively predicted to target ~60% of all genes and each miRNA is expected to repress hundreds of target genes. miRNAs are a vital part of genetic regulation and exhibit a wide range of biological functions including cell differentiation, proliferation, apoptosis, metabolism, and self-renewal [4]. Recent studies have established a direct correlation between miRNA regulation and aging in worms (*Caenorhabditis elegans*), mice, and humans [5,6]. Lin-4 is the first miRNA identified that is highly related to life span in *C. elegans* [3,7]. A number of other miRNAs including the miR-29 family, miR-34 family, miR-15/16, miR-17-92 cluster, miR-146a/b, and miR-200 family are all known to be involved in networks regulating cell senescence and death [8–10].

Approximately one-fourth of known mouse miRNAs are expressed in the inner ear of mice [11–13]. Many of these miRNAs are associated with proliferation, differentiation, and morphological/functional development of auditory sensory epithelia [14–16]. For example, miR-124 and the miR-183 family are necessary for neurosensory cell fate determination [14,15,17]. Other studies have shown that miR-181a and the let-7 family play important roles in hair cell regeneration in chicken and newt [18–20]. Although miRNAs are known to affect cellular proliferation, differentiation, and growth in the inner ear, the role of miRNAs in aging of the OC has not been examined. The goal of our study was to identify miRNAs that were differentially expressed in the OC between younger and older mice. Identification of which miRNAs are indicated in aging is a first step in the effort to elucidate the roles of miRNAs and their regulatory networks in age-related degeneration of the OC.

We reasoned that miRNAs that are involved in the age-related degeneration of the OC should be differentially expressed before and after the onset of ARHL. GeneChip miRNA microarray was used to examine miRNA expression in the OC at three different ages in two mouse strains, C57BL/6J and CBA/J. We then used quantitative real-time PCR (q-PCR) to validate the expression profiles of four individual miRNAs that were indicated by microarray analysis. To compare and correlate differential miRNA expression profiles with functional and morphological changes of hair cells, we also examined hearing thresholds and hair cell morphology at different stages before and after the onset of ARHL.

Materials and Methods

OC Tissue Collection

C57BL/6J and CBA/J mice were used for the study. Both strains were bred in-house after purchase from Jackson Laboratory (Bar Harbor, ME, USA). Care and use of the animals in this study were approved by grants from the National Institutes of Health and by the Institutional Animal Care and Use Committees of Creighton University and Boys Town National Research Hospital.

Cochleae were rapidly dissected in cold phosphate-buffered saline (PBS; 10 mM Na_2HPO_4, 1.7 mM KH_2PO_4, 137 mM NaCl, 2.7 mM KCl, pH7.4) after the mice were euthanized. The basilar membrane together with the OC was isolated. Tissue from ten cochleae from five mice was pooled as one group for each GeneChip microarray analysis. Three groups for each age and mouse strain were prepared using C57 mice at postnatal day 21 (P21), 3 months (3 m) and 9 months (9 m), and CBA mice at P21, 9 m, and 16 months (16 m). Isolated tissues were stored at −20°C in RNAlater stabilization reagent (Ambion, Austin, TX, USA). Total RNA including miRNAs was isolated using the mirVana miRNA Isolation Kit (Ambion) and dissolved into 20–30 μl of RNase-free water. RNA concentration was determined by UV spectrophotometry (Nanodrop ND-1000), and RNA quality was examined by measuring the ratio of 28S to 18S rRNA using an Agilent 2100 BioAnalyzer.

GeneChip Microarray of miRNAs

The miRNA gene expression profile of each OC tissue sample was determined by GeneChip microarray analysis (Affymetrix, Santa Clare, CA, USA) using approximately 250 ng of total RNA obtained from each group. Synthesis of cDNA, hybridization to chips, and washes were performed according to the manufacture's protocol. GeneChips were scanned at 3 μm density with a GeneArray Scanner (Affymetrix). Images were inspected to ensure that all chips had low background but bright hybridization signals. Mean fluorescence signal intensity for each probe was quartile normalized. The average of three mean signals for each miRNA probe was normalized to that for an added control oligonucleotide and was log2 transformed. Each miRNA probe was assessed for expression based on a Wilcoxon Rank-Sum test of the miRNA probe set signals compared to the distribution of signals from the background. The Student's t-test was used to determine significant differences in miRNA expression between P21 and older-aged groups, where $p<0.05$ was interpreted as significant.

Quantitative Real-time PCR

For quantitative real-time PCR (q-PCR) analysis of miRNAs, the apical turn of the cochlea from five additional animals for each group from different ages of C57 and CBA mice was obtained. q-PCR detection of miRNAs was performed using mirVana q-PCR miRNA Primer sets (Ambion). 100 ng total RNA from each group was reverse transcribed using SuperScript Reverse Transcriptase (Invitrogen) in a 20 μl reaction to produce cDNA. q-PCR was performed using a 7500 Fast Real-Time PCR System (Applied Biosystems) to analyze triplicate reactions (20 μl) containing 2× SYBR Green PCR Master Mix (Applied Biosystems), a 10-fold dilution of mirVana q-PCR Primer Set, and cDNA. After incubation at 95°C for 20 seconds, PCR products were analyzed throughout 40 cycles consisting of an incubation at 95°C for 3 s and 60°C for 30 s. U6 RNA was detected as an internal relative control for each group. The threshold cycle (C_T) was defined as the PCR cycle number at which the fluorescence intensity was appreciably above the background level but was still in the early exponential phase of amplification. The change in C_T between a given miRNA and U6 RNA for each reaction was defined as ΔC_T and averaged for each group. The change in ΔC_T between two groups was defined as $\Delta\Delta C_T$, which represented a relative difference in expression of miRNA. Fold difference in miRNA expression between groups was calculated as $2^{-\Delta\Delta CT}$. We compared the ΔCT values for each miRNA from older groups with those for the P21 group using the Student's t-test, where $p<0.05$ was interpreted as significant.

Hearing Threshold Measurement Using Auditory Brainstem Responses (ABR)

Five animals for each mouse strain were used for ABR recordings. The mouse was anesthetized with mixture of ketamine/xylazine (ketamine 100 mg/kg; xylazine 15 mg/kg; ip), and supplemented as needed. ABRs were recorded in response to tone bursts of 2, 2.8, 4, 5.6, 8, 11, 16, 22, 32, 40, 50, and 60 kHz using standard procedures previously described [21]. Tone bursts with 1 ms rise cosine on/off ramps were generated digitally using a clock rate of 125 kHz and 16-bit D/A converters. Stimulus levels were calibrated using a 1/8″ Brüel and Kjær microphone (Model 4138) and were presented in sound pressure level in decibel (dB SPL: referenced to 20 μPa). ABR signals were collected with subcutaneous platinum needle electrodes placed at the vertex, mastoid prominence, and shoulder. Response signals were amplified (100,000×), filtered, and acquired by TDT Workstations (Tucker-Davis Technologies). Each averaged response was based on 200 stimulus repetitions. During the procedure, the body temperature was maintained at 38°C with a heating pad. All records were obtained in a sound-attenuating chamber.

Hair Cell Counting

The cochleae of CBA (at the age of P21, 9 m, and 16 m) and C57 mice (at P21, 3 m, and 9 m) were perfused with 4% paraformaldehyde (PFA) after transcardiac perfusion and maintained in the fixative at 4°C overnight. The basilar member including the OC was dissected and cut into two (apical and basal) segments. The tissue was blocked for 1 hour with 0.25% normal goat serum in PBS containing 0.01% Triton-X-100 for 1 hour. Primary antibody for Myo VIIa (Invitrogen) was diluted 1:200 and incubated for 24 hours at 4°C. After several washes with PBS, secondary antibody (1:500) (Alexa fluor molecular probe 488; Invitrogen) was added and incubated overnight at 4°C. Tissues were washed with PBS and mounted on slides with antifade solution (5-ml PBS, 5-ml glycerol, 0.1-g n-propyl gallate). Images were captured using a LSM 510 META confocal scanning system with three lasers mounted on a Zeiss AxioPlan 2IE MOT motorized upright microscope (Carl Zeiss International). Hair cell counts from two areas (400 μm in length) at the basal and apical turns were obtained from confocal images offline.

Results

1.Hearing Thresholds of C57 and CBA Mice

The CBA and C57 strains are the most widely used mouse models of ARHL [22,23]. The CBA strain has a slow, progressive hearing loss that occurs near 18 months after birth [22–26]. The C57 strain possesses a mutation in the *Ahl* gene that leads to deficiencies in the cadherin 23 protein [27,28], an important component of the transduction apparatus in the stereocilia of hair cells [29–31]. The C57 mice have an accelerated ARHL, as reflected in rapid deterioration in ABR thresholds and declines in distortion product otoacoustic emission levels that start in the higher frequencies (basal turn) and progress to lower frequencies (apical turn) with aging [24,32,33]. We measured ABR-based hearing thresholds of C57 and CBA mice to determine when hearing loss began in these two strains. Although ABR thresholds of these two strains were previously examined [22,24,26], we used a wider range of frequencies to determine thresholds at higher frequencies. ABR thresholds were measured at the ages of P21, 3 m, and 9 m for C57 mice, and at P21, 9 m, and 16 m for CBA mice. Five animals from each strain were used. Figure 1 shows the thresholds (presented as means ± sd) obtained from C57 and CBA mice using tone bursts with frequencies varied from 2 to 60 kHz. For comparison, thresholds of CBA mice at P21 are also presented in Figure 1A, along with the audiograms of C57 mice. C57 and CBA mice showed some difference at the low and high frequency ends. C57 mice had a threshold elevation of approximately 30 dB at the frequency of 60 kHz at P21 compared to the threshold of CBA mice at the same age (Fig. 1A). At the age of 3 m, C57 mice exhibited a significant elevation of the threshold at 50 and 60 kHz. Hearing loss extended toward middle and low frequencies during aging, and by 9 m hearing loss greater than 50 dB was observed at 22 kHz and greater. In contrast, the ABR thresholds of CBA mice remained unchanged between P21 and 16 m (Fig. 1B). The ABR audiogram indicates that C57 mice displayed an onset and rapid progression of hearing loss starting from high frequencies as early as 3 months after birth, whereas CBA mice exhibit minimal hearing loss even at 16 m.

2.Hair Cell Counting

We examined hair cell loss at two cochlear locations at different ages for the two mouse strains. The total length of the basilar membrane of the mouse cochlea is approximately 5.8 mm (measured from middle point of the basilar membrane) based on a study by Müller et al. [34]. The locations where hair cell count were taken were approximately 0.5–0.9 and 5.0–5.4 mm from the basal end of the basilar membrane, representing two regions in the basal and apical turns with best frequencies of 55–45 and 2–3 kHz, respectively [34]. As shown in Figure 2A, there was no apparent hair cell loss in this near-hook region in the basal turn at P21 for C57 mice, despite a 30-dB deficit compared to the threshold of CBA mice at 60 kHz. Thus, the threshold elevation might be either inherent to C57 mice or due to ultrastructural changes in the hair cells that could not be detected upon gross morphological examination. At the age of 3 m, sporadic outer hair cell loss was observed in the basal region of the C57 mice. However, no significant hair cell loss was detected in the apical region. By 9 m, a complete loss of outer hair cells and 96% loss of inner hair cells were observed in the basal turn region (Fig. 2B and 2C). In the apical turn region, there was less than 10% loss of outer hair cells and no significant loss of inner hair cells. For CBA mice, no significant hair cell loss was detected in either of the two regions at the age of 9 m (Fig. 2D). At 16 m, the apical turn region exhibited no significant hair cell loss, whereas a 5% loss of inner hair cells and an 8% loss of outer hair cells were observed in the basal region. Thus, hearing loss and hair cell loss observed in 3-month-old C57 mice were greater than those of 16-month-old CBA mice.

3.Differential Expression of miRNAs in the OC during Aging

The expression profiles of miRNAs presented in this study represented 3 repeats for each age/species for the GeneChip microarray. The raw data of miRNA array can be downloaded from the National Center for Biotechnology Information-Gene Expression Omnibus (GEO) (GEO submissions number: GSE45026). A total of 45,930 miRNA genes were probed in the OC tissues, including 7788 probe sets that covered a variety of other species. Our analyses were performed on all known mouse miRNAs (mmu-miRNAs). There were 609 probes of mmu-miRNAs. Two criteria were used for identifying differentially expressed miRNAs between younger and older mice: first, the miRNA had to be "expressed" in each of the two samples for each age group; second, the expression level of the miRNAs had to be significantly different from that of the younger group ($p<0.05$, student's t-test). miRNAs that met the two criteria are presented in Figures 3 and 4.

P21 mice were selected as reference for screening miRNAs that were differentially expressed during aging for both strains. At this age, the OC is known to be structurally and functionally adult-like while no hair cell loss is detected. We examined miRNA differential expression between P21 and 3 m as well as between P21 and 9 m in C57 mice. The selection of 3- and 9-month-old mice as the older groups for C57 mice was based on the fact that onset of high frequency hearing loss began in the basal turn at 3 m, and by 9 m hearing loss and hair cell loss were extended to mid-frequencies. Thus, these two ages represent the onset and progression of ARHL in C57 mice. Figure 3 presents differential expression profiles of miRNAs from the OC of C57 mice between P21 and 3 m (in blue), as well as between P21 and 9 m (in red). A total of 111 miRNAs were identified as significantly differentially expressed. Among them, ninety-eight (88%) miRNAs showed changes in the same direction (upregulation or downregulation) at the two different ages. miRNAs that were downregulated during aging outnumbered upregulated miRNAs by a ratio of approximately 4.4:1 (80/18). Sixteen miRNAs had their expression level downregulated by more than 50%, whereas 10 miRNAs were upregulated by more than twofold.

ABR-based threshold measurements showed that CBA mice did not have significant high frequency hearing loss even at 16 months after birth. We compared miRNA expression of CBA mice between P21 and 9 m, as well as between P21 and 16 m. Comparison between P21 and 9 m allowed us to determine whether changes in the expression profile of miRNAs start much earlier than any morphological and functional changes are detected. As shown in Figure 4, 71 miRNAs were found to be differentially expressed. Fifty-nine (83%) miRNAs exhibited expression-level changes in the same directions in the two age groups. Similar to the trend seen in C57 mice, downregulated miRNAs eclipsed upregulated miRNAs by a ratio of approximately 7.5:1 (52/7). This ratio was substantially greater than that seen for C57 mice.

C57 and CBA mice have different genetic backgrounds, which might contribute to different miRNA expression. The early onset and rapid progression of hearing loss seen in C57 mice is due to *Ahl* gene mutation [27,28,35]. Thus, some differences in miRNA expression are likely associated with the *Ahl* mutation that may cause early degeneration of stereocilia and the mechanotranduc-

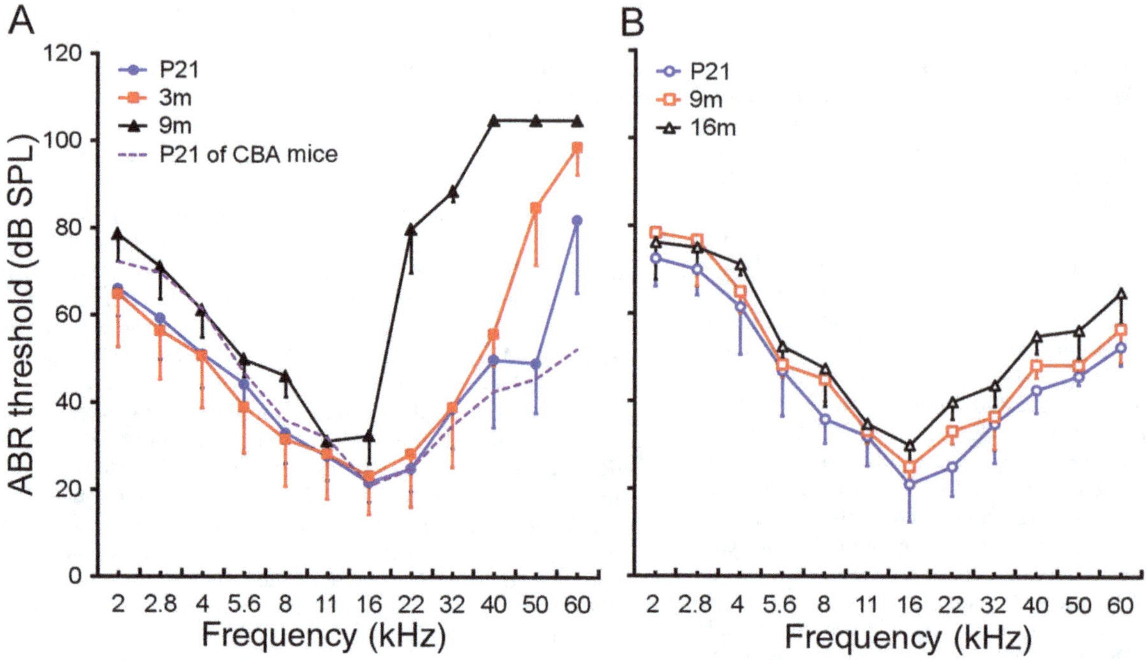

Figure 1. ABR thresholds of C57 and CBA mice. A: ABR thresholds of C57 mice at the ages of P21, 3 m, and 9 m. The dotted lines are the ABR threshold of CBA mice at P21. **B**: ABR thresholds of CBA mice at the ages of P21, 9 m, and 16 m.

tion apparatus, leading to hair cell apoptosis. We thus examined and compared the miRNA expression profile of C57 mice with that of CBA mice. Forty-nine miRNAs were found to be differentially expressed only in C57 mice (Fig. 5). Among the list, twelve miRNAs were significantly up-regulated, while thirty-seven miRNAs were significantly down-regulated.

Despite the differences between C57 and CBA mice, these two strains should share some common miRNAs that are associated with hair cell apoptosis and degeneration of the OC. To identify common miRNAs that were involved in ARHL in both strains, we also identified miRNAs that were present in both C57 and CBA mice. Figure 6 depicts 44 miRNAs that were present in both strains. Among this list, forty miRNAs showed significant down-regulation whereas four miRNAs, miR-29a, miR-29b, miR-34a and miR-124, were up-regulated.

4.Validation by q-PCR Analyses

We used q-PCR assays to validate differential expression of some of the miRNAs identified by microarray analyses. Two upregulated and two downregulated miRNAs were selected for q-PCR analyses. The two upregulated miRNAs, miR-29a and miR-34a, are known to regulate apoptosis pathways [36–38]. The two downregulated miRNAs, miR-181 and miR-183, are important for proliferation and differentiation, respectively [39–42]. The OC from the apical turn was selected for q-PCR analyses since the apical turn had minimal hair cell loss during aging, even for C57 mice. Using U6 RNA as an internal control, the change in miRNA expression was determined comparing older groups to P21. Figure 7 exhibits changes in expression of four different miRNAs during aging using q-PCR. For comparison, the change in expression of these four miRNAs from microarray analyses is also presented. As shown, the expression levels of miR-183 and miR-181 were significantly downregulated, while miR-29a and miR-34a were upregulated with aging compared to P21. These changes in expression are consistent with the trends seen in microarray analyses.

Discussion

The analysis of miRNAs that are differentially expressed in tissues from younger and older organisms has led to the discovery of numerous miRNAs that are important for controlling aging processes in previous studies [5,6,8,9,43]. We used high-throughput microarray analysis to identify miRNAs that were up- or downregulated in the OC in two strains of mice during aging. We show that approximately 111 and 71 miRNAs exhibit differential expression in C57 and CBA mice. Many miRNAs indicated by our microarray analyses (Figures 3 and 4) were previously known to be involved in differentiation, proliferation, growth, and apoptosis in other tissues and organs [44–47]. The precise functions and specific targets of these miRNAs in regulating cellular senescence and aging are yet to be revealed. However, changes in expression levels during aging suggest that these miRNAs are directly and/or indirectly involved in regulatory processes that contribute to degeneration of the OC.

The majority of miRNAs identified in the present study can be classified into two categories by their perceived functions in the aging process: anti-apoptotic (or pro-growth) and pro-apoptotic. Most miRNAs that are significantly upregulated with aging in the OC are pro-apoptotic, while most downregulated miRNAs are pro-growth. The miRNAs in the pro-apoptotic category include miR-29a/b/c, miR-34a/b/c, let-7a/b/c/e/f/g/i, miR-141, miR-146, miR-203, miR-429, and several others. The anti-apoptotic category of miRNAs includes miR-17, miR-181a/b/d, and miR-182/183 [45]. These miRNAs can work through different pathways to directly or indirectly affect apoptosis through multiple transcript factors and functional proteins such as p53, the Bcl2 family, p27, the TNF receptors super family, caspases and caspase regulators. We summarize the known functions and regulatory mechanisms of these anti- and pro-apoptotic miRNAs in Table S1.

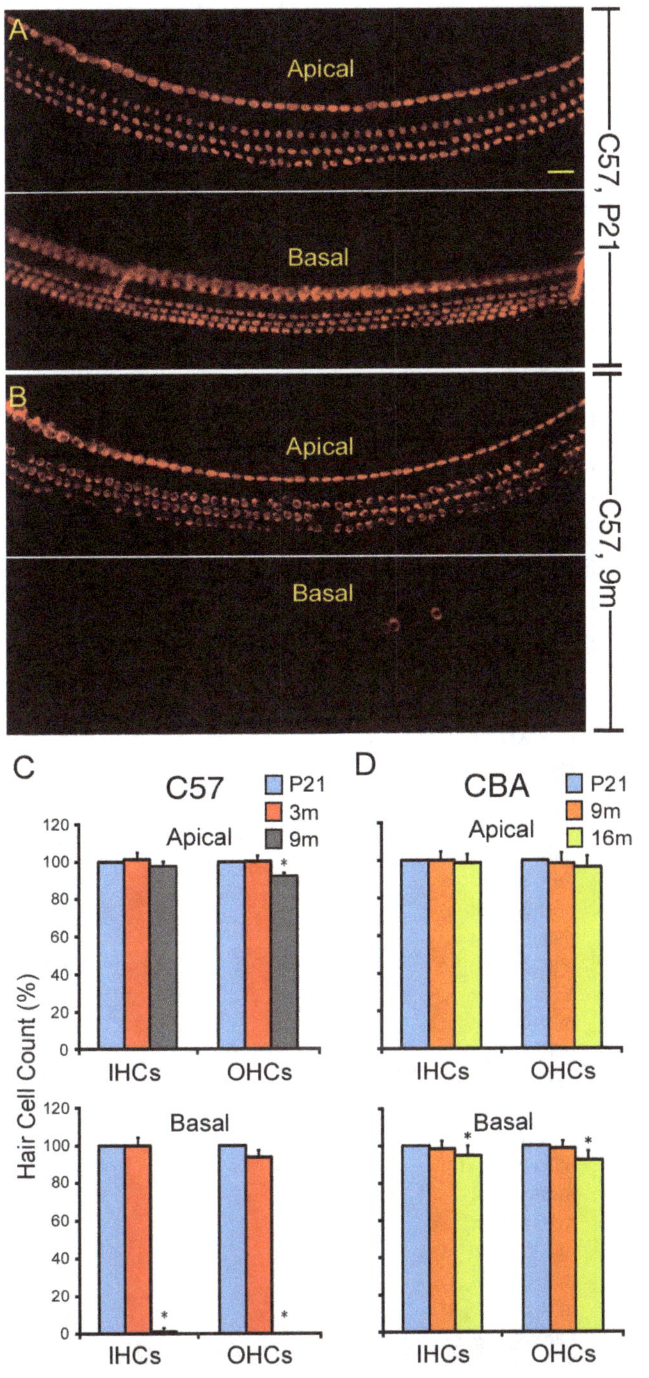

Figure 2. Hair cell counts from the OC of C57 and CBA mice. A, B: Representative confocal images of myo7a-labeled hair cells at the apical and basal turns of C57 mice at P21 (A) and 9 m (B). **C, D:** Hair cell counts obtained from two representative cochlear locations from C57 (C) and CBA (D) mice at different ages. The two locations were approximately 0.5–0.9 and 5.0–5.4 mm from the basal end of the basilar membrane. IHCs and OHCs were counted from each location. Three animals for each strain and age were included in the counts. The average numbers of IHCs and OHCs at each location are normalized to those of P21 mice (100%). Asterisks indicate statistically significant differences ($p<0.05$, Student's t-test) compared to P21.

miRNAs that showed approximately 2-fold upregulation include members of the miR-29 family and miR-34 family, which have been demonstrated to be involved in cellular senescence and apoptosis in cell lines, tissues, and organisms during aging [48–51]. Both miR-29 and miR-34 can affect genes that activate or enhance p53 pathways. Therefore, these two miRNAs are generally considered to be pro-apoptotic [48,49]. miR-29 can suppress several important genes that drive cell survival (e.g. Cdc42, p85a, Mcl1, and Tcl1). miR-29 family members indirectly upregulate p53 levels and induce apoptosis in a p53-dependent manner by suppressing p85a (the regulatory subunit of PI3Kinase) and CDC42 (a Rho family GTPase), both of which negatively regulate p53 [52]. Studies have also shown that miR-29a is able to revert DNA methylation by targeting DNA methyltransferases 3A (Dnmt 3a) and 3B (Dnmt3b) [53]. Overexpression of miR-29 family members inhibits cell proliferation [50]. High levels of miR-29 may render the cells more susceptible to p53-dependent stress responses [54]. miR-29a and miR-29b were significantly upregulated in both strains of mice in our study. The increased expression of miR-29 during aging and the pro-apoptotic nature of this family indicate miR-29 is likely involved in the degeneration of the OC.

Another p53-relevant miRNA indicated in the process of ARHL in our study is miR-34a. miR-34 family members participate in downstream signaling of the p53 pathway [55]. The level of miR-34a expression may affect the decision between apoptosis and cell-cycle arrest. Studies have shown that p53 can bind directly to the promoter and activate miR-34 genes in response to DNA damage and oncogenic stress. miR-34 mediates the downstream effects of p53 by suppressing a number of genes including CDK4/6, Cyclin E2, MET, and Bcl-2, thereby promoting apoptosis [56,57]. One recent study showed that miR-34a expression in the inner ear was drastically upregulated during the course of damage induced by ototoxic drugs [58]. In the present study, the highest expression level of miR-34a appeared amid the progression of ARHL. Whereas miR-29 regulates genes upstream of p53 pathways and miR-34a regulates genes downstream of p53 pathways, the results suggest that miRNAs contribute to p53-dependent apoptosis in degeneration of the OC in the inner ear. The role of p53 in hair cell apoptosis and ARHL has been demonstrated in a number of studies [59–64].

miRNAs that were significantly downregulated include members of the miR-181 and miR-183 families. The miR-181 family is known to mediate proliferation in many cells [54,65,66]. Previous studies have shown that transfection of miR-181b in HeLa and HCT-116 tumor cells regulates a large number of genes, inducing those related to cell growth. miR-181a has been specifically shown to have a proliferative effect in human myeloid leukemia cells [67]. This effect appears to be mediated in part by downregulation of the p27 pathway [39]. In the inner ear, miR-181a is upregulated during regeneration of the sensory epithelium in the basilar papilla of chicken, suggesting that miR-181a is involved in mechanisms that control proliferation and differentiation in the auditory sensory epithelium [19]. Among all the family members, miR-181a/b/d exhibited significant downregulation in the OC of both strains in our microarray analyses and q-PCR validation.

miR-183 family members include miR-96, miR-182, and miR-183. This family regulates genes that are associated with differentiation, proliferation, and growth in various types of normal and cancer cells [68,69]. The family is abundantly expressed in sensory neurons and hair cells into adulthood in the inner ear, and it is important for cell specification and hair cell fate determination [12]. Recent studies show that two single-base mutations in the seed region of miR-96 result in autosomal dominant, progressive hearing loss in both humans and mice [70,71]. The mutation alters the function of miR-96 and gene

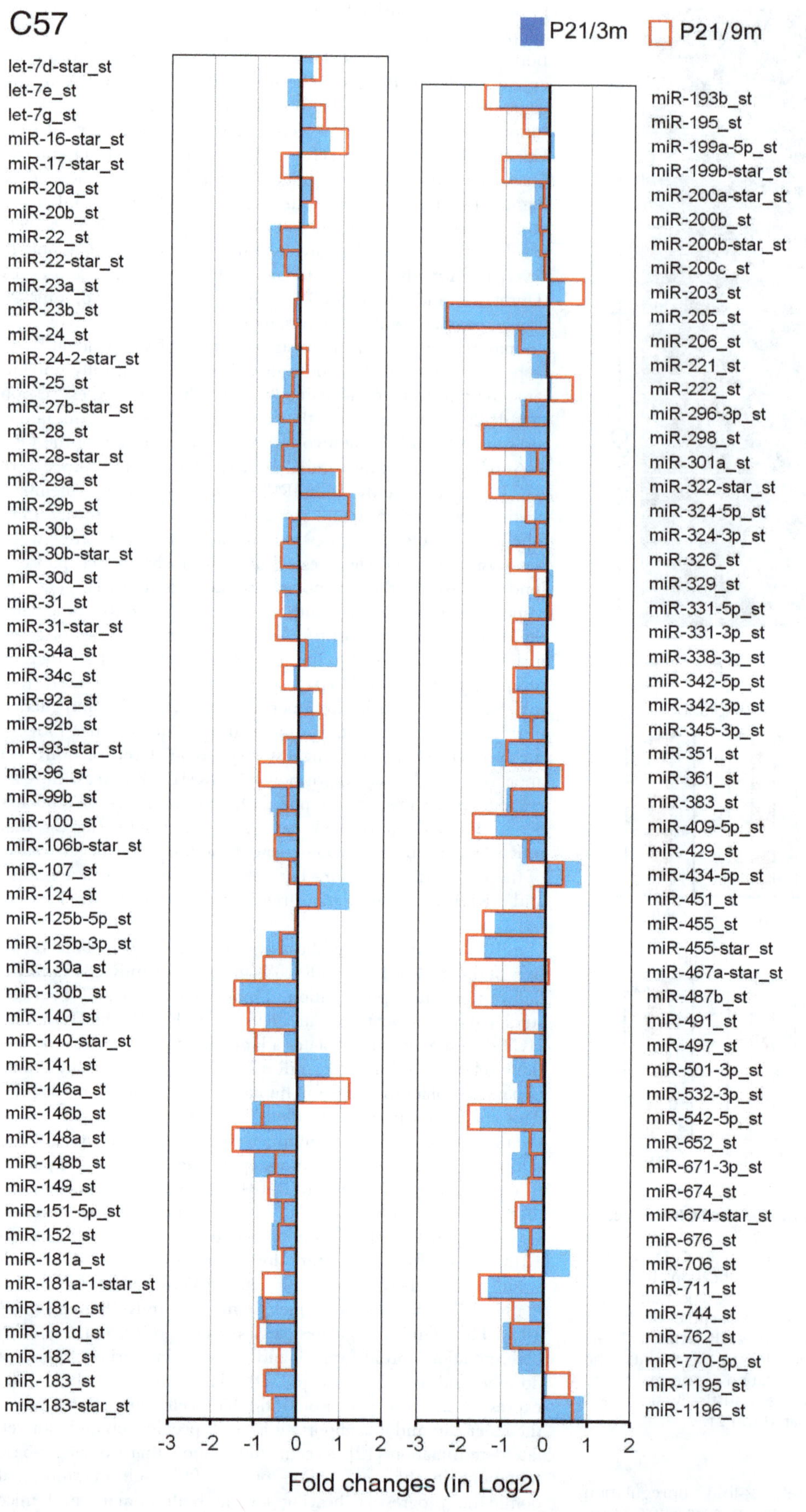
C57
P21/3m
P21/9m
let-7d-star_st
let-7e_st
let-7g_st
miR-16-star_st
miR-17-star_st
miR-20a_st
miR-20b_st
miR-22_st
miR-22-star_st
miR-23a_st
miR-23b_st
miR-24_st
miR-24-2-star_st
miR-25_st
miR-27b-star_st
miR-28_st
miR-28-star_st
miR-29a_st
miR-29b_st
miR-30b_st
miR-30b-star_st
miR-30d_st
miR-31_st
miR-31-star_st
miR-34a_st
miR-34c_st
miR-92a_st
miR-92b_st
miR-93-star_st
miR-96_st
miR-99b_st
miR-100_st
miR-106b-star_st
miR-107_st
miR-124_st
miR-125b-5p_st
miR-125b-3p_st
miR-130a_st
miR-130b_st
miR-140_st
miR-140-star_st
miR-141_st
miR-146a_st
miR-146b_st
miR-148a_st
miR-148b_st
miR-149_st
miR-151-5p_st
miR-152_st
miR-181a_st
miR-181a-1-star_st
miR-181c_st
miR-181d_st
miR-182_st
miR-183_st
miR-183-star_st
miR-193b_st
miR-195_st
miR-199a-5p_st
miR-199b-star_st
miR-200a-star_st
miR-200b_st
miR-200b-star_st
miR-200c_st
miR-203_st
miR-205_st
miR-206_st
miR-221_st
miR-222_st
miR-296-3p_st
miR-298_st
miR-301a_st
miR-322-star_st
miR-324-5p_st
miR-324-3p_st
miR-326_st
miR-329_st
miR-331-5p_st
miR-331-3p_st
miR-338-3p_st
miR-342-5p_st
miR-342-3p_st
miR-345-3p_st
miR-351_st
miR-361_st
miR-383_st
miR-409-5p_st
miR-429_st
miR-434-5p_st
miR-451_st
miR-455_st
miR-455-star_st
miR-467a-star_st
miR-487b_st
miR-491_st
miR-497_st
miR-501-3p_st
miR-532-3p_st
miR-542-5p_st
miR-652_st
miR-671-3p_st
miR-674_st
miR-674-star_st
miR-676_st
miR-706_st
miR-711_st
miR-744_st
miR-762_st
miR-770-5p_st
miR-1195_st
miR-1196_st
-3 -2 -1 0 1 2
-3 -2 -1 0 1 2
Fold changes (in Log2)

Figure 3. Differentially expressed miRNAs in the OC of C57 mice during aging. The X-axis relates Log2 transformed fold change in miRNA expression at 3 m (in blue) and 9 m (in red) compared to P21. Only those miRNAs which showed a statistically significant different in expression ($p<0.05$, Student's t-test) compared to P21 are shown.

expression profiles in mouse OC. Moreover, hair cell gene expression required for normal function is considerably perturbed. Five genes, *Ocm* [72], *Pitpnm1* [73], *prestin* [74], *Ptprq* [75], and *Gfi1* [76], are among disregulated genes in the mutant mice. All of these genes are specifically expressed in hair cells, and mutations in each of the latter three genes are known to result in deafness and hair cell degeneration [77–79]. We observed a significant downregulation of miR-182 and miR-183 in the two strains. Interestingly, miR-96 downregulation was only detected in C57 mice at 9 m. No significant change of miR-96 was detected in CBA and C57 mice at 3 m. The fact that miR-96 did not show a significant change in the early stage of degeneration of the OC suggests that significant change of miR-96 might only occur during the later stage of ARHL.

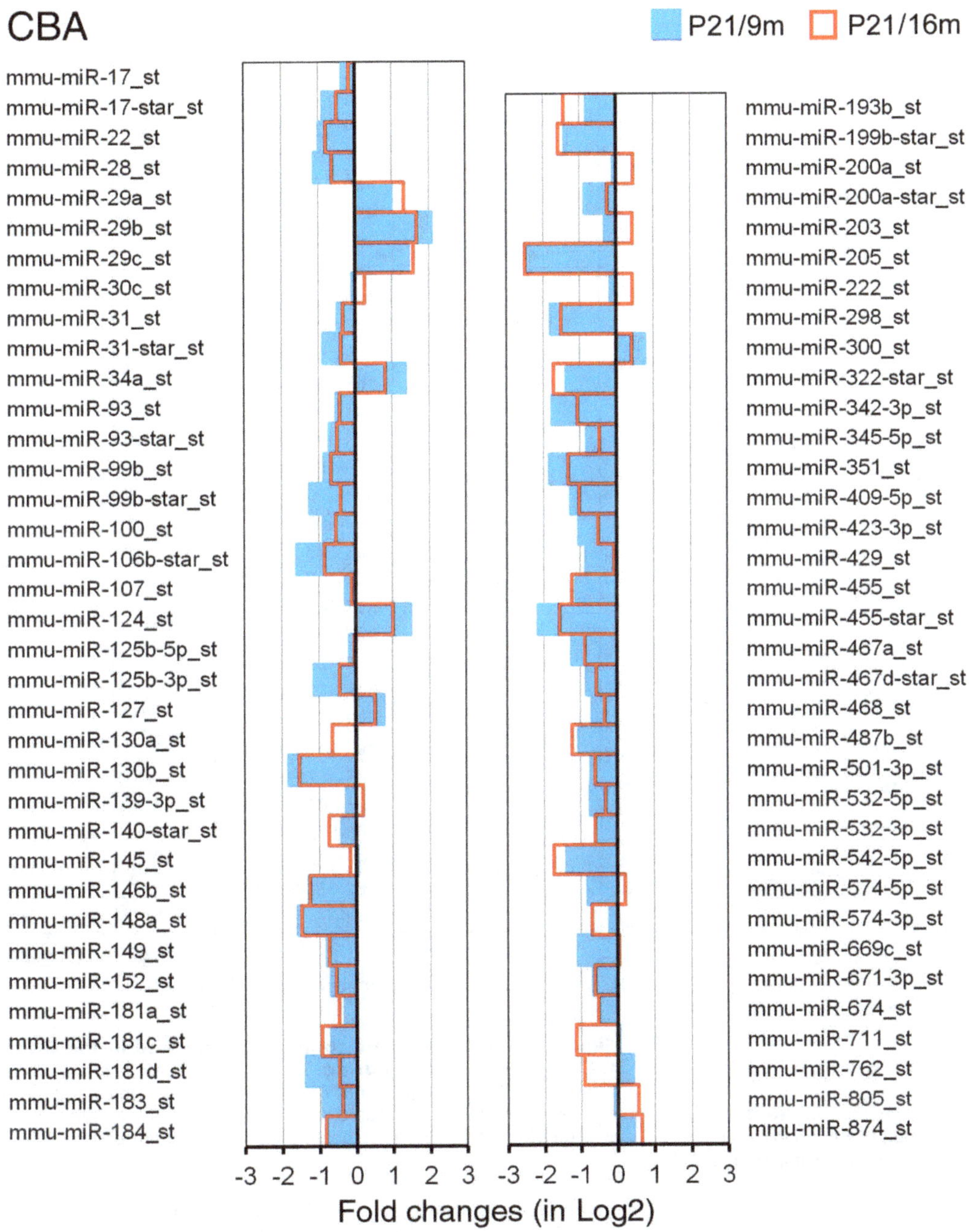

Figure 4. Differentially expressed miRNAs in the OC of CBA mice during aging. The X-axis relates Log2 transformed fold change in miRNA expression at 9 m (in blue) and 16 m (in red) compared to P21. Only those miRNAs which showed a statistically significant different in expression ($p<0.05$, Student's t-test) compared to P21 are shown.

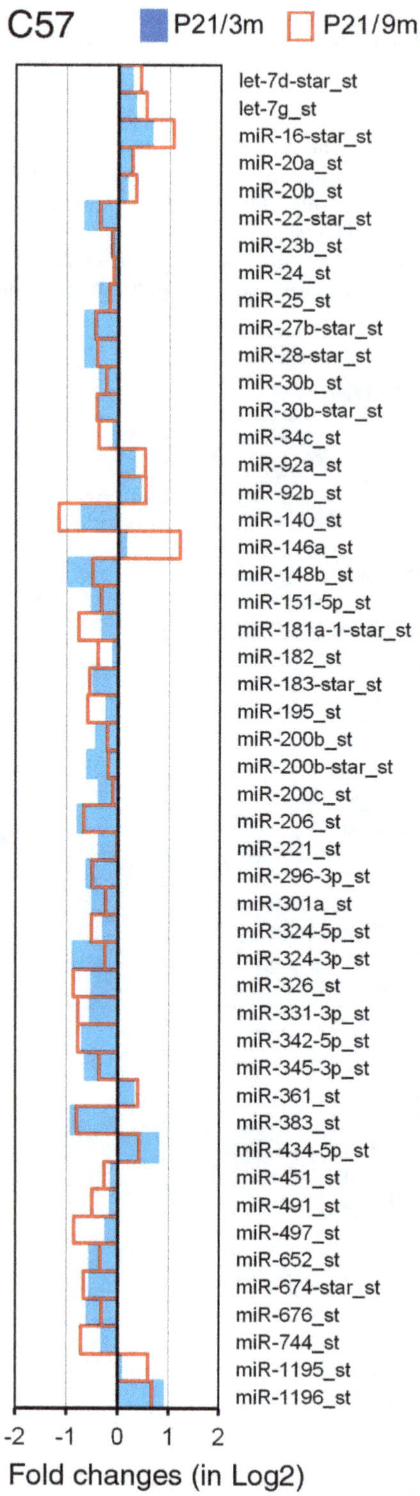

Figure 5. miRNAs that are uniquely expressed in the OC of C57 mice during aging. The X-axis relates Log2 transformed fold change in miRNA expression 3 m (in blue) and 9 m (in red) compared to P21.

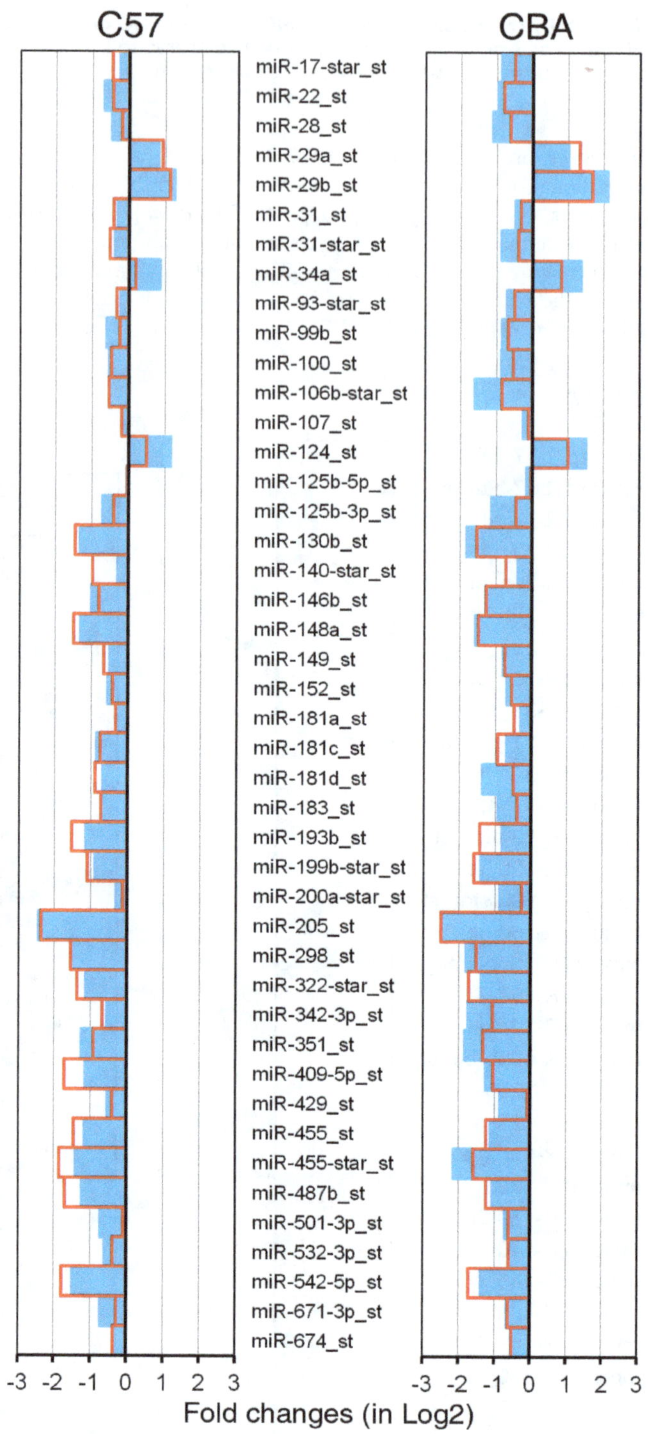

Figure 6. miRNAs that are commonly expressed in the OC of C57 and CBA mice during aging. The X-axes relate Log2 transformed fold change in miRNA expression for C57 mice at 3 m (in blue) and 9 m (in red) compared to P21 (left panel), and for CBA mice at 9 m (in blue) and 16 m (in red) compared to P21 (right panel).

Weston et al. [12] examined miRNA expression in the mouse inner ear during development between P0 and P100 by microarray analyses. Their study uncovered 76 miRNAs expressed in the whole inner ear including ganglion neurons, the basilar membrane, and the cochlear lateral wall. The present study identified more miRNAs despite the fact that the tissue collected only contained the basilar membrane containing the OC. Comparison of the two studies shows that most miRNAs indicated in the miRNA expression profile of Weston et al. [12] are also present in our study. The majority of miRNAs that are present in

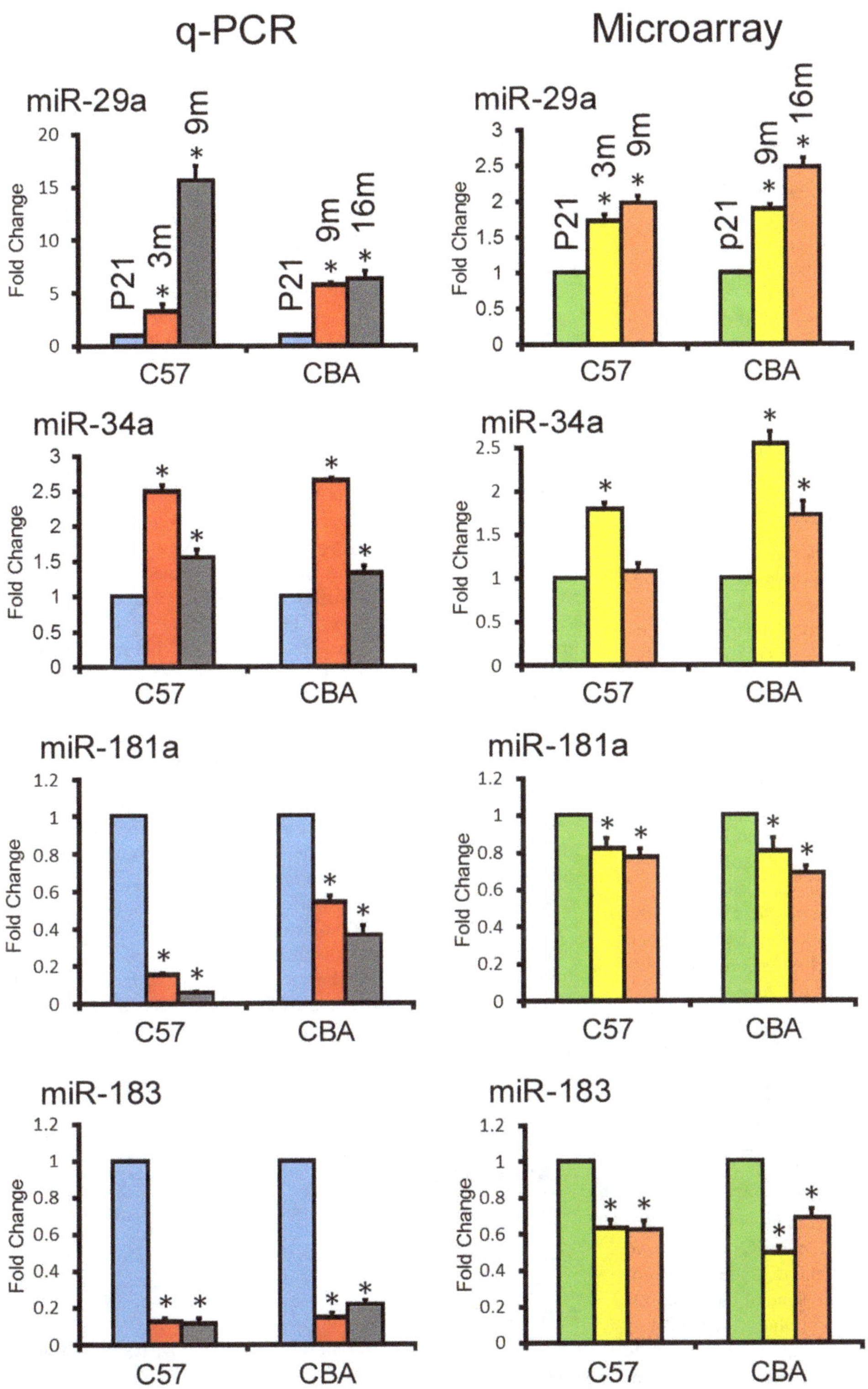

Figure 7. Comparison of changes in miRNA expression detected by q-PCR versus microarray analyses for four miRNAs in the OC of C57 and CBA mice. Asterisks indicate statistically significant differences ($p<0.05$, Student's t-test) compared to P21. Each q-PCR plot represents means from three repeats.

their profile and absent in our analysis are those important for proliferation and differentiation. These miRNAs include miR-135, miR-143/145, miR-189, and miR-204. One miRNA worthy of mention is the miR-143/145 cluster. This cluster has been shown to be involved in cardiac morphogenesis and smooth muscle fate determination [80]. The miR-143/145 cluster has also been implicated in tumorgenesis of various types of carcinoma by suppressing the RAS, c-Myc, and human telomerase (hTERT) signaling pathways [81,82]. We note that most miRNAs that are not in the miRNA profile in the study by Weston et al. [12] are miRNAs that were not available in the oligonucleotide microarray in 2006. These miRNAs include miR-652, miR-711, miR-744, and miR-762, all of which are downregulated during aging. The functions and regulatory mechanisms of these miRNAs in the auditory system are not known. However, recent studies have revealed their involvement in age-related diseases, such as heart disease, hypertension, and age-related metabolic syndrome [83]. For example, miR-652 is upregulated, whereas miR-744 is downregulated in older hearts. miR-744 is also found differentially expressed in senescent cell lines and mesenchymal stem cells. Short-term overexpression of miR-744 results in enhanced cell proliferation, while long-term expression causes chromosomal instability and tumor suppression *in vivo* [84].

One of the important findings of our study is that the majority of expressed miRNAs decline in relative abundance during aging. Downregulated miRNAs outnumbered upregulated miRNAs by a wide margin. This global decline of miRNA during aging is consistent with the trend observed in other studies [85]. For example, in the aging brain, 85 miRNAs are downregulated while only 8 miRNAs are upregulated [85]. The vast majority of *C. elegans* miRNAs that are differentially expressed during aging are also downregulated [7]. Interestingly, the majority of miRNAs that are in decline are known regulators for differentiation, proliferation, and growth, whereas those miRNAs that are upregulated are all known pro-apoptotic regulators. Our study likewise suggests that age-related degeneration of the OC is a complex process that involves a shift in the balance of pro-growth and differentiation miRNAs and factors toward pro-apoptotic miRNAs and factors.

Hair cell loss was observed initially in the basal end of the OC during aging; hair cell loss occurred as early as 3 months in C57 mice. Loss of hair cells and supporting cells can lead to global decline of miRNAs in the older tissue when compared to the younger tissue. However, it is unlikely that loss of hair cells and supporting cells is the reason behind the decline of some miRNAs in the older tissue for the following reasons: first, changes in miRNA expression were observed even before hair cell loss occurred. In CBA mice, hair cell loss did not occur until 16 months, while downregulation of many miRNAs was already observed at 9 months (blue color in Fig. 4); second, although there was some hair cell loss at 3 months (in C57 mice) and 16 months (in CBA mice), the loss was limited to the basal region and accounted for less than 10% of the hair cells (Fig. 2). This limited reduction would translate to less than 2–3% of total hair cell populations in the whole cochlea. Such nominal loss of hair cells is unlikely to account for the significant decline of miRNAs observed in our microarray analyses. Finally, we validated four different types of miRNAs using q-PCR. To avoid the issue of hair cell loss, the tissue was collected from the apical turn where hair cell loss was insignificant at all ages (top panels in Fig. 2C,D). Our q-PCR analyses were consistent with the expression patterns observed in microarray analyses. Taken together, we conclude that it is unlikely that hair cell loss is responsible for reduced expression of the majority of miRNAs observed in the aging cochlea.

We observed substantial differences in the number and amount of miRNA expression between C57 and CBA mice. The extent and amount of miRNA changes depend on the molecular mechanisms and the stage of aging. Different genetic backgrounds of the two strains may also contribute to different miRNA expression. The early onset and rapid progression of hearing loss seen in C57 mice is due to *Ahl* gene mutation [27,28,35]. Thus, some differences in miRNA expression are likely associated with the *Ahl* mutation.

We examined miRNA expression at different stages during aging for the two strains of mice. These different time points represent different phases before and after the onset of ARHL. For C57 mice, high frequency hearing loss accompanied by some hair cell loss in the basal end of the cochlea already occurred at 3 months. Thus, comparison of miRNA expression at P21 with those at 3 m and 9 m reveals miRNAs involved in progression of ARHL. For CBA mice, the hearing function was normal and no significant hair cell loss was detected at 9 months. However, significant reduction of pro-growth miRNAs and upregulation of pro-apoptotic miRNAs was already detectible at this age. This suggests that changes in miRNA expression precede morphological and functional changes. The fact that the shift from pro-growth to pro-apoptotic processes starts well before the onset of ARHL suggests that miRNAs are contributing factors to the onset and progress of ARHL.

In conclusion, our study for the first time demonstrates the extent and specificity of miRNA expression during aging in the mammalian inner ear. We show that the underlying process and regulatory mechanism of aging in the auditory sensory epithelium involve repression of miRNAs important for proliferation and differentiation and enhancement of miRNAs that promote apoptosis. Such change in the miRNA expression profile takes place well before morphological changes and hearing loss are detected. The present work is the first step in an effort to elucidate the roles of miRNAs and their regulatory networks in age-related degeneration of the OC. It also lays the groundwork for future experiments that can explore whether suppression or overexpression of some miRNAs can slow the onset and progression of ARHL.

Acknowledgments

We thank Barbara Bittner for critical reading of the manuscript.

Author Contributions

Conceived and designed the experiments: DH QZ GS. Performed the experiments: QZ HL. Analyzed the data: QZ JM EW GS DH. Wrote the paper: QZ DH.

References

1. Gilad O, Glorig A (1979a) Presbycusis: The aging inner ear. Part I. J Am Audit Soc 4: 195–206.
2. Gilad O, Glorig A (1979b) Presbycusis: The aging ear. Part II. J Am Audit Soc 4: 207–217.
3. Lee RC, Feinbaum RL, Ambros V (1993) The C. elegans heterochronic gene lin-4 encodes small RNAs with antisense complementarity to lin-14. Cell 75: 843–854.
4. Bartel DP (2004) MicroRNAs: genomics, biogenesis, mechanism and function. Cell 116: 281–297.
5. Kato M, Slack FJ (2008) microRNAs: small molecules with big roles – C. elegans to human cancer. Biol Cell 100: 71–81.
6. Bates DJ, Li N, Liang R, Sarojini H, An J, et al. (2010) MicroRNA regulation in Ames dwarf mouse liver may contribute to delayed aging. Aging Cell 9: 1–18.
7. Boehm M, Slack F (2005) A developmental timing microRNA and its target regulate life span in *C. elegans*. Science 310: 1954–1957.

8. Cimmino A, Calin GA, Fabbri MV, Iorio M, Ferracin M, et al. (2005) miR-15 and miR-16 induce apoptosis by targeting BCL2. Proc Natl Acad Sci USA 102: 13944–13949.
9. Hwang HW, Mendell JT (2006) MicroRNAs in cell proliferation, cell death, and tumorigenesis. British Journal of Cancer 94: 776–780.
10. Hermeking H (2010) The miR-34 family in cancer and apoptosis. Cell Death Differ 17: 193–199.
11. Wienholds E, Kloosterman WP, Miska E, Alvarez-Saavedra E, Berezikov E, et al. (2005) MicroRNA expression in zebrafish embryonic development. Science 309: 310–311.
12. Weston MD, Pierce ML, Rocha-Sanchez S, Beisel KW, Soukup GA (2006) MicroRNA gene expression in the mouse inner ear. Brain Res 1111: 95–104.
13. Pierce ML, Weston MD, Fritzsch B, Gabel HW, Ruvkun G, et al. (2008) MicroRNA-183 family conservation and ciliated neurosensory organ expression. Evol Dev 10: 106–113.
14. Soukup GA (2009) Little but loud: small RNAs have a resounding affect on ear development. Brain Res 1277: 104–114.
15. Friedman LM, Dror AA, Mor E, Tenne T, Toren G, et al. (2009) MicroRNAs are essential for development and function of inner-ear hair cells in vertebrates. Proc Natl Acad Sci USA 106: 7915–7920.
16. Li H, Fekete DM (2010) MicroRNAs in hair cell development and deafness. Curr Opin Otolaryngol Head Neck Surg 18: 459–465.
17. Li H, Kloosterman W, Fekete DM (2010) MicroRNA-183 family members regulate sensorineural fates in the inner ear. J Neurosci 30: 3254–3263.
18. Frucht CS, Uduman M, Duke JL, Kleinstein SH, Santos-Sacchi J, et al. (2010) Gene expression analysis of forskolin treated basilar papillae identifies microRNA181a as a mediator of proliferation. PLoS One 5: e11502.
19. Frucht CS, Santos-Sacchi J, Navaratnam DS (2011) MicroRNA181a plays a key role in hair cell regeneration in the avian auditory epithelium. Neurosci Lett 493: 44–48.
20. Tsonis PA, Call MK, Grogg MW, Sartor MA, Taylor RR, et al. (2007) MicroRNAs and regeneration: Let-7 members as potential regulators of dedifferentiation in lens and inner ear hair cell regeneration of the adult newt. Biochem Biophys Res Commun 362: 940–945.
21. Song L, McGee J, Walsh EJ (2008) Development of cochlear amplification, frequency tuning, and two-tone suppression in the mouse. J Neurophysiol 99: 344–355.
22. Spongr VP, Flood DG, Frisina RD, Salvi RJ (1997) Quantitative measures of hair cell loss in CBA and C57BL/6 mice throughout their life spans. J Acoust Soc Am 101: 3546–3553.
23. Willott JF (1986) Effects of aging, hearing loss, and anatomical location on thresholds of inferior colliculus neurons in C57BL/6 and CBA mice. J Neurophysiol 56: 391–408.
24. Willott JF, Parham K, Hunter KP (1991) Comparison of the auditory sensitivity of neurons in the cochlear nucleus and inferior colliculus of young and aging C57BL/6J and CBA/J mice. Hear Res 53: 78–94.
25. Guimaraes P, Zhu X, Cannon T, Kim S, Frisina RD (2004) Sex differences in distortion product otoacoustic emissions as a function of age in CBA mice. Hear Res 192: 83–89.
26. Sha SH, Kanicki A, Dootz G, Talaska AE, Halsey K, et al. (2008) Age-related auditory pathology in the CBA/J mouse. Hearing Res 243: 87–94.
27. Johnson KR, Erway LC, Cook SA, Willott JF, Zheng QY (1997) A major gene affecting age-related hearing loss in C57BL/6J mice. Hear Res 114: 83–92.
28. Noben-Trauth K, Zheng QY, Johnson KR (2003) Association of cadherin 23 with polygenic inheritance and genetic modification of sensorineural hearing loss. Nat Genet 35: 21–23.
29. Boëda B, El-Amraoui A, Bahloul A Goodyear R, Daviet L, et al. (2002) Myosin VIIa, harmonin and cadherin 23, three Usher I gene products that cooperate to shape the sensory hair cell bundle. EMBO J 21: 6689–6699.
30. Siemens J, Lillo C, Dumont RA, Reynolds A, Williams DS, et al. (2004) Cadherin 23 is a component of the tip link in hair-cell stereocilia. Nature 428: 950–955.
31. Kazmierczak P, Sakaguchi H, Tokita J, Wilson-Kubalek EM, Milligan RA, et al. (2007) Cadherin 23 and protocadherin 15 interact to form tip-link filaments in sensory hair cells. Nature 449: 87–91.
32. Henry KR, Chole RA (1980) Genotypic differences in behavioral, physiological and anatomical expressions of age-related hearing loss in the laboratory mouse. Audiology 19: 369–383.
33. Jimenez AM, Stagner BB, Martin GK, Lonsbury-Martin BL (1999) Age-related loss of distortion product otoacoustic emissions in four mouse strains. Hear Res 138: 91–105.
34. Müller M, von Hünerbein K, Hoidis S, Smolders JW (2005) A physiological place-frequency map of the cochlea in the CBA/J mouse. Hear Res 202: 63–73.
35. Johnson KR, Zheng QY, Erway LC (2000) A major gene affecting age-related hearing loss is common to at least ten inbred strains of mice. Genomics 70: 171–180.
36. Wojakowski W, Tendera M, Cybulski W, Zuba-Surma EK, Szade K, et al. (2012) Effects of intracoronary delivery of allogenic bone marrow-derived stem cells expressing heme oxygenase-1 on myocardial reperfusion injury. Thromb Haemost 108(3): 464–475.
37. Rivetti di Val Cervo P, Tucci P, Majid A, Lena AM, Agostini M, et al. (2009) p73, miR106b, miR34a, and Itch in chronic lymphocytic leukemia. Blood 113: 6498–6499.
38. Kumamoto K, Spillare EA, Fujita K, Horikawa I, Yamashita T, et al. (2008) Nutlin-3a activates p53 to both down-regulate inhibitor of growth 2 and up-regulate mir-34a, mir-34b, and mir-34c expression, and induce senescence. Cancer Res 68: 3193–3203.
39. Wang X, Gocek E, Liu CG, Studzinski GP (2009) MicroRNAs181 regulate the expression of p27Kip1 in human myeloid leukemia cells induced to differentiate by 1,25-dihydroxyvitamin D3. Cell Cycle 8: 736–741.
40. Cichocki F, Felices M, McCullar V, Presnell SR, Al-Attar A, et al. (2011) Cutting edge: microRNA-181 promotes human NK cell development by regulating Notch signaling. J Immunol 187: 6171–6175.
41. Weeraratne SD, Amani V, Teider N, Pierre-Francois J, Winter D, et al. (2012) Pleiotropic effects of miR-183/96/182 converge to regulate cell survival, proliferation and migration in medulloblastoma. Acta Neuropathol 123: 539–552.
42. Soukup GA, Fritzsch B, Pierce ML, Weston MD, Jahan I, et al (2009) Residual microRNA expression dictates the extent of inner ear development in conditional Dicer knockout mice. Dev Biol 328: 328–341.
43. Provost P (2010) Interpretation and applicability of microRNA data to the context of Alzheimer's and age-related diseases. Aging 2: 166–169.
44. Ambros V (2004) The functions of animal microRNAs. Nature 431: 350–355.
45. Xu P, Guo M, Hay BA (2004) MicroRNAs and the regulation of cell death. Trends Genet 20: 617–624.
46. Karp X, Ambros V (2005) Developmental biology. Encountering microRNAs in cell fate signaling. Science 310: 1288–1289.
47. O'Donnell KA, Wentzel EA, Zeller KI, Dang CV, Mendell JT (2005) c-Mycregulated microRNAs modulate E2F1 expression. Nature 435: 839–843.
48. Mott JL, Kobayashi S, Bronk SF, Gores GJ (2007) miR-29 regulates Mcl-1 protein expression and apoptosis. Oncogene 26: 6133–6140.
49. Tarasov V, Jung P, Verdoodt B, Lodygin D, Epanchintsev A, et al. (2007) Differential regulation of microRNAs by p53 revealed by massively parallel sequencing: miR-34a is a p53 target that induces apoptosis and G1-arrest. Cell Cycle 6: 1586–1593.
50. Wang H, Garzon R, Sun H, Ladner KJ, Singh R, et al. (2008) NF-kB-YY1-miR-29 regulatory circuitry in skeletal myogenesis and rhabdomyosarcoma. Cancer Cell 14: 369–381.
51. Chen J, Wang L, Matyunina LV Hill CG, McDonald JF (2011) Overexpression of miR-429 induces mesenchymal-to-epithelial transition (MET) in metastatic ovarian cancer cells. Gynecol Oncol 121: 200–205.
52. Park SY, Lee JH, Ha M, Nam JW, Kim VN (2009) miR-29 miRNAs activate p53 by targeting p85a and CDC42. Nat Struct Mol Biol 16: 23–29.
53. Fabbri M, Garzon R, Cimmino A, Liu Z, Zanesi N, et al. (2007) MicroRNA-29 family reverts aberrant methylation in lung cancer by targeting DNA methyltransferases 3A and 3B. Proc Natl Acad Sci USA 104: 15805–15810.
54. Pekarsky Y, Santanam U, Cimmino A, Palamarchuk A, Efanov A, et al. (2006) Tcl1 expression in chronic lymphocytic leukemia is regulated by miR-29 and miR-181. Cancer Res 66: 11590–11593.
55. Welch C, Chen Y, Stallings RL (2007) MicroRNA-34a functions as a potential tumor suppressor by inducing apoptosis in neuroblastoma cells. Oncogene 26: 5017–5022.
56. Bommer GT, Gerin I, Feng Y, Kaczorowski AJ, Kuick R, et al. (2007) p53-mediated activation of miRNA34 candidate tumor-suppressor genes. Curr Biol 17: 1298–1307.
57. Raver-Shapira N, Marciano E, Meiri E, Spector Y, Rosenfeld N, et al. (2007) Transcriptional activation of miR-34a contributes to p53-mediated apoptosis. Mol Cell 26: 731–743.
58. Yu L, Tang H, Jiang XH, Tsang LL, Chung YW, et al. (2010) Involvement of calpain-I and microRNA34 in kanamycin-induced apoptosis of inner ear cells. Cell Biol Int 34: 1219–1225.
59. Zhang M, Liu W, Ding D, Salvi R (2003) Pifithrin-alpha suppresses p53 and protects cochlear and vestibular hair cells from cisplatin-induced apoptosis. Neuroscience 120: 191–205.
60. Riva C, Donadieu E, Magnan J, Lavieille JP (2007) Age-related hearing loss in CD/1 mice is associated to ROS formation and HIF target proteins up-regulation in the cochlea. Exp Gerontol 42: 327–336.
61. Laine H, Doetzlhofer A, Mantela J, Ylikoski J, Laiho M, et al. (2007) p19(Ink4d) and p21(Cip1) collaborate to maintain the postmitotic state of auditory hair cells, their codeletion leading to DNA damage and p53-mediated apoptosis. J Neurosci 27: 1434–1444.
62. Tadros SF, D'Souza M, Zhu X, Frisina RD (2008) Apoptosis-related genes change their expression with age and hearing loss in the mouse cochlea. Apoptosis 13: 1303–1321.
63. Hu BH, Cai Q, Manohar S, Jiang H, Ding D, et al. (2009) Differential expression of apoptosis-related genes in the cochlea of noise-exposed rats. Neuroscience 161: 915–925.
64. Yang WP, Guo WW, Liu HZ, Xu Y, Chen L, et al. (2012) Age-related changes in the ratio of Mcl-1/Bax expression in the rat cochlea. Acta Otolaryngol 132: 123–132.
65. Ouyang YB, Lu Y, Yue S, Giffard RG (2012) miR-181 targets multiple Bcl-2 family members and influences apoptosis and mitochondrial function in astrocytes. Mitochondrion 12: 213–219.
66. Zhao J, Gong AY, Zhou R, Liu J, Eischeid AN, et al. (2012) Downregulation of PCAF by miR-181a/b provides feedback regulation to TNF-α-induced transcription of proinflammatory genes in liver epithelial cells. J Immunol 188: 1266–1274.

67. Marcucci G, Radmacher MD, Maharry K, Mrózek K, Ruppert AS, et al. (2008) MicroRNA expression in cytogenetically normal acute myeloid leukemia. N Engl J Med 358: 1919–1928.
68. Kuhn S, Johnson SL, Furness DN, Chen J, Ingham N, et al. (2011) miR-96 regulates the progression of differentiation in mammalian cochlear inner and outer hair cells. Proc Natl Acad Sci USA 108: 2355–2360.
69. Lin H, Dai T, Xiong H, Zhao X, Chen X, et al. (2010) Unregulated miR-96 induces cell proliferation in human breast cancer by downregulating transcriptional factor FOXO3a. PLoS ONE 5: e15797.
70. Mencía A, Modamio-Høybjør S, Redshaw N, Morín M, Mayo-Merino F, et al. (2009) Mutations in the seed region of human miR-96 are responsible for nonsyndromic progressive hearing loss. Nat Genet 41: 609–613.
71. Lewis MA, Quint E, Glazier AM, Fuchs H, De Angelis MH, et al. (2009) An ENU-induced mutation of miR-96 associated with progressive hearing loss in mice. Nat Genet 41: 614–618.
72. Gillen MF, Banville D, Rutledge RG, Narang S, Seligy VL, et al. (1987) A complete complementary DNA for the oncodevelopmental calcium-binding protein, oncomodulin. J Biol Chem 262: 5308–5312.
73. Rubboli F, Bulfone A, Bogni S, Marchitiello A, Zollo M, et al. (1998) A mammalian homologue of the Drosophila retinal degeneration B gene: implications for the evolution of phototransduction mechanisms. Genes Funct 1: 205–213.
74. Zheng J, Shen W, He DZ, Long KB, Madison LD, et al. (2000) Prestin is the motor protein of cochlear outer hair cells. Nature 405: 149–155.
75. Schraders M, Oostrik J, Huygen PL, Strom TM, van Wijk E, et al. (2010) Mutations in PTPRQ are a cause of autosomal-recessive nonsyndromic hearing impairment DFNB84 and associated with vestibular dysfunction. Am J Hum Genet 86: 604–610.
76. Bell DW, Taguchi T, Jenkins NA, Gilbert DJ, Copeland NG, et al. (1995) Chromosomal localization of a gene, GF1, encoding a novel zinc finger protein reveals a new syntenic region between man and rodents. Cytogenet Cell Genet 70: 263–267.
77. Liberman MC, Gao J, He DZ, Wu X, Jia S, et al. (2002) Prestin is required for electromotility of the outer hair cell and for the cochlear amplifier. Nature 419: 300–304.
78. Goodyear RJ, Legan PK, Wright MB, Marcotti W, Oganesian A, et al. (2003) A receptor-like inositol lipid phosphatase is required for the maturation of developing cochlear hair bundles. J Neurosci 23: 9208–9219.
79. Wallis D, Hamblen M, Zhou Y, Venken KJ, Schumacher A, et al. (2003) The zinc finger transcription factor Gfi1, implicated in lymphomagenesis, is required for inner ear hair cell differentiation and survival. Development 130: 221–232.
80. Long X, Miano JM (2011) Transforming growth factor-beta1 (TGF-beta1) utilizes distinct pathways for the transcriptional activation of microRNA 143/145 in human coronary artery smooth muscle cells. J Biol Chem 286: 30119–30129.
81. Akao Y, Nakagawa Y, Naoe T (2006) MicroRNAs 143 and 145 are possible common onco-microRNAs in human cancers. Oncol Rep 16: 845–850.
82. Bonifacio LN, Jarstfer MB (2010) MiRNA profile associated with replicative senescence, extended cell culture, and ectopic telomerase expression in human foreskin fibroblasts. PLoS One 5: e12519.
83. Zhang X, Azhar G, Wei JY (2012) The expression of microRNA and microRNA clusters in the aging heart. PloS One 7: e34688.
84. Huang V, Place RF, Portnoy V, Wang J, Qi Z, et al. (2012) Upregulation of Cyclin B1 by miRNA and its implications in cancer. Nucleic Acids Res 40: 1695–1707.
85. Inukai S, de Lencastre A, Turner M, Slack F (2012) Novel microRNAs differentially expressed during aging in the mouse brain. PloS One 7: e40028.

Novel Compound Heterozygous *TMC1* Mutations Associated with Autosomal Recessive Hearing Loss in a Chinese Family

Xue Gao[1,2,3☯], Yu Su[1☯], Li-Ping Guan[4☯], Yong-Yi Yuan[1], Sha-Sha Huang[1], Yu Lu[1], Guo-Jian Wang[1], Ming-Yu Han[1,2], Fei Yu[1], Yue-Shuai Song[1,2], Qing-Yan Zhu[4], Jing Wu[5], Pu Dai[1,2*]

1 Department of Otorhinolaryngology, Head and Neck Surgery, PLA General Hospital, Beijing, P. R. China, **2** Department of Otorhinolaryngology, Hainan Branch of PLA General Hospital, Sanya, P. R. China, **3** Department of Otorhinolaryngology, the Second Artillery General Hospital, Beijing, P. R. China, **4** BGI-Shenzhen, Beishan Industrial Zone, Yantian District, Shenzhen, P. R. China, **5** BGI-Tianjin, Tianjin, P. R. China

Abstract

Hereditary nonsyndromic hearing loss is highly heterogeneous and most patients with a presumed genetic etiology lack a specific diagnosis. It has been estimated that several hundred genes may be associated with this sensory deficit in humans. Here, we identified compound heterozygous mutations in the *TMC1* gene as the cause of recessively inherited sensorineural hearing loss by using whole-exome sequencing in a family with two deaf siblings. Sanger sequencing confirmed that both siblings inherited a missense mutation, c.589G>A p.G197R (maternal allele), and a nonsense mutation, c.1171C>T p.Q391X (paternal allele), in *TMC1*. We also used DNA from 50 Chinese familial patients with ARNSHL and 208 ethnicity-matched negative samples to perform extended variants analysis. Both variants co-segregated in family 1953, which had the hearing loss phenotype, but were absent in 50 patients and 208 ethnicity-matched controls. Therefore, we concluded that the hearing loss in this family was caused by novel compound heterozygous mutations in *TMC1*.

Editor: Andreas R. Janecke, Innsbruck Medical University, Austria

Funding: This work was supported by grants from the Project of the National Natural Science Foundation of China (Grant Nos. 30801285, 31071099, 81230020, 81200751, 81070792, 81000414, 81070792, 81000415), a grant from State 863 High Technology R&D Key Project of China (2011AA02A112), a grant from Natural Science Foundation of Beijing (Grant No 7122172), a grant from Minister of Science and Technology of China (2012BAI09B02) and a grant from Minister of Health of China (201202005). The funders had no role in study design, data collection and analysis, decision to publish, or preparation of the manuscript.

Competing Interests: The authors have declared that no competing interests exist.

* E-mail: daipu301@vip.sina.com

☯ These authors contributed equally to this work.

Introduction

Hearing loss is a common sensory defect that can significantly impact quality of life, and the majority of congenital cases of hearing loss are attributable to genetic factors [1]. Non-syndromic hereditary forms, in which the hearing loss is the only clinical sign, are genetically heterogeneous. Autosomal recessive nonsyndromic hearing loss (ARNSHL) is the most common type and accounts for ~80% of cases of inherited hearing loss. To date, 61 genes and more than 100 genetic loci have been implicated in ARNSHL (http://hereditaryhearingloss.org/). The marked heterogeneity of genetic hearing loss can be explained by the complexity of the auditory system, which requires coordination of multiple processes involving the inner ear and nervous system. A defect in any part of this complex chain of events can lead to hearing impairment. However, despite previous intensive linkage analysis and candidate gene screening, a large proportion of ARNSHL remain genetically unexplained.

Next-generation sequencing, in particular whole-exome sequencing (WES) involving the targeted sequencing of the protein-coding subset of the human genome, has become a highly efficient strategy for identifying novel causative genes and mutations involved in heritable disease. Both simple nonsyndromic and complex syndromic forms of hearing loss can be resolved efficiently using WES, especially small families with distinct and interesting phenotypes that are too small to map [2,3]. To date, nine syndromic or nonsyndromic deafness genes have been identified using targeted genomic enrichment and next-generation sequencing including *TPRN*, *GPSM2*, *CEACAM16*, *SMPX*, *HSD17B4*, *HARS2*, *MASP1*, *DNMT1*, *TSPEAR* [4,5,6,7,8,9,10,11,12].

TMC1 is predicted to be involved in the functional maturation of cochlear hair cells [13]. The precise function of the TMC1 protein in the inner ear is unknown although its expression is localized to outer hair cells of the mouse inner ear after P3 [14]. Mutations in this gene at the DFNA36 and DFNB7/11 loci have previously been reported to cause nonsyndromic autosomal dominant and recessive hearing loss, respectively [15]. *TMC1* mutations are the sixth most common causes of ARNSHL in populations from North Africa, the Middle East, and India [16,17,18,19]. To date, 35 recessive mutations in *TMC1* were shown to be associated with ARNSHL at the DFNB7/11 locus in more than 40 families worldwide (Table 1). However, these mutations were not found in Chinese populations. Almost all reported recessive cases showed a similar phenotype characterized by prelingual severe-to-profound hearing loss.

Table 1. Overview of all *TMC1* mutations identified to date.

Origin	MutationDNA	Protein	Exon(E)/Intron(I)	Type of variant	Inheritance pattern	Reference
North Ameirica	c. 1714 G>A	p. D572N	E19	Missense	AD	[15,24,29]
North Ameirica	c. 1714 G>C	p. D572H	E19	Missense	AD	[30]
China	c.589G>A	p.G197R	E11	Missense	AR	Present study
China	c.1171C>T	p.Q391X	E15	Nonsense	AR	Present study
PakistanTunisia Lebanon JordanTurkey	c. 100 C>T	p. R34X	E7	Nonsense	AR	[15,19,24,30,31]
Pakistan	c. IVS3_IVS5	n.d.	E5	Deletion	AR	[15]
PakistanIndia	c. 295_296 delA	n.d.	E8	Deletion	AR	[15]
Pakistan	c. IVS10-8T>A	n.d.	I10	Splice site mutation	AR	[15]
Pakistan	c. IVS13+1G>A	n.d.	I13	Splice site mutation	AR	[15,32]
Turkey	c. 776 A>G	p. Y259C	E13	Missense	AR	[25]
Turkey	c.821C>T	p.P274L	E13	Missense	AR	[25]
Turkey	c. 1083_1087delCAGAT	p.R362P*fs*X6	E15	Deletion	AR	[25]
TurkeyPakistan	c. 1334 G>A	p. R455H	E16	Missense	AR	[25,32]
Pakistan	c. 1534C>T	p. R512X	E17	Nonsense	AR	[15]
India	c.1960A>G	p.M654V	E20	Missense	AR	[15]
Pakistan	c.884+1G>A		E13	Splice site mutation	AR	[15]
Pakistan	c.830A>G	p.Y277C	E13	Missense	AR	[32]
Pakistan	c.536-8T>A		E11	Splice site mutation	AR	[32]
Pakistan	c.1114G>A	p.V372M	E15	Missense	AR	[32]
Pakistan	c.2004T>G	p.S668R	E21	Missense	AR	[32]
Pakistan	c.2035G>A	p.E679K	E21	Missense	AR	[32]
SudanTunisiaLebanonJordan	c.1165C>T	p.R389X	E15	Nonsense	AR	[18,24,31]
Sudan	c.IVS19+5G>A	n.d.	I19	Splice site mutation	AR	[18]
Pakistan	c. 1541C>T	p.P514L	E17	Missense	AR	[17]
Pakistan	c.1543T>C	p.C515R	E17	Missense	AR	[17]
Pakistan	c.IVS5+1G>T	Splice Site	I5	Splice site mutation	AR	[17]
Greece	c.2350C>T	p.R604X	E20	Nonsense	AR	[24]
Iran	c.776+1G>A	Splice Site	E7	Splice site mutation	AR	[24]
Turkey	c.767delT	p.F255FfsX14	E13	Deletion	AR	[24]
Turkey	c.1166G>A	p.R389Q	E15	Missense	AR	[24]
Tunisia	c.1764G>A	p.W588X	E19	Nonsense	AR	[31]
Turkey	c.1330G>A	p.G444R	E16	Missense	AR	[19]
Turkey	c.1333C>T	p.G445R	E16	Missense	AR	[19]
Turkey	c.2030T>C	p.I667T	E21	Missense	AR	[19]
Turkey	c.IVS6+2T>A	Splice Site	I6	Splice site mutation	AR	[19]
Turkey	c.1685_2280 del		E19–24	Deletion	AR	[19]
The Netherlands	c.1763+3A>G	p.W588WfsX81	I19	Splice site mutation	AR	[16]

AD, Autosomal Dominant; AR, Autosomal Recessive.

Here, we report a family with two siblings affected by sensorineural hearing loss. Mutations in *GJB2* and *SLC26A4* were excluded previously. As the family is small and non-consanguineous, neither linkage analysis nor homozygosity mapping would have been informative in identifying the causative gene. Therefore, we used WES to identify the gene responsible for the disease in this family. WES was carried out in two affected siblings, followed by validation in the family. The results identified two compound heterozygous disease-segregating mutations, c.589G>A (p.G197R) and c.1171C>T (p.Q391X), in the *TMC1* gene. To exclude the possibility that these mutations were polymorphisms, DNA samples of 50 affected and 208 unaffected individuals were also analyzed.

Materials and Methods

Clinical Data

Family 1953 is a two-generation Chinese family with autosomal recessive prelingual non-syndromic sensorineural hearing loss. To screen for candidate mutations, we used 208 ethnicity-matched controls and 50 affected DNA samples from the Department of Otolaryngology, Head and Neck Surgery, Chinese PLA General Hospital. The fifty affected individuals were from families presenting with ARNSHL and in whom mutations of *GJB2* and *SLC26A4* had been excluded previously. Fully informed written consent was attained from each subject or their guardians. The study was approved by the Chinese PLA General Hospital Research Ethics Committee. Medical histories of the members of family 1953 were obtained using a questionnaire regarding the following aspects of this condition: subjective degree of hearing loss, age at onset, progression, symmetry of the hearing impairment, use of hearing aids, presence of tinnitus, medication, noise exposure, pathological changes in the ear, and other relevant clinical manifestations. Otoscopy, physical examination, and pure tone audiometric examination (at frequencies from 250 to 8000 Hz) were performed to identify the phenotype. Immittance testing was applied to evaluate middle-ear pressure, ear canal volumes, and tympanic membrane mobility. Unaffected phenotype status was defined by threshold lower than age- and gender-matched 50th percentile values for all frequencies measured. Computed tomography (CT) scan of the temporal bone was performed. The diagnosis of profound sensorineural hearing impairment was made according to the ICD-10 criteria based on audiometric examination. Tandem gait and Romberg tests were performed to evaluate balance.

All genomic DNA was extracted from peripheral blood using a blood DNA extraction kit according to the protocol provided by the manufacturer (TianGen, Beijing, China).

Targeted Gene Capture and Sequencing

Approximately 99.71% of CCDS exons or 99.62% of RefSeq exons from 6 μg of genomic DNA were captured using the NimblegenSeqCap EZ Library (44 Mb for II:1 and II:2). Genomic DNA sample was randomly fragmented by Covaris; the size of the library fragments was distributed mainly between 250 and 300 bp. Then, adapters were ligated to both ends of the resulting fragments. Extracted DNA was then amplified by ligation-mediated PCR (LM-PCR), purified, and hybridized to the NimblegenSeqCap EZ Library for enrichment; non-hybridized fragments were then washed out. Both non-captured and captured LM-PCR products were subjected to quantitative PCR to estimate the magnitude of enrichment. Each captured library was then loaded onto the Illumina Hiseq2000 platform, and we performed high-throughput sequencing for each captured library to ensure that each sample met the desired average sequencing depth. Raw image files were processed by Illumina base calling Software 1.7 for base calling with default parameters and the sequences of each individual were generated as 90-bp pair-end reads.

Reads, Mapping, and Variant Detection

SNP detection was performed as follows: (i) SOAPaligner (version 2.21) [20] was used to align the high-quality reads to the human reference genome (hg19, NCBI build 37.1); (ii) for paired-end reads with duplicated start and end sites, only one copy with the highest quality was retained, and the reads with adapters were removed; (iii) SOAPsnp (version 1.05) [21] was used to assemble the consensus sequence and call genotypes. For SNP quality control, low-quality SNPs that met one of the four following criteria were filtered out: (i) genotype quality less than 20; (ii) sequencing depth of less than 4 for the site; (iii) estimated copy number more than 2; (iv) distance from the adjacent SNPs less than 5 bp. Small indel detection was performed using the UnifiedGenotyper tool from GATK (version v1.0.4705) [22] after all the high-quality reads were aligned to the human reference genome using BWA (version 0.5.9-r16) [23]. SNP and indel detection were performed only on the targeted exome regions and flanking regions within 200 bp.

Filtering and Annotation

The detected variants were annotated and filtered based on four databases; *i.e.*, NCBI CCDS (http://www.ncbi.nlm.nih.gov/CCDS/CcdsBrowse.cgi), RefSeq (http://www.ncbi.nlm. nih.-gov/RefSeq/), Ensembl (http://www.ensembl.org), and Encode (http://genome.ucsc.edu/ENCODE). Four major steps were taken to prioritize all the high-quality variants: (i) variants within intergenic, intronic, and UTR regions and synonymous mutations were excluded from downstream analysis; (ii) variants in dbSNP132 (http://www.ncbi.nlm.nih.gov/projects/SNP/), 1000 Genome project (ftp://ftp.1000genomes.ebi.ac.uk/vol1/ftp), YH Database (http://yh. genomics.org.cn/), and HapMap Project (ftp://ftp.ncbi.nlm.nih.gov/hapmap) were excluded; (iii) Possible impacts of variants were predicted by SIFT (http://sift.bii. a-star.edu.sg/) and Polyphen2 (http://genetics.bwh.harvard.edu/pph2/); (iv) Gene Ontology (http://www. geneontology.org) and KEGG Pathway Annotations (http://www.ebi.ac.uk./clustalw) were used.

Mutation Validation

After filtering against multiple databases, Sanger sequencing was used to determine if any of the potential novel mutations in known causative genes of ARNSHL co-segregated with the disease phenotype in this family. Direct polymerase chain reaction (PCR) products were sequenced using Bigdye terminator v3.1 cycle sequencing kits (Applied Biosystems, Foster City, CA) and analyzed using an ABI 3700XL Genetic Analyzer.

Mutational Analysis

Segregation of the mutations was studied in all family members. In addition, 208 negative samples and 50 ARNSHL families were also screened for the mutations by direct sequencing. Genotyping for c.589G>A and c.1171C>T was performed by PCR (primer sequences are available on request) and detected by bidirectional sequencing of the amplified fragments using an automated DNA sequencer (ABI 3100, Applied Biosystems). Nucleotide alteration(s) were identified by sequence alignment with the *TMC1*GenBank sequence using Genetool software.

Multiple Sequence Alignment

Multiple sequence alignment was performed using Homologene with the default settings and the sequences NP_619636.2 (*H. sapiens*), XP_001093188.2 (*M. mulatta*), XP_528322.2 (*P. troglodytes*), XP_002689695.1 (*B. taurus*), XP_541284.3 (*C. lupus*), NP_083229.1

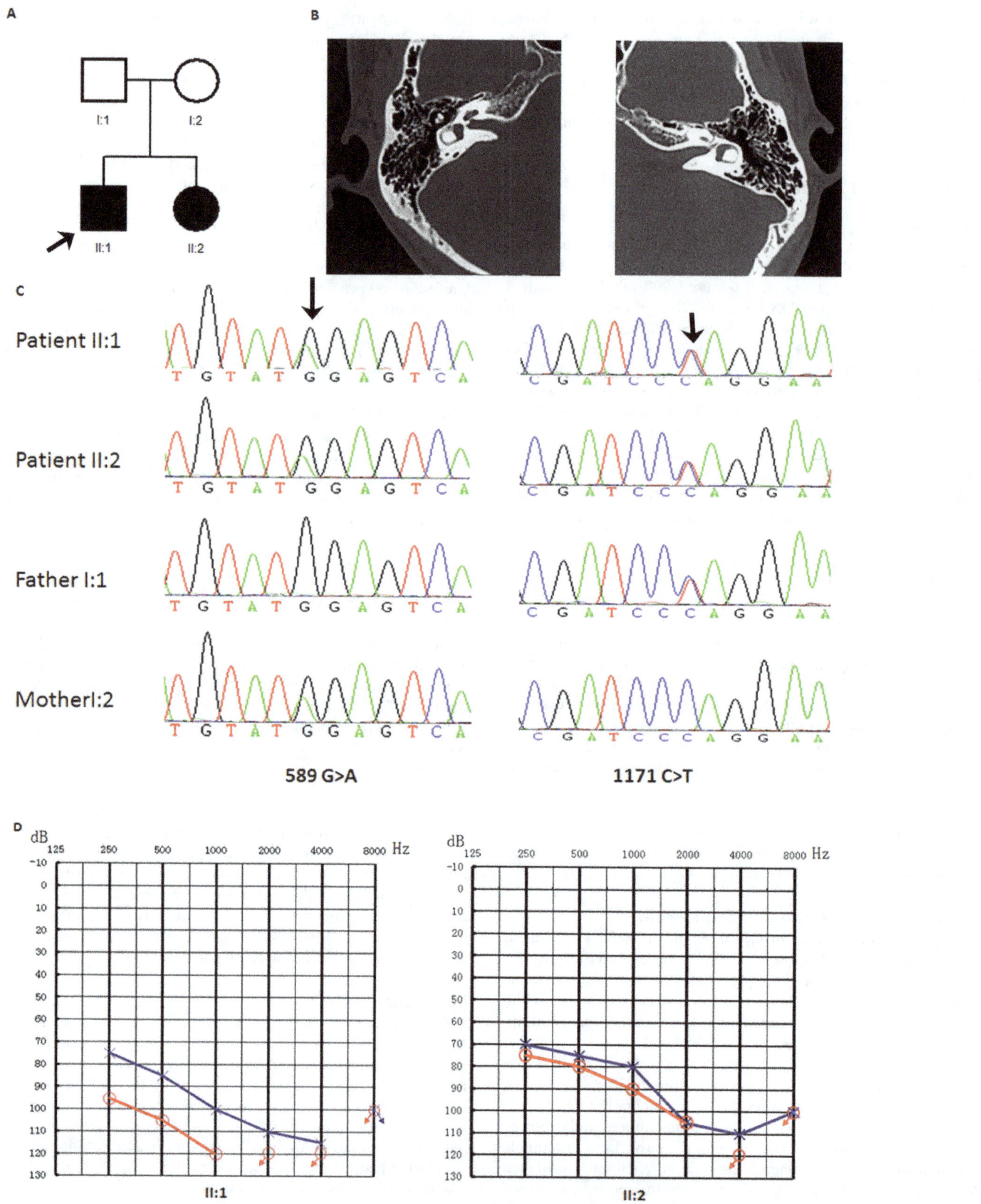

Figure 1. Combined figure. A. Pedigree of Family 1953 with ARNSHL Affected subjects are denoted in black. Arrow indicates the proband; B. temporal bone CT of the II:1 shows no structural change; C. Electropherograms analysis of TMC1 in family 1953 showing the compound heterozygous mutations (c.589G>A and c.1171C>T) co-segregated with the phenotype. D. Audiogram of affected subjects showed hearing loss ranged from severe to profound.

Table 2. Candidate SNP calls identified in 2 affected siblings.

Chr:Position	Gene	Mutation	Mode	Mutation type	Maternal allele	Paternal allele	SIFT/Polyphen2	Expressed in inner ear	Deafness gene	frequencies in the Exome variant Server
1:16354325	CLCNKA	791c>a	heterozygous	missense		Yes	Damaging/Benign	Yes	N/A	N/A
1:16360198	CLCNKA		heterozygous	5'-UTR	Yes		N/A	Yes	N/A	N/A
16:21747633	OTOA	2353a>c	heterozygous	missense	Yes		Tolerated/Benign	Yes	Yes	N/A
16:21747639	OTOA	2359g>t	heterozygous	nonsense	Yes		Damaging/possibly damaging	Yes	Yes	N/A
9:75366819	TMC1	589g>a	heterozygous	missense	Yes		Damaging/possibly damaging	Yes	Yes	N/A
9:75404180	TMC1	1171c>t	heterozygous	nonsense		Yes	Damaging/possibly damaging	Yes	Yes	N/A

(*M. musculus*), NP_001101991.1 (*R. norvegicus*), NP_001006580.1 (*G. gallus*), and XP_695621.3 (*D. rerio*). (http://www.ncbi.nlm.nih.gov/homologene?cmd = Retrieve&dopt = MultipleAlignment&list_uids = 23670).

Results

Clinical Presentation of Family 1953

We analyzed a two-generation ARNSHL family (family 1953) including two affected siblings (16 and 24 years old) and unaffected parents (Figure 1A). Audiograms of the two affected siblings showed that the hearing loss was bilateral, severe to profound, with some residual hearing at low frequency (Figure 1D). The stable nature of hearing loss was reported by the affected individuals but was not verified with audiograms. Immittance testing demonstrated normal and bone conduction values equal to the air conduction measurements, suggesting a sensorineural hearing impairment. Affected individuals did not have delays in gross motor development; neither did they have balance problems, vertigo, dizziness, nor spontaneous and positional nystagmus. Tandem walking was normal and Romberg test was negative. CT scan of the temporal bone in the proband excluded inner-ear malformations (Figure 1B). The parents reported no history of stillbirth or miscarriage. Physical examination of all members revealed no signs of systemic illness or dysmorphic features. The remaining examination results were completely normal. Affected individuals did not have delayed gross motor development. This phenotype is consistent with that reported previously for DFNB7/11 [15,19,24]. To exclude mutations in the genes commonly known to be associated with hereditary hearing loss, *SLC26A4* and *GJB2* were sequenced in the proband (patient II:1 in Figure 1A). No mutations were found in these genes and we proceeded to sequence the whole exomes of the two patients.

Whole-exome Sequencing

By WES of the proband II:1 and proband II:2, we generated 6.4 and 5.9 billion bases of sequence with mean target region depths of 61.93 and 66.68, respectively. Approximately 99% and 98.98% (2739 Mb and 2942 Mb in length, respectively) of the targeted bases were covered sufficiently to pass our thresholds for calling SNPs and short insertions or deletions (indels). The rates of nucleotide mismatch were 0.37% and 0.36%, respectively. After identification of variants, we focused only on non-synonymous variants (NS), splice acceptor and donor site mutations (SS), and frameshift coding insertions of deletions (indels), which were more likely to be pathogenic than others, especially those in homozygous or multiple heterozygous mode.

In II:1 and II:2, we separately identified 12192 and 12395 SNPs in the coding regions (11975 and 12171 missense, 72 and 74 readthrough, 145 and 150 nonsense), 2527 and 2557 variants in introns that may affect splicing (within 10 bp of the intron/exon junction), respectively. Then we compared these variants in two affected members with the dbSNP135, HapMap project, 1000 Genome Project, and YH database. Under the autosomal recessive model, we identified 113 genes with homozygous or multiple heterozygous variants (216 SNPs and 59 indels) common to both affected siblings. Then, we compared these variants with reported Nonsyndromic Hereditary Hearing Loss genes (http://hereditaryhearingloss. org/), in which six mutations were found in previously reported deafness-related genes (Table 2).

Mutation Detection and Analysis

SIFT and Polyphen2 were used as a first-pass filter to predict how the identified amino acid substitutions would affect protein

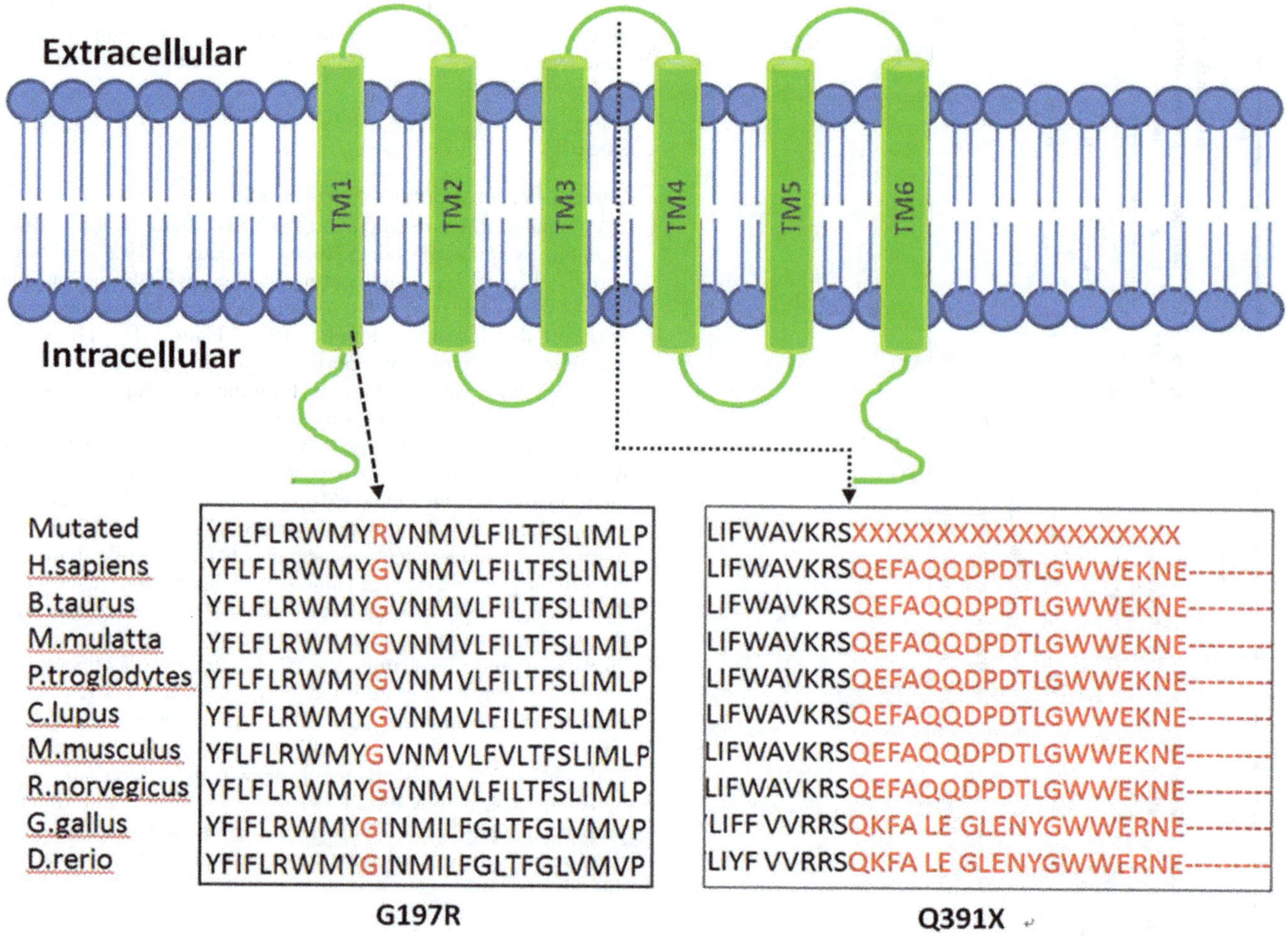

Figure 2. Schematic structure of TMC1 and Conservation analysis. G197R occur in the second TMhelix, Q391X occur extracellular between TM3 and TM4. Protein alignment showed conservation of residues TMC1 G197 and Q391 across nine species. These two mutations occur at an evolutionarily conserved amino acid (in red).

function taking into account sequence homology and the physical properties of amino acids. Two novel mutations in the previously described pathogenic gene *TMC1* were predicted to be damaging: *TMC1* c.589G>A (G197R) and *TMC1* c.1171G>A (Q391X) (according to GenBank accession number NM_138691.2). The mutation c.589G>A located within exon 11 and predicted to lie within hydrophobic transmembrane domains changes a hydrophilic glycine to a hydrophobic alanine at position 197, and may lead to a change in protein tertiary structure. Mutation c.1171G>A located within exon 15 results in the nonsense mutation Q391X, and the premature stop codon is likely to activate the nonsense-mediated mRNA decay response, thus leading to a decrease in TMC1 mRNA expression.

Both amino acid changes affect highly preserved residues (Figure 2). Sanger sequencing validated the two affected siblings' mutations and demonstrated that the parents were unaffected carriers of G197R (mother) and Q391X (father) deletion, showing complete co-segregation of the mutations with the phenotype (Figure 1C).

By direct sequencing, 208 ethnicity-matched negative controls and 50 Chinese familial patients with ARNSHL were genotyped to screen for the mutations. The two mutations described above were absent in 208 negative samples and in 50 ARNSHL families.

These data, together with the clinical presentation of the two affected siblings, indicate clearly that *TMC1* mutations were responsible for ARNSHL in this family.

We used TMHMM2.0 to predict the TMC1 protein with six membrane-spanning regions and cytoplasmic N- and C-termini. The result indicated that G197R occurs in the second TM helix, while Q391X occurs in the extracellular region between TM3 and TM4 (Figure 2). This predicted model of TMC1 membrane topology was similar to those of ion channels or transporters.

Discussion

For many decades, linkage analysis has been the most powerful and widely used strategy to identify the gene defects responsible for inherited disorders. However, this approach is time consuming, and requires the availability of cohorts of homogeneous and informative families. Homozygosity mapping is a potentiated version of linkage analysis, which makes possible the identification of several dozens genes responsible for autosomal recessive diseases, but it requires the availability of informative, possibly large, consanguineous families. As the molecular basis of deafness in most of our Chinese probands was unsolved, we predict that many new hearing loss genes and mutations remain to be identified. Next-generation sequencing can now be performed rapidly and at minimal cost, allowing analysis of the coding regions (exome) of the human genome in single individuals or small families, including patients in whom a clear genotype-phenotype correlation is absent or for clinically and genetically heterogeneous conditions. WES provides unprecedented opportunities to identify causative DNA mutations in rare heritable disorders.

This represents the first report of novel compound heterozygous mutations in the *TMC1* gene as a cause of ARNSHL. The *TMC1* gene on chromosome 9q12 contains 24 exons, including four exons encoding sequence upstream of a methionine codon in exon 5, and normally encodes a product of 760 amino acids. *TMC1* mutations seem to be rather common causes of recessive deafness in India, Pakistani, Turkish, and Tunisian families [15,19,25].

TMC1 is predicted to contain six transmembrane domains, and both C- and N-termini are located intracellularly; this protein exhibits no apparent amino acid sequence similarity to any other proteins of known function. Expression analysis of *TMC1* resulted in detection of transcripts in human fetal cochlea and mouse inner and outer cochlear hair cells as well as in neurosensory epithelia of the vestibular organs [15], and is required for postnatal hair cell development and maintenance [14].

Tmc1 deficiency in the recessive deafness mouse mutant *dn* leads to complete deafness and hair cell degeneration, suggesting that *Tmc1* is necessary for maturation and survival of hair cells in the murine cochlea.

Mouse models with the *Tmc1* defect [14,15] support a role for Tmc1 in the inner and outer hair cells, either in proper trafficking of other membrane proteins in these cells or in regulating the differentiation of immature hair cells into fully functional auditory receptors [13]. This model suggested that mechanical forces brought about by bending of stereocilia and tension on the tip links directly activate ion channels. If TMC1 is an ion channel that is mainly localized in the IHC, then it may be involved in the most basic auditory process of hair cell transduction.

The predicted structure of TMC1 bears similarity to that of the α-subunit of voltage-dependent K^+ channels, which have six α-helical TM segments and intracellular N- and C-termini [26]. TMC1 has been predicted to be an ion channel or transporter that mediates K^+ homeostasis in the inner ear [27]. Ion channels serve many functions, including the transport of ions and water, the control of electrical excitability, and the regulation of ionic homeostasis. The first four TM domains of the K^+ channel α-subunit act as voltage sensors for activation gating [28], whereas the intervening segment between TM5 and TM6 appears to confer channel selectivity [26]. *TMC1* c.589G>A (G197R) lies in TM2 and c.1171G>A (Q391X) lies between TM3 and TM4 extracellularly, and the mutations may affect an ion channel function in hair cells.

The stop codon in exon 15 (c.1171G>A [Q391X]) identified in this study is close to the previously reported mutation c.1165G>A [Q389X], and is predicted to result in formation of a truncated protein with impaired function [18].

In summary, we have reported the clinical and genetic characteristics of a non-consanguineous Chinese family with ARNSHL by WES. A major challenge for mutation discovery by WES is determining which variants are potentially causative and which are likely to be benign. To identify pathogenic variants, we consecutively filtered these variants by subjecting them to an analytical pipeline for high-confidence variant calling and annotation and identified novel compound heterozygous mutations in *TMC1*. The identification of additional mutations in *TMC1* further confirms its crucial role in auditory function. These results support sequence analysis of *TMC1* in clinical diagnostic testing of individuals with ARNSHL, as families with an affected child both parents of which are carriers have a 25% risk of recurrence. Moreover, pre-implantation genetic diagnosis is possible.

The English in this document has been checked by at least two professional editors, both native speakers of English. For a certificate, please see: http://www.textcheck.com/certificate/KuK2Ub.

Acknowledgments

We sincerely thank all the family members for their participation and cooperation in this study. We are also grateful to Dr. Guangchun Bai of Albany Medical College, New York State Department of Health for his valuable comments and suggestions.

Author Contributions

Conceived and designed the experiments: PD XG. Performed the experiments: XG YS SSH YL. Analyzed the data: XG LPG QYZ JW YYY. Contributed reagents/materials/analysis tools: GJW MYH FY YSS. Wrote the paper: XG PD.

References

1. Morton CC, Nance WE (2006) Newborn hearing screening–a silent revolution. N Engl J Med 354: 2151–2164.
2. Shearer AE, Hildebrand MS, Sloan CM, Smith RJ (2011) Deafness in the genomics era. Hear Res 282: 1–9.
3. Brownstein Z, Bhonker Y, Avraham KB (2012) High-throughput sequencing to decipher the genetic heterogeneity of deafness. Genome Biol 13: 245.
4. Delmaghani S, Aghaie A, Michalski N, Bonnet C, Weil D, et al. (2012) Defect in the gene encoding the EAR/EPTP domain-containing protein TSPEAR causes DFNB98 profound deafness. Hum Mol Genet 21: 3835–3844.
5. Li Y, Pohl E, Boulouiz R, Schraders M, Nurnberg G, et al. (2010) Mutations in TPRN cause a progressive form of autosomal-recessive nonsyndromic hearing loss. Am J Hum Genet 86: 479–484.
6. Walsh T, Shahin H, Elkan-Miller T, Lee MK, Thornton AM, et al. (2010) Whole exome sequencing and homozygosity mapping identify mutation in the cell polarity protein GPSM2 as the cause of nonsyndromic hearing loss DFNB82. Am J Hum Genet 87: 90–94.
7. Zheng J, Miller KK, Yang T, Hildebrand MS, Shearer AE, et al. (2011) Carcinoembryonic antigen-related cell adhesion molecule 16 interacts with alpha-tectorin and is mutated in autosomal dominant hearing loss (DFNA4). Proc Natl Acad Sci U S A 108: 4218–4223.
8. Schraders M, Haas SA, Weegerink NJ, Oostrik J, Hu H, et al. (2011) Next-generation sequencing identifies mutations of SMPX, which encodes the small muscle protein, X-linked, as a cause of progressive hearing impairment. Am J Hum Genet 88: 628–634.
9. Pierce SB, Walsh T, Chisholm KM, Lee MK, Thornton AM, et al. (2010) Mutations in the DBP-deficiency protein HSD17B4 cause ovarian dysgenesis, hearing loss, and ataxia of Perrault Syndrome. Am J Hum Genet 87: 282–288.
10. Pierce SB, Chisholm KM, Lynch ED, Lee MK, Walsh T, et al. (2011) Mutations in mitochondrial histidyl tRNA synthetase HARS2 cause ovarian dysgenesis and sensorineural hearing loss of Perrault syndrome. Proc Natl Acad Sci U S A 108: 6543–6548.
11. Sirmaci A, Walsh T, Akay H, Spiliopoulos M, Sakalar YB, et al. (2010) MASP1 mutations in patients with facial, umbilical, coccygeal, and auditory findings of Carnevale, Malpuech, OSA, and Michels syndromes. Am J Hum Genet 87: 679–686.
12. Klein CJ, Botuyan MV, Wu Y, Ward CJ, Nicholson GA, et al. (2011) Mutations in DNMT1 cause hereditary sensory neuropathy with dementia and hearing loss. Nat Genet 43: 595–600.
13. Marcotti W, Erven A, Johnson SL, Steel KP, Kros CJ (2006) Tmc1 is necessary for normal functional maturation and survival of inner and outer hair cells in the mouse cochlea. J Physiol 574: 677–698.
14. Vreugde S, Erven A, Kros CJ, Marcotti W, Fuchs H, et al. (2002) Beethoven, a mouse model for dominant, progressive hearing loss DFNA36. Nat Genet 30: 257–258.
15. Kurima K, Peters LM, Yang Y, Riazuddin S, Ahmed ZM, et al. (2002) Dominant and recessive deafness caused by mutations of a novel gene, TMC1, required for cochlear hair-cell function. Nat Genet 30: 277–284.
16. de Heer AM, Collin RW, Huygen PL, Schraders M, Oostrik J, et al. (2011) Progressive sensorineural hearing loss and normal vestibular function in a Dutch

DFNB7/11 family with a novel mutation in TMC1. Audiol Neurootol 16: 93–105.
17. Kitajiri SI, McNamara R, Makishima T, Husnain T, Zafar AU, et al. (2007) Identities, frequencies and origins of TMC1 mutations causing DFNB7/B11 deafness in Pakistan. Clin Genet 72: 546–550.
18. Meyer CG, Gasmelseed NM, Mergani A, Magzoub MM, Muntau B, et al. (2005) Novel TMC1 structural and splice variants associated with congenital nonsyndromic deafness in a Sudanese pedigree. Hum Mutat 25: 100.
19. Sirmaci A, Duman D, Ozturkmen-Akay H, Erbek S, Incesulu A, et al. (2009) Mutations in TMC1 contribute significantly to nonsyndromic autosomal recessive sensorineural hearing loss: a report of five novel mutations. Int J Pediatr Otorhinolaryngol 73: 699–705.
20. Li R, Yu C, Li Y, Lam TW, Yiu SM, et al. (2009) SOAP2: an improved ultrafast tool for short read alignment. Bioinformatics 25: 1966–1967.
21. Li R, Li Y, Fang X, Yang H, Wang J, et al. (2009) SNP detection for massively parallel whole-genome resequencing. Genome Res 19: 1124–1132.
22. McKenna A, Hanna M, Banks E, Sivachenko A, Cibulskis K, et al. (2010) The Genome Analysis Toolkit: a MapReduce framework for analyzing next-generation DNA sequencing data. Genome Res 20: 1297–1303.
23. Li H, Durbin R (2010) Fast and accurate long-read alignment with Burrows-Wheeler transform. Bioinformatics 26: 589–595.
24. Hilgert N, Alasti F, Dieltjens N, Pawlik B, Wollnik B, et al. (2008) Mutation analysis of TMC1 identifies four new mutations and suggests an additional deafness gene at loci DFNA36 and DFNB7/11. Clin Genet 74: 223–232.
25. Kalay E, Karaguzel A, Caylan R, Heister A, Cremers FP, et al. (2005) Four novel TMC1 (DFNB7/DFNB11) mutations in Turkish patients with congenital autosomal recessive nonsyndromic hearing loss. Hum Mutat 26: 591.
26. Hanlon MR, Wallace BA (2002) Structure and function of voltage-dependent ion channel regulatory beta subunits. Biochemistry 41: 2886–2894.
27. Keresztes G, Mutai H, Heller S (2003) TMC and EVER genes belong to a larger novel family, the TMC gene family encoding transmembrane proteins. BMC Genomics 4: 24.
28. Li-Smerin Y, Hackos DH, Swartz KJ (2000) alpha-helical structural elements within the voltage-sensing domains of a K(+) channel. J Gen Physiol 115: 33–50.
29. Makishima T, Kurima K, Brewer CC, Griffith AJ (2004) Early onset and rapid progression of dominant nonsyndromic DFNA36 hearing loss. Otol Neurotol 25: 714–719.
30. Kitajiri S, Makishima T, Friedman TB, Griffith AJ (2007) A novel mutation at the DFNA36 hearing loss locus reveals a critical function and potential genotype-phenotype correlation for amino acid-572 of TMC1. Clin Genet 71: 148–152.
31. Tlili A, Rebeh IB, Aifa-Hmani M, Dhouib H, Moalla J, et al. (2008) TMC1 but not TMC2 is responsible for autosomal recessive nonsyndromic hearing impairment in Tunisian families. Audiol Neurootol 13: 213–218.
32. Santos RL, Wajid M, Khan MN, McArthur N, Pham TL, et al. (2005) Novel sequence variants in the TMC1 gene in Pakistani families with autosomal recessive hearing impairment. Hum Mutat 26: 396.

21

Non-Syndromic Hearing Impairment in India: High Allelic Heterogeneity among Mutations in *TMPRSS3, TMC1, USHIC, CDH23* and *TMIE*

Aparna Ganapathy[1], Nishtha Pandey[1], C. R. Srikumari Srisailapathy[2], Rajeev Jalvi[3], Vikas Malhotra[4], Mohan Venkatappa[1], Arunima Chatterjee[1], Meenakshi Sharma[1], Rekha Santhanam[1], Shelly Chadha[4], Arabandi Ramesh[2], Arun K. Agarwal[4], Raghunath R. Rangasayee[3], Anuranjan Anand[1]*

1 Molecular Biology and Genetics Unit, Jawaharlal Nehru Centre for Advanced Scientific Research, Bangalore, India, **2** Department of Genetics, Dr. ALM Post Graduate Institute of Basic Medical Sciences, Chennai, India, **3** Department of Audiology, Ali Yavar Jung National Institute for the Hearing Handicapped, Mumbai, India, **4** Department of ENT, Maulana Azad Medical College, New Delhi, India

Abstract

Mutations in the autosomal genes *TMPRSS3, TMC1, USHIC, CDH23* and *TMIE* are known to cause hereditary hearing loss. To study the contribution of these genes to autosomal recessive, non-syndromic hearing loss (ARNSHL) in India, we examined 374 families with the disorder to identify potential mutations. We found four mutations in *TMPRSS3*, eight in *TMC1*, ten in *USHIC*, eight in *CDH23* and three in *TMIE*. Of the 33 potentially pathogenic variants identified in these genes, 23 were new and the remaining have been previously reported. Collectively, mutations in these five genes contribute to about one-tenth of ARNSHL among the families examined. New mutations detected in this study extend the allelic heterogeneity of the genes and provide several additional variants for structure-function correlation studies. These findings have implications for early DNA-based detection of deafness and genetic counseling of affected families in the Indian subcontinent.

Editor: Jörg D. Hoheisel, Deutsches Krebsforschungszentrum, Germany

Funding: Funds for this work were provided by Department of Biotechnology, New Delhi (BT/PR4449/Med/12/172/2003) and JNCASR, Bangalore. AG and NP received research fellowships from Council of Scientific and Industrial Research, New Delhi. The funders had no role in study design, data collection and analysis, decision to publish, or preparation of the manuscript.

Competing Interests: The authors have declared that no competing interests exist.

* E-mail: anand@jncasr.ac.in

Introduction

Hearing impairment is the most common sensory defect in humans, occurring at a frequency of about one in 1000 live births, of which 50% are due to genetic causes [1]. About 70% of hereditary hearing loss is non-syndromic, wherein hearing impairment is not associated with any additional clinical phenotype. To date, 65 genes for non-syndromic hearing loss (NSHL) have been identified (http://hereditaryhearingloss.org/) [2]. Mutations in *TMPRSS3* (transmembrane serine protease 3) [3], *TMC1* (transmembrane cochlear-expressed gene 1) [4], *USHIC* (Usher 1C) [5], *CDH23* (cadherin 23) [6] and *TMIE* (transmembrane inner ear) [7] are known to play a causative role in NSHL. Indeed, *TMPRSS3* [3], *TMC1* [4] and *TMIE* [7], were identified in studies involving a few multi-affected families from the Indian subcontinent. However, a detailed study evaluating the contribution of these genes has not been carried out for Indian populations. In this study, we describe the spectrum of mutations in *TMPRSS3, TMC1, USHIC, CDH23* and *TMIE* in 374 families with ARNSHL from India.

Materials and Methods

Subjects

A total of 1739 individuals from 374 families with at least two members affected with recessive, prelingual, severe-to-profound NSHL were included in this study. Of these 316 were families with two affected sibs, 54 with three affected sibs and 4 with four or more affected sibs. These families had been ruled out for mutations in *Cx26* (connexin 26, *GJB2*), which is known to be the most common cause of hereditary hearing loss in India [8]. A detailed clinical history of each affected member was collected to ensure that hearing loss was not due to infections, ototoxic drugs, trauma or premature birth and was not accompanied by any apparent ear, eye, head, neck, skin, skeletal or neurological abnormalities. The degree of hearing loss was ascertained by audiological evaluation involving pure tone audiometry, which included bone conduction. Hearing thresholds were obtained between 250–8000 Hz in a sound-treated room. Ten milliliters of venous blood was collected from members of the families. Fifty-four healthy unaffected individuals, above 20 years of age without any apparent family history of hearing impairment, were also included in this study as controls to estimate allele frequencies of the sequence variants found during the course of this work. Genomic DNA was extracted using the phenol-chloroform method [9]. This study was approved by the Institutional Human Bioethics and Biosafety Committees of the four institutes involved in the work and informed written consent was obtained from all participating individuals and from the parents of those affected individuals who were younger than 18 years of age.

Genetic analysis

To identify families that may harbour mutations in *TMPRSS3*, *TMC1*, *USHIC* and *CDH23*, we carried out concordance/discordance tests using polymorphic microsatellite markers flanking the genes (Table 1) in 374 families. These markers were amplified using the polymerase chain reaction (PCR) with 50 ng of genomic DNA, 25 pmol primers, 1.5 mM $MgCl_2$ and 2.5 U *Taq* DNA polymerase. PCR was carried out using a GeneAmp PCR 9700 and genotyping using an ABI PRISM 3730 DNA Analyzer (Applied Biosystems, USA). Allele sizing was done using GENEMAPPER v3.7 (Applied Biosystems). For the families that could not be excluded on the basis of marker discordance among affected siblings, complete *TMPRSS3* (13 exons), *TMC1* (24 exons), *USH1C* (28 exons) and *CDH23* (70 exons) transcript structures, comprising exonic and flanking intronic regions, were analyzed by direct sequencing. For *TMIE* (DFNB6), direct sequencing of its four exons and flanking intronic regions for an affected member, in each of the 374 families, was carried out. The primers for sequencing were designed using PRIMER3 (http://primer3.ut.ee) [10]. PCR was performed and the amplified products were purified by Montage PCR96 Cleanup reagents (Millipore). Cycle sequencing was performed using 20 ng of purified PCR products, 3.2 pmol of each primer and ABI PRISM BigDye Terminator cycle sequencing reagents. Following cycle sequencing, the samples were loaded onto an ABI PRISM 3730 DNA Analyzer. Each amplicon was sequenced in both directions and analyzed using DNASTAR SeqmanII 5.01.

Bioinformatic analysis

The amino acid and nucleotide residue conservations across species were examined using NCBI BLAST (http://www.ncbi.nlm.nih.gov/BLAST/) and conservation across protein or gene families using ClustalW (http://www.ebi.ac.uk/clustalw/) [11] and ConSeq (consurf.tau.ac.il/) [12]. Splice site prediction was done using NetGene2 (http://www.cbs.dtu.dk/services/NetGene2) [13]; disulphide bond prediction, using DISULFIND (http://disulfind.dsi.unifi.it/) [14]. The possible pathogenic effect of protein-coding variants was examined using two prediction tools: SIFT (http://sift.jcvi.org/) [15] and Polyphen-2 (http://genetics.bwh.harvard.edu/pph2/) [16].

Results

Pathogenic and apparently benign variants in *TMPRSS3*, *TMC1*, *CDH23*, *USH1C* and *TMIE*

For the aforementioned genes, concordance/discordance test were carried out in the 374 ARNSHL families. Based on this test, the possibility for mutation could not be excluded in 48 families for *TMPRSS3*, in 50 families for *TMC1*, in 24 families for *CDH23* and in 46 families for *USH1C*. Further analysis of one affected member in each of the families revealed 12 variants in *TMPRSS3*, 20 in *TMC1*, 36 in *USH1C* and 44 in *CDH23*. In *TMIE*, 11 variants were identified. To assess their pathological potential, these variants were evaluated for (i) segregation among additional affected members of the families, (ii) evolutionary conservation of nucleotide or amino acid residue and (iii) frequency among individuals with apparently normal hearing. These criteria helped identify 33 potential mutations: four in *TMPRSS3*, eight in *TMC1*, ten in *USH1C*, eight in *CDH23* and three in *TMIE* (Table 2, Figure 1 and 2). Additionally, 90 apparently benign gene variants were found, which included 77 known polymorphisms (http://www.ncbi.nlm.nih.gov/) and 13 new ones. Of the new ones, five were in *TMC1*, two in *USH1C*, two in *CDH23* and four in *TMIE*. The variants classified as benign satisfied one or more of the following criteria: (i) allele frequency of 0.01 or more among the control individuals; (ii) lack of segregation with the deafness phenotype; (iii) poor evolutionary conservation and (iv) apparently no effect on transcript or protein function (Table S1).

Exonic mutations

Among the mutations likely to affect protein structure or function were the nonsense mutations: p.R34X in TMC1 and p.Q362X in USH1C and, 20 missense mutations: p.V116M, p.G243R and p.C386R in TMPRSS3; p.G267E, p.V372M and p.R445C in TMC1; p.R63W, p.R89H, p.G200S, p.R620C, p.A804T and p.A871T in USH1C; p.V139I, p.D918N, p.D990N, p.E1701K, p.T1887I and p.S2527L in CDH23; p.E31G and p.R84W in TMIE. In addition, a deletion, p.I210del in TMC1 and two insertions: CDH23, c.189_190insC and TMIE, c.125_126insCGCC were also identified. Several of the substitution mutations (p.V116M, p.G243R, p.C386R, p.V372M, p.R445C, p.R63W, p.R89H, p.R620C, p.D918N, p.E1701K, p.S2527L, p.E31G and p.R84W) were predicted to have severe detrimental effects by SIFT and POLYPHEN analysis (Table 2). Further, many of the identified coding mutations (p.V116M, p.G243R, p.C386R, p.I210del, p.V372M, p.R445C, p.R620C, p.A804T, p.V139I, p.D918N, p.D990N, p.E1701N and p.T1887I) reside in structurally or functionally important protein domains (Table 2, Figure 3). Upon sequence comparison across species and protein families, a high degree of evolutionary-conservation was observed for the amino acid residues at the mutation sites (Figure 1 and 2). For example, in TMPRSS3, p.G243R and p.C386R mutations occur in the highly conserved catalytic serine protease domain. Disulfide bond prediction and available crystal structure of the extracellular region of Hepsin (TMPRSS1, pdb 1z8g) suggest the presence of a disulfide bridge involving Cys386 and Cys370 in TMPRSS3, similar to the disulphide bond of corresponding Cys338 and Cys322 in Hepsin

Table 1. Genes and locations of microsatellite markers used in the concordance/discordance tests.

Gene (locus)	Polymorphic microsatellite markers and their locations
TMPRSS3 (DFNB8/10)	D21S1260 (900 kb centromeric), D21S1225 (128 kb centromeric), D21S49 (83 kb telomeric) and D21S1411 (344 kb telomeric)
TMC1 (DFNB7/11, DFNA36)	D9S789 (1.3 Mb centromeric), D9S1822 (300 kb telomeric) and D9S1876 (an intragenic marker).
USH1C (DFNB18)	D11S902 (25 kb telomeric), D11S4130 (180 kb centromeric), D11S1888, (190 kb centromeric) and D11S4138 (175 kb centromeric)
CDH23 (DFNB12)	D10S537 (1 Mb centromeric), D10S1688 (860 kb centromeric), D10S412 (147 kb centromeric) and D10S218 (300 kb telomeric).

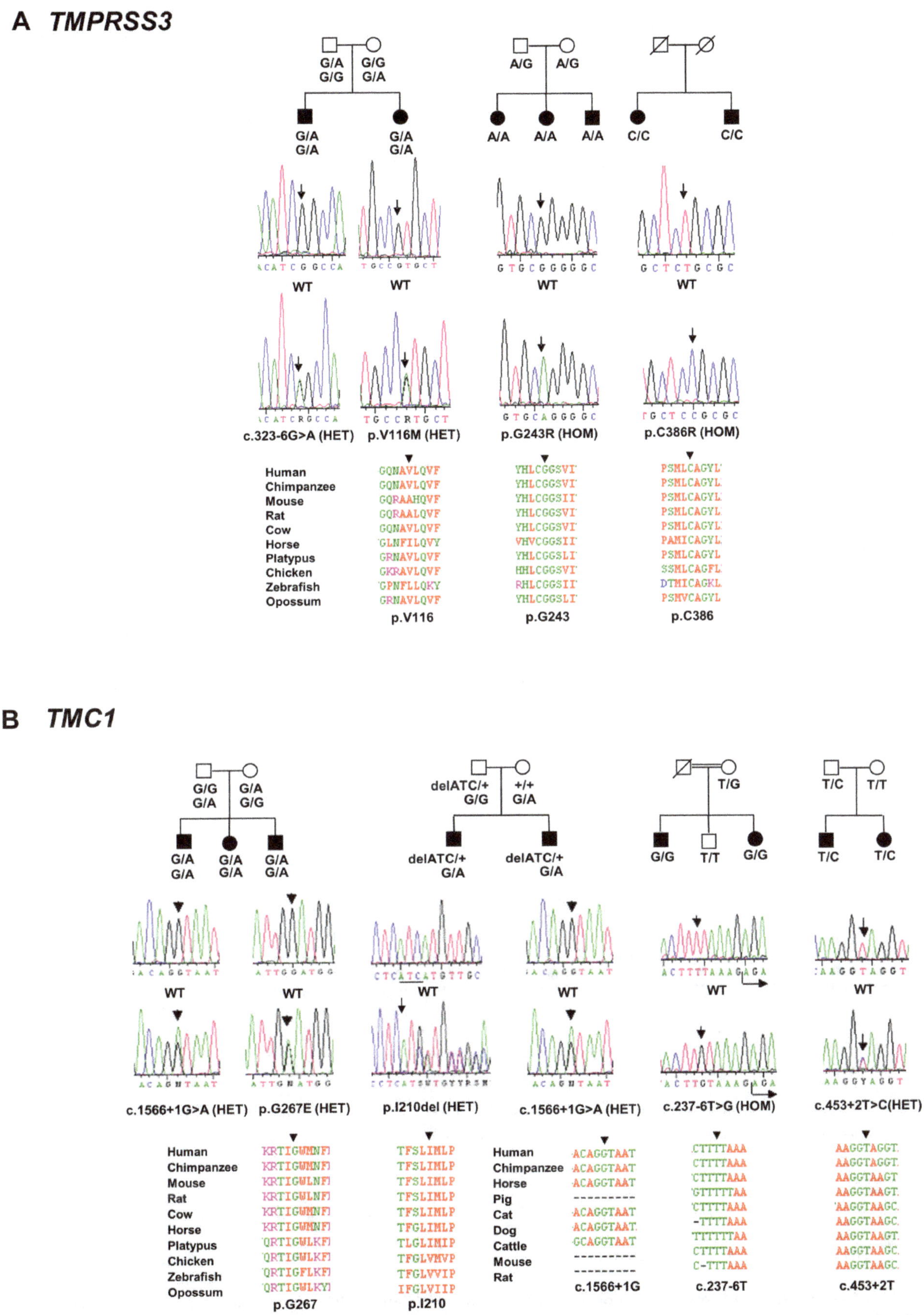
A TMPRSS3
WT
c.323-6G>A (HET)
p.V116M (HET)
p.G243R (HOM)
p.C386R (HOM)
Human
Chimpanzee
Mouse
Rat
Cow
Horse
Platypus
Chicken
Zebrafish
Opossum
p.V116
p.G243
p.C386
B TMC1
WT
c.1566+1G>A (HET)
p.G267E (HET)
p.I210del (HET)
c.1566+1G>A (HET)
c.237-6T>G (HOM)
c.453+2T>C(HET)
Human
Chimpanzee
Mouse
Rat
Cow
Horse
Platypus
Chicken
Zebrafish
Opossum
p.G267
p.I210
Human
Chimpanzee
Horse
Pig
Cat
Dog
Cattle
Mouse
Rat
c.1566+1G
c.237-6T
c.453+2T

Figure 1. Analysis of segregation and conservation of novel variants in *TMPRSS3* and *TMC1*. A) *TMPRSS3* and B) *TMC1*. Top panel shows the family structure and segregation of the variants; in cases where the variants were seen in more than one family, a single representation is provided; middle panel shows the electropherogram and lower panel shows the conservation of the mutated residue.

[17]. Mutation p.V116M, is predicted to be a damaging substitution in the SRCR domain involved in binding of TMPRSS3 to the cell surface and in its interaction with the extracellular molecules [18]. In p.I210del, conservation analysis by ConSeq, showed that the deleted isoleucine is located in a stretch of conserved and buried hydrophobic residues of the first transmembrane domain of TMC1. Mutation p.A804T resides in the third PDZ domain and, mutation p.A871T in the C-terminal

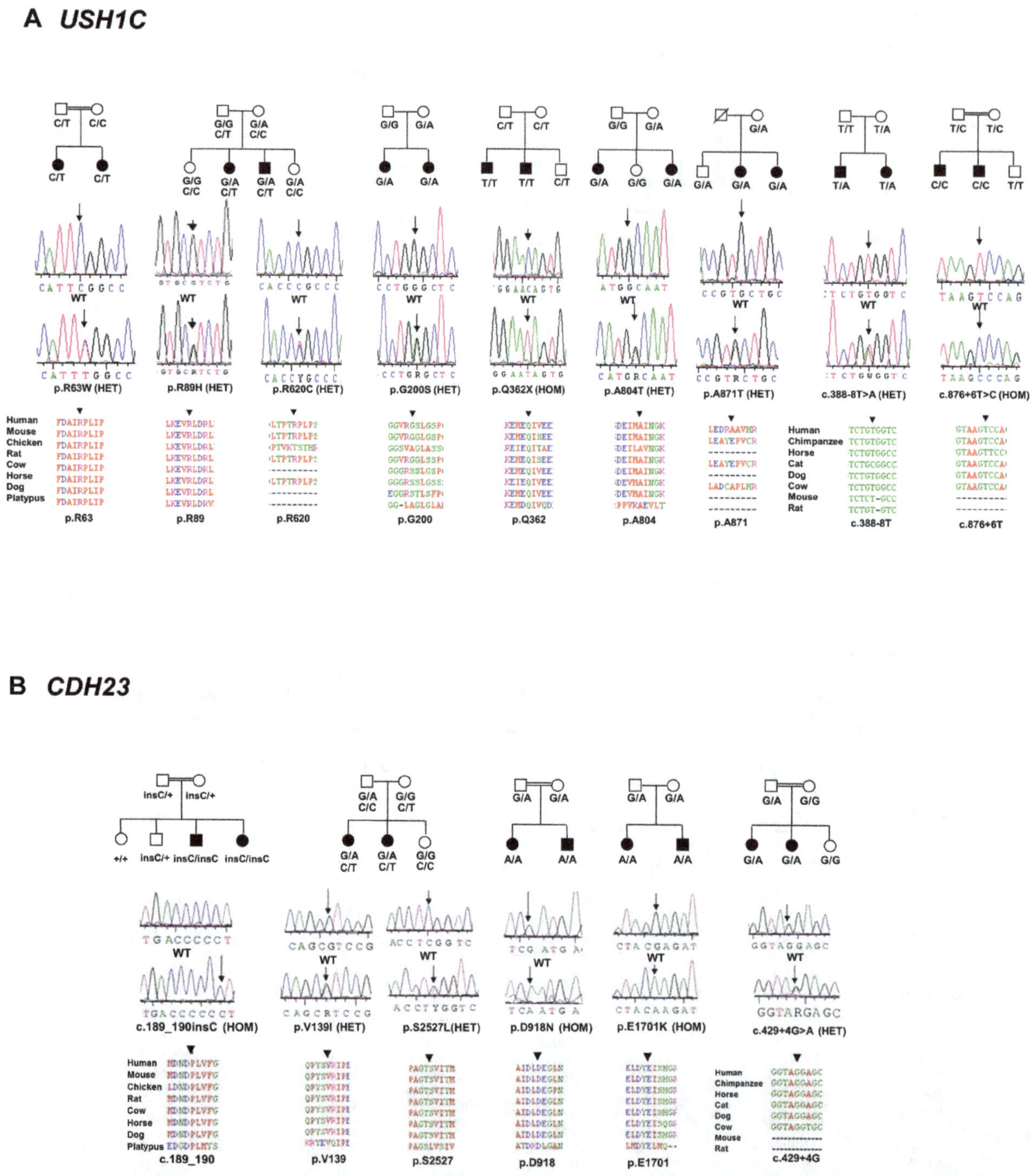

Figure 2. Analysis of segregation and conservation of novel variants in *USH1C* and *CDH23*. A) *USHIC* and B) *CDH23*. Top panel shows the family structure and segregation of the variants; in cases where the variants were seen in more than one family, a single representation is provided; middle panel shows the electropherogram and lower panel shows the conservation of the mutated residue.

Table 2. Mutations in the *TMPRSS3, TMC1, USH1C, CDH23* and *TMIE* genes.

Gene sequence variant	Location	Domain	Possible effect on gene or protein	SIFT	PolyPhen-2	Hom/Het	Number of families: samples per family	Novel or known	dbSNP Accession	Frequency in control chromosomes
A. ***TMPRSS3***										
c.323-6G>A	Intron 4	-	Splice site regulation	-	-	Hom + ompound het	3+1:4,4,3+4	Known[3]	-	-
c.346G>A	Exon 5	SRCR	p.V116M	Damaging	Probably damaging	Compound het	1:4	Novel	rs200090033[a]	0/102
c.727G>A	Exon 8	Serine Protease	p.G243R	Damaging	Probably damaging	Hom	1:5	Novel	-	0/108
c.1156T>C	Exon 11	Serine Protease	p.C386R	Damaging	Probably damaging	Hom	1:2	Novel	-	0/108
B. ***TMC1***										
c.100C>T	Exon 7	N-TERM	p.R34X	-	-	Hom	1:4	Known[4]	rs121908073[a]	-
c.237-6T>G	Intron 7	-	Splice site regulation	-	-	Hom	1:4	Novel	-	0/100
c.453+2T>C[b]	Intron 9	-	Splice site regulation	-	-	Het	1:4	Novel	-	0/102
c.628_630del	Exon 11	TM1	p.I210del	-	-	Compound het	1:4	Novel	-	0/102
c.800G>A	Exon 13	EC1-LOOP	p.G267E	Tolerated	Probably damaging	Compound het	1:5	Novel	-	0/108
c.1114G>A	Exon 15	TM3	p.V372M	Damaging	Probably damaging	Hom	2:6,6	Known[26]	-	-
c.1333C>T	Exon 16	TM4	p.R445C	Damaging	Probably damaging	Hom	1:2	Known[27]	-	0/108
c.1566+1G>A	Intron 17	-	Splice site regulation	-	-	Compound het	2:4,5	Novel	-	0/106
C. ***USH1C***										
c.187C>T[b]	Exon 3	N-TERM	p.R63W	Damaging	Probably damaging	Het	1:4	Novel	-	0/100
c.267G>A	Exon 4	N-TERM	p.R89H	Damaging	Probably damaging	Compound het	1:6	Novel	-	0/100
c.388-8T>A[b]	Intron 4	-	Splice site regulation	-	-	Het	1:4	Novel	-	0/100
c.496+1G>A	Intron 5	-	Splice site regulation	-	-	Hom	1:5	Known[20]	-	0/100
c.598G>A[b]	Exon 8	Proximal to PDZ	p.G200S	Tolerated	Benign	Het	1:4	Novel	-	0/100
c.876+6T>C	Intron 11	-	Splice site regulation	-	-	Hom	1:5	Novel	-	0/100
c.1084C>T	Exon 13	CC1	p.Q362X	-	-	Hom	1:5	Novel	-	0/100
c.1858C>T	Exon 19	PST	p.R620C	Damaging	Probably damaging	Compound het	1:6	Novel	rs143160805[a]	0/100
c.2410G>A[b]	Exon 25	PDZ3	p.A804T	Tolerated	Probably damaging	Het	1:5	Novel	rs 150593932[a]	0/100
c.2611G>A[b]	Exon 27	C-TERM	p.A871T	Tolerated	Benign	Het	1:4	Novel	rs56165709[a]	0/100
D. ***CDH23***										
c.189_190insC	Exon 4	EC1	Frameshift	-	-	Hom	2:6,5	Novel	-	0/96
c.415G>A	Exon 6	Between EC1 and EC2	p.V139I	Tolerated	Benign	Compound het	1:5	Novel	-	0/96
c.429+4G>A[b]	Intron 6	-	Splice site regulation	-	-	Het	1:5	Novel	-	0/96
c.2752G>A	Exon 25	EC9	p.D918N	Damaging	Probably damaging	Hom	1:4	Novel	-	0/96
c.2968G>A	Exon 26	EC9	p.D990N	Tolerated	Probably damaging	Hom	1:4	Known[28]	-	-
c.5101G>A	Exon 40	EC16	p.E1701K	Damaging	Probably damaging	Hom	1:4	Novel	-	0/96

Table 2. Cont.

Gene sequence variant	Location	Domain	Possible effect on gene or protein	SIFT	PolyPhen-2	Hom/Het	Number of families: samples per family	Novel or known	dbSNP Accession	Frequency in control chromosomes
c.5660C>T[b]	Exon 43	EC18	p.T1887I	Tolerated	Probably damaging	Het	2:4,3	Known[29]	-	0/96
c.7580C>T	Exon 54	EC24 proximal	p.S2527L	Damaging	Probably damaging	Compound het	1:5	Novel	-	0/96
E. *TMIE*										
c.92A>G	Exon 1	EC-LOOP	p.E31G	Damaging	Probably damaging	Hom	2:4,5	Known[30]	-	-
c.125_126insCGCC	Exon 2	EC-LOOP	Frameshift	-	-	Hom	4:6,6, 4,5	Known[7]	-	-
c.250C>T	Exon 3	C-TERM	p.R84W	Damaging	Probably damaging	Hom	2:5,6	Known[7]	rs28942097	-

[a]Allele frequency in the range of 0.000– 0.003 is observed for the variant in the dbSNP137 database. Gene sequence variants shown are either almost certainly pathogenic alleles, or [b]potentially pathogenic. CC: coiled-coiled, C-TERM: C-Terminal, EC-LOOP: Extracellular loop, EC: Cadherin extracellular repeat domain, Hom: Homozygous, Het: Heterozygous, N-TERM: N-Terminal, PDZ: Post synaptic density protein-95, Drosophila disc large tumor suppressor, Zonula occludens-1 domain, PST: Proline-serine-threonine rich region, SRCR: scavenger receptor cysteine-rich, TM: Transmembrane domain.
TMPRSS3: Gene ID: 64699; mRNA: NM_024022; Protein: NP_076927
TMC1: Gene ID: 117531; mRNA: NM_138691; Protein; NP_619636
USH1C: Gene ID: 10083; mRNA: NM_153676; Protein: NP_710142
CDH23: Gene ID: 64072; mRNA: NM_022124.3; Protein: NP_071407.3
TMIE: Gene ID: 259236; mRNA: NM_147196.1; Protein: NP_671729.

tail of USH1C. p.D918N and p.E1701K in CDH23, disrupt the highly conserved peptide motifs, DXD and LDRE, respectively [19]. These motifs are involved in binding of calcium ions for the interdomain rigidification of the cadherin repeat domains. The c.189_190insC insertion mutation causes a frameshift leading to premature termination after an incorporation of 19 unrelated amino acids in CDH23.

Intronic mutations

The following novel intronic mutations were observed: c.237-6T>G, c.453+2T>C and c.1566+1G>A in *TMC1*; c.388-8T>A and c.876+6T>C in *USHIC* and c.429+4G>A in *CDH23*. Potential effects of the intronic variants on regulation of splicing were predicted by using NetGene2 and by examining evolutionary conservation of the nucleotide residues. c.453+2T>C, c.1566+1G>A and c.876+6T>C are predicted to affect the 5′ splice-site donor usage. c.237-6T>G is a change in the conserved polypyrimidine tract flanking 3′ splice acceptor site in intron 7. c.388-8T>A could generate a relatively strong splice acceptor site, which would introduce two additional residues, valine and lysine, at positions 129 and 130 in the conserved stretch of first PDZ domain. *TMPRSS3*, c.323-6G>A [3] and *USH1C*, c.496+1G>A are previously known splice-site mutation observed in this study [20].

Homo-, hetero- and compound hetero- zygotes, and a search of *CDH23* and *USH1C* interacting alleles

In five families with *TMPRSS3* mutations, all affected members were homozygotes and in one family all affected members were compound heterozygotes (p.V116M and c.323-6G>A) (Table 2). In five families with *TMC1* mutations, all affected members were homozygotes, whereas in two families affected members were compound heterozygotes (c.1566+1G>A/p.I210del and c.1566+1G>A/p.G267E). In one family with a *TMC1* mutation, heterozygotes were affected. For *USH1C* mutations, affected individuals were homozygotes in three families, compound heterozygotes (p.R620C/p.R89H) in one family and heterozygotes in five families. In case of *CDH23* mutations, affected members in five families were homozygotes; in three families they were heterozygotes and in one family they were compound heterozygotes (p.V139I/p.S2527L). For *TMIE*, all eight mutation positive families were homozygous for the observed mutations. Among the 40 families that were mutation positive, 26 were homozygous for the mutation; five, compound heterozygous and in nine families, the mutation occurred in a heterozygous condition. For five *USHIC* and three *CDH23* families carrying heterozygous potentially pathogenic alleles, we examined sequences of the genes known to interact with *USHIC* and *CDH23*, for the possibility of the presence of a second mutation. Families carrying heterozygous variants in *USHIC* (Table 2C) were analyzed for the *MYO7A* [21], *CDH23* [6] and *SANS* [22] genes. Similarly, *USH1C*, which is known to interact with *CDH23*, was analyzed in the three families carrying heterozygous changes in *CDH23* (Table 2D). In the five *USHIC* families studied, six new changes (p.V66V, p.R412H, p.A1425V, p.N1667K, c.9510+13C>T and p.D3253A) were observed as heterozygous variants in addition to several known polymorphisms in *CDH23*. p.R412H, p.A1425V and p.N1667K did not segregate with the phenotype in the families studied; and p.V66V, c.9510+13C>T and p.D3253A were present in control chromosomes of unaffected individuals, implying that these changes were unlikely to be pathogenic. In an analysis of 48 exons of *MYO7A* in the families heterozygous for *USH1C* mutations, one new intronic variant c.736-73C>T was observed in four out of the five families examined. This change did not

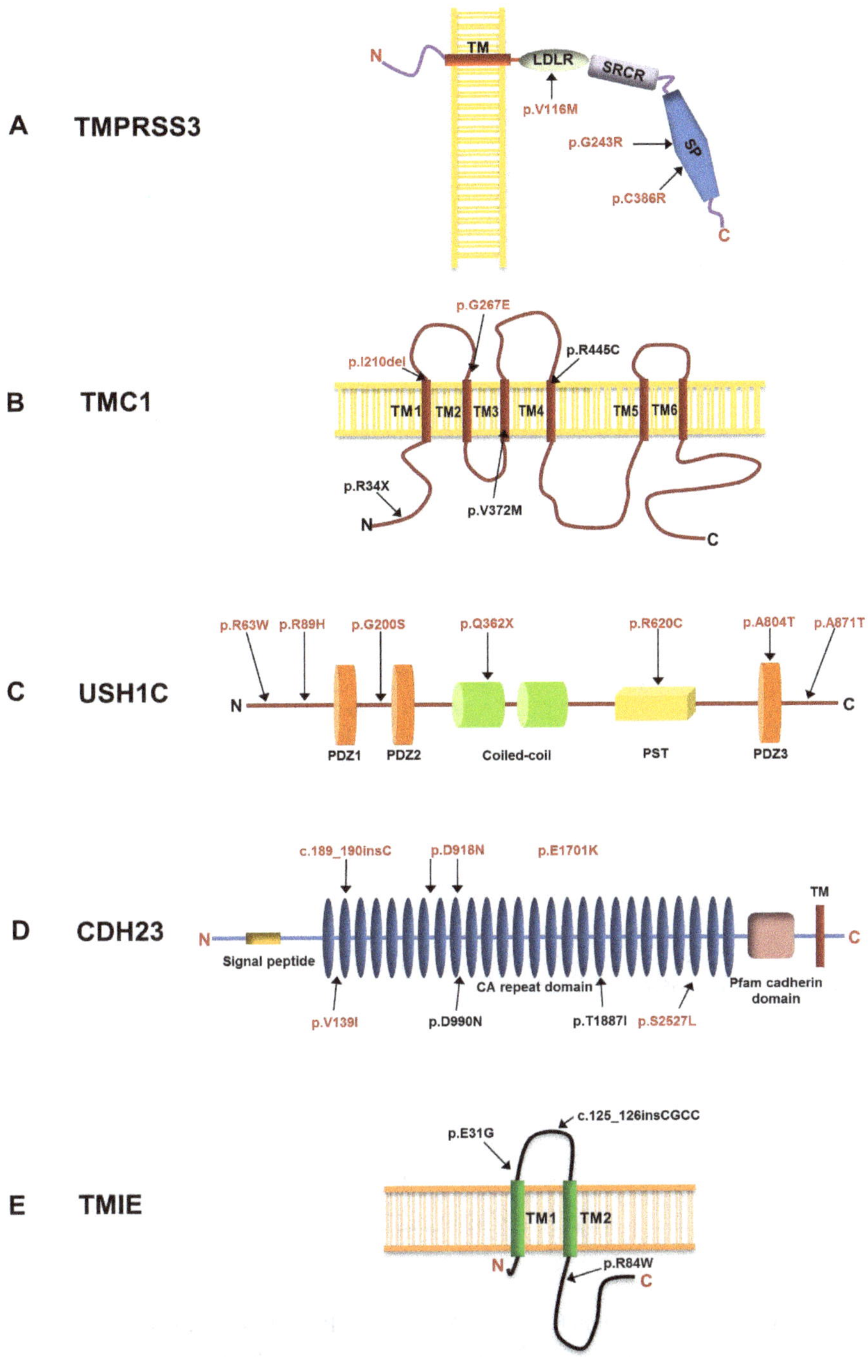

Figure 3. Schematic representation of TMPRSS3, TMC1, USH1C, CDH23 and TMIE. A) TMPRSS3, B) TMC1, C) USH1C, D) CDH23 and E) TMIE. Arrows point to the location of the mutations. Shown in red are the mutations identified in the study.

segregate with the phenotype. No variant was observed in the three exons of *SANS*. Similarly, no novel potentially pathogenic *USHIC* alleles were detected, in the three families with the heterozygous *CDH23* variants.

Discussion

The contribution of mutations to ARNSHL has been found to be variable among populations from different parts of the world. Population-specific social parameters such as marriage among persons with hearing loss and consanguinity may affect the prevalence of a mutation, leading to certain mutations becoming common in one population and rare in another. Therefore, population-specific studies are necessary to understand the contribution of mutations to the genetic load. Studies carried out earlier on Indian families with ARNSHL have revealed that mutations in *Cx26* are the most common cause of the disorder and account for about 25% of severe-to-profound hereditary hearing loss in India [8]. However, data on families from the Indian

Table 3. Genetic epidemiology of the *TMPRSS3, TMC1, USH1C, CDH23* and *TMIE* genes.

Population	Subjects	Prevalence/Mutation Positives	Reference
TMPRSS3			
Caucasian	448 NSHL probands negative for *Cx26*, 35delG	0.45%	[31]
Pakistan	159 NSHL families, 449 ARNSHL families, 353 ARNSHL families	2.5%, 1.8%, 10 families	[32], [33], [34]
Turkey	49 NSHL families negative for *Cx26* two *Cx30* genomic deletions and a mitochondrial mutation in *MTRNR1*, 1555A>G, 86 ARNSHL families negative for *Cx26*, 25 ARNSHL families	1.7%, 8%	[35], [36]
Tunisia	39 ARNSHL families	2 families	[37]
Korea	40 ARNSHL subjects	2.5%	[38]
India	374 ARNSHL families negative for *Cx26*	1.2%	This study
TMC1			
Pakistan and India	230 ARNSHL families, 168 ARNSHL families negative for *Cx26*, 557 ARNSHL large families	5.4%, 4.4%, 3.4%	[4], [26], [23]
Turkey	65 ARNSHL families negative for *Cx26*, 49 NSHL families negative for *Cx26*, two *Cx30* genomic deletions and a mitochondrial mutation in *MTRNR1*, 1555A>G, 86 ARNSHL families negative for *Cx26*	6%, 6.6%, 8.1%	[39], [27], [35]
Iran	54 ARNSHL families	1 family	[40]
India	374 ARNSHL families negative for *Cx26*	1.6%	This study
USH1C			
China	32 recessive NSHL families	1 family	[41]
Caucasian	16 NSHL sib pairs + 2 NSHL families	0%	[42]
CDH23			
America, Sweden, Dutch, German, Spain, Pakistan, South Africa, France, Italy, Ireland	38 recessive NSHL families negative for *Cx26* and *MYO7A*	5%	[29]
Japan	64 ARNSHL probands negative for *Cx26*, 919 probands from ARNSHL families	5%, 5.4%	[43], [44]
Turkey	49 NSHL families negative for *Cx26*, two *Cx30* genomic deletions and a mitochondrial mutation in *MTRNR1*, 1555A>G	3.3%	[35]
India	374 ARNSHL families negative for *Cx26*	1.8%	This study
TMIE			
Pakistan	168 ARNSHL families negative for *Cx26*	1.7%	[30]
Turkey	49 NSHL families negative for *Cx26*, two *Cx30* genomic deletions and a mitochondrial mutation in *MTRNR1*, 1555A>G	6.6%	[35]
Taiwan	250 NSHL subjects	1 subject	[45]
India	374 ARNSHL families negative for *Cx26*	1.6%	This study

subcontinent have not been available previously for the genes examined in this study.

In TMPRSS3 three novel mutations, p.G243R, p.C386R and p.V116M, were detected. As mentioned earlier, Gly243 and Cys386 are located in the highly conserved catalytic serine protease domain of the protein. Glycine is a small amino acid, usually known to play a crucial role in protein structure. In p.G243R, the uncharged glycine is substituted by a large polar residue, arginine, which may affect protein-folding and, therefore, TMPRSS3 function. Six conserved cysteine residues, C242, C258, C370, C386, C397 and C425, present in the serine protease domain of TMPRSS3, are likely to form intra subunit disulfide bonds [17]. p.C386R is possibly altering the secondary structure of the serine protease domain of TMPRSS3 protein and affecting its function. In TMC1, nonsense mutation, p.R34X is known to occur at a high frequency in Pakistan and may be due to a founder effect: an SNP marker c.45C>T (rs2589615) was observed in all the families with p.R34X from Pakistan [23]. Interestingly, in this study c.45C>T was also observed in the family in which p.R34X was found. The age of this mutation has been estimated to be between 1075 and 1900 years [24]. In *TMC1*, two mutations, c.237-6T>G and c.453+2T>C, are likely to affect splicing. p.I210del in TMC1 occurs in the first transmembrane domain. Deletion of isoleucine in the conserved region of the first transmembrane domain might affect its topology. A highly conserved uncharged glycine is mutated to an acidic amino acid glutamic acid in the extracellular region of TMC1 in p.G267E, which is likely to affect protein structure. Two intronic mutations, c.1566+1G>A and c.453+2T>C, in *TMC1* are proposed to affect splicing, leading to a frameshift and formation of a non-functional protein. In *TMC1*, c.237-6T>G, a transition of thiamine to guanine, 4 bases before the splice acceptor site in intron 7, is likely to affect the polypyrimidine tract. The polypyrimidine tract is one of the *cis*-acting elements in the splicing machinery that is recognized by several protein factors to form a functional spliceosome [25]. In CDH23, five out of the eight mutations reside in the calcium-binding EC domains. EC domains are thought to have a critical role in rigidification, linearization and dimerization of cadherin proteins.

A total of 123 variants were observed in this study, of which 10 are known deafness mutations, 23 are previously unreported mutations, and 90, apparently neutral variants. Further, functional validation of the variants identified in this study is likely to result in a better understanding of their pathogenic potential. Before sequencing transcript structures of the *TMC1*, *TMPRSS3*, *CDH23* and *USH1C* genes, we examined concordance/discordance of the microsatellite markers tightly linked to the gene of interest. Those families which showed a clear discordance of the markers among affected siblings were excluded from further analysis of the gene. However, families which showed marker-concordance as well as the ones which were uninformative for the markers, were examined for mutations by sequencing all known exonic and flanking intronic regions of the genes. We may have missed a mutation due to an intragenic recombination event, genetic heterogeneity, or when the mutation is present in deep intronic regions or *cis*-regulatory regions of the gene. Large exonic deletions or in/dels as well as those second site mutations which occur in heterozygous carriers may have also gone undetected.

Among the sequence variants found in this study, eight were found to occur in a heterozygous condition. These were rare variants and were present at conserved locations. Five of these were in *USHIC*, two in *CDH23* and one in *TMC1* (Table 2). These changes seem potentially pathogenic. It is possible that individuals with these variants are hearing impaired due to another unknown mutation at these genes or another gene.

Mutational survey of *TMPRSS3*, *TMC1*, *USH1C*, *CDH23* and *TMIE* genes have been carried out in certain world populations. These data suggest that the contribution of these genes to ARNSHL is not the same in all population and varies from 0.5-5% (Table 3). Our observations suggest that the overall contribution of *TMPRSS3*, *TMC1*, *USH1C*, *CDH23* and *TMIE* mutations for ARNSHL is low in India: 1.2% of the hearing impaired examined showed mutations in *TMPRSS3*, 1.6% in *TMC1*, 1.8% in *USH1C*, 1.8% in *CDH23* and 1.6% in *TMIE*. Unlike mutations in the *Cx26* gene, which are the most common cause of hereditary impairment in India, the contribution of mutations in these five genes is rather small. The spectra of alleles in the *TMPRSS3*, *TMC1*, *USH1C* and *CDH23* genes in Indian populations seem to be quite different from those observed for other world populations; among the 33 mutations observed in our study 23 were not reported in other populations. These studies have implications for early detection of hearing loss, genetic counseling, and for implementation of suitable early intervention strategies.

Acknowledgments

We thank members of all the families who participated in this study. We thank Karen Avraham (Tel Aviv University) for her contribution to the early stages of the project. We thank Sharat Chandra for critical reading of the manuscript and helpful discussions.

Author Contributions

Conceived and designed the experiments: AA. Performed the experiments: AG NP MV AC MS RS. Analyzed the data: AA AG NP. Contributed reagents/materials/analysis tools: CRSS RJ VM SC AKA AR RRR. Wrote the paper: AA AG NP.

References

1. Morton NE (1991) Genetic epidemiology of hearing impairment. Ann N Y Acad Sci 630: 16–31.
2. Yan D, Liu XZ (2008) Cochlear molecules and hereditary deafness. Front Biosci 13: 4972–4983.
3. Scott HS, Kudoh J, Wattenhofer M, Shibuya K, Berry A, et al. (2001) Insertion of beta-satellite repeats identifies a transmembrane protease causing both congenital and childhood onset autosomal recessive deafness. Nat Genet 27: 59–63.
4. Kurima K, Peters LM, Yang Y, Riazuddin S, Ahmed ZM, et al. (2002) Dominant and recessive deafness caused by mutations of a novel gene, TMC1, required for cochlear hair-cell function. Nat Genet 30: 277–284.
5. Verpy E, Leibovici M, Zwaenepoel I, Liu XZ, Gal A, et al. (2000) A defect in harmonin, a PDZ domain-containing protein expressed in the inner ear sensory hair cells, underlies Usher syndrome type 1C. Nat Genet 26: 51–55.
6. Bolz H, von Brederlow B, Ramirez A, Bryda EC, Kutsche K, et al. (2001) Mutation of CDH23, encoding a new member of the cadherin gene family, causes Usher syndrome type 1D. Nat Genet 27: 108–112.
7. Naz S, Giguere CM, Kohrman DC, Mitchem KL, Riazuddin S, et al. (2002) Mutations in a novel gene, TMIE, are associated with hearing loss linked to the DFNB6 locus. Am J Hum Genet 71: 632–636.
8. Ramshankar M, Ganapathy A, Jalvi R, Srikumari Srisailapathy CR, Malhotra V, et al. (2008) Functional consequences of novel connexin 26 mutations associated with hereditary hearing loss. Eur J Hum Genet 10: 502–509.
9. Sambrook J, Russell DW (2001) Molecular cloning: a laboratory manual. Cold Spring Harbor, New York: Cold Spring Harbor Laboratory Press.
10. Rozen S, Skaletsky HJ (2000) Primer3 on the WWW for general users and for biologist programmers. In: Krawertz S, Misener S Bioinformatics Methods and Protocols: Methods in Molecular Biology, New Jersey: Humana Press pp. 365–386.
11. Thompson JD, Higgins DG, Gibson TJ (1994) CLUSTAL W: improving the sensitivity of progressive multiple sequence alignments through sequence weighting, position specific gap penalties and weight matrix choice. Nucleic Acids Res 22: 4673–4680.
12. Berezin C, Glaser F, Rosenberg Y, Paz I, Pupko T, et al. (2004) ConSeq: The Identification of Functionally and Structurally Important Residues in Protein Sequences. Bioinformatics 20: 1322–1324.
13. Hebsgaard SM, Korning PG, Tolstrup N, Engelbrecht J, Rouze P, et al. (1994) Splice site prediction in Arabidopsis thaliana DNA by combining local and global sequence information. Nucleic Acids Res 24: 3439–3452.
14. Ceroni A, Passerini A, Vullo A, Frasconi P (2001) DISULFIND: A Disulfide Bonding State and Cysteine Connectivity Prediction Server. Nucleic Acids Res 34: W177–W181.
15. Ng PC, Henikoff S (2001) Predicting deleterious amino acid substitutions. Genome Res 11:863–874.
16. Adzhubei IA, Schmidt S, Peshkin L, Ramensky VE, Gerasimova A, et al. (2010) A method and server for predicting damaging missense mutations. Nat Methods 7: 248–249.
17. Herter S, Piper DE, Aaron W, Gabriele T, Cutler G, et al. (2005) Hepatocyte growth factor is a preferred in vitro substrate for human hepsin, a membrane-anchored serine protease implicated in prostate and ovarian cancers. Biochem J 390: 125–136.
18. Guipponi M, Antonarakis SE, Scott HS (2008) TMPRSS3, a type II transmembrane serine protease mutated in nonsyndromicautosomal recessive deafness. Front Biosc 13: 1557–1567.
19. Nollet F, Kools P, van Roy F (2009) Phylogenetic analysis of the cadherin superfamily allows identification of six major subfamilies besides several solitary members. J Mol Biol 299: 551–572.
20. Ahmed ZM, Smith TN, Riazuddin S, Makishima T, Ghosh M, et al. (2002) Nonsyndromic recessive deafness DFNB18 and Usher syndrome type IC are allelic mutations of USHIC. Hum Genet 110: 527–531.
21. Weil D, Blanchard S, Kaplan J, Guilford P, Gibson F, et al. (1995) Defective myosin VIIA gene responsible for Usher syndrome type 1B. Nature. 374: 60–61.
22. Weil D, El-Amraoui A, Masmoudi S, Mustapha M, Kikkawa Y, et al. (2003) Usher syndrome type IG (USH1G) is caused by mutations in the gene encoding SANS, a protein that associates with the USH1C protein, harmonin. Hum Mol Genet. 12: 463–471.

23. Kitajiri S, McNamara R, Makishima T, Husnain T, Zafar AU, et al. (2007) Identities, frequencies and origins of TMC1 mutations causing DFNB7/B11deafness in Pakistan. Clin Genet 72: 546–550.
24. Ben Saïd M, Hmani-Aifa M, Amar I, Baig SM, Mustapha M, et al. (2010) High frequency of the p.R34X mutation in the TMC1 gene associated with nonsyndromic hearing loss is due to founder effects. Genet. Test Mol Biomarkers. 14: 307–300.
25. Wagner EJ, Garcia-Blanco MA (2001) Polypyrimidine tract binding protein antagonizes exon definition. Mol Cell Biol 21: 3281–3288.
26. Santos RL, Wajid M, Khan MN, McArthur N, Pham TL, et al. (2005) Novel sequence variants in the TMC1 gene in Pakistani families with autosomal recessive hearing impairment. Hum Mutat 26: 396–404.
27. Sirmaci A, Duman D, Oztürkmen-Akay H, Erbek S, Incesulu A, et al. (2009) Mutations in TMC1 contribute significantly to nonsyndromic autosomal recessive sensorineural hearing loss: a report of five novel mutations. Int J Pediatr Otorhinolaryngol 73: 699–705.
28. Bork JM, Peters LM, Riazuddin S, Bernstein SL, Ahmed ZM, et al. (2001) Usher syndrome 1D and nonsyndromic autosomal recessive deafness DFNB12 are caused by allelic mutations of the novel cadherin-like gene CDH23. Am J Hum Genet 68: 26–37.
29. Astuto LM, Bork JM, Weston MD, Askew JW, Fields RR, et al. (2002) CDH23 mutation and phenotype heterogeneity: a profile of 107 diverse families with Usher syndrome and nonsyndromic deafness. Am J Hum Genet 71: 262–275.
30. Santos RL, El-Shanti H, Sikandar S, Lee K, Bhatti A, et al. (2006) Novel sequence variants in the TMIE gene in families with autosomal recessive nonsyndromic hearing impairment. J Mol Med 84: 226–231.
31. Wattenhofer M, Di Iorio MV, Rabionet R, Dougherty L, Pampanos A, et al. (2002) Mutations in the TMPRSS3 gene are a rare cause of childhood nonsyndromic deafness in Caucasian patients. J Mol Med 80: 124–131.
32. Ben-Yosef T, Wattenhofer M, Riazuddin S, Ahmed ZM, Scott HS, et al. (2001) Novel mutations of TMPRSS3 in four DFNB8/B10 families segregating congenital autosomal recessive deafness. J Med Genet 38: 396–400.
33. Ahmed ZM, Li XC, Powell SD, Riazuddin S, Young TL, et al. (2004) Characterization of a new full length TMPRSS3 isoform and identification of mutant alleles responsible for nonsyndromic recessive deafness in Newfoundland and Pakistan. BMC Med Genet 5: 24.
34. Lee K, Khan S, Islam A, Ansar M, Andrade PB, et al. (2012) Novel TMPRSS3 variants in Pakistani families with autosomal recessive non-syndromic hearing impairment. Clin Genet 82: 56–63.
35. Duman D, Sirmaci A, Cengiz FB, Ozdag H, Tekin M (2011) Screening of 38 genes identifies mutations in 62% of families with nonsyndromic deafness in Turkey Genet Test Mol Biomarkers 15: 29–33.
36. Wattenhofer M, Sahin-Calapoglu N, Andreasen D, Kalay E, Caylan R, et al. (2005) A novel TMPRSS3 missense mutation in a DFNB8/10 family prevents proteolytic activation of the protein. Hum Genet 117: 528–535.
37. Masmoudi S, Antonarakis SE, Schwede T, Ghorbel AM, Gratri M, et al. (2001) Novel missense mutations of TMPRSS3 in two consanguineous Tunisian families with nonsyndromic autosomal recessive deafness. Hum Mutat 18: 101–108.
38. Lee JW, Baek JI, Choi JY, Kim UK, Lee SH, et al. (2013) Genetic analysis of TMPRSS3 gene in the Korean population with autosomal recessive nonsyndromic hearing loss. Gene pii: S0378-1119.
39. Kalay E, Karaguzel A, Caylan R, Heister A, Cremers FP, et al. (2005) Four novel TMC1 (DFNB7/DFNB11) mutations in Turkish patients with congenital autosomal recessive nonsyndromic hearing loss. Hum Mutat 26: 591–598.
40. Davoudi-Dehaghani E, Zeinali S, Mahdieh N, Shirkavand A, Bagherian H, et al. (2013) A transversion mutation in non-coding exon 3 of the TMC1 gene in two ethnically related Iranian deaf families from different geographical regions; evidence for founder effect. Int J Pediatr Otorhinolaryngol 77: 821–826.
41. Ouyang XM, Xia XJ, Verpy E, Du LL, Pandya A, et al. (2002) Mutations in the alternatively spliced exons of USH1C cause non-syndromic recessive deafness. Hum Genet 111: 26–30.
42. Blaydon DC, Mueller RF, Hutchin TP, Leroy BP, Bhattacharya SS, et al. (2003) The contribution of USH1C mutations to syndromic and non- syndromic deafness in the UK. Clin Genet 63: 303–307.
43. Wagatsuma M, Kitoh R, Suzuki H, Fukuoka H, Takumi Y, et al. (2007) Distribution and frequencies of CDH23 mutations in Japanese patients with nonsyndromic hearing loss. Clin Genet 72: 339–344.
44. Miyagawa M, Nishio SY, Usami S (2012) Prevalence and clinical features of hearing loss patients with CDH23 mutations: a large cohort study. PLoS One 7: e40366.
45. Yang JJ, Su MC, Chien KH, Hsin CH, Li SY (2010) Identification of novel variants in the TMIE gene of patients with nonsyndromic hearing loss. Int J Pediatr Otorhinolaryngol. 74: 489–493.

Independent Validation of an Existing Model Enables Prediction of Hearing Loss after Childhood Bacterial Meningitis

Rogier C. J. de Jonge[1,2*], **Marieke S. Sanders[1,3,4]**, **Caroline B. Terwee[5]**, **Martijn W. Heymans[5]**, **Reinoud J. B. J. Gemke[6]**, **Irene Koomen[7]**, **Lodewijk Spanjaard[8]**, **A. Marceline van Furth[1]**

1 Department of Pediatric Infectious Diseases - Immunology, and Rheumatology, VU University Medical Center, Amsterdam, The Netherlands, **2** Department of Neonatology, Erasmus MC - Sophia Children's Hospital, Rotterdam, The Netherlands, **3** Department of Medical Microbiology, Laboratory for Immunogenetics, VU University Medical Center, Amsterdam, The Netherlands, **4** Department of General Medicine, Antonius Hospital, Nieuwegein, The Netherlands, **5** Department of Epidemiology and Biostatistics and the EMGO Institute for Health and Care Research, VU University Medical Center, Amsterdam, The Netherlands, **6** Department of Pediatrics, VU University Medical Center, Amsterdam, The Netherlands, **7** Department of Pediatrics, Westfriesgasthuis, Hoorn, The Netherlands, **8** Department of Medical Microbiology, Netherlands Reference Laboratory for Bacterial Meningitis, Academic Medical Center, Amsterdam, The Netherlands

Abstract

Objective: This study aimed external validation of a formerly developed prediction model identifying children at risk for hearing loss after bacterial meningitis (BM). Independent risk factors included in the model are: duration of symptoms prior to admission, petechiae, cerebral spinal fluid (CSF) glucose level, *Streptococcus pneumoniae* and ataxia. Validation helps to evaluate whether the model has potential in clinical practice.

Study design: 116 Dutch school-age BM survivors were included in the validation cohort and screened for sensorineural hearing loss (>25 dB). Risk factors were obtained from medical records. The model was applied to the validation cohort and its performance was compared with the development cohort. Validation was performed by application of the model on the validation cohort and by assessment of discrimination and goodness of fit. Calibration was evaluated by testing deviations in intercept and slope. Multiple imputation techniques were used to deal with missing values.

Results: Risk factors were distributed equally between both cohorts. Discriminative ability (Area Under the Curve, AUC) of the model was 0.84 in the development and 0.78 in the validation cohort. Hosmer-Lemeshow test for goodness of fit was not significant in the validation cohort, implying good fit concerning the similarity of expected and observed cases. There were no significant differences in calibration slope and intercept. Sensitivity and negative predicted value were high, while specificity and positive predicted value were low which is comparable with findings in the development cohort.

Conclusions: Performance of the model remained good in the validation cohort. This prediction model might be used as a screening tool and can help to identify those children that need special attention and a long follow-up period or more frequent auditory testing.

Editor: Helene F. Rosenberg, NIAID, United States of America

Funding: There are no current external funding sources for this study.

Competing Interests: The authors have declared that no competing interests exist.

* E-mail: r.c.j.dejonge@erasmusmc.nl

These authors contributed equally to this work.

Introduction

Due to successful vaccination programs, and to spontaneous decline in *Neisseria meningitidis* serogroup B infections, the incidence of bacterial meningitis (BM) in childhood is decreasing in the Western world. Still, BM ranks among the top ten causes of death in children younger than 14 years in high-income countries. Further, developing countries account for 98% of the estimated 5.6 million disability-adjusted life years attributed to meningitis globally [1,2]. Sensorineural hearing loss is the most common severe consequence of BM, with an incidence in children of 7–31% [3,4,5,6,7,8,9]. Hearing loss after BM is probably multicausal. Bacterial labyrinthitis due to dissemination of the infection from the subarachnoid space in combination with toxic or serous labyrinthitis, direct nerve fiber damage and secondary ischemic damage are thought to be part of the mechanism [10].

Especially in (young) children even mild impairment in hearing abilities may impair auditory, linguistic, communication and learning skills. Early identification of hearing loss is indispensable for effective treatment resulting in the acquisition of normal linguistic development [11,12]. Further, cochlear ossification may complicate cochlear implantation making early diagnosis even more essential. [13,14].

The actual incidence of post-meningitis hearing loss is probably underestimated because audiometric testing is only performed in clinical suspected cases. Many cases are late or never diagnosed [9]. For that reason, routine hearing evaluation is recommended in the standard follow-up program of childhood BM aiming to achieve more timely intervention [8,14].

To support the recognition of patients at high risk for hearing loss after BM, Koomen *et al.* developed a clinical prediction rule (figure 1) [6]. Clinical prediction rules are (regression) models that use three or more variables from patient history, clinical course or diagnostic tests to calculate a probability of an outcome measure. These rules are potentially strong tools that are currently used in clinical decision-making [15]. The model constructed by Koomen et al. included the following independent predictors for hearing loss: duration of symptoms prior to admission, absence of petechiae, cerebral spinal fluid (CSF) glucose level, *Streptococcus pneumoniae* as causative pathogen and ataxia.

In general a prediction model does not perform well in a different cohort than the one it was constructed in. For that reason external validation in an independent cohort is essential before implementation in practice [16,17,18]. The aim of this study was to externally validate the existing model for hearing loss after childhood BM in a validation cohort of Dutch school-age BM survivors in order to evaluate the potential for usage in clinical practice.

Methods

The study was approved by the medical ethics committee of the VU University Medical Center in Amsterdam. Written informed consent was obtained from the parents or guardians of all children and from the children themselves if they were at least 12 years of age.

Development Cohort

The construction of the prediction rule was described in the original publication by Koomen *et al.* [6]. Files of the Netherlands Reference Laboratory for BM (NRLBM) were searched for children born between January 1986 and December 1994 who survived BM between January 1990 and December 1995. The NRLBM receives approximately 90% of the isolates of Dutch meningitis patients [19]. The diagnosis BM was based on the isolation of bacteria in the CSF. Exclusion criteria included a complex onset of meningitis (defined as: meningitis secondary to immunodeficiency states, CNS surgery, cranial trauma, CSF shunt infections of relapsing meningitis), pre-existent cognitive or behavioral problems, and diseases developed after BM, which could have caused cognitive or behavioral problems. These last 2 exclusion criteria were used while the cohort was also constructed for a study on academic or behavioral problems after BM [20].

Sixteen hundred and five children were eligible for inclusion and their pediatricians were approached to send the parents a letter requesting participation. Six hundred and twenty-eight children were included, and their medical records were investigated for risk factors and for perceptive hearing loss of >25 dB. Hearing loss was found in forty-three children (7%) and by reviewing medical records; information was collected on all potential risk factors for this hearing loss. Predictors univariably associated with the outcome ($p \leq 0.10$) were included and a prediction model was developed using multivariable logistic regression. Five risk factors for hearing loss were found to be independent determinants: duration of symptoms prior to admission longer than two days, the absence of petechiae, CSF glucose level ≤0.6 mmol/L, *S. pneumoniae* as causative pathogen and the presence of ataxia during the illness. After internal validation using bootstrapping techniques and shrinkage of regression coefficients this model was transformed into a clinical prediction rule as presented in figure 1. The scores and the matching probability of hearing loss were visually presented in a nomogram for use in clinical practice. [6].

Validation Cohort

In 2005, the files of the NRLBM were searched again for Dutch children born between January 1993 and December 1999 who suffered from non-*Haemophilus influenzae* type b (Hib) BM between January 1997 and December 2001. The exclusion criteria were identical to those used in the original study [6]. One thousand and thirty-six children were eligible for inclusion, and the pediatricians were requested to send the parents (or guardians) an invitation letter to participate in the study. After informed consent the parents were sent screening questionnaires regarding health, learning and behavior. Three hundred and fifty eight children were included in the cohort used for validation of this model. Parallel to the approach used in the development study of Koomen *et al.* in which a prediction rule for academic and behavioral problems after BM was constructed, a nested cohort approach was used [20]. In this design only a subset of cases and controls are selected for further analysis, which decreases the necessary time and financial resources resulting in an improved efficiency [20,21].

In the total cohort of 358 children a nested cohort of 160 children were randomly selected and invited to visit our department for academic and neuropsychological testing and for the completion of questionnaires regarding behavior and health. Forty-four of the invited children did not participate in this part of the study.

Again, the outcome measure "hearing loss" was defined as a unilateral or bilateral perceptive loss of >25 dB and was based on findings in these records and on parental information provided in the questionnaires about the children's health (Dutch versions of the Child Health Questionnaire (CHQ) and the Health Utilities Index (HUI) mark 2&3) [22,23]. Information on the risk factors for hearing loss was also collected by reviewing medical records of the pediatrician and the otolaryngologist after permission from the parents. Conductive hearing loss was not included. Finally,

Risk score (max 100 points) =

10 * symptoms >2 days + 27 * absence of petechiae + 15 * CSF glucose level ≤0.6 mmol/L

+ 12 * *S. pneumoniae* as causative pathogen + 36 * ataxia as a symptom of BM

Figure 1. clinical prediction rule for the prediction of hearing loss after childhood BM, as presented by Koomen *et al.*

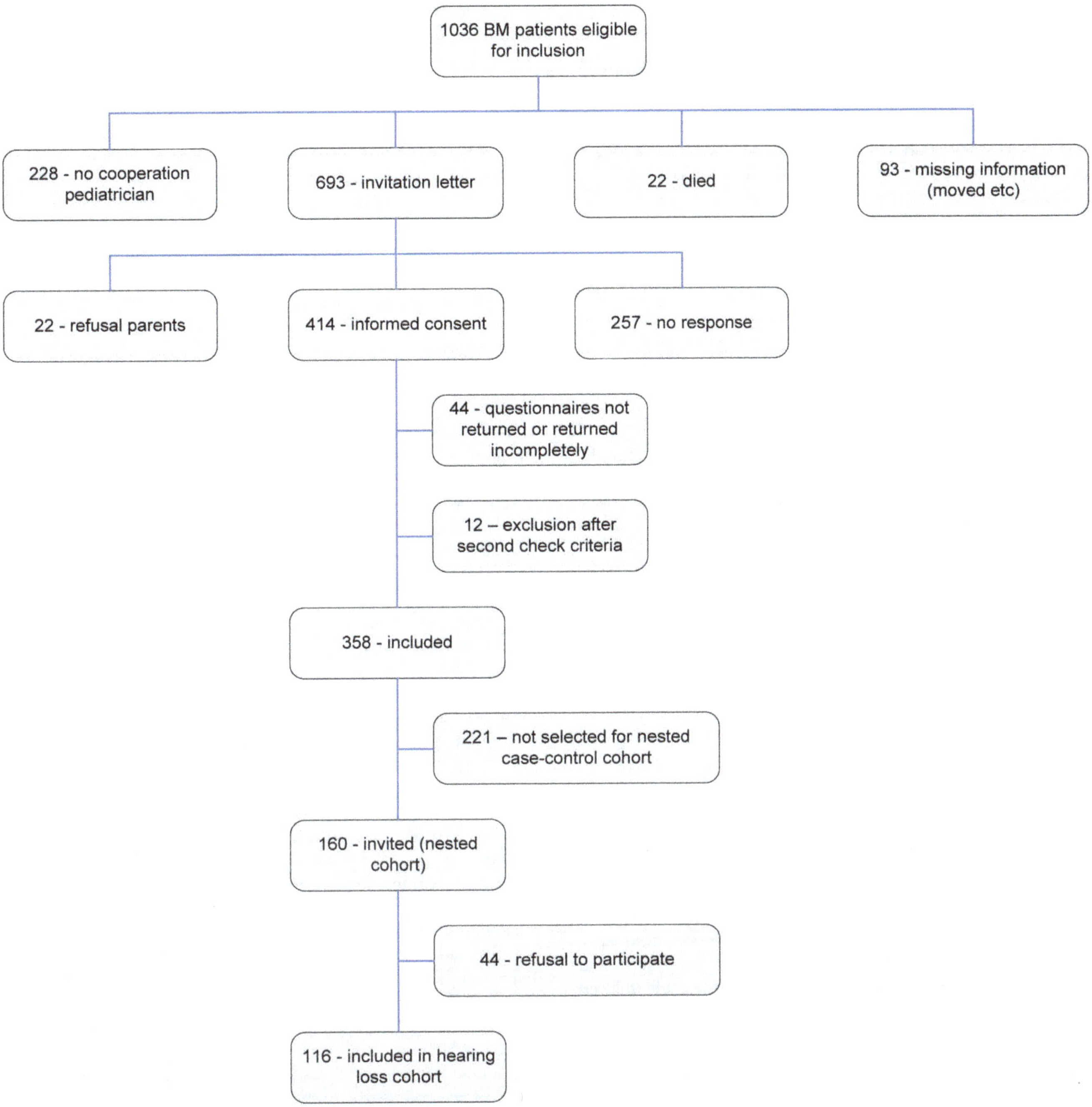

Figure 2. Flow chart of patient inclusion.

information about hearing loss was retrieved from 116 children. Figure 2 presents a flow chart of patient inclusion.

The risk factors evaluated for this study were the five aforementioned independent predictors included in the original model.

Data analysis. Univariate comparison of the distribution of patient characteristics and clinical data in the development and the validation cohort was performed by independent sample t-tests for continuous and χ^2-tests for nominal data. Fisher's Exact test was used if the data did not meet the criteria for a χ^2-test. Statistical significance was considered with 2-tailed p-values of ≤ 0.05.

Missing Data

In both the development and the validation cohort multiple imputation techniques were used for substitution of missing variables. In the development cohort a maximum of 20% of the data was missing per variable [6]. In the validation cohort no more than 5% of the data was missing per variable, resulting in 9.5% missing cases for the whole model. Imputation was repeated five times, resulting in five different datasets [24,25,26].

External Validation

For external validation the discriminative ability of the model in both cohorts was compared. In all sets the model with the original regression coefficients was applied on the data of each individual child. Receiver operating characteristic (ROC) curves of all imputated datasets were constructed for these results predicting the outcome measure "hearing loss". An average area under the curve (AUC) was calculated and compared with the average AUC of the ROC curves of the development cohort. The fit of the model in the validation cohort was tested with the Hosmer-Lemeshow test for goodness of fit. For this test the patients were grouped by decile of predicted probability and differences between expected and observed outcome in the ten groups were tested using χ^2-tests. The five results of these χ^2-tests of the imputated datasets were pooled [27].

The intercept in a logistic regression model results in equal averages of the predicted probabilities and the outcomes when the model is applied in the validation cohort ("calibration in the large"). The slope reflects that the regression coefficients are correctly estimated and that they yield the correct predictions in the validation cohort. We also assessed more specifically whether calibration was successful by separately testing deviations in the intercept and calibration slope when the model was applied in the validation cohort [27].

For each child in the validation cohort the individual risk score was calculated. The distribution of the number of subjects across categories according to these scores were compared between the development and the validation cohort. Positive and negative predictive value, sensitivity and specificity were calculated for different cut-off points and were compared for their clinical value with those composed with the original prediction model.

All data was analyzed using SPSS Statistics 18.0 (IBM Corporation, Somers, NY) and R (The R Project for Statistical Computing).

Results

Table 1 presents the distribution of the patient characteristics, independent predictors and the outcome measure "hearing loss" in the development and the validation cohort. Differences in distribution of characteristics between the two cohorts were observed for the duration of symptoms before admission, consciousness, presentation of the child with meningeal irritation at admission, (duration of) dexamethasone prescription, number of children mechanically ventilated, duration of hospitalization, duration of anti-epileptic therapy and the number of children with focal neurological deficits. There were no significant differences in the distributions of the five predictors of the prediction rule. The incidence of hearing loss was 6.8% in the development cohort and 12.1% in the validation cohort.

External Validation of the Prediction Rule

The average AUC of the ROC curves of the validation cohort was 0.78 (95% CI 0.64–0.92). In the development cohort, the reported AUC was 0.84 (95% CI 0.78–0.91) [6]. The pooled result of the Hosmer-Lemeshow test for goodness of fit of the five datasets was not significant (p-value 0.10), indicating good fit of the model in the validation cohort concerning the similarity of expected and observed cases of hearing loss. When the original model was applied in the validation cohort there was no significant deviation in intercept ($p = 0.07$–0.11) and calibration slope ($p = 0.14$–0.34).

Comparison of the Distribution of Risk Score Categories

Table 2 shows the numbers of subjects across categories of the score for both the development and the validation cohort. Children without hearing loss had an average risk score of 19.6 and children with hearing 45.3. In both cohorts approximately 40% of children without hearing loss score zero points, while only 1 child of all children with hearing loss has a score of 0. While most of the children with hearing loss had a higher score, children without hearing loss were in the groups with high scores as well. Table 3 presents positive and negative predictive value, sensitivity and specificity for the different cut-off points. Using a cut-off point of zero, the sensitivity is 100% while at a score of 1–25 the negative predicted value is 97.8%. At a maximum score on the risk score the specificity is 96.1%, but decreases rapidly at a lower score. The positive predictive value is low (60%). The conclusion of these tables is that sensitivity and negative predictive value are good, but specificity and positive predictive value are poor.

Discussion

In this study, the prediction model for hearing loss after childhood BM was validated successfully in a new independent cohort of school-age children. This is the first validated model for the identification of children at high risk for hearing loss after BM. Our recommendation is that at least the patients who are positive at one or more risk score should achieve timely and frequent hearing evaluation. It is not a replacement for standard hearing tests, but an addition to these tests, to estimate the risk for hearing loss in an early stage of disease.

Despite increasing awareness and recommendation of routine hearing evaluation in the standard follow-up of childhood BM, the amount of children whom hearing is not tested or hearing loss is even missed could be up to 25–30% [6,14]. Relatively little is known about the clinical course of hearing loss after BM. It is not always noticeable or present directly after the infection and fluctuation and deterioration of hearing later in time might occur [28,29,30]. Modern follow-up protocols therefore include a prolonged period of hearing loss evaluation. The only current treatment option in complete and profound hearing loss is cochlear implantation, which may only be possible in a critical period. A good opportunity for hearing restoration could disappear within weeks since labyrinthitis ossificans makes implantation extremely difficult or even impossible [14,31]. This prediction model can be used as a screening tool and can help to identify those children that need special attention and a long follow-up period or more frequent auditory testing even when the first test is negative.

For clinical practice the optimal cut-off point of the risk score has to be defined. Conform Koomen *et al.* we state that hearing loss should not be missed at all and therefore propose a low cut-off value of zero points [6]. In this study it was confirmed that this is the optimal cut-off point. The risk score reaches excellent sensitivity and negative predictive value at this cut-off point. Unfortunately, as one increased the sensitivity of a rule, its specificity tends to decrease (and vice versa). In clinical practice, this indicates that our prediction rule has to be used to select the children at high risk, accepting the fact that a relatively high number of children without hearing impairment will be selected as well. Although with a low cut-off point sensitivity is high, in the validation cohort one child with a score of zero points did have hearing loss, while in the construction cohort no case was missed. We conclude that at least those patients who are positive at one or more factor score should achieve timely and frequent hearing evaluation. In the lower risk group, hearing must be evaluated as well, but it may be considered to perform auditory tests less frequently of for a shorter time period. This may improve the balance between costs and benefit. It can create awareness of the

Table 1. Patient characteristics of the development and validation cohort.

Characteristics	Validation cohort (n = 116)			Development cohort (n = 628)			*p*-value[f] (development vs validation cohort)
	No[a]			No[a]			
Age at infection (years)[b]	116	2.5	(1.8)	628	2.4	(2.0)	0.58
Male gender[c]	116	57	(49.1%)	628	356	(56.7%	0.13
Patient history and physical examination at admission							
Duration of symptoms prior to admission (days)[b]	113	2.4	(1.4)	621	1.9	(1.8)	0.001
Duration of symptoms >2 days[c]	113	36	(31.9%)	621	146	(23.5%)	0.059
Seizures prior to admission[c]	116	8	(6.9%)	628	57	(9.1%)	0.45
Seizures ad admission[c]	116	4	(3.4%)	628	59	(9.4%)	0.035
Decreased consciousness[c]	106	53	(50.0%)	590	401	(68.0%)	<0.001
Rectal temperature (°C)[b]	100	39.1	(1.2)	583	39.1	(1.0)	0.64
Rectal temperature ≥38°C[c]	112	94	(83.9%)	583	502	(86.1%)	0.55
Meningeal irritation[c]	109	78	(71.6%)	628	511	(81.4%)	0.018
Petechiae[c]	115	65	(56.5%)	618	336	(54.4%)	0.67
Focal neurological deficits[c, d]	115	6	(5.2%)	628	58	(9.2%)	0.16
Middle ear infection[c]	93	13	(14.0%)	514	48	(9.3%)	0.17
Laboratory tests							
CSF leukocyte count (/uL)[b]	111	3827	(6778)	548	3736	(6719)	0.90
CSF glucose (mmol/l)[b]	110	2.2	(1.9)	543	2.2	(1.8)	0.94
CSF glucose ≤0.6 mmol/l[c]	110	33	(30.0%)	543	165	(30.4%)	0.94
CSF protein level (g/l)[b]	104	1.8	(1.5)	508	1.8	(1.7)	0.89
Causative pathogen in CSF: (total)	116			628			
N. meningitides		92	(79.3%)		495	(78.8%)	0.91
S. pneumonia		22	(19.0%)		103	(16.4%)	0.50
S. agalactie (group B)		2	(1.7%)		18	(2.9%)	0.76
E. coli		0	(0%)		10	(2.9%)	0.38
L. monocytogenes		0	(0%)		2	(0.3%)	1.0
Bloodculture positive for BM causing pathogen	116	49	(42.2%)	628	300	(47.8%)	0.27
Serum leukocyte count (x1ô9)[b]	116	16.2	(9.4)	613	17.8	(10.7)	0.15
Therapy and clinical course							
Dexamethasone prescribed[c]	110	19	(17.3%)	628	170	(27.1%)	0.029
Duration dexamethasone therapy (days)[b]	110	0.6	(1.5)	602	0.9	(1.8)	0.025
Mechanical ventilation[c]	116	14	(12.1%)	627	39	(6.2%)	0.025
Duration of hospitalization (days)[b]	115	12.9	(8.0)	618	14.7	(9.4)	0.046
Seizures during hospitalization[c]	115	8	(7.0%)	628	64	(10.2%)	0.28
Duration of anti-epileptic therapy (days)[b]	112	0.6	(2.6)	610	1.4	(5.7)	0.011
Focal neurological deficits[c, d]	114	7	(6.1%)	627	94	(15.0%)	0.011
(transient) ataxia[c,e]	115	3	(2.6%)	628	16	(2.5%)	0.97
Outcome measure							
Hearing loss	116	14	(12.1%)	628	43	(6.8%)	0.052

[a]Number of subjects the variable was obtained.
[b]Mean (standard deviation).
[c]Number of subjects (%).
[d]Focal neurological deficits are defined as cranial nerve deficits, increased or decreased reflexes of arms or legs, increased or decreased tonus of arms or legs, focal convulsions and ataxia.
[e](Transient) ataxia was defined as signs of ataxia, which lasted at least until discharge from the hospital, as documented in the medical records.
[f]P-value: independent sample t-test for continuous data; χ^2-test for nominal data, or Fisher's Exact test if the data does not meet the criteria for χ^2-test.
Abbrevations: No. = number, CSF = cerebrospinal fluid.

Table 2. Distribution of children with and without hearing loss across categories of the risk score.

Risk score	Children in the cohort				Children with hearing loss				Children without hearing loss			
	Development (n = 628)		Validation (n = 116)		Development (n = 43)		Validation (n = 14)		Development (n = 585)		Validation (n = 102)	
	cumulative		cumulative		cumulative		cumulative		cumulative		cumulative	
	n (%)	n (%)	n (%)	n (%)	n (%)	n (%)	n (%)	n (%)	n (%)	n (%)	n (%)	n (%)
Score 0	236 (38)		45 (39)		0 (0)		1 (7)		236 (40)		44 (43)	
Score 1–24	86 (14)	322 (51)	14 (12)	59 (51)	2 (5)	2 (5)	2 (14)	3 (21)	84 (14)	320 (55)	12 (12)	56 (55)
Score 25–36	87 (14)	409 (65)	15 (13)	74 (64)	5 (11)	7 (16)	1 (7)	4 (29)	82 (14)	402 (69)	14 (14)	70 (69)
Score 37–63	197 (31)	606 (96)	32 (27)	106 (91)	24 (56)	31 (72)	4 (29)	8 (57)	173 (30)	575 (98)	28 (27)	98 (96)
Score ≥64	22 (3)	628 (100)	10 (9)	116 (100)	12 (28)	43 (100)	6 (43)	14 (100)	10 (2)	585 (100)	4 (4)	102 (100)

importance of hearing evaluation in clinicians and the parents in an early stage of disease.

Further, BM and subsequent morbidity is considerably more prevalent in developing countries where adequate follow-up, hearing tests, financial resources and support in case of auditory deficits are scarcely available [32]. Prediction models should be developed these countries as well and may help to select and at least test the group that urgently needs to achieve hearing evaluation.

This study has several strengths. This is the first model developed and externally validated that predicts hearing loss after BM in childhood. In the last decade, many prediction models have been designed and presented in literature. Before implementation in practice is possible, external validation is an essential step [16,17,18]. However, the majority of proposed models have never been validated [18,33]. Therefore, successful validation of our model is an important step forward in the development of a complete protocol for the follow-up of children who suffered from BM.

In general, the discrimination of a prediction model is interpreted to be fair, good or excellent when the AUC is or 0.7–0.8, 0.8–0.9 or 0.9–1.0, respectively. This model has an AUC of 0.84 in the development cohort and an AUC of 0.78 in the validation cohort, thus can be at least considered as fair.

Further, state of the art methodology is used and described clearly. Therefore it may be easily to reproduce in a wide range of future studies.

The validation cohort was constructed using the nested cohort approach while in the development of the rule the total initial cohort was used [6,20]. From the 1036 patients selected from the NRLBM database, 116 were included. Most children were excluded in the first step because approached pediatricians or parents refused participation or because the parents could not be contacted due to missing or incorrect address data. From the resulting 361 children 116 were included for validation of the hearing loss model. This nested cohort design, in which only a subset of cases and controls are randomly selected for further analysis, is a known and appreciated methodology that results in more efficiency with reference to time and financial resources [21]. This stepwise construction may lead to differences in case mix between de development cohort and the validation cohort due to selection. The incidence of sensorineural hearing loss was 6.8% in the development versus 12.1% in the validation cohort (p-value = 0.052). This difference may be explained by the fact that in the development cohort 27% of the children were not tested for hearing loss, resulting in underestimation of the incidence [6]. Further, an increase in awareness in the period of approximately seven years between the two studies might have resulted in increased follow-up and incidence of hearing loss. Last, the selection process of the nested cohort described above may also be responsible.

Case mix differences were also found in patient characteristics and risk factors, such as: duration of symptoms >2 days, meningeal irritation, dexamethasone therapy, mechanical ventilation, duration of anti-epileptic therapy and focal neurological deficits. These differences could have been responsible for a smaller spread in the risk of hearing loss (0–91% in the development versus 2–70% in the validation cohort). This may in turn be responsible for the small drop in discrimination of the model in the validation cohort. Because the differences in case mix

Table 3. Positive and negative predictive value, sensitivity and specificity for the different cut-off points of the prediction rule.

Risk score cut-off point	Positive predictive value (%)		Negative predictive value (%)		Sensitivity (%)		Specificity (%)	
	Development	Validation	Development	Validation	Development	Validation	Development	Validation
Score ≥0	6.8	12.1			100.0	100.0	0.0	0.0
Score ≥1	11.0	18.3	100.0	97.8	100.0	92.9	40.3	43.1
Score ≥25	13.4	19.3	99.4	94.9	95.3	78.6	54.7	54.9
Score ≥37	16.4	23.8	98.3	94.6	83.7	71.4	68.7	68.6
Score ≥64	54.5	60.0	94.9	92.5	27.9	42.9	98.3	96.1

may partly be explained by the selection processes, we must be careful to draw conclusions from the comparison of the incidence of hearing loss and risk factors, while some selection bias may have occurred.

Though, for the external validation selection bias is not a major issue: the development cohort appeared to be a representative sample of the pediatric BM population of that time: The NRLBM receives approximately 90% of the isolates of Dutch BM patients, and the 628 children included where very similar compared with the 1605 eligible children regarding, sex, age, and causative pathogens [6].

Validation samples may differ from development samples in predictor (patient) characteristics and in outcome frequency. These differences may, as we discussed, also occur during the selection of patients in the development sample and not only depend on selection of patients in the validation sample. Differences between samples may be caused by sampling variability or true differences, and not by selection bias per se. The goal of external validation is to investigate to what extend these differences influence the generalizability of the prediction model. Sampling variability (or working with smaller validation samples) will often show a small influence on the performance of the prediction model. We showed that at low and high risk score categories, which are most important for clinical practice, the model performed equally well in the validation as in the development sample [16,18,34,35].

Information bias may have occurred. Risk factors and the outcome were determined retrospectively, with a risk of bias and missing data. To minimize the chance of bias, collection and interpretation of clinical data from the medical files was performed in a standardized w ay, and consensus meetings were held when there was any doubt about how to interpret the medical files. The diagnosis "perceptive hearing loss of >25 dB" is made in the Netherlands by clinicians or audiologists by standard tests. Multiple imputation techniques were used for substitution of missing data, which is currently the most reliable strategy to deal with missing information on covariates [26,36,37,38].

Further, sample size of the validation cohort was small. A frequently used general rule in the development of clinical prediction models is that the ratio events per variable (EVP) should be approximately 10 [39]. In the development cohort there were 43 events for 5 predictors included in the model, resulting in an EVP of 8.6. For external validation new insights in sample size issues are developed in recent years. It has been suggested that to detect minor changes in discrimination and calibration, and prevent type II error (the Null hypothesis of equal model performance is falsely not rejected), the validation cohort should contain at least 100 events and 100 non-events [40]. The sample size of our validation cohort is limited, and therefore small differences in calibration might have been missed.

Future Perspectives

It is hypothesized that the distribution of BM pathogens has changed since the introduction of these vaccines and therefore the model will not perform well in the contemporary population. Since the development of the prediction rule two new vaccines against *N. meningitidis* serogroup C and high frequency serotypes of *S. pneumoniae* were introduced in the Netherlands and other western countries: Accompanied by a spontaneous decrease of *N. meningitidis* serogroup B infections this resulted in a dramatic decrease in incidence of BM. Serotype replacement with increasing incidence of infections has not yet occurred for *N. meningitidis*, but new outbreaks with non-vaccine-serotypes are possible and have occurred in history [41,42,43]. For *S. pneumoniae* there is a net reduction of invasive infections but an increase in infections with non-vaccine-serotypes is observed [44]. Therefore, we should be careful expecting BM to become and stay a rare disease, and prediction rules for sequelae remain valuable. In a recent study our group simulated a population without the seven serotypes of *S. pneumoniae* included in the vaccine, and showed that the model remains stable in this situation [45]. To investigate whether the long-term consequences of vaccination have impact on the performance of the model, another validation study in children that were infected more recently is planned.

Another important development is the rapidly increasing knowledge on the influence of genetics on the course of diseases. This also applies for BM and hearing loss, and in recent publications an effort was made to disclose the influence of genetic variation in the immune response and the course of the disease in children. Van Well *et al.* described a strong association between host genetic polymorphisms in pathogen recognition receptors and hearing loss after BM extracted from both development and validation cohort described in this study [46]. Additional analyses will be performed to study whether our model can be extended with genetic factors to predict post-meningitis hearing loss even more accurately.

We conclude that we created and externally validated a clinical useful tool in addition to regular auditory testing for the identification of children at high risk for hearing loss after BM. In the future larger development and validation studies must be performed, in which hearing loss is measured prospectively and genetic risk factors are included in the construction of the prediction model. In our opinion, international cooperation is the answer to the problem of decreasing incidence in the development of prediction models.

Author Contributions

Supervision of the analyses: CBT RJBJG AMVF. Revising the manuscript: RJBJG CBT LS AMVF. Conceived and designed the experiments: RCJJ IK RJBJG AMVF. Performed the experiments: RCDJ IK. Analyzed the data: RCJJ MSS CT MWH. Contributed reagents/materials/analysis tools: LS. Wrote the paper: RCJJ MSS CBT MWH IK AMVF.

References

1. McIntyre PB, O'Brien KL, Greenwood B, van de Beek D (2012) Effect of vaccines on bacterial meningitis worldwide. Lancet 380: 1703–1711.
2. Organization WH (2008) The global burden of disease: 2004 update. Geneva: Department of Health Statistics and Informatics in the Information, Evidence and Research Cluster of WHO.
3. Fortnum H, Davis A (1993) Hearing impairment in children after bacterial meningitis: incidence and resource implications. Br J Audiol 27: 43–52.
4. Baraff LJ, Lee SI, Schriger DL (1993) Outcomes of bacterial meningitis in children: a meta-analysis. Pediatr Infect Dis J 12: 389–394.
5. Husain E, Chawla R, Dobson S, Dele Davies H (2006) Epidemiology and outcome of bacterial meningitis in Canadian children: 1998–1999. Clin Invest Med 29: 131–135.
6. Koomen I, Grobbee DE, Roord JJ, Donders R, Jennekens-Schinkel A, et al. (2003) Hearing loss at school age in survivors of bacterial meningitis: assessment, incidence, and prediction. Pediatrics 112: 1049–1053.
7. Oostenbrink R, Maas M, Moons KG, Moll HA (2002) Sequelae after bacterial meningitis in childhood. Scand J Infect Dis 34: 379–382.
8. Wellman MB, Sommer DD, McKenna J (2003) Sensorineural hearing loss in postmeningitic children. Otology & neurotology : official publication of the American Otological Society, American Neurotology Society [and] European Academy of Otology and Neurotology 24: 907–912.
9. Worsoe L, Caye-Thomasen P, Brandt CT, Thomsen J, Ostergaard C (2010) Factors associated with the occurrence of hearing loss after pneumococcal meningitis. Clin Infect Dis 51: 917–924.

10. Fortnum HM (1992) Hearing impairment after bacterial meningitis: a review. Arch Dis Child 67: 1128–1133.
11. Moeller MP, Tomblin JB, Yoshinaga-Itano C, Connor CM, Jerger S (2007) Current state of knowledge: language and literacy of children with hearing impairment. Ear and hearing 28: 740–753.
12. Yoshinaga-Itano C (1999) Benefits of early intervention for children with hearing loss. Otolaryngologic clinics of North America 32: 1089–1102.
13. Dodds A, Tyszkiewicz E, Ramsden R (1997) Cochlear implantation after bacterial meningitis: the dangers of delay. Arch Dis Child 76: 139–140.
14. Merkus P, Free RH, Mylanus EA, Stokroos R, Metselaar M, et al. (2010) Dutch Cochlear Implant Group (CI-ON) Consensus Protocol on Postmeningitis Hearing Evaluation and Treatment. Otol Neurotol.
15. Laupacis A, Sekar N, Stiell IG (1997) Clinical prediction rules. A review and suggested modifications of methodological standards. JAMA 277: 488–494.
16. Altman DG, Vergouwe Y, Royston P, Moons KG (2009) Prognosis and prognostic research: validating a prognostic model. Bmj 338: b605.
17. Bleeker SE, Moll HA, Steyerberg EW, Donders AR, Derksen-Lubsen G, et al. (2003) External validation is necessary in prediction research: a clinical example. Journal of clinical epidemiology 56: 826–832.
18. Toll DB, Janssen KJ, Vergouwe Y, Moons KG (2008) Validation, updating and impact of clinical prediction rules: a review. J Clin Epidemiol 61: 1085–1094.
19. Netherlands Reference Laboratory for Bacterial Meningitis (AMC/RIVM) (2011) Bacterial meningitis in the Netherlands: annual report 2010. Amsterdam: University of Amsterdam.
20. Koomen I, Grobbee DE, Roord JJ, Jennekens-Schinkel A, van der Lei HD, et al. (2004) Prediction of academic and behavioural limitations in school-age survivors of bacterial meningitis. Acta Paediatr 93: 1378–1385.
21. Biesheuvel CJ, Vergouwe Y, Oudega R, Hoes AW, Grobbee DE, et al. (2008) Advantages of the nested case-control design in diagnostic research. BMC Med Res Methodol 8: 48.
22. Landgraf JM, Abetz L, Ware JE (1996) The CHQ user's manual. Boston. The Health Institute, New England Medical Center. Boston: The Health Institute, New England Medical Center.
23. Raat H, Bonsel GJ, Essink-Bot ML, Landgraf JM, Gemke RJ (2002) Reliability and validity of comprehensive health status measures in children: The Child Health Questionnaire in relation to the Health Utilities Index. J Clin Epidemiol 55: 67–76.
24. Janssen KJ, Vergouwe Y, Donders AR, Harrell FE, Jr., Chen Q, et al. (2009) Dealing with missing predictor values when applying clinical prediction models. Clin Chem 55: 994–1001.
25. Vergouwe Y, Royston P, Moons KG, Altman DG (2009) Development and validation of a prediction model with missing predictor data: a practical approach. J Clin Epidemiol.
26. Moons KG, Donders RA, Stijnen T, Harrell FE, Jr (2006) Using the outcome for imputation of missing predictor values was preferred. J Clin Epidemiol 59: 1092–1101.
27. Marshall A, Altman DG, Holder RL, Royston P (2009) Combining estimates of interest in prognostic modelling studies after multiple imputation: current practice and guidelines. BMC Med Res Methodol 9: 57.
28. Richardson MP, Reid A, Tarlow MJ, Rudd PT (1997) Hearing loss during bacterial meningitis. Arch Dis Child 76: 134–138.
29. Jayarajan V, Rangan S (1999) Delayed deterioration of hearing following bacterial meningitis. J Laryngol Otol 113: 1011–1014.
30. Brookhouser PE, Auslander MC, Meskan ME (1988) The pattern and stability of postmeningitic hearing loss in children. Laryngoscope 98: 940–948.
31. Merkus P, van Furth AM, Goverts ST, Suer M, Smits CF, et al. (2007) [Postmeningitis deafness in young children: action warranted before obliteration of the cochlea]. Ned Tijdschr Geneeskd 151: 1209–1213.
32. van de Beek D (2012) Progress and challenges in bacterial meningitis. Lancet 380: 1623–1624.
33. Maguire JL, Kulik DM, Laupacis A, Kuppermann N, Uleryk EM, et al. (2011) Clinical Prediction Rules for Children: A Systematic Review. Pediatrics.
34. Altman DG, Royston P (2000) What do we mean by validating a prognostic model? Stat Med 19: 453–473.
35. Moons KG, Kengne AP, Grobbee DE, Royston P, Vergouwe Y, et al. (2012) Risk prediction models: II. External validation, model updating, and impact assessment. Heart 98: 691–698.
36. Donders AR, van der Heijden GJ, Stijnen T, Moons KG (2006) Review: a gentle introduction to imputation of missing values. J Clin Epidemiol 59: 1087–1091.
37. Janssen KJ, Donders AR, Harrell FE, Jr., Vergouwe Y, Chen Q, et al. (2010) Missing covariate data in medical research: to impute is better than to ignore. J Clin Epidemiol 63: 721–727.
38. van der Heijden GJ, Donders AR, Stijnen T, Moons KG (2006) Imputation of missing values is superior to complete case analysis and the missing-indicator method in multivariable diagnostic research: a clinical example. J Clin Epidemiol 59: 1102–1109.
39. Steyerberg EW (2009) Clinical Prediction Models: A Practical Approach to Development, Validation, and Updating; Gail M, Krickeberg K, Samet J, Tsiatis A, Wong W, editors. New York: Springer Science+Business Media. 500 p.
40. Vergouwe Y, Steyerberg EW, Eijkemans MJ, Habbema JD (2005) Substantial effective sample sizes were required for external validation studies of predictive logistic regression models. J Clin Epidemiol 58: 475–483.
41. Peltola H (1983) Meningococcal disease: still with us. Rev Infect Dis 5: 71–91.
42. Stephens DS, Greenwood B, Brandtzaeg P (2007) Epidemic meningitis, meningococcaemia, and Neisseria meningitidis. Lancet 369: 2196–2210.
43. Netherlands Reference Laboratory for Bacterial Meningitis (2010) Bacterial meningitis in the Netherlands: annual report 2009. Amsterdam, The Netherlands: AMC/RIVM.
44. Rodenburg GD, de Greeff SC, Jansen AG, de Melker HE, Schouls LM, et al. (2010) Effects of pneumococcal conjugate vaccine 2 years after its introduction, the Netherlands. Emerg Infect Dis 16: 816–823.
45. Commandeur AE, de Jonge RC, Koomen I, Spanjaard L, van Furth AM, et al. (2010) Simulated effect of pneumococcal vaccination in the Netherlands on existing rules constructed in a non-vaccinated cohort predicting sequelae after bacterial meningitis. BMC Infectious Diseases 10: 259.
46. van Well GT, Sanders MS, Ouburg S, van Furth AM, Morre SA (2012) Polymorphisms in Toll-like receptors 2, 4, and 9 are highly associated with hearing loss in survivors of bacterial meningitis. PLoS One 7: e35837.

23

Deafness Gene Expression Patterns in the Mouse Cochlea Found by Microarray Analysis

Hidekane Yoshimura, Yutaka Takumi*, Shin-ya Nishio, Nobuyoshi Suzuki, Yoh-ichiro Iwasa, Shin-ichi Usami

Department of Otorhinolaryngology, Shinshu University School of Medicine, Matsumoto, Nagano, Japan

Abstract

Background: Tonotopy is one of the most fundamental principles of auditory function. While gradients in various morphological and physiological characteristics of the cochlea have been reported, little information is available on gradient patterns of gene expression. In addition, the audiograms in autosomal dominant non syndromic hearing loss can be distinctive, however, the mechanism that accounts for that has not been clarified. We thought that it is possible that tonotopic gradients of gene expression within the cochlea account for the distinct audiograms.

Methodology/Principal Findings: We compared expression profiles of genes in the cochlea between the apical, middle, and basal turns of the mouse cochlea by microarray technology and quantitative RT-PCR. Of 24,547 genes, 783 annotated genes expressed more than 2-fold. The most remarkable finding was a gradient of gene expression changes in four genes (*Pou4f3*, *Slc17a8*, *Tmc1*, and *Crym*) whose mutations cause autosomal dominant deafness. Expression of these genes was greater in the apex than in the base. Interestingly, expression of the *Emilin-2* and *Tectb* genes, which may have crucial roles in the cochlea, was also greater in the apex than in the base.

Conclusions/Significance: This study provides baseline data of gradient gene expression in the cochlea. Especially for genes whose mutations cause autosomal dominant non syndromic hearing loss (*Pou4f3*, *Slc17a8*, *Tmc1*, and *Crym*) as well as genes important for cochlear function (*Emilin-2* and *Tectb*), gradual expression changes may help to explain the various pathological conditions.

Editor: Manuel S. Malmierca, University of Salamanca- Institute for Neuroscience of Castille and Leon and Medical School, Spain

Funding: This study was supported by a Health and Labour Sciences Research Grant for Comprehensive Research on Disability Health and Welfare from the Ministry of Health, Labour and Welfare of Japan (S.U.), and by a Grant-in-Aid for Scientific Research from the (then) Ministry of Education, Science and Culture of Japan (http://www.mext.go.jp/english/) (S.U., Y.T.). The funders had no role in study design, data collection and analysis, decision to publish, or preparation of the manuscript.

Competing Interests: The authors have declared that no competing interests exist.

* E-mail: takumi@shinshu-u.ac.jp

Introduction

The auditory systems of mammalians that perceive sounds are organized based on the separation of complex sounds into their component frequencies (tonotopy). Tonotopy begins at the level of the auditory sensory epithelium where specific frequencies are distributed along the tonotopic axis of the mammalian cochlea [1].

Gradients in morphological and physiological characteristics of the inner ear in different species have also been reported [1]. In addition, gene expression gradients along the tonotopic axis in chicken auditory epithelium have been also reported [2]. However, few reports are available on mammalian gene expression gradients.

Hearing loss that disturbs normal communication is a common sensory disorder worldwide. Most congenital or childhood onset hearing impairments are non syndromic. As of Apr. 2013, 27 dominant, 40 recessive and 3 X-linked genes whose mutations cause non syndromic hearing loss have been reported according to the Hereditary Hearing loss Homepage (http://hereditaryhearingloss.org/).

Interestingly, the audiograms of autosomal dominant non syndromic hearing loss (ADNSHL) can be distinctive, and thus useful to identify the gene responsible [3]. For example, mutations in *WFS1* are found in 75% of families with dominantly inherited hearing loss that initially affects the low frequencies while sparing the high frequencies [4,5]. On the contrary, many of the mutations in ADNSHL, like *KCNQ4*, *DFNA5*, *POU4F3*, and *SLC17A8*, affect the high frequencies [6]. However, the mechanism that accounts for the distinct frequency patterns has not been clarified. We hypothesized that certain gene expression patterns might show a gradient within the cochlea that could, at least in part, correspond with the distinct shapes of audiograms in ADNSHL.

Microarray analysis, which provides whole gene expression data, can be used to analyze differential gene expression among tissues [7]. In this study, to analyze the mechanism of the distinct audiograms in ADNSHL, we examined and compared gradient gene expression profiles, in particular ADNSHL genes, between the apical, middle, and basal turns of the cochlea by microarray technology.

Materials and Methods

Tissue dissection and RNA extraction

Four C57BL/6 mice aged 6 weeks were euthanized by decapitation under deep anesthesia induced by an intraperitoneal injection containing 75 mg/kg Ketamine (Daiichi Sankyo, Tokyo, Japan) and 32.4 mg/kg Pentobarbital Sodium (Kyoritsu, Tokyo, Japan). Inner ears were rapidly extracted from the temporal bone and transferred into RNA*later* solution (Ambion, Austin, TX, USA). After removing the otic capsule, the cochlea including the lateral wall comprising the stria vascularis, spiral ligament, and spiral prominence, the organ of Corti and the spiral ganglion neurons were dissected and separated into the apical, middle and basal turns (Fig. 1). All of these dissections were performed in RNA*later* solution to prevent RNA degradation. Total RNA was were extracted using the QIAGEN RNeasy Mini Kit (QIAGEN, Hilden, Germany) according to the manufacturer's protocol. The quality of the extracted total RNA was assessed with the Agilent 2100 Bioanalyzer (Agilent Technologies, Waldbronn, Germany) and found to be adequate for microarray analysis (data not shown).

RNA labeling and purification

Total RNA (25 ng each) was reverse transcribed with the Low Input Quick Amp Whole Transcriptome Labeling Kit (Agilent Technologies). After reverse transcription process, labeled cRNA was synthesized from cDNA by using T7 RNA polymerase mix and cyanine 3-CTP according to the manufacturer's instructions. Labeled cRNA was purified using the Rneasy Mini kit (QIAGEN).

Microarray hybridization

To analyze gene expression of each cochlea turn, 12 SurePrint G3 Mouse Exon Microarrays (Agilent Technologies), which were spotted with 165,984 exon probes (24,547 genes), were hybridized to labeled cRNA (4 microarrays were used for each turn sample). Prior to the hybridization step, Cyanine 3-labeled cRNAs were fragmented using 25X fragmentation buffer at 60°C in a water bath for 30 min and then hybridized to a microarray slide for 17 hours at 65°C in a hybridization oven and washed using Gene Expression Wash Buffer (Agilent Technologies).

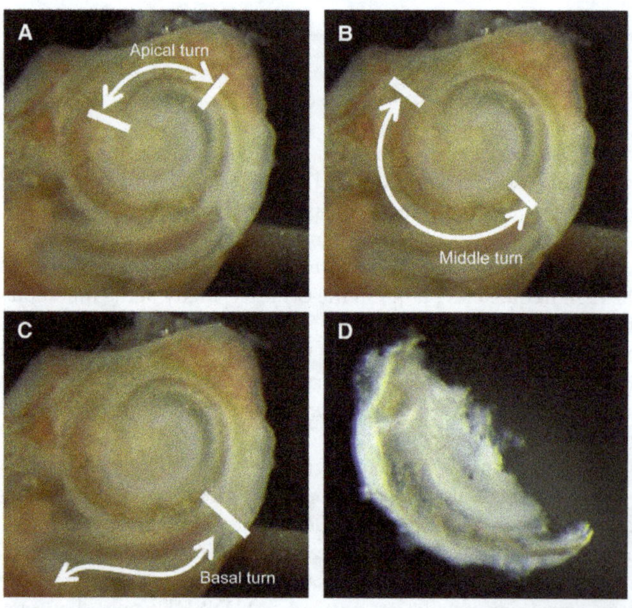

Figure 1. Microscopical image of the mouse cochlea (right ear). Bars indicate the incision points for each turn sample. A: apical turn, B: middle turn, C: basal turn, D: dissection example

Microarray scanning and statistical analysis

Fluorescence intensities were measured with the Agilent Microarray Scanner (Agilent) using the scanning protocols specific for each microarray assay and raw microarray image files were created. The expression data were extracted from raw microarray image files using Agilent Feature Extraction Image Analysis Software (Version 10.7.3.1). The software also generated quality control reports using the protocol specific for the microarray assays as well as data files for analysis with GeneSpring GX (Version 11, Agilent Technologies). Signal intensities for each probe were normalized to the 75th percentile without baseline transformation.

Data for each microarray was analyzed using the manufacturer's workflow in GeneSpring GX. For gene-level analysis, the average expression levels of each exon probe were used. Then averages of four microarray data of each cochlea turn (base, middle, and apex) were used for comparison analysis (one-way analysis of variance (ANOVA)) by using GeneSpring GX. The microarray data have been lodged in the Gene Expression Omnibus (http://www.ncbi.nlm.nih.gov/geo/) as accession number: GSE53863.

Quantitative RT-PCR

To confirm the microarray analysis results, qPCR was performed on 9 deafness genes. Reverse transcription was performed with 4 total RNA samples of each cochlea turn by using High Capacity RNA-to-cDNA Kit (Life Technologies, Foster City, CA, USA) as described in the manufacturer's procedure. The TaqMan probe for each gene was selected from the TaqMan Gene Expression Assay system (https://products.appliedbiosystems.com/ab/en/US/adirect/ab?;cmd=ABGEKeywordSearch,Life Technologies). *Gapdh*, *Actb*, *Rps17*, *Rpl30*, *Atp6*, and *Ipo8* were chosen as internal control genes. The estimated gene expression level (EL) was normalized to the internal control gene expression level and data are presented as the mean of $\log_2$EL.

Ethics Statement

All experimental procedures were performed in accordance with the regulations for animal experimentation of Shinshu University. These experiments were approved by Shinshu University institutional animal care and use committee.

Results

Scatter plot analysis

To confirm the technical stability of cochlear dissection and RNA extraction and to estimate global gene expression change, we performed scatter plot analysis of the gene expression profiles of each cochlear turn. In each comparison of basal, middle and apical cochlear turns, the gene expression patterns were quite similar and most gene expression changes were less than 2-fold (Fig. 2).

In detail, the gene expression profile of the apical turn of the cochlea was more similar to that of the middle turn than the basal turn. The scatter plot of the apical turn vs. basal turn showed lower correlation than the others. From these results, the gene expression of each cochlear turn clearly indicated gradual gene expression change according to the tonotopic axis.

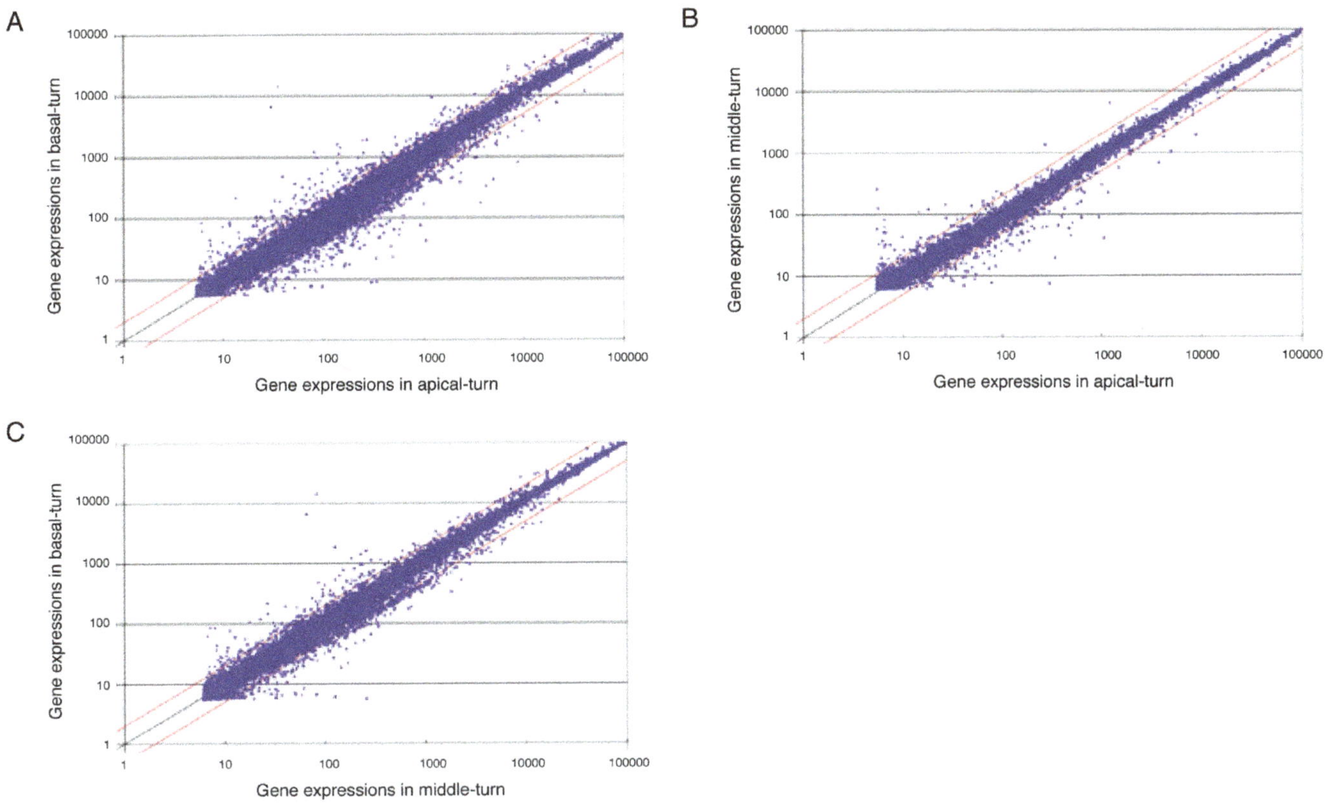

Figure 2. Scatter plot analysis of gene expression profile of each cochlear turn. Black lines indicate equal gene expression and red lines indicate 2-fold gene expression. A: apical turn vs. basal turn, B: apical turn vs. middle turn, C: middle turn vs. basal turn.

Genes indicate differential expression in each cochlear turn

To analyze difference in gene expression, we focused on the genes, which were expressed 2-fold or more in one turn than in the other turn. Each of the gene expression levels was estimated from the average value of four microarray results for independent mouse samples and one-way ANOVA was employed before the comparative analysis as written in the material and methods. Of 24,547 genes, 941 differed more than 2-fold. Of these genes, 783 genes (3.2%: 783/24547) had been annotated and the others were predicted genes (Table S1).

Out of the 783 annotated genes, 747 were differentially expressed between apex and base; 51 were differentially expressed between apex and middle, and 458 genes were differentially expressed between middle and base (some genes were in more than one group) (Table 1). This is consistent with the notion that those genes whose expression changes showed an apical-to-basal gradient along the tonotopic axis. The complete list of differentially expressed genes for each of the three comparisons (i.e., apex vs. base, apex vs. middle, middle vs. base) is indicated as a supporting information file (Tables S2, S3, and S4).

Overall tonotopic expression pattern

Most (96.2%) genes expression changes did not differ and only a limited number of genes showed tonotopic expression pattern.

Tonotopic expression of the genes responsible for hearing loss

The results of gene expression analysis of each cochlear turn showed that 4 ADNSHL genes (*Pou4f3*, *Slc17a8*, *Tmc1*, and *Crym*) and 9 autosomal recessive non syndromic hearing loss genes (*Otof*, *Strc*, *Ush1c*, *Pcdh15*, *Grxcr1*, *Dfnb59*, *Slc26a5*, *Lhfpl5*, and *Ptprq*) were changed 2-fold or more (Table 2). Interestingly, expression of

Table 1. The numbers of differentially expressed genes for apex vs. base, apex vs. middle, middle vs. base.

apex vs. base		**apex vs. middle**		**middle vs. base**	
up in apex	**up in base**	**up in apex**	**up in middle**	**up in middle**	**up in base**
571/783	176/783	38/783	13/783	389/783	69/783
747/783		51/783		458/783	

Table 2. Gene expression levels of corresponding genes for non syndromic hearing loss in each cochlea turn.

Gene Symbol	Gene Name [Mus musculus]	Deafness causing Locus	Microarray						Quantitative RT-PCR		
			Signal Intensity Averages			Fold Change			Fold Change		
			apex	middle	base	middle/base	apex/middle	apex/base	apex/base	middle/base	apex/middle
Pou4f3	POU domain, class 4, transcription factor 3	DFNA15	200.1	167.3	77.9	2.33	1.09	2.52	3.19	2.59	1.23
Slc17a8	solute carrier family 17, member 8	DFNA25	152.3	104.8	47.7	2.36	1.33	3.15	5.07	2.49	2.03
Tmc1	transmembrane channel-like gene family 1	DFNA36, DFNB7	90.4	58.5	35.9	1.78	1.42	2.52	2.01	1.97	1.02
Crym	crystallin, mu	DFNA40	450.5	301.5	140.1	2.29	1.37	3.14	3.83	2.35	1.63
Otof	otoferlin	DFNB9	287.3	210.6	108.8	2.07	1.26	2.61	3.33	2.83	1.18
Strc	stereocilin	DFNB16	134.0	80.8	36.0	2.39	1.52	3.65	N/A	N/A	N/A
Ush1c	Usher syndrome 1C homolog (human)	DFNB18	211.3	146.7	102.5	1.54	1.33	2.04	1.48	1.39	1.07
Pcdh15	protocadherin 15	DFNB23	80.0	50.2	28.6	1.88	1.47	2.76	4.32	1.44	3.00
Grxcr1	glutaredoxin, cysteine rich 1	DFNB25	50.9	31.4	12.7	2.65	1.48	3.93	N/A	N/A	N/A
Dfnb59	deafness, autosomal recessive 59 (human)	DFNB59	216.5	187.2	86.7	2.34	1.07	2.50	N/A	N/A	N/A
Slc26a5	solute carrier family 26, member 5	DFNB61	358.4	201.6	47.0	4.70	1.63	7.65	8.41	5.87	1.86
Lhfpl5	lipoma HMGIC fusion partner-like 5	DFNB67	1228.7	902.1	402.9	2.43	1.26	3.07	4.90	2.63	1.86
Ptprq	protein tyrosine phosphatase, receptor type, Q	DFNB84	125.0	63.2	30.8	2.18	1.83	3.99	N/A	N/A	N/A

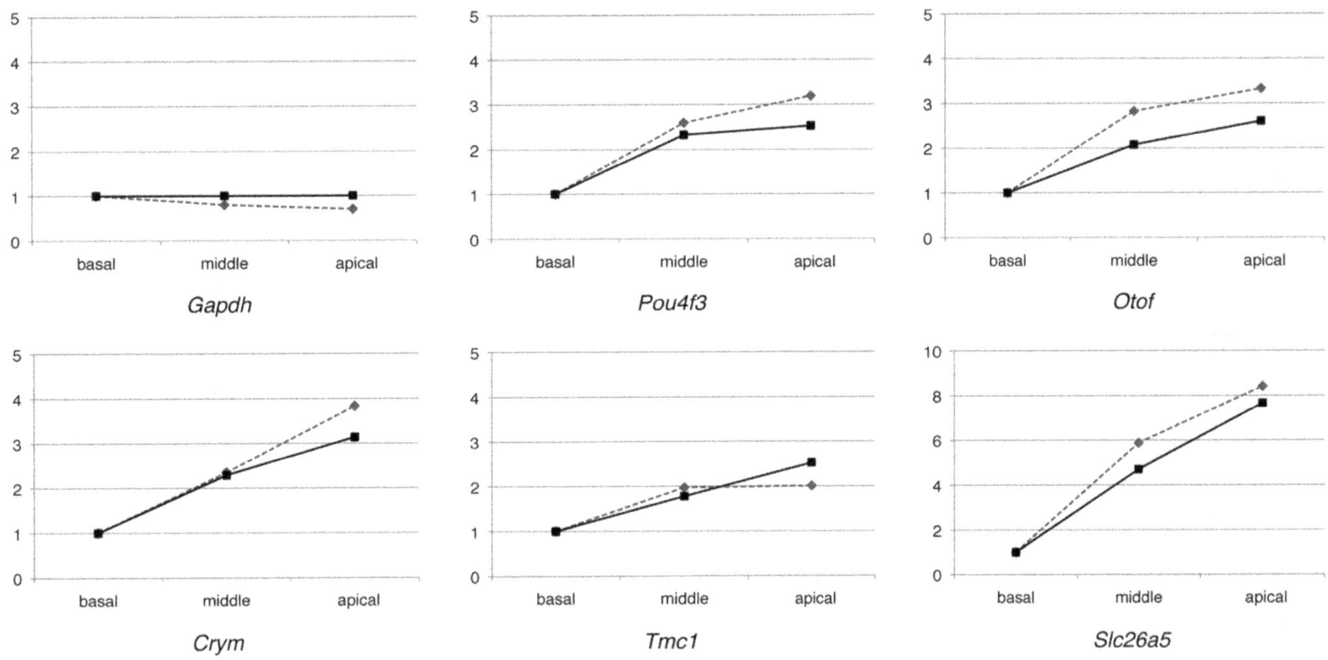

Figure 3. Gene expression patterns found by microarray analysis and quantitative RT-PCR. Values of each gene expression are indicated as a relative value to the basal turn. The expression level of each gene measured by microarray analysis (solid lines) was comparable with the level measured by quantitative RT-PCR (dotted lines).

those was greater in the apex than in the base. However, there were no significant differences in *WFS1* gene expression.

Tonotopic expression of sodium, potassium, and calcium channels

Many sodium, potassium, and calcium channels were differentially expressed between the basal and apical turns. Specifically, expression of most potassium voltage-gated channels (i.e., *Kcna1*, *Kcna2*, *Kcnab2*, *Kcnab3*, *Kcnb2*, *Kcnc1*, *Kcnc3*, *Kcnd2*, *Kcne4*, *Kcnh2*, *Kcnh5*, *Kcnq3*, and *Kcns3*) was greater in the apex. There was also differential expression of voltage-dependent calcium channels (i.e., *Cacna2d3* and *Cacng2* were higher up in the apex while *Cacng4* was higher up in the base basal). Additionally, sodium channels (i.e., *Scn1a*, *Scn4b*, and *Scn8a*) were differentially expressed between the base basal and apex, and expression of those was greater in the apex. These observations suggest important functional roles for some of these channels in the mouse inner ear.

Tonotopic expression of other genes important for cochlear function

Emilin-2, a major component of the cochlear basal membrane (BM), expressed more in the apex (12.58-fold). Additionally, *Tectb*, a glycoprotein that is localized to the tectorial membrane, also expressed more in the apex (23.85-fold).

Quantitative RT-PCR (qPCR) confirms microarray data

To validate the microarray data, qPCR primers were designed for of 15 selected genes. Of them, 9 deafness genes expressed more in the apical turn (*Pou4f3*, *Slc17a8*, *Tmc1*, *Crym*, *Otof*, *Ush1c*, *Pcdh15*, *Slc26a5*, and *Lhfpl5*) and six were internal controls (*Gapdh*, *Actb*, *Rps17*, *Rpl30*, *Atp6*, and *Ipo8*). In all genes, qPCR data was coincident to microarray data. Data of 9 genes together with the control (*Gapdh*) are shown in Figure 3.

Discussion

These data revealed the baseline of gene expression in each mouse cochlear turn. However, we identified only gene expressions in equal amounts of RNA at each cochlear turn rather than in specific tissue (e.g., the lateral wall, the organ of Corti, and hair cells). This data can be utilized as a tool for global gene analysis such as of the biological function of the genes expressed in the inner ear, or in the search for novel hearing loss causative genes. Sato et al. demonstrated differential gene expression profiles along the axis of the mouse cochlea by cDNA microarray [8]. However, some of our results were not consistent with their findings. This difference may be attributed to the number of microarray probes (165,984 exon probes used in our experiments compared to 20,289 gene probes in theirs). In addition, our microarray analysis results were confirmed by qPCR.

The most remarkable finding was gradients of gene expression, being greater in the apex than the base in ADNSHL genes (*Pou4f3*, *Slc17a8*, *Tmc1*, and *Crym*). There are two prevailing theories explaining autosomal dominant diseases [9]. One of these is haploinsufficiency, referring to a lack of sufficient gene function due to reduced wild-type gene copy number. Cook et al. proposed that haploinsufficiency diseases are caused when the gene expression that is essential to maintain biological function falls below some critical level due to a loss-of-function mutation in one of the two homologous gene loci [10]. Many papers supported this theory by quantifying variability in gene expression [9]. If this theory is applied to genes such as *POU4F3*, *SLC17A8*, *TMC1*, and *CRYM*, mutations of these genes would cause reduction of gene products. In such a case, basal turn gene expression may fall below some critical level more rapidly compared with apical turn because of a gradient of gene expression greater in the apex than in the base, resulting in progressive high frequency hearing loss. This speculation is consistent with the reported hearing loss types (such as high frequency progressive) in patients with the

POU4F3 [11,12], *SLC17A8* [13], *TMC1* [14,15], and *CRYM* [16] mutations.

Emilin-2 is a major component of the cochlear BM. The considerably higher level of *Emilin-2* in the cochlea compared to kidney or other tissues suggests a specialized role in the development or biomechanical function of the cochlear BM [17]. Amma et al. considered that if *Emilin-2* confers elasticity on the BM, *Emilin-2* would decrease the rigidity [17] and our results that expression of *Emilin-2* was greater in the apex than in the base may help to explain increased stiffness in BM towards the base.

Tectb mRNA expression was 23-fold in the apical turn compared with the middle and basal turns. *Tectb* encodes β-tectorin, a glycoprotein that is localized to the TM and the absence of which leads to disruption of the TM's core structure [18]. Russell et al. reported that *Tectb*$^{-/-}$ mutant mice, in which exons 1–4 of the gene are deleted, had low frequency hearing loss [19]. Our data that *Tectb* was mainly expressed in the apex, which is sensitive to low frequencies, was consistent with theirs.

In summary, this study demonstrated the gene expression profiles in each mouse cochlear turn. Especially for ADNSHL genes (*Pou4f3*, *Slc17a8*, *Tmc1*, and *Crym*) and other genes important for cochlear function (*Emilin-2* and *Tectb*), gradual expression changes help to explain the findings obtained from previous studies.

Supporting Information

Table S1 Gene list showing at least two-fold change in expression in one turn compared to the other turn.

Table S2 Gene list showing at least two-fold change in expression for apex vs. basal.

Table S3 Gene list showing at least two-fold change in expression for apex vs. middle.

Table S4 Gene list showing at least two-fold change in expression for middle vs. basal.

Acknowledgments

We thank A. C. Apple-Mathews for help in preparing the manuscript.

Author Contributions

Conceived and designed the experiments: SN SU. Performed the experiments: HY YT SN YI NS. Analyzed the data: HY YT SN SU. Wrote the paper: HY YT SN SU.

References

1. Mann ZF, Kelley MW (2011) Development of tonotopy in the auditory periphery. Hear Res 276: 2–15.
2. Frucht CS, Uduman M, Kleinstein SH, Santos-Sacchi J, Navaratnam DS (2011) Gene expression gradients along the tonotopic axis of the chicken auditory epithelium. J Assoc Res Otolaryngol 412: 23–35.
3. Hildebrand MS, Tack D, McMordie SJ, DeLuca A, Hur IA, et al. (2008) Audioprofile-directed screening identifies novel mutations in KCNQ4 causing hearing loss at the DFNA2 locus. Genet Med 10: 797–804.
4. Fukuoka H, Kanda Y, Ohta S, Usami S (2007) Mutations in the WFS1 gene are a frequent cause of autosomal dominant nonsyndromic low-frequency hearing loss in Japanese. J Hum Genet 52: 510–515.
5. Cryns K, Sivakumaran TA, Van den Ouewland JM, Pennings RJ, Cremers CW, et al. (2003) Mutational spectrum of the WFS1 gene in Wolfram syndrome, nonsyndromic hearing impairment, diabetes mellitus and psychiatric disease. Hum Mut 22: 275–287.
6. Smith RJH, Hildebrand MS, Van Camp G (1999) Deafness and Hereditary Hearing Loss Overview. GeneReviews. Available: http://www.ncbi.nlm.nih.gov/books/NBK 1434/#deafness-overview.REF.cryns.2003.275. Accessed 10 Apr 2013.
7. Morris KA, Snir E, Pompeia C, Koroleva IV, Kachar B, et al. (2005) Differential expression of genes within the cochlea as defined by a custom mouse inner ear microarray. J Assoc Res Otolaryngol 6: 75–89.
8. Sato T, Doi K, Hibino H, Kubo T (2009) Analysis of gene expression profiles along the tonotopic map of mouse cochlea by cDNA microarrays. Acta Otolaryngol Suppl 129(Supple 562): 12–17.
9. Bosl WJ, Li R (2010) The role of noise and positive feedback in the onset of autosomal dominant diseases. BMC Syst Biol 4: e93.
10. Cook DL, Gerber AN, Tapscott SJ (1998) Modeling stochastic gene expression: implications for haploinsufficiency. Proc Natl Acad Sci U S A 95: 15641–15646.
11. Lee HK, Park HJ, Lee KY, Park R, Kim UK. (2010) A novel frameshift mutation of POU4F3 gene associated with autosomal dominant non-syndromic hearing loss. Biochem Biophys Res Commun 396: 626–630.
12. de Heer AM, Huygen PL, Collin RW, Kremer H, Cremers CW. (2009) Mild and variable audiometric and vestibular features in a third DFNA15 family with a novel mutation in POU4F3. Ann Otol Rhinol Laryngol 118: 313–320.
13. Ruel J, Emery S, Nouvian R, Bersot T, Amilhon B, et al. (2008) Impairment of SLC17A8 encoding vesicular glutamate transporter-3, VGLUT3, underlies nonsyndromic deafness DFNA25 and inner hair cell dysfunction in null mice. Am J Hum Genet 83: 278–292.
14. Kurima K, Peters LM, Yang Y, Riazuddin S, Ahmed ZM, et al. (2002) Dominant and recessive deafness caused by mutations of a novel gene, TMC1, required for cochlear hair-cell function. Nat Genet 30: 277–284.
15. Hilgert N, Alasti F, Dieltjens N, Pawlik B, Wollnik B, et al. (2008) Mutation analysis of TMC1 identifies four new mutations and suggests an additional deafness gene at loci DFNA36 and DFNB7/11. Clin Genet 74: 223–232.
16. Abe S, Katagiri T, Saito-Hisaminato A, Usami S, Inoue Y, et al. (2003) Identification of CRYM as a candidate responsible for nonsyndromic deafness, through cDNA microarray analysis of human cochlear and vestibular tissues. Am J Hum Genet 72: 73–82.
17. Amma LL, Goodyear R, Faris JS, Jones I, Ng L, et al. (2003) An emilin family extracellular matrix protein identified in the cochlear basilar membrane. Mol Cell Neurosci 23: 460–472.
18. Ghaffari R, Aranyosi AJ, Richardson GP, Freeman DM (2010) Tectorial membrane travelling waves underlie abnormal hearing in Tectb mutant mice. Nat Commun 1: e96
19. Russell IJ, Legan PK, Lukashkina VA, Lukashkin AN, Goodyear RJ, et al. (2007) Sharpened cochlear tuning in a mouse with a genetically modified tectorial membrane. Nat Neurosci 10: 215–223.

24

Prolactin Expression in the Cochlea of Aged BALB/c Mice is Gender Biased and Correlates to Loss of Bone Mineral Density and Hearing Loss

Robert J. Marano[1,2]*, Jennifer Tickner[3], Sharon L Redmond[1,2]

1 Ear Science Institute Australia, Subiaco, Western Australia, Australia, 2 Ear Sciences Centre, School of Surgery, The University of Western Australia, Nedlands, Western Australia, Australia, 3 School of Pathology and Laboratory Medicine, QEII Medical Centre, The University of Western Australia, Nedlands, Western Australia, Australia

Abstract

Prolactin is a versatile hormone with over 300 known functions and predominantly expressed in the pituitary. However, its expression has additionally been found in a number of extrapituitary organs. Recently, we described the expression of prolactin in the inner ear of mice, where it was correlated to age. Previous research has shown prolactin to be linked to abnormal bone metabolism and hearing loss due to changes in morphology of the bony otic capsule. Here we further investigated the relationship between prolactin, hearing loss and cochlea bone metabolism. BALB/c mice were tested for hearing using ABR at 6 and 12 months of age. Bone mineral density of the cochlea was evaluated using microCT scanning. Prolactin expression was calculated using quantitative real time PCR. Expression of the key regulators of bone metabolism, osteoprotegerin and receptor activator of nuclear factor-kappaB ligand were also determined. We found that prolactin expression was exclusive to the female mice. This also correlated to a greater threshold shift in hearing for the females between 6 and 12 months of age. Analyses of the cochlea also show that the bone mineral density was lower in females compared to males. However, no gender differences in expression of osteoprotegerin or receptor activator of nuclear factor-kappaB ligand could be found. Further analysis of cochlea histological sections revealed larger ostocyte lacunae in the females. These results provide a possible mechanism for an age related hearing loss sub-type that is associated with gender and provides clues as to how this gender bias in hearing loss develops. In addition, it has the potential to lead to treatment for this specific type of hearing loss.

Editor: Bernd Sokolowski, University of South Florida, United States of America

Funding: This work was primarily supported by the Garnet Passe and Rodney Williams Memorial Foundation Project Grant (Grant # 2008) and Fellowship Award program and the Ear Science Institute Australia. Further support was provided by the HEARing Cooperative Research Centre (CRC), established and supported under the Australian Government's Cooperative Research Centres Program; the Victorian State Government's Operational Infrastructure Support Program and the Australian Government's National Health and Medical Research Council's (NHMRC) Independent Research Institutes Infrastructure Support Scheme (IRIISS). The funders had no role in study design, data collection and analysis, decision to publish, or preparation of the manuscript.

Competing Interests: The authors have declared that no competing interests exist.

* E-mail: rob.marano@earscience.org.au

Introduction

Prolactin (*PRL*) is a helix bundle peptide hormone predominantly expressed by lactotrophic cells located in the anterior pituitary gland. Since its early discovery associated with promoting lactation in mammals or "crop milk" in birds [1], it is now known to possess over 300 biological activities (more than all the other pituitary hormones combined) and has been the subject of numerous detailed reviews [2–7]. In addition to the pituitary, localised *PRL* expression has been found in a number of other extrapituitary sites including the brain [8–11], reproductive organs, tissue associated with the immune system (lymphocytes, thymus and spleen) [7] and adipocytes [5].

One of the activities of *PRL* is a direct inhibitory effect on osteoblast function [12]. In addition, *PRL* enhances bone resorption by decreasing the expression ratio between osteoprotegerin (OPG) and receptor activator of nuclear factor-kappaB ligand (RANKL) in osteoblasts derived from humans, by both decreasing OPG and increasing RANKL [13]. Further to this, it has been shown that induced hyperprolactinemia in a guinea pig model leads to bone dismorphology of the otic capsule with an associated hearing loss [14].

Recently we conducted a microarray study comparing the relative expression of genes within the cochlea of mice aged between 4 weeks (young) and 45 weeks (old) [15]. Of the 117 genes that displayed differential expression between the young and old mice, *PRL* showed the highest levels of upregulation of 108 fold. However, during validation using qRT-PCR, it was found that *PRL* expression was not detectable in the young mice, but was readily detectable in the old mice. This result was unique in that *PRL* expression in the cochlea had not previously been described in the literature, and the expression was associated with age. In addition to *PRL*, the closely related hormone Growth Hormone (*Gh*) was also highly upregulated, and the potent *PRL* inhibitor calcitonin-a (*CalcA*) was downregulated.

Subsequent histological sectioning of the contralateral cochlea from the same mice, followed by immunostaining with antibodies specific to *PRL*, revealed spiral ganglion cells and marginal cells of the stria vascularis as the sole sites of expression. Further immunostaining using *PRL* receptor (*PRLR*) specific antibodies

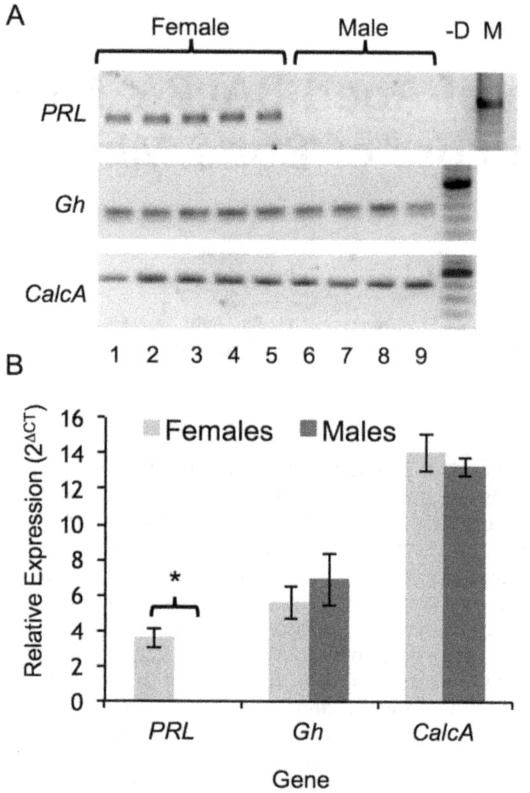

Figure 1. Analysis of gene expression. PCR was used to determine the expression profile of *PRL, Gh* and *CalcA*, which were visualised on an agarose gel (panel A). *PRL* was expressed in the female mice (n = 5) but was absent in the males (n = 4). However, *Gh* and *CalcA* were expressed in both sexes. A control consisting of no DNA template (-D) was also included. Subsequent quantitative analysis (panel B) revealed that the relative expression of *Gh* and *CalcA* were not significantly different between the sexes (p = 0.24 and p = 0.35 respectively). Error bars represent the SEM.

revealed a wide variety of cell types expressing *PRLR*, including osteocytes and bone lining cells (BLC). This provided an indication that *PRL* expression was potentially linked to abnormal bone metabolism or degeneration of other structures within the cochlea leading to an age-related hearing loss (ARHL) pathology.

We hypothesized that localised *PRL* expression in the cochlea leads to bone and/or tissue degeneration resulting in hearing loss. Therefore, in this study we have investigated for the presence of *PRL* and its association to hearing loss in a cohort of BALB/c mice. In addition, we investigated if changes in *Gh* and *CalcA* expression were linked to *PRL* expression as previously found. We also examined the bone mineral density (BMD) of the cochlea to determine if there was a correlation between *PRL* expression and bone dismorphology. Furthermore, the OPG:RANKL ratio was also calculated for each of the mice.

Materials and Methods

Auditory Brainstem Response Testing

Animal experiments were considered and approved by the Walter and Eliza Hall Institute animal ethics committee (project 2011.016) and performed in accordance with the Australian Code of Practice for the Care and Use of Animals for Scientific Purposes (7th ed, 2004). The hearing of BALB/c mice (n = 9; 5 female and 4 male) were assessed with an Auditory Brainstem Response (ABR) test using a Tucker Davis Technologies (TDT) Evoked Potentials Workstation (Tucker Davis Technologies, Alachua, FL, USA) under conditions similar to that reported by Carpinelli *et al.* 2011 [16]. Briefly, the mice were anaesthetized and presented with computer-generated clicks (0–50 KHz spectrum) and pure-tone stimuli of 4, 8, 16 and 32 kHz at maximum intensities of 100 dB peak equivalent SPL from a TDT free-field magnetic speaker (FF1) with a Free Field Frequency response of 108 dB SPL at 10 cm from 1 KHz to 50 KHz using +/−4 V input. The speaker was placed 10 cm from the nose tip of the mouse. Speaker calibration was performed using an ACO model 7016 microphone (ACO Pacific, Inc. Belmont, CA, USA) also placed 10 cm from the speaker. Clicks used had a 100 µsec duration and 100 KHz sampling rate with a null at 10, 20, 30, 40 and 50 KHz. ABRs were averaged from 512 recordings and thresholds were defined as the lowest intensity stimulus that reproducibly elicited a Wave III ABR using a visual detection criterion. Results of the ABR were analyzed using a Wilcoxon Rank Sum/Mann-Whitney U-Test and Repeated Measures ANOVA. Differences were considered significant at $p<0.05$.

RNA Extraction

RNA was extracted from the mice cochlea as previously described [15] using the AllPrep kit (QIAGEN Pty Ltd – Australia, Doncaster, VIC, Australia) as per the manufactures instructions. Briefly, under a dissecting microscope, the cochlea (including the bone) was separated from the vestibular organs and placed into a 1.5 ml microfuge tube (Thermo, Melbourne, VIC, Australia) containing extraction buffer and homogenized using a polypropylene, pellet pestle (Sigma-Aldrich, St Louis, MO, USA). The homogenized mixture was then centrifuged at full speed for five minutes (Eppendorf Centrifuge 5424, Eppendorf South Pacific Pty. Ltd., North Ryde, NSW, Australia) and the supernatant removed and used for the remainder of the extraction protocol. RNA was eluted in 40 µl of RNase free H_2O. The concentration of RNA was measured using a NanoPhotometer™ (IMPLEN, München, Germany).

cDNA Synthesis

Synthesis of first strand cDNA was performed using the SuperScript™ III Reverse Transcriptase (RT) kit (Invitrogen, Mulgrave, Australia) as per the manufactures instructions. Samples of the extracted RNA were used as the template in a final reaction volume of 20 µl with an incubation period of 60 minutes at 55°C. Samples were purified after first strand synthesis using Centri–Spin™-40 columns (Princeton Separations Inc., USA). The cDNA concentration was measured using the NanoPhotometer™ (IMPLEN), and adjusted to 1 ng/µl and stored at −20°C.

Quantitative Real Time PCR (qRT-PCR)

For all experiments, primers were designed using Primer – BLAST (National Library of Medicine) and consist of the following: (sequences given in 5′–3′) PRL Forward GCC CCA CTT CTT CCC TGG CT; Reverse GGG CAA TTT GGC ACC TCA GGA (411 bp); Gh Forward TGC CCA GGC TGC TTT CTG CT, Reverse ACC CGC AGG TAG GTC TCC GC (393 bp); CalcA Forward AGG CGC TGG GAG GCA CAG GAG CCA, Reverse AGG CCT GAA GGT CCC TGC GGC GG (508 bp); OPG Forward AGC ACT GAC CCA GCG GCT GCC TCC T, Reverse GGA GCC CGG GGG ACA GCT CCG GT (429 bp); RANKL Forward AGC GGC CCC GGC GTC CCA CA, Reverse GGC TGG GCC TCA GGC TTG CC TCG C (431 bp) and the housekeeping gene GAPDH Forward CCG CCC CTT CTG CCG ATG CCC CC, Reverse GCA GCC

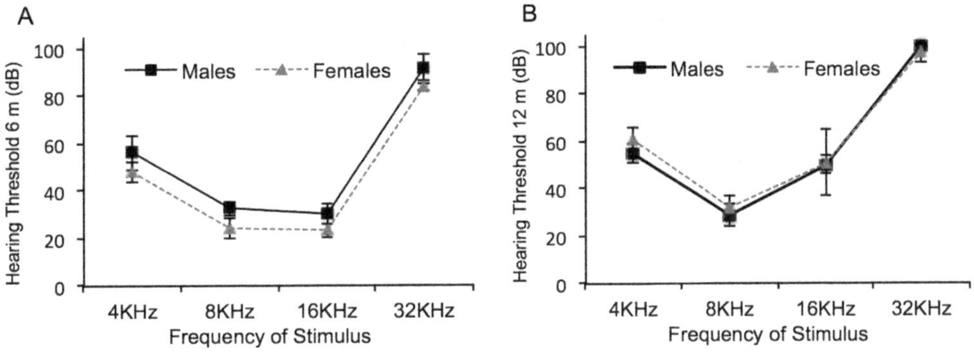

Figure 2. Hearing analysis using ABR. Mice were subjected to ABR analysis at 6 months of age (A) and at 12 months of age (B) to determine their hearing ability. At 6 months, female mice possessed significantly better hearing than males at 8, 16 and 32 KHz. However, at 12 months of age, the hearing of the females had worsened compared to males. Error bars equal the SEM.

CCA CGG CCA TCA CGC C (244 bp). Reaction components per tube were as follows: 10 µl of iQ™ iSYBR Green® supermix (Bio-Rad Laboratories, UK), 1 pmol each forward and reverse primer and 5 ng of template cDNA with the final volume adjusted to 20 µl with ddH_2O. PCR was performed using an iCycler™ MyiQ™ (Bio-Rad) with the cycling conditions consisting of an initial, two-step melt and extension of 95°C for two minutes and 68°C for two minutes respectively. This was followed by 40 cycles of 95°C–15 seconds and 68°C–30 seconds. Technical repeats were performed for each sample and the average C_T values for each gene and gender were used to calculate the relative gene expression for *PRL*, *Gh* and *CalcA* using the Livak Method ($2^{-\Delta CT}$) [17]. The OPG:RANKL ratio was calculated using the $2^{-\Delta\Delta CT}$ method. Samples of the amplicons were also run on a 1.5% agarose gel at 90 V for 45 minutes, visualized on a UV transilluminator and photographed with a digital camera. Statistical analysis of expression levels and ratio's between males and females were analyzed using a Students T-test. Differences were considered significant at $p<0.05$.

Histology and Staining

Mouse cochlea were fixed in 4% paraformaldehyde, pH 8.0 and decalcified at 40°C in a 14% EDTA w/v solution for 48 hours on a rocker shaker (100 rpm) (Ratek, Boronia, VIC, Australia). Cochlea tissue were then routinely processed overnight in a Leica automated tissue processor (model TP1020, Leica, Australia), paraffin embedded and sectioned at 4 µm. Sections were deparaffinised through xylene, graded ethanol and rinsed in tap water before commencement of staining.

Tartrate-resistant acid phosphatase (TRAcP) staining. Sections were immersed in TRAcP stain (pH 5.0) solution at 37°C and monitored every 30 minutes for two hours. Sections were then lightly counterstained in Gill's haematoxylin, washed well and mounted in an aqueous mounting medium.

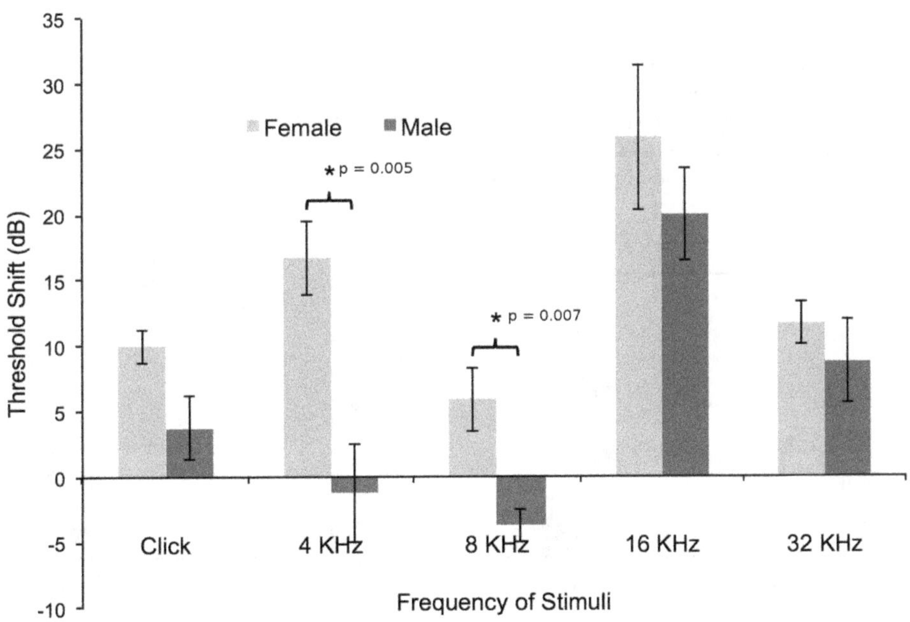

Figure 3. Threshold shift in hearing ability for male and female mice. The change in hearing acuity between 6 and 12 months for female and male mice were calculated for a click response and at various pure tone frequencies. It was found that females displayed a significantly greater shift in hearing threshold compared to males at 4 KHz (p = 0.005) and 8 KHz (p = 0.007). Error bars denote the SEM and * indicates a significance of p<0.05.

Table 1. ABR analysis of mice at 6 and 12 months of age.

	Mean Hearing Threshold (dB) at 6 Months					Mean Hearing Threshold (dB) at 12 Months				
	Male		Female			Male		Female		
Test	Mean	SD	Mean	SD	P	Mean	SD	Mean	SD	P
Click	40	7.07	33	2.74	0.059	43.75	4.79	43	2.45	0.893
4KHz	56.25	7.5	48	4.47	0.076	55	4.08	61	4.9	0.090
8KHz	32.5	2.89	24	4.18	0.023*	28.75	4.79	32	5.1	0.373
16KHz	30	4.08	33	2.74	0.028*	50	4.08	51	13.93	0.711
32KHz	91.25	6.29	84	2.24	0.031*	100	0	97	4	0.180

*denotes a significant p value ($p<0.05$).

Positive control samples were stained in parallel and consisted of mouse femur known to contain active osteoclasts.

Haematoxylin and Eosin (H&E). Sections were deparaffinised through xylene, graded ethanols, rinsed in tap water and placed in Gills haematoxylin for five minutes. Slides were washed well in tap water followed by blueing in saturated lithium carbonate for two minutes. Slides were then washed well in running tap water followed by one minute in 1% alcoholic eosin, dehydration in graded ethanols and xylene. Sections were permanently coverslipped in DePeX mounting media (Sigma-Aldrich, Sydney, Australia). Stained sections were digitally scanned using an Aperio ScanScope XT automated slide scanner (Aperio Technologies Inc., Vista, CA) with a 2× doubler inserted.

Analysis of Bone

Bone Mineral Density (BMD) Measurement. Water controls, cochlea samples, and phantoms were scanned at 6.1 µm resolutions in a Skyscan 1174 microCT instrument (Skyscan, Aartselaar, Belgium). Source voltage was 50 kV, current of 800 µA, rotation step 0.4°, with a 0.5 mm aluminium filter. Scans were reconstructed using NRecon software (cone beam reconstruction algorithm, Skyscan) with a constant global threshold. Reconstructed samples were then imported into CTan software (Skyscan) for 3D analysis. BMD was measured by CTan, which was calibrated using phantoms of known BMD (0.25 g/cm^3 and 0.75 g/cm^3). All water controls, phantoms, and samples were scanned, reconstructed, and analysed under the same conditions, and samples were blinded prior to scanning. Results of BMD measurements were statistically compared between female and male mice using a Students T-test. Results were considered significant at $p<0.05$.

Area of Lacunae. Images from the scanned slides of H&E stained sections were visualised using Aperio ImageScope™ software (v11.2.0.780, Aperio Technologies). A combined total of 100 osteocyte lacuna were randomly chosen from the sections of both female and male mice. The areas of the lacunae were calculated by measuring the diameter of circular lacuna and applying the formula area $= \pi \times \text{radius}^2$. The area of elliptical lacunae was calculated by measuring the length of the major (Maj) and minor axis (Min) and applying the formulae area $= (0.5\times \text{Maj}) \times (0.5\times \text{Min}) \times \pi$. Data were analysed using a Students T-test and were considered significant at $p<0.05$.

Results

Gene Expression

The expression of *PRL*, *Gh* and *CalcA* was analysed using qRT-PCR with samples of the amplicons being visualized on an agarose gel (Figure 1A). *PRL* was detected in the female mice but was absent in the male mice. However, both *Gh* and *CalcA* were detected in the cochlea of both sexes. Subsequent expression analysis revealed no significant differences in *Gh* ($p=0.24$) and *CalcA* ($p=0.35$) between males and females (Figure 1B).

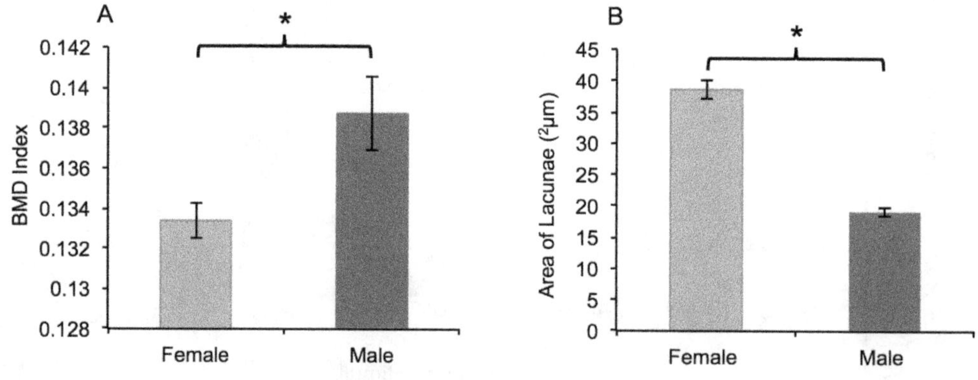

Figure 4. Analysis of cochlea bone. Bone mineral density of the cochlea was calculated for female and male mice using microCT scanning (panel A). Female mice possessed a significantly lower BMD index than male mice ($p=0.014$). Subsequent analysis revealed that the average size of the osteocyte lacunae was significantly larger in the female mice compared to the males ($p<0.001$). Error bars denote the SEM and * indicates a significance of $p<0.05$.

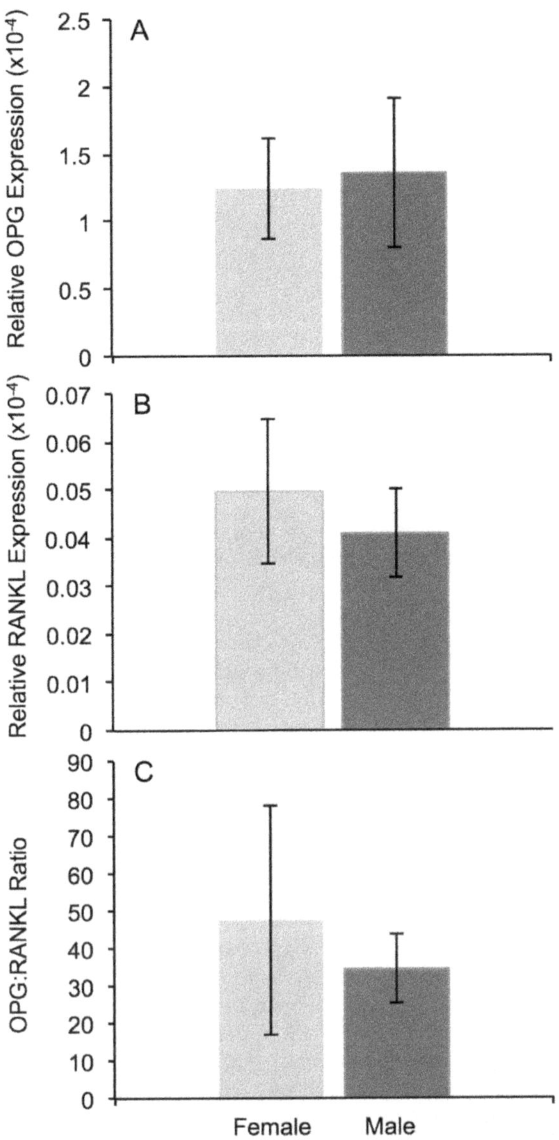

Figure 5. Calculation of expression levels for OPG, RANKL and their ratio. Analysis using qRT-PCR revealed that the relative expression of OPG (panel A) and RANKL (panel B) were not significantly different ($p = 0.38$ and $p = 0.14$ respectively) between females and males. Subsequent analysis of the OPG:RANKL ratio (panel 5C) also did not reveal a gender bias ($p = 0.36$). Error bars denote the SEM.

ABR Hearing Thresholds

Mean ABR thresholds were calculated for male and female mice at 6 months and 12 months of age for a click response and at pure tones. At 6 months of age, both sexes displayed a typical ABR threshold curve (Figure 2A) for this strain of mouse, characterized by substantial hearing loss at the higher frequency of 32 KHz [18]. Additionally, although the shape of the curve was similar, males possessed significantly higher ABR thresholds than females for pure tone stimuli at 8, 16 and 32 KHz (Table 1) when analyzed using the Wilcoxon Rank Sum/Mann-Whitney U-Test. However, at 12 months of age, the situation appeared to reverse with the males recording statistically similar thresholds compared to the females for all corresponding stimuli (Figure 2B). Both sexes essentially recorded complete hearing loss at 32 KHz with thresholds above 95 dB (Table 1). Further analysis calculating the ABR threshold shift between 6 and 12 months revealed significant differences in loss of hearing between females and males (Figure 3) when analyzed using Repeated Measures ANOVA. For a click stimulus it appeared that females suffered a greater threshold shift of 10 dB ±1.29 compared to males, which demonstrated an ABR threshold shift of 3.75 dB ±2.39. However, this was not considered significant ($F = 5.12$; $p = 0.058$). For a pure tone stimulus at 4 KHz, females recorded a significantly ($F = 15.89$; $p = 0.005$) greater increase of ABR threshold of 16.66 dB ±2.79 compared to males, which recorded a reduction of 1.25 dB ±3.75. This result is also reflected in the calculations at 8 KHz, which shows females recording a mean threshold increase of 5.83 dB ±2.39, while the males recorded a threshold reduction of 3.75 dB ±1.25 ($F = 14.44$; $p = 0.007$). No significant difference was detected between females and males at 16 KHz and 32 KHz ($F = 0.881$; $p = 0.380$ and $F = 1.89$; $p = 0.212$ respectively).

Analysis of Bone

Bone Mineral Density. Micro-CT scanning was used to calculate the BMD of cochlea of mice (Figure 4A). The BMD differed significantly ($p = 0.014$) between the female and male mice, which were 0.133±0.009 and 0.139±.002 respectively. This shows female mice possessed a lower BMD.

Area of Lacunae. The mean area of a sample of osteocyte lacunae in the cochlea of female mice was calculated to be 36.62 ^{2}µm ±1.43. The mean area of a sample of osteocyte lacunae in the cochlea of male mice was calculated to be 19.12 ^{2}µm ±0.69 (Figure 4B). A Students T-test revealed that the difference in mean lacunae area was significantly higher in the female mice compared to the males ($p < 0.001$).

OPG:RANKL Ratio

The relative expression of OPG and RANKL were calculated using qRT-PCR and the ratio determined for each of the sexes. A significant difference was not detected between females and males in the expression level of OPG ($p = 0.38$, Figure 5A) and RANKL ($p = 0.14$, Figure 5B). Consequently, the OPG:RANKL ratio (Figure 5C) also did not reveal a gender bias, which was 47.5:1±30.9 for females and 34.6:1±9.2 for males ($p = 0.36$).

Histology and Staining

TRAcP staining for osteoclasts. Cochlea sections of both female and male mice were negative for TRAcP staining in all areas. However, positive controls stained strongly for activated osteoclasts (images not shown).

H&E Staining for changes in bone. Morphological observations of H&E stained sections indicated that the osteocyte lacunae appeared larger in the females compared to the males (Figure 6).

Discussion

We have found that localised *PRL* expression in the cochlea of aged BALB/c mice demonstrated a gender bias, insomuch as it was only detectable in females. The expression of *Gh* and *CalcA* seemed to be independent of *PRL* expression. Additionally, *PRL* expression correlated to an increase in hearing thresholds at certain frequencies. Furthermore, a reduction of cochlea BMD also correlated to *PRL* expression in the female mice. However, our hypothesis that this was due to changes in the RANKL:OPG ratio could not be proven.

ARHL is a broad term used to describe an increase in hearing threshold associated with age. It is a condition that is asynchronous with the age-related condition of other organs of the body, and

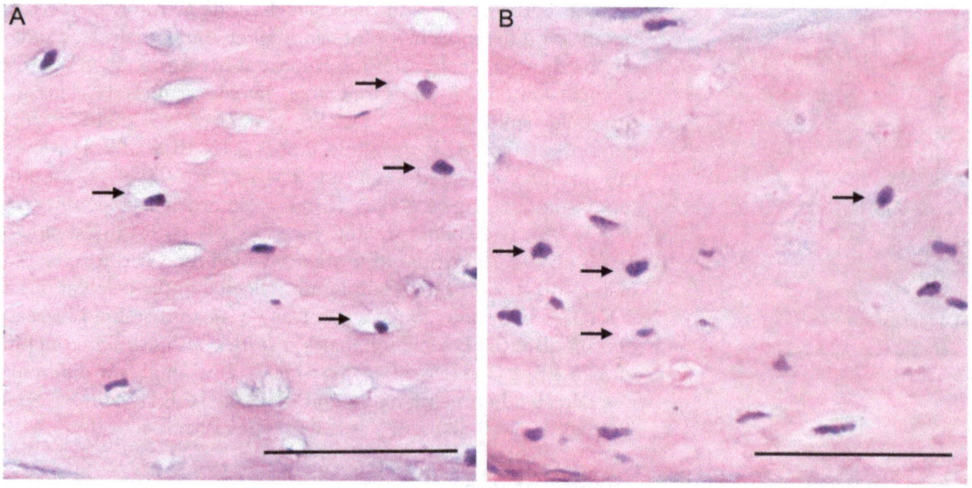

Figure 6. Representative histological sections of cochlea bone for female and male mice. H&E stained sections of cochlea bone revealed that the osteocyte lacunae (arrows) appeared larger in the female mice (panel A) compared to the male mice (pane B). Scale bars equal 50 μm.

singularly interferes with the quality of life [19]. While ARHL is multifactorial in its pathology, there is general agreement there is a genetic component. In C57BL/6J mice, the *cdh23ahl* allele was found to be a major contributing factor for premature hearing loss [20]. However, subsequent studies in a wide variety of inbred strains have found the contribution of this gene to be highly variable and conclude the necessity of other contributing genes [21]. Currently, while there are a large number of publications describing different genes and potential mechanisms in mice, none have so far been proven as a definitive cause for ARHL in the general population. Considering the high volume of contrasting research, it may be true that there is more than one form of ARHL resulting from one of many different types of mechanisms or altered genes as postulated by others [22,23].

We have previously shown *PRL* to be expressed in the cochlea of aged mice, and that this expression was localised to the cells of the spiral ganglion and marginal cells of the stria vascularis [15]. In addition, the expression of *PRL* seemed to correlate to a similar upregulation of growth hormone (*Gh*) and a downregulation of a known *PRL* inhibitor calcitonin (*CalcA*). Furthermore, we also demonstrated that the *PRL* receptor (*PRLR*) was located in most structures of the inner ear. Previous research by others have established a link between hyperprolactinemia and altered bone metabolism [13,24–26]. In addition, hyperprolactinemia has been shown to cause bone related hearing loss [14]. In this present study we have shown that the expression of *PRL* in the cochlea of BALB/c mice seems independent of *Gh* and *CalcA* expression. In the pituitary, which is the primary site of *PRL* expression, these genes are regulated by the same mechanism [2]. However, at extrapituitary sites, *PRL* expression is predominantly controlled by elements within the superdistal promoter. This regulation is disassociated with *Gh* and *CalcA* expression, in addition to being independent of *PRL* production in the pituitary [27]. Our current results of *PRL* expression within the cochlea are is in keeping with these findings. However, *PRL* expression did correlate to gender (where it was only expressed in female mice), an increase in the ABR hearing threshold and a reduction of the BMD of the otic capsule.

These results seem to compare favorably with clinical ARHL in humans. In terms of ARHL progression, recent research has correlated the severity of hearing loss to the extent of degeneration of many inner ear structures, including the stria vascularis, ganglion cells, inner and outer hair cells [28]. Additionally, for humans, there is a gender bias in rates of hearing loss similar to that of the BALB/c mice used in our study [29]. Briefly, the research by Sharashenidze et al demonstrated that in the relatively early ages of 30–59 years, threshold elevations appear more rapid in males than in females. Thereafter, in the latter ages of 60–79 years, the threshold shifts become steeper in females. As a result, the gender differences in hearing become smoothed. However, the cause of the degeneration and the reported gender bias has yet to be determined. The results seen in our study support both of these previous findings. That is, female mice possess lower hearing thresholds than males at 6 months of age, but exhibit an accelerated loss of hearing compared to males between 6 and 12 months at a number of frequencies. Additionally, the relative abundance of *PRLR* in most areas of the cochlea indicates the potential for adverse metabolic change in the presence of hyper-expressed *PRL* as seen in other pathologies [25,30,31]. Furthermore, as stated earlier, we have shown that the sites of *PRL* expression in the cochlea are restricted to spiral ganglion cells and marginal cells of the stria vascularis [15]. These are the same cell types that exclusively possess estrogen receptors (ER) α and ERß respectively [32]. In addition, loss of ERß has also been linked to a hearing loss pathology [33]. The relationship between estrogen as an effector of *PRL* expression has been well documented [34–36]. This provides a strong indication that estrogen may play a role in the expression of cochlea *PRL*, and provides a clue as to why there is a gender bias in its expression. However, the mechanism by which *PRL* may be regulated by estrogen in this instance is yet to be determined.

As mentioned earlier, research has shown that estrogen-induced hyperprolactinemia is correlated with bone-related hearing loss in a guinea pig model [14]. However, the role reduced BMD has in the loss of hearing was one aspect of our study that was less clear. The BMD of the bony otic capsule was significantly reduced in female mice compared to males. However, the reduction was small and it is unclear if it would have a significant effect on hearing. Furthermore, the use of qRT-PCR was unable to detect any significant differences in the OPG:RANKL expression ratio, which were high for both sexes. Subsequent TRAcP staining also failed to reveal activation of osteoclasts in either female or male mice. Therefore, the possibility exists that BMD reduction is due to other mechanisms. One such mechanism may be osteocytic osteolysis, a process whereby osteocytes directly mobilise bone minerals for metabolic use (reviews by [37,38]). The evidence for this occurring lies in the significantly larger lacunae seen in the female mice compared to the males. However, as other bones within the mice were not available, it is unknown if this process was due to *PRL* expression in the cochlea, or a function of other hormonal changes specific to female mice.

A limitation of this study was the lack of expression, BMD and histological data from mice at 6 months of age or less, that could be correlated to corresponding audiological data. However, this does not detract from the fact that *PRL* is only detectable in females and correlated to differences in bone mineral density and hearing function compared to males of the same age.

In conclusion, we have found *PRL* to be exclusively expressed in the cochlea of aged, female, BALB/c mice. This expression correlated to an increase in the hearing threshold between 6 and 12 months of age and a loss of BMD. However, we were not able to show a relationship between reduced BMD and a decrease in the OPG:RANKL ratio as hypothesized.

Acknowledgments

The authors would like to thank Dr Rachel Burt, Dr Marina Carpinelli and Ms Anne Cooray from the Murdoch Children's Research Institute and the Walter and Eliza Hall Institute of Medical Research, Parkville 3052 VIC, Australia for their assistance in obtaining the ABR data. The authors also wish to acknowledge the facilities, scientific and technical assistance of the Australian Microscopy & Microanalysis Research Facility at the Centre for Microscopy, Characterisation and Analysis, The University of Western Australia, a facility funded by the University, State and Commonwealth Governments.

Author Contributions

Conceived and designed the experiments: RJM JT SLR. Performed the experiments: RJM JT SLR. Analyzed the data: RJM SR JT. Contributed reagents/materials/analysis tools: RJM JT SLR. Wrote the paper: RJM JT SLR.

References

1. Riddle O, Bates RW, Dykshorn SW (1933) The preparation, identification and assay of prolactin – a hormone of the anterior pituitary. American Journal of Physiology 105: 191–216.
2. Ben-Jonathan N, Mershon JL, Allen DL, Steinmetz RW (1996) Extrapituitary prolactin: distribution, regulation, functions, and clinical aspects. Endocr Rev 17: 639–669.
3. Ben-Jonathan N, LaPensee CR, LaPensee EW (2008) What can we learn from rodents about prolactin in humans? Endocr Rev 29: 1–41.
4. Bole-Feysot C, Goffin V, Edery M, Binart N, Kelly PA (1998) Prolactin (PRL) and its receptor: actions, signal transduction pathways and phenotypes observed in PRL receptor knockout mice. Endocr Rev 19: 225–268.
5. Brandebourg T, Hugo E, Ben-Jonathan N (2007) Adipocyte prolactin: regulation of release and putative functions. Diabetes Obes Metab 9: 464–476.
6. Egli M, Leeners B, Kruger TH (2010) Prolactin secretion patterns: basic mechanisms and clinical implications for reproduction. Reproduction 140: 643–654.
7. Freeman ME, Kanyicska B, Lerant A, Nagy G (2000) Prolactin: structure, function, and regulation of secretion. Physiol Rev 80: 1523–1631.
8. Emanuele NV, Jurgens JK, Halloran MM, Tentler JJ, Lawrence AM, et al. (1992) The rat prolactin gene is expressed in brain tissue: detection of normal and alternatively spliced prolactin messenger RNA. Mol Endocrinol 6: 35–42.
9. Ramesh R, Kuenzel WJ, Buntin JD, Proudman JA (2000) Identification of growth-hormone- and prolactin-containing neurons within the avian brain. Cell Tissue Res 299: 371–383.
10. Roselli CE, Bocklandt S, Stadelman HL, Wadsworth T, Vilain E, et al. (2008) Prolactin expression in the sheep brain. Neuroendocrinology 87: 206–215.
11. Torner L, Maloumby R, Nava G, Aranda J, Clapp C, et al. (2004) In vivo release and gene upregulation of brain prolactin in response to physiological stimuli. Eur J Neurosci 19: 1601–1608.
12. Charoenphandhu N, Teerapornpuntakit J, Methawasin M, Wongdee K, Thongchote K, et al. (2008) Prolactin decreases expression of Runx2, osteoprotegerin, and RANKL in primary osteoblasts derived from tibiae of adult female rats. Can J Physiol Pharmacol 86: 240–248.
13. Seriwatanachai D, Thongchote K, Charoenphandhu N, Pandaranandaka J, Tudpor K, et al. (2008) Prolactin directly enhances bone turnover by raising osteoblast-expressed receptor activator of nuclear factor kappaB ligand/osteoprotegerin ratio. Bone 42: 535–546.
14. Horner KC, Cazals Y, Guieu R, Lenoir M, Sauze N (2007) Experimental estrogen-induced hyperprolactinemia results in bone-related hearing loss in the guinea pig. Am J Physiol Endocrinol Metab 293: E1224–32.
15. Marano RJ, Tickner J, Redmond SL (2012) Age related changes in gene expression within the cochlea of C57BL/6J mice. Aging Clin Exp Res 24: 603–611.
16. Carpinelli MR, Wise AK, Burt RA (2011) Vitamin D-deficient diet rescues hearing loss in Klotho mice. Hear Res 275: 105–109.
17. Livak KJ, Schmittgen TD (2001) Analysis of relative gene expression data using real-time quantitative PCR and the 2(-Delta Delta C(T)) Method. Methods 25: 402–408.
18. Willott JF, Turner JG, Carlson S, Ding D, Seegers Bross L, et al. (1998) The BALB/c mouse as an animal model for progressive sensorineural hearing loss. Hear Res 115: 162–174.
19. Ohlemiller KK (2009) Mechanisms and genes in human strial presbycusis from animal models. Brain Res 1277: 70–83.
20. Johnson KR, Erway LC, Cook SA, Willott JF, Zheng QY (1997) A major gene affecting age-related hearing loss in C57BL/6J mice. Hear Res 114: 83–92.
21. Johnson KR, Zheng QY, Erway LC (2000) A major gene affecting age-related hearing loss is common to at least ten inbred strains of mice. Genomics 70: 171–180.
22. Liu XZ, Yan D (2007) Ageing and hearing loss. J Pathol 211: 188–197.
23. Fetoni AR, Picciotti PM, Paludetti G, Troiani D (2011) Pathogenesis of presbycusis in animal models: a review. Exp Gerontol 46: 413–425.
24. Colao A, Di Somma C, Loche S, Di Sarno A, Klain M, et al. (2000) Prolactinomas in adolescents: persistent bone loss after 2 years of prolactin normalization. Clin Endocrinol (Oxf) 52: 319–327.
25. Meaney AM, O'Keane V (2003) Reduced bone mineral density in patients with schizophrenia receiving prolactin raising anti-psychotic medication. J Psychopharmacol 17: 455–458.
26. Seriwatanachai D, Charoenphandhu N, Suthiphongchai T, Krishnamra N (2008) Prolactin decreases the expression ratio of receptor activator of nuclear factor kappaB ligand/osteoprotegerin in human fetal osteoblast cells. Cell Biol Int 32: 1126–1135.
27. Berwaer M, Martial JA, Davis JR (1994) Characterization of an up-stream promoter directing extrapituitary expression of the human prolactin gene. Mol Endocrinol 8: 635–642.
28. Nelson EG, Hinojosa R (2006) Presbycusis: a human temporal bone study of individuals with downward sloping audiometric patterns of hearing loss and review of the literature. Laryngoscope 116: 1–12.
29. Sharashenidze N, Schacht J, Kevanishvili Z (2007) Age-related hearing loss: gender differences. Georgian Med News 14–18.
30. Abraham G, Paing WW, Kaminski J, Joseph A, Kohegyi E, et al. (2003) Effects of elevated serum prolactin on bone mineral density and bone metabolism in female patients with schizophrenia: a prospective study. Am J Psychiatry 160: 1618–1620.
31. Misra M, Papakostas GI, Klibanski A (2004) Effects of psychiatric disorders and psychotropic medications on prolactin and bone metabolism. J Clin Psychiatry 65: 1607–18; quiz 1590, 1760–1.
32. Stenberg AE, Wang H, Fish Jr, Schrott-Fischer A, Sahlin L, et al. (2001) Estrogen receptors in the normal adult and developing human inner ear and in Turner's syndrome. Hear Res 157: 87–92.
33. Simonoska R, Stenberg AE, Duan M, Yakimchuk K, Fridberger A, et al. (2009) Inner ear pathology and loss of hearing in estrogen receptor-beta deficient mice. J Endocrinol 201: 397–406.
34. Adamson AD, Friedrichsen S, Semprini S, Harper CV, Mullins JJ, et al. (2008) Human prolactin gene promoter regulation by estrogen: convergence with tumor necrosis factor-alpha signaling. Endocrinology 149: 687–694.
35. Duan R, Ginsburg E, Vonderhaar BK (2008) Estrogen stimulates transcription from the human prolactin distal promoter through AP1 and estrogen responsive elements in T47D human breast cancer cells. Mol Cell Endocrinol 281: 9–18.
36. Horiguchi K, Naito J, Ishida M, Harigaya T (2007) The effect of estrogen on phosphorylation of prolactin in the mouse pituitary gland. J Reprod Dev 53: 515–523.
37. Atkins GJ, Findlay DM (2012) Osteocyte regulation of bone mineral: a little give and take. Osteoporos Int 23: 2067–2079.
38. Qing H, Bonewald LF (2009) Osteocyte remodeling of the perilacunar and pericanalicular matrix. Int J Oral Sci 1: 59–65.

High Fibrinogen in Peripheral Blood Correlates with Poorer Hearing Recovery in Idiopathic Sudden Sensorineural Hearing Loss

Sho Kanzaki[1]*, Masafumi Sakagami[2], Hiroshi Hosoi[3], Shingo Murakami[4], Kaoru Ogawa[1]

1 Department of Otorhinolaryngology, Head and Neck Surgery, Keio University, School of Medicine, Shinjuku, Tokyo, Japan, 2 Department of Otorhinolaryngology, Hyogo College of Medicine, Nishinomiya, Hyogo, Japan, 3 Department of Otorhinolaryngology, Nara Medical University, Kashihara, Nara, Japan, 4 Department of Otorhinolaryngology, Graduate School of Medical Sciences, Nagoya City University, Mizuho, Nagoya, Aichi, Japan

Abstract

Objectives: We used hearing tests and peripheral blood sample analyses to characterize the pathology of idiopathic sudden sensorineural hearing loss (ISSNHL) and to identify possible prognostic factors for predicting recovery of hearing loss.

Study Design: A retrospective, multicenter trial was conducted.

Methods: Two hundred three patients examined within 7 days after the onset of ISSNHL received prednisone with lipo-prostaglandin E1. Pure-tone auditory tests were performed before and after treatment with these drugs. Blood tests were performed on blood samples collected during the patients' initial visit to our clinic.

Results: In all patients, elevated white blood cell (WBC) counts, fasting blood sugar levels, HgbA1c, and erythrocyte sedimentation rate (ESR) significantly correlated with high hearing threshold measurements obtained on the initial visit. High fibrinogen levels, WBC counts, ESR, and low concentrations of fibrinogen degradation products (FDP) were associated with lower hearing recovery rates. Additionally, different audiogram shapes correlated with different blood test factors, indicating that different pathologies were involved.

Conclusions: High fibrinogen levels measured within seven days after ISSNHL onset correlated with poorer hearing recovery. This may be a consequence of ischemia or infections in the inner ear. The high WBC counts also observed may therefore reflect an immune response to inner ear damage induced by ischemic changes or infections. Our data indicate that therapeutic strategies should be selected based on the timing of initial treatment relative to ISSNHL onset.

Editor: Jonathan I. Matsui, Harvard University, United States of America

Funding: The authors have no support or funding to report.

Competing Interests: The authors have declared that no competing interests exist.

* Email: skan@a7.keio.jp

Introduction

Idiopathic sudden sensorineural hearing loss (ISSNHL) is characterized by a sudden onset of hearing loss and generally presents unilaterally [1]. Little is known about the pathogenesis of ISSNHL. However, a diversity of treatments has been proposed to cover all the possible underlying mechanisms of the disease, such as those related to viruses, the immune system, and vascular injury [2,3].

Many studies have identified factors that predict which patients possess a favorable prognosis and require minimal or no treatment. However, only a few studies have determined the probability of whether a patient's hearing will recover by using prognostic models that incorporate probability data [4]. Several reports have investigated the prognostic value of certain factors, such as the timing of initial treatment, initial hearing levels, absence or presence of accompanying vertigo, and audiogram profiles [4,5,6,7,8]. Beginning treatment earlier, soon after diagnosis results in a better prognosis and decreases patients' likelihood of acquiring irreversible damage from inner ear pathologies. Audiogram profiles may also indicate different pathologies that lead to cochlear lesions as well as different prognoses.

Other researchers have tested various blood indices as potential prognostic factors for ISSNHL. Analyses of peripheral blood samples from patients who experience ISSNHL revealed they present with certain vascular risk factors, such as elevated plasma and whole blood viscosity [9],[10], prothrombotic genes [11,12,13,14], and elevated fibrinogen levels [3,15]. This suggests that these factors are involved in the pathology of ISSNHL. As these factors were not correlated with hearing recovery, we did not consider them as candidates for potential prognostic factors.

Table 1. Diagnostic criteria for idiopathic sudden sensorineural hearing loss (ISSNHL)*.

Main symptoms	
1	Sudden onset of hearing loss
2	Sensorineural hearing loss, usually severe
3	Unknown cause
Accessory symptoms	
1	May be accompanied by tinnitus
2	May be accompanied by vertigo, nausea, and/or vomiting without recurrent episodes
3	No cranial nerve symptoms (other than from cranial nerve XIII)

*ISSNHL was defined according to criteria described by the Sudden Deafness Research Committee of the Japanese Ministry of Health and Welfare [23]. Patients were diagnosed with *definite ISSNHL* if they presented with all the listed symptoms, or with *probable ISSNHL* if they presented mainly with only symptoms 1 and 2.

It is well known that vascular risk factors can affect inner ear function by compromising the vascular endothelium, leading to functional disruption [11]. Studies indicate that ISSNHL patients have higher levels of circulating adhesion molecules [16,17]. Other studies on immunologic factors in ISSNHL show that anti-heat shock protein (HSP) 70 autoantibodies correlate well with a good prognosis [18]. Antinuclear antibody (ANA) titer and erythrocyte sedimentation rate (ESR) are two other blood parameters that are significantly elevated in ISSNHL patients compared to normal individuals [19].

White blood cell (WBC) count is another potential prognostic factor. High WBC counts are frequently found in ISSNHL patients [20]. Guided by cytokines and other soluble molecules, WBCs migrate to vascular epithelial cells [16]. WBCs are usually involved in tissue damage after cardiac ischemic changes [21] and stroke [22]. Thus, they may similarly contribute to the inner ear tissue damage seen in ISSNHL.

In this study, we performed hearing tests and analyzed peripheral blood samples to characterize the pathology of ISSNHL and to identify prognostic factors for predicting hearing recovery.

Subjects and Methods

Subjects were 203 patients with unilateral ISSNHL (Table 1), who were seen at different hospitals between January 2005 and May 2012. The hospitals were all registered to participate in the present study. This study, which involved using retrospective data, was approved by the ethical committees of Keio University School of Medicine, Hyogo College of Medicine, Nara Medical University, and Nagoya City University (International Clinical Trials Registry JPRN-UMIN000008356). No new data were obtained for this study. The patients consented that their data could be used for future studies. The authors were involved in the initial collection of the data. The university hospitals stated in the original, written informed consent that any patient data obtained initially could be used in future studies. Data was anonymized at the time of collection.

The study was conducted according to the principles expressed in the Declaration of Helsinki. Inclusion criteria were as follows: (1) hearing loss appeared acutely, without recognizable cause; (2) hearing loss was sudden, sensorineural in origin, and untreated; (3) patients were seen at our clinics within 7 days of onset; (4) patients followed up until their hearing recovered; (5) patients presenting with hearing loss of more than a 30 dB hearing level (HL), affecting at least three frequencies; (6) normal hearing in the contralateral ear (air conduction pure-tone average [PTA] at 0.25, 0.5, 1, 2, 4, and 8 kHz frequencies were <40 dB HL); (7) negative history of hearing loss or ear surgery in the affected ear; (8) lack of impairment of the cranial nerves (except cranial nerve VIII); and (9) gadolinium-enhanced magnetic resonance image verifying negative cranial nerve VIII pathology. All patients affected by Ménière's disease, noise-induced hearing loss, and other known causes of inner ear disease (including viral infection) were excluded (Figure 1) (Protocol S1).

On the patients' initial visit to one of our clinics, a complete clinical history was obtained and standard audiovestibular exams were performed. These consisted of pure-tone testing and MRI of the internal auditory canal and posterior cranial fossa. Peripheral blood samples for chemistry and hematological tests were collected from the patients after informed consent was obtained but before treatment was given. All patients were then subjected to the same treatment protocol, which consisted of intravenous prednisone (60 mg tapered to 20 mg), Lipo PGE1 (vasodilators), ATP, and vitamin B12 for 7 days. Hearing improvement was evaluated using the following improvement rate criterion described by Ogawa et al. [23]. Soon after the patients' hearing stabilized, recovery was evaluated as follows:

$$\begin{aligned}&\text{Recovery rate}(\%)\\&\quad = (\text{initial PTA} - \text{final PTA of the affected ear}\\&\quad\quad / \text{initial PTA} - \text{PTA of the opposite ear}) \times 100.\end{aligned}$$

Blood samples were analyzed. Clinical chemistry determinations were made for glucose, hemoglobin A1c (Hgb A1c), total cholesterol, high-density lipoprotein (HDL), low-density lipoprotein (LDL), and serum triglyceride levels. Hematology determinations were made for WBCs, red blood cells (RBCs), thrombocytes, hemoglobin, hematocrit, and ESR. Hemostasis determinations were made for prothrombin time (PT %), activated partial thromboplastin time (APTT %), fibrinogen, and fibrinogen degradation products (FDPs).

We examined whether initial hearing or hearing recovery rate correlated with the above-mentioned blood data values. All results were expressed as mean values ± standard deviation. Statistical analysis was performed using parametric and nonparametric tests (SPSS 17.0, Chicago, IL, USA).

Results

The data obtained from patients with ISSNHL were summarized and tabulated. Table 2–6 presents the patients' clinical characteristics. There were no significant differences in the prognoses of male and female subjects (Table 2). Total deafness and having a high-pitch, sloping audiogram shape translated to poorer recovery rate (Table 3). On average, blood test data were not abnormal (Table 4). Subjects with vertigo exhibited a poorer hearing recovery rate. Only 13 patients with tinnitus, ear fullness, and vertigo had a poor hearing recovery rate (Table 5). Time of initial treatment relative to ISSNHL onset (1–7 days) did not correlate with hearing recovery rate (Table 6).

High WBC counts 1–7 days after the onset of sensorineural hearing loss correlated with hearing recovery rate (Table 7). In subjects who received treatment within seven days of ISSNHL onset, hearing recovery rate correlated with high WBC counts,

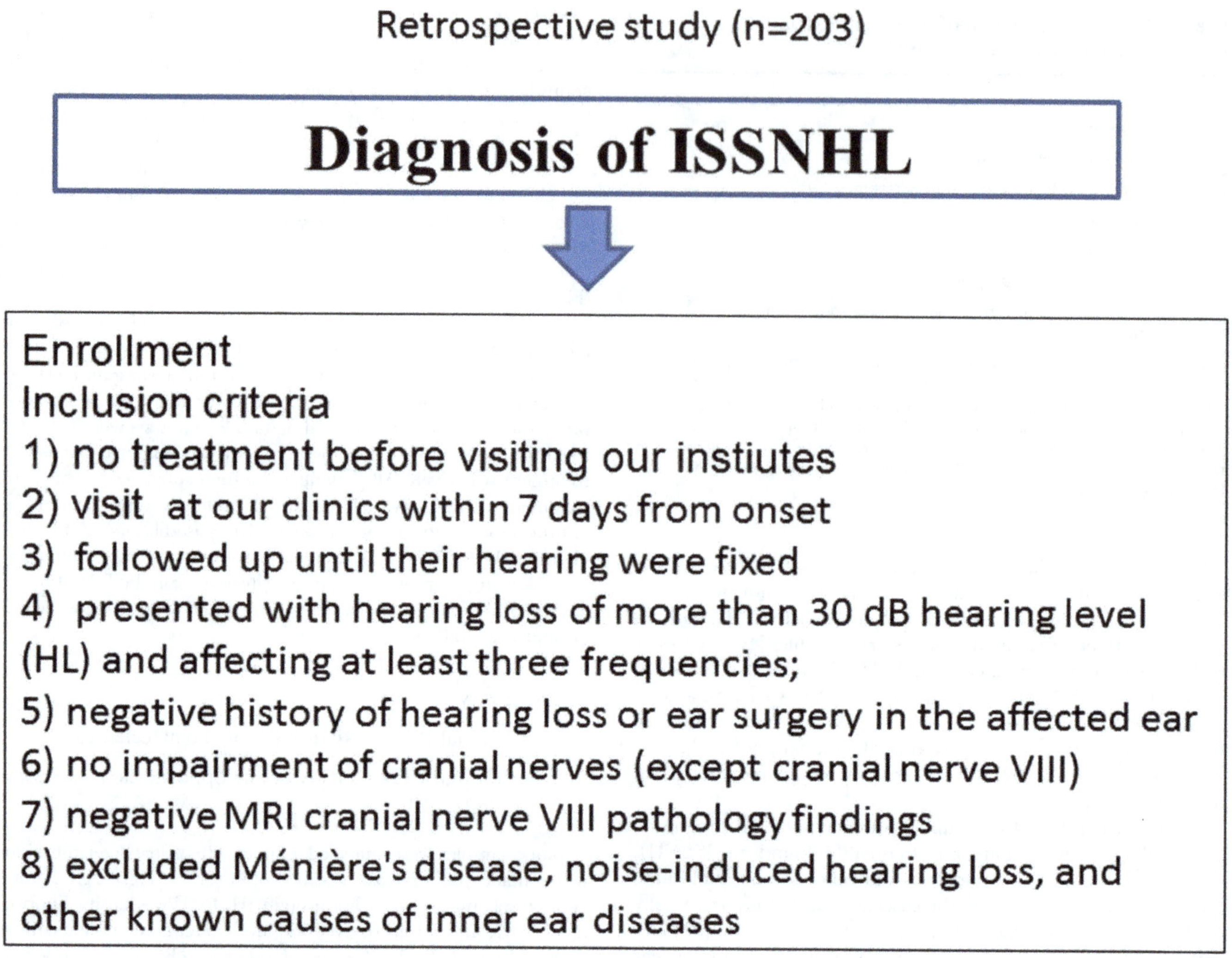

Figure 1. Flowchart showing patient inclusion criteria.

elevated fibrinogen levels, and elevated ESR (Table 8). Taken together, our data indicate that hearing recovery rate was correlated with the patients' hearing and fibrinogen levels at the time they first sought hospital treatment for their hearing loss (i.e., 1–7 days after onset).

We also classified several types of audiogram shapes and analyzed their correlation with prognostic factors (see Table 9). We used simple linear regression analysis, with fibrinogen as the only factor (RR = 146.376–0.270 * fibrinogen ($p = 0.026$) ($R = 0.274$, $R^2 = 0.075$, Adjusted $R^2 = 0.060$). Multivariate analyses (multiple regression) failed to identify any relevant factors.

Table 2. Gender and hearing recovery rate.

Gender	No. of cases	Hearing recovery rate	HL at initial visit (dB)
Male	87	70.1%	67.99
Female	116	58.4%	67.94
Total	203	63.4%	67.96

Discussion

Here, we report results from an ongoing multicenter clinical trial evaluating prognostic factors for ISSNHL. In all 203 patients included in this study, elevated fibrinogen levels and WBC counts correlated with poorer hearing recovery rates and poorer prognosis. Higher ESR values and WBC counts obtained during

Table 3. Audiogram shape and hearing recovery rate.

Audiogram shape	No. of cases	Recovery rate (%)	Hearing level at initial exam (dB)
Flat	48	62.5%	73.21
High	35	48.5%	50.49
Total	31	54.7%	99.71
Low and high	8	65.6%	48.63
Mid	25	82.2%	63.00
Other	53	69.4%	61.62
Unknown	3	73.2%	64.67

Table 4. Average hearing level data and laboratory blood test values.

	Average	Standard deviation
*Initiation of treatment relative to ISSNHL onset (days)	2.3	1.8
Initial hearing (dB)	68.0	23.0
Hearing recovery rate (%)	63.4	56.5
WBC	6.6	2.1
RBC	4.6	0.5
Plt	224.7	52.6
Hct (%)	40.9	4.6
PT (%)	19.9	25.8
APTT (%)	26.8	4.1
Fibrinogen	286.8	55.5
FDP	5.4	17.0
FBS	119.7	38.0
HgbA1c	5.6	1.3
Total cholesterol	214.6	35.7
LDL	129.1	30.9
TG	119.4	85.3
ESR	13.1	14.2

the patients' initial hospital visit significantly correlated with higher hearing thresholds (average threshold measured at five frequencies).

It remains unclear whether ESR is a reliable prognostic factor for ISSNHL, as some researchers consider it to convey a poor prognosis [2], while others consider it to have no prognostic value at all [7]. In the present study, elevated ESR values obtained 1–7 days after disease onset correlated not only with the patients' initial hearing levels but also with disease outcome in ISSNHL. Indeed, ESR values correlated positively with fibrinogen levels ($r = 0.435$, $P = 0.0001$). We speculate that increased levels of fibrinogen increase ESR; thus, the elevated ESR observed in our patients may represent a secondary reaction to fibrinogen. Elevated fibrinogen and ESR values occur in response to inflammation, tissue damage, viral infection, autoimmune disease, and ischemic changes [24].

Table 5. Correlation of symptoms with initial hearing levels and recovery rate.

	No. of cases	Recovery rate (%)	Hearing level at initial exam (dB)
Tinnitus	126	60.7%	67.60
Vertigo	62	46.2%	74.95
Fullness	81	63.2%	64.52
Tinnitus and vertigo	24	43.6%	75.00
Tinnitus, vertigo, and fullness	13	33.2%	77.08
Vertigo and fullness	7	47.9%	60.14
Tinnitus and fullness	34	67.5%	64.65

Table 6. Treatment timing and hearing recovery rate.

Timing (days)*	No. of cases	Recovery rate (%)	Hearing level at initial exam (dB)
0	28	63.6%	78.69
1	55	70.1%	69.49
2	40	65.4%	67.33
3	35	68.7%	63.26
4	16	49.9%	69.81
5	12	56.9%	61.25
6	11	34.5%	60.45
7	6	59.5%	57.83

APTT, activated partial thromboplastin time; ESR, erythrocyte sedimentation rate; FBS, fasting blood sugar; FDP, fibrinogen degradation products; Hct, hematocrit; HgbA1c, hemoglobin A1c; LDL, low-density lipoprotein cholesterol; Plt, platelets; PT, prothrombin time; RBC, red blood cell count; TG, triglycerides; WBC, white blood cell count.

*Initiation of treatment relative to ISSNHL onset; zero day is baseline value.

As previously reported, ANA titer and ESR are two parameters that are significantly more elevated in ISSNHL patients than in normal individuals [19]. Nevertheless, the significance of these parameters remains controversial [19].

The elevated WBC counts in our patients may be due to an immune response to more extensive tissue damage in the inner ear. This hypothesis is consistent with our finding that higher WBC counts negatively correlates with hearing recovery rates in patients having a "total deafness" audiogram shape and in patients with severe hearing loss (Table 9).

Higher WBC counts did correlate with hearing level measured during the initial visit and hearing recovery of patients that sought treatment within 1–7 days after onset (Tables 7 and 8). Myocardial infarct size has been shown to be directly correlated with increased WBC counts [25]. The same may also apply to cases involving inner ear damage.

As mentioned, within 1–7 days of ISSNHL onset, fibrinogen levels correlate negatively with hearing recovery rate, and elevated ESR correlates with the patients' hearing level at the initial visit. The finding that fibrinogen levels measured one day after ISSNHL onset correlates with hearing recovery rate indicates that, at ISSNHL onset, blood viscosity is high and thus blood supply to affected areas is decreased. We surmised that a few days thereafter, inner ear tissue damage further progresses due to

Table 7. Correlation between patient hearing levels measured during the initial exam with blood test values of patients treated within 7 days of ISSNHL onset.

	R	P value
WBC	0.166	0.019*
FBS	0.255	0.001**
HgbA1c	0.168	0.039*
ESR	0.307	0.005**

WBC, white blood cell count; FBS, fasting blood sugar; ESR, erythrocyte sedimentation; rate; R, rate.

*$p<0.05$; **$p<0.01$.

Table 8. Correlation between patient hearing recovery rate and blood test values of patients treated within 7 days of ISSHNL onset.

	R	P value
WBC	−0.202	0.005**
Fibrinogen	−0.264	0.004**
FDP	0.204	0.029*
ESR	−0.259	0.020*
Initial hearing	−0.226	0.001**

WBC, white blood cell count; ESR, erythrocyte sedimentation rate; FDP, fibrinogen degradation products; R, rate.
*p<0.05; ** p<0.01.

WBCs being drawn to the site by adhesion molecules expressed by local blood vessels.

From the start of this study in 2005, we have used vasodilators to treat ISSHL, even though their use for this purpose remains unsubstantiated due to the poor hearing outcome. However, one of our co-authors (K. Ogawa) has observed marked hearing improvement at higher frequencies and significant improvement of tinnitus in patients receiving PGE1 compared to placebo (44% versus 13%), even though no significant differences were observed in the overall hearing gain or in the rate of hearing improvement between the PGE1 and placebo groups of patients [23]. Nevertheless, we chose to treat our ISSHL patients with the vasodilator lipoPGE1, even though sufficient evidence supporting its use in this patient population is lacking at this time.

The time course of molecular factors, such as adhesion molecules, contributing to inner ear damage might be influenced by transcriptional factors. Indeed, nuclear factor kappa B (NFkB), a transcriptional factor that activates cytokines and adhesion molecules, may be involved in inner ear damage or sensorineural hearing loss [26]. In animal models of inner ear damage, such as acoustic trauma, NFkB and cytokines have been shown to promote inner ear damage just a few hours after the delivery of acoustic trauma (noise) [27,28]. Macrophages migrate into the cochlea a few days later [29].

Table 9. Correlation between various potential prognostic blood factors and audiogram shape and hearing recovery rate.

Audiogram shape	Hearing recovery rate		
	Factors	**R**	**P value**
Flat	None	–	–
High-pitch sloping	Fibrinogen	−0.406	0.04
	ESR	−0.639	0.01
Total deafness	WBC	−0.397	0.03
	FBS	−0.447	0.03
	LDL	−0.655	0.02
	Hct	+0.661	0.00
Low and high	None	–	–
Middle-pitch notch	Fibrinogen	−0.625	0.01
	TG	+0.563	0.01
Other	WBC	−0.312	0.02

+, Positive correlation; –, negative correlation; ESR, erythrocyte sedimentation rate; FBS, fasting blood sugar; Hct, hematocrit; LDL, low-density lipoprotein cholesterol; Plt, platelets; PT, prothrombin time; TG, triglycerides; WBC, white blood cell count.

We also demonstrated that audiogram shape varies across different pathological backgrounds that require different prognostic factors for blood tests.

Our data demonstrate that patients with higher LDL values have lower hearing recovery rates. High LDL and high cholesterol levels increase atherosclerosis and blood viscosity. Cholesterol, however, is not prognostic factor for ISSHL. This may induce extensive inner ear ischemia, which could be responsible for the "total deafness" audiogram pattern observed in some of our patients.

Canis et al. recommended fibrinogen and LDL apheresis in patients presenting with high fibrinogen and LDL levels [30]. Our data demonstrate that apheresis treatment may be indicated in patients with middle-pitch notch, higher-pitch sloping, or total deafness audiogram shapes.

In the present study, we propose a novel therapeutic concept for the treatment of ISSNHL, in which treatment choice depends on the timing and type of audiogram obtained.

We demonstrated that high fibrinogen levels (measured one day after ISSNHL onset) correlate with poorer hearing recovery in ISSNHL. High fibrinogen levels may indicate ischemic changes in the inner ear [30]. High WBC counts may reflect an immune response to inner ear damage induced by ischemic changes or infections. Thus, elevated WBC counts suggest that several causative factors may contribute to ISSNHL pathology. Our data have also led us to conclude that the time course of ISSNHL (i.e., progression of tissue damage after onset) and audiogram shape dictate different therapeutic strategies. Additional prospective studies are necessary to further elucidate the precise mechanisms underlying ISSNHL pathology.

Supporting Information

Table S1 Data of all the patients in this study.

Checklist S1 TREND checklist.

Protocol S1 We provided the protocol (English version and Japanese original version).

Acknowledgments

We thank Professor Toshio Yoshihara (Department of Otolaryngology, Tokyo Women's Medical University, Tokyo, Japan) for helpful comments.

Author Contributions

Conceived and designed the experiments: SK MS HH SM KO. Performed the experiments: SK MS HH SM KO. Analyzed the data: SK. Contributed reagents/materials/analysis tools: SK. Wrote the paper: SK. Discussion regarding data: SK MS HH SM KO. Responses from reviewers: KO SK.

References

1. Schweinfurth JM, Parnes SM, Very M (1996) Current concepts in the diagnosis and treatment of sudden sensorineural hearing loss. Eur Arch Otorhinolaryngol 253: 117–121.
2. Fetterman BL, Saunders JE, Luxford WM (1996) Prognosis and treatment of sudden sensorineural hearing loss. Am J Otol 17: 529–536.

3. Suckfull M, Wimmer C, Reichel O, Mees K, Schorn K (2002) Hyperfibrinogenemia as a risk factor for sudden hearing loss. Otol Neurotol 23: 309–311.
4. Cvorovic L, Deric D, Probst R, Hegemann S (2008) Prognostic model for predicting hearing recovery in idiopathic sudden sensorineural hearing loss. Otol Neurotol 29: 464–469.
5. Byl FM Jr (1984) Sudden hearing loss: eight years' experience and suggested prognostic table. Laryngoscope 94: 647–661.
6. Mattox DE, Lyles CA (1989) Idiopathic sudden sensorineural hearing loss. Am J Otol 10: 242–247.
7. Chang NC, Ho KY, Kuo WR (2005) Audiometric patterns and prognosis in sudden sensorineural hearing loss in southern Taiwan. Otolaryngol Head Neck Surg 133: 916–922.
8. Narozny W, Kuczkowski J, Kot J, Stankiewicz C, Sicko Z, et al. (2006) Prognostic factors in sudden sensorineural hearing loss: our experience and a review of the literature. Ann Otol Rhinol Laryngol 115: 553–558.
9. Ohinata Y, Makimoto K, Kawakami M, Haginomori S, Araki M, et al. (1994) Blood viscosity and plasma viscosity in patients with sudden deafness. Acta Otolaryngol 114: 601–607.
10. Ciuffetti G, Scardazza A, Serafini G, Lombardini R, Mannarino E, et al. (1991) Whole-blood filterability in sudden deafness. Laryngoscope 101: 65–67.
11. Capaccio P, Cuccarini V, Ottaviani F, Fracchiolla NS, Bossi A, et al. (2009) Prothrombotic gene mutations in patients with sudden sensorineural hearing loss and cardiovascular thrombotic disease. Ann Otol Rhinol Laryngol 118: 205–210.
12. Capaccio P, Ottaviani F, Cuccarini V, Ambrosetti U, Fagnani E, et al. (2005) Methylenetetrahydrofolate reductase gene mutations as risk factors for sudden hearing loss. Am J Otolaryngol 26: 383–387.
13. Capaccio P, Ottaviani F, Cuccarini V, Ambrosetti U, Fagnani E, et al. (2005) Sudden hearing loss and MTHFR 677C>T/1298A>C gene polymorphisms. Genet Med 7: 206–208.
14. Capaccio P, Ottaviani F, Cuccarini V, Bottero A, Schindler A, et al. (2007) Genetic and acquired prothrombotic risk factors and sudden hearing loss. Laryngoscope 117: 547–551.
15. Rudack C, Langer C, Stoll W, Rust S, Walter M (2006) Vascular risk factors in sudden hearing loss. Thromb Haemost 95: 454–461.
16. Ramunni A, Quaranta N, Saliani MT, Fallacara RA, Ria R, et al. (2006) Does a reduction of adhesion molecules by LDL-apheresis have a role in the treatment of sudden hearing loss? Ther Apher Dial 10: 282–286.
17. Quaranta N, Ramunni A, Brescia P, D'Elia A, Vacca A, et al. (2008) Soluble intercellular adhesion molecule 1 and soluble vascular cell adhesion molecule 1 in sudden hearing loss. Otol Neurotol 29: 470–474.
18. Gross M, Eliashar R, Ben-Yaakov A, Ulmansky R, Elidan J (2008) Prevalence and clinical significance of anticardiolipin, anti-beta2-glycoprotein-1, and anti-heat shock protein-70 autoantibodies in sudden sensorineural hearing loss. Audiol Neurootol 13: 231–238.
19. Suslu N, Yilmaz T, Gursel B (2009) Utility of anti-HSP 70, TNF-alpha, ESR, antinuclear antibody, and antiphospholipid antibodies in the diagnosis and treatment of sudden sensorineural hearing loss. Laryngoscope 119: 341–346.
20. Mattox DE, Simmons FB (1977) Natural history of sudden sensorineural hearing loss. Ann Otol Rhinol Laryngol 86: 463–480.
21. Smit JJ, Ottervanger JP, Slingerland RJ, Kolkman JJ, Suryapranata H, et al. (2008) Comparison of usefulness of C-reactive protein versus white blood cell count to predict outcome after primary percutaneous coronary intervention for ST elevation myocardial infarction. Am J Cardiol 101: 446–451.
22. Balestrino M, Partinico D, Finocchi C, Gandolfo C (1998) White blood cell count and erythrocyte sedimentation rate correlate with outcome in patients with acute ischemic stroke. J Stroke Cerebrovasc Dis 7: 139–144.
23. Ogawa K, Takei S, Inoue Y, Kanzaki J (2002) Effect of prostaglandin E1 on idiopathic sudden sensorineural hearing loss: a double-blinded clinical study. Otol Neurotol 23: 665–668.
24. Timmer JR, Ottervanger JP, Hoorntje JC, De Boer MJ, Suryapranata H, et al. (2005) Prognostic value of erythrocyte sedimentation rate in ST segment elevation myocardial infarction: interaction with hyperglycaemia. Journal of internal medicine 257: 423–429.
25. Chia S, Nagurney JT, Brown DF, Raffel OC, Bamberg F, et al. (2009) Association of leukocyte and neutrophil counts with infarct size, left ventricular function and outcomes after percutaneous coronary intervention for ST-elevation myocardial infarction. Am J Cardiol 103: 333–337.
26. Merchant SN, Adams JC, Nadol JB Jr (2005) Pathology and pathophysiology of idiopathic sudden sensorineural hearing loss. Otol Neurotol 26: 151–160.
27. Masuda M, Nagashima R, Kanzaki S, Fujioka M, Ogita K, et al. (2006) Nuclear factor-kappa B nuclear translocation in the cochlea of mice following acoustic overstimulation. Brain Res 1068: 237–247.
28. Fujioka M, Kanzaki S, Okano HJ, Masuda M, Ogawa K, et al. (2006) Proinflammatory cytokines expression in noise-induced damaged cochlea. J Neurosci Res 83: 575–583.
29. Hirose K, Discolo CM, Keasler JR, Ransohoff R (2005) Mononuclear phagocytes migrate into the murine cochlea after acoustic trauma. J Comp Neurol 489: 180–194.
30. Canis M, Heigl F, Suckfuell M (2012) Fibrinogen/LDL apheresis is a promising rescue therapy for sudden sensorineural hearing loss. Clinical research in cardiology supplements 7: 36–40.

26

Efficacy of Individual Computer-Based Auditory Training for People with Hearing Loss

Helen Henshaw*, Melanie A. Ferguson

NIHR Nottingham Hearing Biomedical Research Unit, Nottingham, United Kingdom

Abstract

Background: Auditory training involves active listening to auditory stimuli and aims to improve performance in auditory tasks. As such, auditory training is a potential intervention for the management of people with hearing loss.

Objective: This systematic review (PROSPERO 2011: CRD42011001406) evaluated the published evidence-base for the efficacy of individual computer-based auditory training to improve speech intelligibility, cognition and communication abilities in adults with hearing loss, with or without hearing aids or cochlear implants.

Methods: A systematic search of eight databases and key journals identified 229 articles published since 1996, 13 of which met the inclusion criteria. Data were independently extracted and reviewed by the two authors. Study quality was assessed using ten pre-defined scientific and intervention-specific measures.

Results: Auditory training resulted in improved performance for trained tasks in 9/10 articles that reported on-task outcomes. Although significant generalisation of learning was shown to untrained measures of speech intelligibility (11/13 articles), cognition (1/1 articles) and self-reported hearing abilities (1/2 articles), improvements were small and not robust. Where reported, compliance with computer-based auditory training was high, and retention of learning was shown at post-training follow-ups. Published evidence was of very-low to moderate study quality.

Conclusions: Our findings demonstrate that published evidence for the efficacy of individual computer-based auditory training for adults with hearing loss is not robust and therefore cannot be reliably used to guide intervention at this time. We identify a need for high-quality evidence to further examine the efficacy of computer-based auditory training for people with hearing loss.

Editor: Joel Snyder, UNLV, United States of America

Funding: This research was funded by the National Institute for Health Research (NIHR). The funders had no role in study design, data collection and analysis, decision to publish, or preparation of the manuscript.

Competing Interests: The authors have declared that no competing interests exist.

* E-mail: helen.henshaw@nottingham.ac.uk

Introduction

Background

The World Health Organization [1] reported in 2004 that over 275 million people worldwide had a significant hearing impairment. Adult-onset hearing loss is highly prevalent, whereby 27% of males and 24% of females aged 45 years and over experience mild hearing loss (defined as a pure-tone hearing threshold of 26 decibels (dB) average across 0.5, 1, 2, 4 k Hz) or greater in the better hearing ear. Hearing loss is currently estimated to be the 13th most common disease burden worldwide, and it has been predicted that by 2030 adult-onset hearing loss will be the seventh leading disease burden, above diabetes and HIV [1]. Hearing loss can lead to additional difficulties with employment, depression, social isolation, and reduced quality of life [2]. Untreated hearing loss has a substantial social impact on the person with hearing loss and for those with whom they communicate [3,4].

For adults who gradually acquire a hearing loss, their first complaint is unlikely to be 'I cannot hear'. More often they report 'I can hear but I cannot understand what is being said', particularly in noisy listening environments [5]. Hearing aids are the most common management option for people with hearing loss, yet uptake is low, with just 20% of people with hearing loss in the UK [6,7], and just under 30% in the US [8] owning them. Furthermore, of those who do own hearing aids, between 15% and 30% do not wear them regularly [6,9]. It has become apparent over the last decade that the challenges faced by people with hearing loss cannot be explained by the audiogram alone [5,10]. Difficulties in hearing may be exacerbated by, or masquerade as, reductions in cognitive ability such as problems in remembering or comprehending speech [11,12]. Although hearing aids may help people with hearing loss *hear* speech, their ability to *listen to* and *make sense of* speech may still be sub-optimal. Cognitive function plays a significant role in listening, whereby greater working memory capacity is associated with improved language comprehension [13], and selective attention has been shown to be central to following multi-speaker conversations (see [14] for a review).

The 2012 British Society of Audiology guidance for adult hearing rehabilitation [15] states that successful rehabilitation should be based upon, 'identifying individual needs, setting specific goals, making shared informed decisions and supporting self-management – steps that are important for helping the client to overcome his/her difficulties in everyday life' [15]. To enable this, clinicians may need to consider interventions that are complementary or alternative to the provision of hearing aids (or cochlear implants where hearing loss is severe to profound). Auditory training is one such clinical intervention, which promotes self-management of hearing difficulties, and is aimed at improving speech intelligibility through the development of auditory perceptual skills. Typically, listeners learn to make perceptual distinctions between sounds presented systematically [16]. Studies of auditory perceptual learning demonstrate the potential for training to improve auditory perceptual skills over the course of an adult's lifespan (see [17] for a review).

Auditory Training as an Intervention for People with Hearing Loss

Historically, a distinction has been made between bottom-up sensory refinement (analytic training) and top-down improvement of spoken language comprehension (synthetic training) [18]. In 2005, Sweetow and Palmer published a systematic review of studies that assessed the efficacy of individual auditory training for adults with hearing loss [18]. These studies assessed clinician-delivered training, an intervention which is time-, resource-, and cost-intensive. Six articles, published between 1970 and 1996 [19–24], met the criteria for inclusion, which were; *Participants:* adults with hearing loss with or without hearing aids, who were not cochlear implant users; *Intervention*: analytic or synthetic auditory training, or combination of the two; *Controls:* with or without a control group comparison; *Outcomes*; one or more measure relating to communication skills (e.g. understanding speech, self-perception of ability); *Study designs:* randomized controlled trials, nonrandomized controlled trials, cohort and repeated measures designs with or without a control group. The authors concluded that speech recognition skills, particularly in noise, may be improved by synthetic training, whereas the contribution of analytic training remains uncertain. Yet, more recently, bottom-up (analytic) auditory training using phoneme discrimination has also shown improvements in top-down cognitive processing, which may offer additional benefit to people with hearing loss, particularly in adverse listening situations [25]. Finally, a meta-analysis of six studies assessing the benefits of (primarily clinician-delivered) auditory training for people with hearing loss published between 1970 and 2009, (including those reviewed by Sweetow & Palmer [18]), suggested a reliable but small post-training improvements in speech recognition performance (Cohen's $d = .352$) [26].

Over the last two decades, the emergence of individual (non-clinician delivered), computer-based auditory training (CBAT) packages has resulted in a resurgence of interest in auditory training as an intervention for people with hearing loss. The key benefits of CBAT include home-delivery, the potential to tailor training packages to individual needs, and the ability to remotely monitor and capture trainee data over the internet. Thus, CBAT is an intervention that is time-, resource- and cost-effective, and can be conveniently accessed by the user [27]. There are several key considerations in using individual CBAT as an intervention to improve speech intelligibility for people with hearing loss. First and foremost, the intervention should be demonstrated to be effective, whereby any on-task learning should generalise to functional benefits in real-world listening ability. Improvements in behavioural measures of speech intelligibility in noise are typically considered by researchers and clinicians to be the ultimate aim of CBAT, as this is the most common complaint of people with hearing loss. However, as speech intelligibility has been shown to be mediated by cognition, particularly where the speech signal is degraded, training-related improvements in cognition (e.g. attention and working memory) are also likely to reflect functional real-world benefits to listening. Second, for auditory training to be accepted by an individual and therefore undertaken, the individual must be able to identify tangible benefits from the training. Thus, improvements in self-reported communication abilities are also important to the success of CBAT. Nevertheless, evidence from studies of alternative interventions suggest that improvements in self-reported outcomes alone may simply reflect expectations created as a result of receiving an intervention [28,29]. Ideally, any improvements in self-reported outcomes should therefore be accompanied by functional benefits, as indexed by behavioural tasks of speech intelligibility or cognitive performance. Third, for auditory training to be a successful intervention for people with hearing loss, any CBAT related improvements should persist over time. Finally, individuals must comply with CBAT, as an intervention can only be effective when individuals conform. This final point is of particular importance where CBAT is used as an unsupervised, home-based intervention.

Research Aims

A systematic review aims to identify, appraise and synthesize all the empirical evidence that meets pre-specified eligibility criteria in order to answer a given research question [30]. The primary aim of the present review was to examine the evidence for individual CBAT as an effective intervention for people with hearing loss. The evidence-base in the published literature was evaluated for both on-task learning for trained stimuli, and generalisation of learning to improvements in untrained measures of speech intelligibility, cognition and communication. Secondary aims sought to examine the feasibility of individual CBAT as an intervention for people with hearing loss by examining (i) the long-term retention of training-related improvements, and (ii) levels of compliance with CBAT programmes.

Specific Research Questions

1. Does evidence exist to support improvements in trained and untrained measures of speech intelligibility, cognition or communication (either behavioural or self-reported outcomes) as a result of individual computer-based auditory training (CBAT) in people with hearing loss?
2. Do any improvement(s) in communication, speech intelligibility or cognitive abilities remain for people with hearing loss after CBAT has ceased (retention of learning)?
3. What are the levels of compliance with individual CBAT?

To address these questions, data from 13 published articles that met the criteria for inclusion were reviewed and quality assessed. Evidence for the efficacy of CBAT for people with hearing loss was extracted from included articles and the quality of evidence examined. Findings are presented together with recommendations for future research.

Methods

The Centre for Reviews and Dissemination, University of York [31], part of the National Institute for Health Research (NIHR), and the Preferred Reporting Items for Systematic Reviews and

Meta-analyses (PRISMA) statement [32], which offer guidance for undertaking and reporting of systematic reviews in health care, were used to inform the methodology, the systematic search procedure, and the reporting of this systematic review (Checklist S1).

Systematic Search Strategy and Study Selection

Methods of data extraction, data analysis, and inclusion and exclusion criteria were pre-specified and documented within the systematic review protocol. This is important in providing transparency in the review process by ensuring that the objectives of the systematic review and methods of data identification and extraction are clearly defined prior to any data being collected. Details of the systematic review protocol have been registered with PROSPERO, the International prospective register of systematic reviews. The protocol is available online at: http://www.crd.york.ac.uk/prospero/display_record.asp?ID = CRD42011001406. Inclusion criteria were formed using the *Participants*, *Intervention*, *Control*, *Outcomes*, and *Study designs* (PICOS) strategy [33]. PICOS inclusion criteria are presented in Table 1. Exclusion criteria included articles that were published prior to 1996 (i.e. those included in the previous review of auditory training for people with hearing loss by Sweetow and Palmer, [18]), studies presenting pilot data, studies that were not peer reviewed and those not available in English.

Study identification. Eight electronic databases (Embase, Medline, Pubmed, Web of Science, Applied Social Sciences Index and Abstracts (ASSIA), Science Direct,/Cumulative Index to Nursing and Allied Health (CINAHL) and PsychINFO) were initially searched in August 2011 using the terms hearing loss OR hearing aid* OR hearing impair* OR cochlear implant* AND auditory training OR auditory learning OR perceptual training OR perceptual learning. Search terms were always combined in an attempt to limit identified papers to those reporting adult subjects with hearing loss. An example search string is provided (Example Search Terms S1). Additional articles were identified through the systematic snowballing of all 349 articles reference lists, and a related article search for each author of an article which met the PICOS criteria for inclusion. Three further articles were identified through ongoing hand-searches of audiology journals, up to the date of first submission of this article (December 2012), to ensure an up-to-date review.

Screening. The database searches returned a total of 349 articles. A further 27 articles were identified through the additional journal searches. A total of 229 articles of potential relevance remained after the removal of duplicate articles (n = 147). Abstracts of the 229 identified articles were independently assessed by the two authors relative to the PICOS criteria for inclusion (Figure 1), of which, 201 failed to meet the inclusion criteria. In cases where insufficient detail was available in the abstract to make a decision, the full-text of the article was retrieved and assessed against the PICOS criteria. A total of 28 abstracts either met the PICOS criteria for inclusion, or contained insufficient information from which to make a judgement, and progressed to a second stage of screening where the full-text articles were obtained.

Eligibility. A second stage of assessment, a full-text review of the 28 potentially relevant articles, revealed 15 articles that failed to meet the PICOS criteria for inclusion. For cases where multiple publications arose from the same participant data, only the first publication was included in line with the Centre for Reviews and Dissemination guidelines [31]. A total of 13 articles were eligible for inclusion in the systematic review.

Data Extraction and Data Synthesis

Data to be extracted were pre-specified within a data extraction and quality assessment form, piloted by the two authors and amended as necessary. Final study data extraction was conducted independently by the same two authors and included details of study design, participants (number, age, sex and hearing loss), training stimuli, amount of training and training duration, outcome measures, main findings (both trained and untrained), compliance and follow-up. Where any instances of non-agreement on the extracted data occurred, the article was jointly revisited until a consensus was reached.

Study Quality and Potential Sources of Study Bias

Scientific study quality and potential sources of study bias were assessed using five independent measures; randomisation, controls, sample size and power calculation, blinding, and outcome measure reporting. Low scores on these measures indicate less information, thus a higher potential for bias in results. Five additional measures, which were all highly specific to training intervention studies, aimed to capture the quality of the intervention study designs. Measures included; generalisation of learning to functional benefits in real-world listening (outcome selection), training feedback, which has been previously shown to maximise auditory learning in auditory training [33,34], ecological validity, compliance with training protocols, and long-term follow-up of improvements. Scores for each of the study quality measures ranged from 0–2. A score of 0 indicated flawed or no information from which to make a judgement, a score of 1 indicated weak information or lack of detail and a score of 2 indicated appropriate use and reporting.

Individual measure scores were summed to form an overall study quality score that was then used to inform the level of evidence attributed to each study. Levels of evidence were adapted from the 2004 Grading of Recommendations Assessment, Development and Evaluation (GRADE) Working Group guidelines [35] and provide an indication of confidence in the estimation of effect (Table 2). Studies that represent a low-level

Table 1. PICOS criteria for inclusion.

Participants	Adult (18+ years) humans with any degree of hearing loss
Intervention	Individual computer-based auditory training.
Control	Comparison with a control group or repeated measures [pre- and post-training comparison].
Outcomes	1+ outcome measure(s) related to speech intelligibility, cognition or communication (either behavioural measures or self-reported outcomes).
Study designs	Randomised controlled trials, non-randomised controlled trials, cohort studies (with a control comparison), and repeated measures (pre- and post-training comparisons).

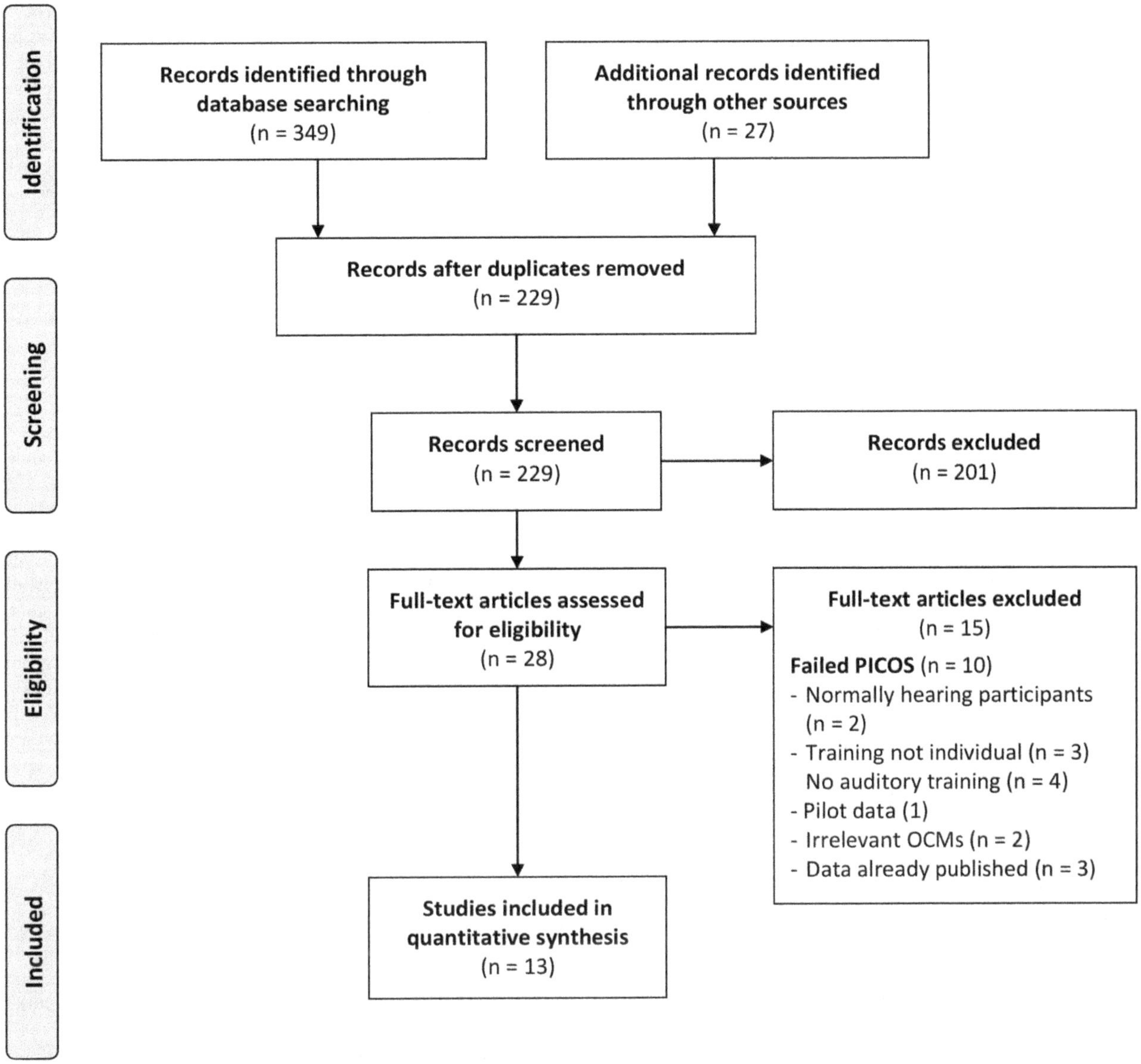

Figure 1. Flow diagram of the study identification, eligibility, and inclusion process.

of evidence offer results that are likely to vary should the experiment be repeated, whereas a study offering a high-level of evidence provides greater confidence that the data are representative of valid results.

A meta-analysis of results from comparable studies was not possible due to the heterogeneity between studies in terms of differences in participant samples (people with hearing loss, hearing aid users, and cochlear implant users), training stimuli, training protocols, and outcome measures adopted. As such, study

Table 2. Level of evidence by study quality score (Adapted from the GRADE Working Group, 2004 [35]).

Study quality score	Level of evidence	Confidence in estimation of effect
0–5	Very low	The estimation of effect is uncertain
6–10	Low	Further evidence is very likely to impact on our confidence in the estimation of effect and are likely to change the estimate
11–15	Moderate	Further evidence is likely to impact on our confidence in the estimation of effect and may change the estimate
16–20	High	Further evidence is very unlikely to change our confidence in the estimation of effect

findings and study quality were incorporated within a narrative synthesis to aid interpretation of findings and to examine any differences in outcomes across the 13 articles included in the systematic review.

Results

Table 3 summarises the data extracted from each of the 13 articles. Where publications reported more than one study or training protocol these are presented separately in the table.

Study Characteristics

Data extracted from the 13 articles are presented in terms of the PICOS criteria (*Participants, Intervention, Controls, Outcome measures, Study designs*).

Participants. Participant samples included people with hearing loss without hearing aids or cochlear implants [37,40,42], new [38] and existing hearing aid users [38,41,46], experienced cochlear implant users [36, 41 43–45, 47], and bimodal (cochlear implant plus hearing aid) users [48]. However, samples were not always consistent. Participants in the study by Burk et al. [37] were not all regular hearing aid users, and the participant sample in Sweetow and Henderson-Sabes [39] included nine participants who reported difficulty understanding speech in adverse listening environments, but did not use hearing aids. Participant sample sizes ranged from n = 3 [44] (Experiment 1) to n = 69 [46], with a median sample of 9.5 (mean = 17.75, SD = 20.33).

Intervention. Training stimuli, training frequency, and training duration varied substantially between studies. Several studies trained participants on small parts of speech, such as phonemes [36], monosyllabic words, vowels or consonants [37,40,42,47,48], spondee words [44], and nonsense syllables [38,41]. Other studies trained participants using digits [45], words or sentences [41,43]. The remaining studies trained their participants using hybrid communication training packages such as the Listening and Communication Enhancement (LACE) program [39], which included a variety of listening and cognitive tasks alongside interactive communication strategies, and 'I hear what you mean' [46], that comprised several listening comprehension tasks. Training sessions ranged from 30 minutes [39] to 2 hours per session [41], and occurred daily to twice-weekly. Training duration ranged from four days [47] to three months [44].

Controls. Ideally a systematic review would assess only high-level evidence arising from randomised controlled trials as randomisation, rather than between-group differences, substantially increases our confidence that any observed effects are attributable to the intervention. Nevertheless, inclusion of only randomised controlled trials in this review would have served to eliminate the majority of published evidence assessing the efficacy of auditory training for people with hearing loss. As such, other study designs were considered. However, only studies that reported direct comparisons between control and trained groups, or between control and trained periods within a subject group, were included in the review. Repeated measures design (where participants act as their own controls) was the most commonly identified study type.

Outcome measures. There were no outcome measures that were common to all training studies. The majority of studies assessed measures of speech intelligibility using validated speech tests such as the Hearing in Noise Test (HINT) [68], the Revised Speech in Noise test (R-SPIN) [71], IEEE sentences [64], and the Nonsense Syllables Test (NST) [70]. The study by Sweetow and Henderson-Sabes [39] also included behavioural measures of cognition (working memory: Listening Span [11], and attention: Stroop Task [75]) and self-report of hearing (either the Hearing Handicap Inventory for the Elderly (HHIE) [67] or the Hearing Handicap Inventory for Adults (HHIA) [67], and the Communication Scale for Older Adults (CSOA] [60]). The study by Ingvalson et al. [47] was the only other study to include a self-report measure of hearing (Speech and Spatial Qualities of Hearing Scale (SSQ) [74]), whereas Stacey et al. [43] assessed self-report of health status using the Glasgow Benefit Inventory (GBI) [65].

Study designs. Some articles reported more than one study. There were 11 repeated measures designs [36–38,40,42–48], two non-randomised controlled trials [37,44] and three randomised controlled trials [38,39,41].

On-task Learning

On-task learning was defined as any improvement in performance on a task or stimulus that had been directly trained. This was almost always reported in studies assessing the efficacy of auditory training for people with hearing loss (10/13). Nine articles reported significant on-task learning for trained stimuli. Despite trends towards improvement, Stacey et al. [43] did not show significant on-task learning for trained words in a group of 10 cochlear implant users. Barcroft et al. [46], Ingvalson et al. [47] and Zhang et al. [48] did not report any on-task learning results.

Burk and colleagues were the only authors to report multiple outcomes from variations in training protocols using the same word training stimuli. Humes et al. [42] reported significant and considerably smaller improvements (20%) in open-set word recognition for trained words presented in larger sets (600 words) than Burk and Humes, (40–55%) who presented words in smaller (150 words) sets [40].

Generalisation of On-task Learning

Generalisation of learning was defined as an improvement in performance on a task or stimulus not directly trained. Outcomes that measured the generalisation of learning were divided into three sub-groups; improvements in speech intelligibility, cognition and self-report of communication.

Speech Intelligibility. All studies reported at least one measure of speech intelligibility. Table 4 provides a summary of these outcomes and any significant post-training improvement. Results are presented for untrained speech stimuli only, thus generalisation to improvements in performance for trained stimuli produced by different talkers is not considered here (refer to Table 3).

A number of studies reporting untrained speech intelligibility measures identified measures that had a degree of overlap between the lexical content of the trained and outcome stimuli. For example, Burk et al. [37] reported a 6–9% overlap and tested trained word recognition embedded in untrained sentences. Humes et al. [42] reported substantially greater overlap between the lexical content of trained and outcome stimuli of 50–80%. For some studies the degree of overlap was unclear, for example, the 'Four Choice Discrimination Task' reported by Barcroft et al. [46] appears to be very similar in nature to a trained exercise, although no details about any lexical overlap are provided.

Results revealed mixed findings for all participant groups, training stimuli, and study designs, whereby generalisation of learning to untrained measures of speech intelligibility did not always occur. For example, Burk et al. [37] reported that training on words generalised to improvements in untrained words and to trained words by untrained speakers, but did not generalise to

Table 3. Descriptive summary of extracted data from the 13 included articles.

Study	Design	Participants		Training			Outcomes	Main findings		Compliance and follow-up
		Hearing loss and hearing device	n, age and sex	Stimuli	Frequency and duration	Laboratory- or home-based training?	(bold indicates trained stimuli)	Trained stimuli	Untrained stimuli	
Fu et al. 2004 [36]	Repeated measures	7 pre-lingually and 3 post-lingually deafened adults. Existing cochlear implant users.	n = 10. 25–60 years, mean = 42.4 years. 4 male, 6 female.	Phonetic (vowel and consonant contrast) training with monosyllabic word, tailored to baseline performance.	1×1–2 hour sessions per day, 5 days per week, duration not reported.	Home	**Consonant and vowel recognition,** voice gender discrimination, HINT sentences.	Improvements for vowel (14.4%***, 10/10 participants tested) and consonant (13.0%**, 7/10 tested) recognition. No improvement in voice gender recognition (0.3%, 7/10 tested).	Improvements in open set word-in-sentence recognition on HINT (27.9%**, 3/10 participants tested).	Compliance not reported. No follow-up assessment.
Burk et al. 2006 Experiment 2 [37]	Repeated measures	Mild to moderate bilateral SNHL.	n = 7. 65–75 years, mean = 69.6 years. 3 male, 4 female.	Right ear only, (open- or closed-set) monosyllabic AB words in noise (0 dB SNR), adjusted for audibility relative to individuals audiogram.	7×1 hour sessions in total over approx. 2 weeks (max. 3 days between s essions).	Laboratory	**Trained AB word recognition,** untrained AB word recognition.	Improvements in open-set (45.3%***) and closed-set (11.0%*) trained AB word recognition. No significant generalisation to trained AB words presented by untrained talkers.	Improvements in open-set untrained AB word recognition (6.9%*), no improvement for closed-set untrained AB word recognition (average improvement = 5.3%, *ns*). No significant generalisation to untrained AB words presented by a trained talker.	Compliance not reported. 5/7 participants returned 6 months post-training (Experiment 3). Performance remained significantly improved from baseline for trained open-set AB words (25.3%*), yet significantly worse than immediate post-training levels.
Burk et al. 2006 Experiment 3 [37]	Non-randomised controlled trial (control group = 9 young listeners, normally hearing.	Mild to moderate bilateral SNHL (5/7 participants from Experiment 2).	n = 5. 68–75 years, mean = 71.0 years. 2 male, 3 female.	Right ear only, (open- or closed-set) monosyllabic AB words in noise (0 dB SNR), adjusted for audibility relative to individuals audiogram.	Less than 1 hour (top-up training).	Laboratory	**Trained AB words recognition, trained AB words** in TIMIT sentences, untrained AB words in TIMIT sentences.	Trained AB words returned to within 95% critical difference of immediate post-training scores (Experiment 2). No significant improvements in trained AB words in TIMIT sentences.	No improvements in untrained AB words in TIMIT sentences.	Compliance not reported. No follow-up assessment.
Stecker et al. 2006 Experiment 1 [38]	Randomised controlled trial crossover (control group trained second).	Mild to moderate bilateral SNHL. New hearing aid users.	n = 23. 50–80 years, mean = 69.0 years. 23 male, 0 female. Immediate training (IT) n = 12. Delayed training (DT) n = 11.	Adaptive nonsense syllable (NST) identification in noise.	5×35–70 minute sessions per week for 8 weeks.	Home	**NST**, R-SPIN.	IT group: Improvement of 10.6%*** in NST identification. DT group: 8.8%*** improvement. Trained NST improvements were shown to generalise to untrained voices ($p<.001$). Significant improvement in performance for trained NST presented by untrained talkers***.	5 subjects from the IT group and 6 from the DT group were tested on the R-SPIN. Average improvement of 3.3% (*ns*) attributed to lack of power.	92.5% average compliance reported. Participants completed 29–44 days of training out of a required 40 days. Mean training days = 37, mode = 40. No significant decrement (−1.1%, *ns*) from post-training performance for NST syllable identification at an 8 week follow-up assessment.

Table 3. Cont.

Study	Design	Participants		Training			Outcomes	Main findings		Compliance and follow-up
		Hearing loss and hearing device	n, age and sex	Stimuli	Frequency and duration	Laboratory- or home-based training?	(bold indicates trained stimuli)	Trained stimuli	Untrained stimuli	
Stecker et al. 2006 Experiment 2 [38]	Repeated measures	Mild-moderate bilateral SNHL. Existing hearing aid users.	n = 8. 61–75 years, mean = 67.7 years. Sex not reported.	Adaptive nonsense syllable (NST) identification in noise.	5×35–70 minute sessions per week for 8 weeks.	Home	**NST.**	Improvement (p<.01) in NST identification, although to a lesser degree than new hearing aid users in Experiment 1.	-	Compliance not reported. No significant decrease in performance for NST syllable identification at a 2 months post-training follow-up.
Sweetow and Henderson-Sabes, 2006 [39]	Randomised controlled trial crossover (control group trained second).	Normal hearing to severe SNHL. n = 56 existing hearing aid users.	n = 89. 28–85 years. Immediate training group (IT) n = 56, mean age = 63.2 years, sex not reported. Delayed training group (DT) n = 33, mean age = 64.2 years, sex not reported.	Listening and Communication Enhancement (LACE).	5×30 min sessions per week for 4 weeks.	Home	**LACE,** QuickSIN, HINT sentences, Listening Span, Stroop, HHIA/E, CSOA.	Improvements shown for all LACE measures overall: Speech/Babble, Time Compression, Competing Speaker, Auditory Memory and Missing Word (all p<.05). Non hearing aid users (n = 9) only improved significantly in Speech/Babble and Competing Speaker (p<.05).	Improvements in the trained group (Group 1, n = 38) for QuickSIN 45 dB (−2.2 dB SNR***) QuickSIN 70 dB (−1.5 dB SNR***), Listening Span (.5 sentences*), Stroop (7.5 points**), HHIA/E (7.5 points/17%**) and CSOA (.14**). No significant improvement in HINT (where the control group also showed improvement).	73% compliance (65/89 participants enrolled completed the training, immediate training group n = 38/56, delayed training group n = 27/33). Improvements are maintained for participants tested on QuickSIN and HINT (n = 42/65 tested), HHIA/E and CSOA (n = 31/65 tested) 1 month post-training. No statistical tests reported.
Burk and Humes, 2008 [40]	Repeated measures	Mild to moderate SNHL.	n = 8. 58–78 years, mean = 69.5 years. 4 male, 4 female.	Right ear only - Recognition of 75 lexically hard and 75 lexically easy CVC monosyllabic words (difficulty switched at training mid-point), presented in noise and adjusted for audibility relative to the audiogram.	20–24 sessions (average 3 per week), for approx. 12 weeks.	Laboratory	**Trained CVC word recognition,** untrained CVC word recognition, VAST sentences.	Improvement in exically hard trained words for open-set (47.4%***) and closed-set recognition (16.4%***). Lexically easy words also improved for both open-set (40.4%***) and closed-set recognition (17.2%***). Improvements for hard words (40.2%***) and easy words (35.0%***) when presented by unfamiliar talkers.	No improvements were shown for recognition of untrained words. Some individual but no group improvements on trained words embedded within VAST sentences.	Compliance not reported. Improvements in trained word recognition were maintained across weekly follow-up assessments beginning 7 weeks post-training and lasting for 7–8 weeks (no statistical tests reported).

Table 3. Cont.

Study	Design	Participants		Training			Outcomes	Main findings		Compliance and follow-up
		Hearing loss and hearing device	**n, age and sex**	**Stimuli**	**Frequency and duration**	**Laboratory- or home-based training?**	**(bold indicates trained stimuli)**	**Trained stimuli**	**Untrained stimuli**	
Miller et al. 2008 [41]	Randomised controlled trial (hearing aid users: n = 8 trained, n = 4 controls. cochlear implant users: n = 8 trained, n = 8 controls).	Existing hearing aid users: n = 11 SNHL, n = 1 mixed loss at low frequencies. Existing cochlear implant users: n = 10 adult onset, n = 6 child onset deafness.	n = 28. n = 12 hearing aid users: 26–90 years, mean = 76.3 years. Sex not reported. n = 16 cochlear implant users: 35–81 years, mean = 55.5 years. Sex not reported.	Speech perception assessment and training system (SPATS): Syllable constituents and sentences (in quiet and in babble).	2×2 hour sessions per week for 6 weeks.	Laboratory	**SPATS,** HINT sentences, CST-AV, CST-A, CID sentences, W22 words, CNC.	Improvements in SPATS (nuclei and onset) in quiet and for hearing aid users (average 8% improvement), and for cochlear implant users (average 6% improvement). Improvement for pooled hearing aid and cochlear implant trained participants of 11% (average 7% improvement in quiet and 15% in noise), relative to controls.	Improvements in CST-AV, CID W22, CNC for hearing aid users (when HINT and CST-A data removed) of around 10%. Averaged over all measures, trained hearing aid users improved by 8% compared to controls. Improvements in all measures for cochlear implant users, with greatest gains for HINT in quiet. Overall, trained cochlear implant users improved by 13% relative to controls. Pooled trained participants improved on average 10% on untrained outcomes relative to controls. Statistical tests not presented for individual outcome measures.	Compliance not reported. No follow-up assessment.
Humes et al. 2009 [42]	Repeated measures	Older adults with hearing impairment n = 10 trained using protocol 1: High frequency pure-tone average (HfPTA) across 1, 2, 4 k Hz mean = 31 dB HL, SD 9.6. n = 6 trained using protocol 2: HfPTA mean = 26.4 dB HL, SD 14.1.	n = 16. Protocol 1: n = 10. Mean age = 70.2, SD = 6.8 years. 7 male, 3 female. Protocol 2: n = 6. Mean age = 72.8, SD = 7.6 years. 5 male, 1 female.	Closed set word identification training in noise (4 speakers). Protocol 1: repeated in blocks of 2400, Protocol 2: repeated in blocks of 600.	24×75–90 minute sessions over 8–12 weeks.	Laboratory	**Trained frequent word recognition,** CID sentences, VAST sentences, Frequent phrases.	Significant improvements shown for frequent word identification of around 18 rationalised arcsine unites (RAUs)*.	Significant improvements in CID sentences, VAST sentences and frequent phrases. Average improvements of between 12–20 RAUs*.	81% compliance reported (13/16 participants completed the requested training duration) across two training protocols. Non-complaint participants retained in main analyses. No follow-up assessment.

Table 3. Cont.

Study	Design	Participants		Training			Outcomes	Main findings		Compliance and follow-up
		Hearing loss and hearing device	n, age and sex	Stimuli	Frequency and duration	Laboratory- or home-based training?	(bold indicates trained stimuli)	Trained stimuli	Untrained stimuli	
Stacey et al. 2010 [43]	Repeated measures	n = 2 pre-lingual, n = 10 post-lingual, n = 1 pre/post-lingually deafened adults. Existing cochlear implant users.	n = 11. 23–71 years, mean = 54.8 years. 6 male, 5 female.	2-AFC discrimination of words presented acoustically from options presented visually.	1 hour per day for 3 weeks.	Home	**Trained word and sentence (IEEE/SPIN) recognition,** IEEE sentences, BKB sentences, Consonant test, Vowel test, GBI.	No improvement in trained stimuli (trend for improvement in trained sentences identified with polynomial contrasts).	Improvement in consonant test (8.06%*).	73% compliance reported (8/11 participants completed the requested training duration). Three participants excluded having completed just five hours of the requested 15 hours training. No follow-up assessment.
Tyler et al. 2010 Experiment 1 [44]	Repeated measures	Post-lingually deafened adults. Existing cochlear implant users.	n = 3. 43–63 years, mean = 60.3 years. 1 male, 2 female.	8-loudspeaker presentation of sound localization and Spondee words in babble.	1–3 months. Details of training sessions not reported.	Home	**Spondee word recognition, Sound localization,** CNC, CUNY sentences, HINT sentences.	Improvement in sound localisation for subject 1 (reduction in RMS error of 7°***). Improvements in the adaptive spondee-in-noise test for subject 1 ($p<.01$–$p<.001$) and subject 2 ($p<.001$)	Improvement in HINT (32%***) for subject 1. Improvements in CNC in noise recognition (4%*) and HINT sentences (36%***) for subject 2.	Compliance not reported. Retention of improvements in sound localisation and HINT at 2 and 7 months post-training for subject 1, other participants not tested. No statistical tests reported.
Tyler et al. 2010 Experiment 2 [44]	Non-randomised controlled trial	Post-lingually deafened adults. Existing cochlear implant users.	n = 9. Trained: n = 3. 63–77 years, mean = 68.7 years. 1 male, 2 female. Controls: n = 6. Age not reported. 3 male, 3 female.	2-loudspeaker presentation of sound localization and Spondee words in babble.	1–3 months.	Home	**Sound localization, Spondee word recognition.**	Improvements in localization scores were shown for subjects 1 ($p<.001$) and 2 ($p<.01$). Significant improvements in recognition scores were shown for subject 1 ($p<.05$) and subject 3 ($p<.05$).	-	Compliance not reported. No follow-up assessment.
Oba et al. 2011 [45]	Repeated measures	Post-lingually deafened. Existing cochlear implant users.	n = 10. 46–78 years, mean = 66.4 years. 4 male, 6 female.	Sound Express: Digits-in-noise (speech babble and steady noise).	5×30 minute sessions per week for 4 weeks.	Home	**Digit-in-noise (babble),** HINT sentences, IEEE sentences.	Improvements in digits-in-noise (steady noise) SRT of −2.8** dB and digits-in-noise (babble) of −4 dB***.	Improvements for HINT sentences in babble (−2.9 dB SRT**) and IEEE sentences in steady noise (improvement in % correct of 1.5%*) and in babble (9.2%*).	100% compliance reported. Performance remained significantly improved from baseline at a 1 month post-training follow-up for all improved measures ($p<.001$).

Table 3. Cont.

Study	Design	Participants		Training			Outcomes	Main findings		Compliance and follow-up
		Hearing loss and hearing device	n, age and sex	Stimuli	Frequency and duration	Laboratory- or home-based training?	(bold indicates trained stimuli)	Trained stimuli	Untrained stimuli	
Barcroft et al. 2011 [46]	Repeated measures	Mild-moderate bilateral SNHL. Existing hearing aid users.	n = 69. Multi-talker training group (MTG): n = 35, 18 male, 17 female. Males: 18–87 years, mean = 67 years. Females: 23–89 years, mean = 62 years. Single-talker training group (STG): n = 34, 21 male, 13 female. Males: 46–89 years, mean = 70 years. Females: 22–87 years, mean = 64 years.	I hear what you mean – listening comprehension activities in four-talker babble.	12×1 hour sessions, twice a week for 6 weeks.	Laboratory	Iowa consonant test, Build-a-sentence test, Four-choice discrimination test.	-	Improvement in four-choice discrimination test (13.7% points***), with scores for the single talker version significantly greater than those on the multi-talker version (p>.001). No effect of STG/MTG training group. Results from other outcomes not reported.	Compliance not reported. No follow-up assessment.
Ingvalson et al. 2012 [47]	Repeated measures	Post-lingually deafened. Existing cochlear implant users.	n = 5. 50–85 years, mean = 71.4 years. 2 male, 3 female.	Seeing and Hearing Speech program (vowel and consonant identification in words, sentences and phrases in multi-speaker babble).	4×1 hour sessions spread over four days.	Laboratory	**Vowel and consonant recognition in words, phrases and sentences,** SSQ, QuickSIN, HINT.	-	Improvement in HINT in quiet**, HINT at +15 dB SNR** and QuickSIN*.	Compliance not reported. Improvements in HINT and QuickSIN maintained at a 4-day post-training follow-up assessment.
Zhang et al. 2012 [48]	Repeated measures	Post-lingually deafened. Existing bimodal hearing aid and cochlear implant users.	n = 7. 51–78 years, mean = 64 years. 2 male, 5 female.	Sound Express: phoneme contrast training (vowels and consonants), for six subjects and monosyllabic word identification in multi-speaker babble for one subject.	1 hour per day, 5 days a week for 4 weeks.	Home	Vowel and consonant recognition, CNC words, AzBio sentences, Voice gender and emotion identification.	-	Improvements for six out of seven participants for speech recognition: Vowel (8.6%*) and consonant (9.8%*) identification, CNC words (14.9%*). No improvements were shown for AzBio s entences (8.3%, *ns*), nor for pitch-related performance (voice gender and emotion identification)	100% compliance reported. Improvements largely maintained at a one-month follow-up (vowel, consonant and CNC word recognition follow-up scores were significantly greater (p<.05) than baseline scores at the follow-up assessment).

Data for normally hearing participants are omitted from this table [42].

– = no data reported, *p<.05, **p<.01, ***p<.001. MSB = multi-speaker babble, SNHL = sensorineural hearing loss; SNR = signal to noise ratio, SRT = speech reception threshold, RAU = rationalised arcsine unit [49]; Adaptive spondee words in babble test [50]; Adaptive 12-choice spondee words with multiple jammers test [51]; AzBio sentences [52]; BKB = Bamford-Kowal-Bench sentence lists [53]; Build-a-sentence test [54]; CID Everyday Sentences = Central Institute for the Deaf everyday sentences [55]; CID W22 = Central Institute for the Deaf word lists [56]; CNC = consonant-vowel nucleus-consonant monosyllables [57]; CNC words [58]; Consonant recognition [59]; CSOA = Communication Scale for Older Adults [60]; CST-A = Connected Speech [audio] test [61]; CST-AV = Connected Speech [audio-visual] test [61]; CUNY = City University of New York sentences [62]; Everyday sounds localization test [63]; IEEE Sentences [64] Four-choice discrimination test [46]; GBI = Glasgow benefit inventory [65]; HHIA = Hearing handicap inventory for adults [66]; HHIE = Hearing handicap inventory for the elderly [67]; HINT = Hearing in noise test [68]; Iowa consonant test [69]; LACE = Listening and Communication Enhancement, [39]; Listening span test [11]; NST = Nonsense syllable test [70]; QuickSIN [70]; R-SPIN = Revised speech perception noise test [71]; SPATS = [72]; SPIN = Speech perception in noise test [73]; SSQ = Speech, Spatial and Qualities of Hearing Scale [74]; Stroop Color Word test [75]; TIMIT sentences [76]; VAST = Verb and sentence test [77]; Vowel recognition [78].

Table 4. Improvements in untrained measures of speech intelligibility by participant type.

	Study	Training stimulus	Outcome measures	Outcome stimulus	Laboratory- or home- based training?	Significant improvement?
A.	**People with hearing loss**					
	Burk et al. 2006 [37]	Monosyllabic words	Word recognition	(SSN) Untrained monosyllabic AB words	Laboratory	**Y**
			TIMIT	(SSN) (Untrained AB) keywords in sentences		N
	Burk and Humes, 2008 [40]	Monosyllabic words	Word recognition	(SSN) Untrained monosyllabic CVC words	Laboratory	N
			VAST	(SSN) (Trained CVC) keywords in sentences		N
	Humes et al. 2009 [42]	Frequent words	CID Everyday Sentences	(ICRA 6) Sentences	Laboratory	**Y**
			VAST sentences	(ICRA 6) Sentences		**Y**
			Frequent phrases	(ICRA 6) Sentences		**Y**
B.	**Hearing aid users**					
	Stecker et al. 2006 [38], Experiment 1	Nonsense syllables	R-SPIN	(MSB) Final keyword in sentences	Home	N
	Sweetow and Henderson Sabes, 2006 [39]	*LACE*	QuickSIN	(MSB) Sentences	Home	**Y**
			HINT	(SSN) Sentences		N
	Miller et al. 2008 [41]	*SPATS* syllables	HINT	(Q) and (SSN) Sentences	Laboratory	N
			CST-A	(Q) and (MSB) Sentences		N
			CST-AV	(Q) and (MSB) Sentences		N
			CID-W22	(Q) and (MSB) Words		N
			CNC	(Q) and (MSB) Monosyllables		N
	Barcroft et al. 2011 [46]	*I hear what you mean* listening comprehension	Four-choice discrimination test	(MSB) Words	Laboratory	**Y**
C.	**Cochlear implant users**					
	Fu et al. 2004 [36]	Phonemes	HINT	(SSN) Sentences	Home	**Y**
	Miller et al. 2008 [41]	*SPATS* syllables	HINT	(Q) and (SSN) Sentences	Laboratory	N
			CST-A	(Q) and (MSB) Sentences		N
			CST-AV	(Q) and (MSB) Sentences		N
			CID-W22	(Q) and (MSB) Words		N
			CNC	(Q) and (MSB) Monosyllables		**Y**
	Stacey et al. 2010 [43]	Words	Vowel test	(Q) h-vowel-d words	Home	N
			Consonant test	(Q) a-consonant-a nonsense words		**Y**
			BKB	(Q) Sentences		N
			IEEE	(Q) Sentences		N
	Tyler et al. 2010 [44] Experiment 1	Spondee words	CNC	(Q) CNC monosyllabic words	Home	N
			CUNY	(MSB) Sentences		N
			HINT	(SSN) Sentences		**Y**
	Oba et al. 2011	*Sound Express* digits	HINT	(SSN) and (MSB) Sentences	Home	**Y**
			IEEE	(SSN) and (MSB) Sentences		**Y**
	Ingvalson et al. 2012 [47]	*Seeing and Hearing Speech* monosyllabic words	QuickSIN	(MSB) Sentences	Laboratory	**Y**
			HINT	(MSB) Sentences		**Y**

Table 4. Cont.

	Study	Training stimulus	Outcome measures	Outcome stimulus	Laboratory- or home- based training?	Significant improvement?
D.	**Bimodal (cochlear implant and hearing aid) users**					
	Zhang et al. 2012 [48]	*Sound Express* phonemes monosyllabic words	Vowel recognition	(MSB) h-vowel-d words	Home	Y
			Consonant recognition	(MSB) a-consonant-a nonsense words		Y
			CNC words	(MSB) Words		Y
			AzBio sentences	(MSB) Sentences		N

Significant improvement **Y** = yes, N = no. (Q) stimuli presented in quiet; (SSN) stimuli presented in speech-shaped noise; (ICRA 6) stimuli presented in ICRA (track 6) two-talker noise-vocoded competition; (MSB) stimuli presented in multi-speaker babble.

trained words embedded in TIMIT [77] sentences. Similarly Zhang et al. [48] showed post-training improvements in the intelligibility of untrained vowels, consonants and words, but no improvements in performance for untrained sentences. Typically, where improvements were reported, the magnitude of improvement for people with hearing loss was small. For example, older hearing impaired listeners in Burk et al. [37] improved on untrained word recognition by an average of 6.9% compared to 45.3% in younger normally hearing listeners. Average improvement in untrained measures of speech intelligibility in people with hearing loss, ranged from 3.3% for sentences [38], to 14.9% average for words [48]. Sweetow and Henderson-Sabes, [39] were the only authors to report effect sizes for improvements in speech outcomes for people with hearing loss following training using LACE. Despite small reported effect sizes (*ES*) for an untrained measure of speech intelligibility, (QuickSIN: improvement of −1.5 dB signal to noise ratio (SNR) when presented at 70 dB, $ES = 0.23$, improvement of −2.2 dB SNR when presented at 45 dB, $ES = 0.31$) [70], the authors suggested that 46% of participants achieved clinically significant post-training improvements (defined as an improvement of −1.6 dB or greater in the SNR). No significant improvements were shown for HINT sentences, which the authors attributed to improvements also being shown in the control group, suggesting likely test-retest improvement effects.

Cognition. The study by Sweetow and Henderson-Sabes [39] was the only study to include cognitive outcome measures. Significant post-training improvements were shown for measures of attention (Stroop, 7.5 points) and working memory (Listening Span, 0.5 sentences). However, unlike the results for speech intelligibility measures in the same study, effect sizes were not presented for these cognitive outcomes. Furthermore, due to the hybrid (auditory-cognitive) nature of the training stimuli, it is not clear which element(s) of LACE contributed to the improvements in cognition.

Self-reported communication. Sweetow and Henderson-Sabes [39] demonstrated significant post-training improvements in self-reported hearing handicap using the HHIE and HHIA [67] and the CSOA [60], with effect sizes of around.4. However, Ingvalson et al. [47] did not report statistically significant post-training improvements for the SSQ [74].

Retention of Learning

Retention of learning was defined as (i) the maintenance of a significant improvement from pre-training baseline performance, or (ii) a non-significant decrease in post-training performance, at a delayed post-training follow-up assessment. Follow-up assessments were reported in 8/13 articles, ranging from 4 days to 7 months post-training.

Retention of on-task learning. Burk et al. [37] reported that trained word-recognition performance at baseline (37.6%) was significantly improved six months post-training (62.9%, $p<.05$), but significantly worse than immediate post-training performance (83.5%, $p<.05$). The authors reported that participants were returned to peak post-training performance levels with as little as one hour of top-up training, although no additional follow-up was conducted to identify for how long peak performance was maintained. Stecker et al. [38] reported that Nonsense Syllable Test (NST) scores for new hearing aid users, showed no significant decrement from immediate post-training performance (9.8%) at an eight week follow-up (8.7%). For existing hearing aid users, the same was true, despite a smaller post-training improvement. Burk and Humes [40] tested participants on the same outcomes once a week for seven weeks after completion of two training protocols (easy and hard words), with no significant reduction in performance over the seven week period (Table 3). Tyler et al. [44] reported retention of trained sound localization and spondee-in-noise performance at two and seven months post-training, although no statistical tests are reported due to the small sample size. Finally, Oba et al. [45] reported retention of trained digit recognition performance at a one-month post-training that was significantly better than pre-training baseline, with no significant reduction from post-training performance levels.

Retention of generalised improvements in untrained outcomes. Sweetow and Henderson-Sabes [39] reported that at the time of publication, 65% (42/65) of trained participants had completed both QuickSIN and HINT sentences, and 48% (31/65) of participants had completed the HHIE, HHIA and the CSOA questionnaires, at a four-week follow-up. Post-training improvements were reported to be maintained for all measures, although no statistical analyses were presented. Tyler et al. [44] reported retention of improvements for HINT sentences seven months post-training for subject 1 (of 3) only. However, the authors also reported a gradual improvement in performance over time at pre-training assessments for subject 1, suggesting that some degree of post-training improvement in this measure may be attributable to

Table 5. Study validity criteria, study quality scores and levels of evidence for included articles.

Article	Scientific study validity criteria					Training-specific study validity criteria					Study quality score	Level of evidence[1]
	Randomisation	Control group	Power calculation	Blinding	Outcome measure reporting	Outcome measure selection[2]	Training feedback	Ecological validity	Reporting of compliance	Follow-up		
Fu et al. (2004) [36]	0	0	0	0	1	2	2	2	0	0	**7**	low
Burk et al. (2006) [37]	0	1	0	0	2	1	2	0	0	2	**8**	low
Stecker et al. (2006) [38]	1	2	0	0	1	1	2	2	1	2	**12**	moderate
Sweetow and Sabes, (2006) [39]	1	2	0	0	2	2	2	2	1	1	**13**	moderate
Burk and Humes (2008) [40]	0	0	0	0	2	2	2	0	0	1	**7**	low
Miller et al. (2008) [41]	0	2	0	0	2	2	0	0	0	0	**6**	low
Humes et al. (2009) [42]	0	0	0	0	2	2	2	0	2	0	**8**	low
Stacey et al. (2010) [43]	0	0	0	0	2	2	2	2	2	0	**10**	low
Tyler et al. (2010) [44]	0	1	0	0	1	1	2	1	0	1	**7**	low
Oba, Fu and Galvin, (2011) [45]	0	0	0	0	2	2	2	2	2	2	**12**	moderate
Barcroft et al. (2011) [46]	1	0	0	0	0	0	0	0	0	0	**1**	very low
Ingvalson et al. (2012) [47]	0	0	0	0	0	2	0	0	0	1	**3**	very low
Zhang et al. (2012) [48]	0	0	0	0	2	2	2	2	1	2	**11**	moderate

Criteria scoring: 0 = flawed or no information from which to make a judgement, 1 = weak information, incorrect use or lack of detail from which to make a judgement, 2 = appropriate use and reporting. Study quality score = sum of scores for scientific and training-specific study validity criteria. 1. Level of evidence: Study quality score of 0–5 = very low, 6–10 = low, 11–15 = moderate, 16–20 = high (adapted from GRADE Working Group, 2004 [35]). 2. Outcome measure selection: to assess generalisation of learning to untrained measure(s) of speech intelligibility, cognition or communication.

test-retest improvement effects. Oba et al. [45] reported retention at one month post-training was significantly greater than pre-training baseline performance for both HINT and IEEE sentences (in steady noise and in babble) with no significant change between immediate post-training and follow-up performance. Ingvalson et al. [47] reported no significant performance differences four days post-training for HINT and QuickSIN sentences. Zhang et al. [48] reported maintenance of a significant increase from pre-training baseline at a one month post-training assessment, for measures of vowel, consonant and CNC word recognition. However, no information was provided as to whether performance on these measures was significantly reduced from immediate post-training levels.

Compliance with training

Compliance was defined as the percentage of participants completing the requested training duration in each study. Compliance was reported in less than half of the articles (6/13) and the method of identifying those participants who did not achieve 100% compliance differed between studies. Stecker et al. [38] reported that on average, participants achieved 37 of the requested 44 days of training (92.5%). Sweetow and Henderson-Sabes [39] reported overall compliance of 73% (65/89 participants completed the training) although no details of training duration were provided for those who had completed. Humes et al. [42] reported that 13/16 participants (81%) completed the requested training duration. The remaining three participants completed 92%, 75% and 50% of the requested training. As these participants did not significantly differ in performance on the post-training outcomes compared with fully-compliant participants (CID Everyday Sentences [55], frequent words and phrases [42], and VAST sentences [78]), data from these low-compliant participants were included in the main analysis. In the article by Stacey et al. [43], compliance was 73% and three participants who completed only five of the requested 15 hours of training were excluded from the main analysis. Oba et al. [45] reported that 100% of participants achieved the required training duration of 600 minutes, despite reported training durations ranging from 583–767 minutes. Similarly, Zhang et al. [48] stated that 100% of participants completed the 20 hours requested training, but reported a mean training duration of 18 hours (range 15.4–21.2 hours).

Quality Assessment

Study quality was assessed using five measures of scientific study validity, and five training-specific study quality criteria (each scoring 0–2), resulting in a possible maximum study quality score of 20. Table 5 shows individual study validity ratings and overall study quality scores for each of the 13 articles. Overall study quality ranged from very low (lowest score for Barcroft et al. [46], scoring 1/20) to moderate study quality (highest score for Sweetow and Henderson-Sabes, [39], scoring 13/20).

Scientific study quality. Out of a maximum 10 points for the scientific study quality, the highest scoring article achieved a total of five points [39]. None of the included articles reported participant or tester blinding, or a power calculation to determine the required participant sample size. Where participant randomisation was used, there was often a lack of detail on how randomisation was conducted [38,39,46]. However, more than half the articles (8/13) scored 2 points for the adequate reporting of all included outcome measures in their studies.

Training intervention-specific study quality. The majority of articles (10/13) reported the use of performance feedback in their training protocols. Reporting of participant compliance with training regimens occurred in almost half of the included articles (6/13). However, definitions of non-compliance varied. For example, some studies reported this as the number of participants remaining in the study irrespective of whether they had completed the requested amount of training, e.g. [39]. Others considered this to mean to completion of the requested training duration, e.g. [43]. Follow-up assessments were reported in 8/13 articles, and ranged from repeated testing of participants at weekly intervals [40] to single follow-up assessments [37–39,44,45,47,48]. Training in the participant's home environment occurred in approximately half of the studies [36,38,39,43–45,48], while the remaining studies delivered training in the laboratory [37,40–42,46,47]. Although the majority of studies (11/13) assessed and reported the generalisation of learning to untrained measures of speech intelligibility, some to cognition or communication, outcome measures were not always reported in adequate detail [37,38,44]. Furthermore, there were frequent reports of test administration inconsistencies whereby not all participants were administered all outcome measures [36,38,46], training stimuli varied between participants [48], and findings from some outcome measures were omitted from the results [46,47].

Risk of funding bias. Sweetow and Henderson-Sabes [39] acknowledged a potential conflict of interest in funding. They reported a financial interest in Neurotone, Inc., the company licenced by the University of California, San Franscisco to produce LACE training software.

Discussion

The primary aim of this systematic review was to examine the evidence for individual computer-based auditory training (CBAT) as an effective intervention for people with hearing loss. Secondary aims sought to examine the feasibility of individual CBAT as an intervention for people with hearing loss by examining (i) the long-term retention of auditory training-related improvements at post-training follow-ups, and (ii) levels of participant compliance with individual CBAT protocols.

Efficacy of Individual Computer-based Auditory Training as an Intervention for People with Hearing Loss

Following a program of individual CBAT, significant improvements on the trained task (on-task learning) were shown for all but one of the articles that reported on-task outcomes [9/10]. However, evidence for the generalisation of learning to functional benefits (i.e. speech intelligibility) for people with hearing loss was mixed. A narrative synthesis and quality assessment of included articles suggested that evidence was not robust, and a number of confounding factors contributed to the inconsistency in reported effects. First and foremost, a lack of homogeneity in training protocols (training stimuli, duration or frequency), outcome measures, participant samples (sample size, hearing loss) and study designs may have resulted in variations in reported outcomes. Second, where generalisation of learning was shown to untrained measures, improvements were often highly variable between trained individuals [36,42,43,48] and not everyone was shown to benefit from auditory training [39–41,44,45,48]. Previous research into the neurophysiological changes resulting from auditory perceptual learning for normally hearing adults suggests that although the auditory system is responsive to training, there is a substantial degree of variability across individuals in their ability to make use of physiological cues [79].

In a previous review of the efficacy of auditory training for adults with hearing loss [18], the authors concluded there was little evidence for real-world effectiveness, but some evidence for within-study efficacy, of individual auditory training for people with hearing loss. A more recent meta-analysis of six (predominantly clinician-delivered) auditory training studies published between 1970 and 2009 [26] suggested reliable but small improvements in speech recognition (Cohen's $d = .352$). Findings from the present review are similar in that on-task learning nearly always occurred for people with hearing loss following individual CBAT. Furthermore, there was some evidence for the generalisation of that on-task learning to untrained measures of speech intelligibility, cognition and self-reports of communication. However, the magnitude of improvement for untrained outcomes is small, and reported improvements are shown to be inconsistent across different studies, and within studies across individual trainees.

Feasibility of Individual Computer-based Auditory Training as an Intervention for People with Hearing Loss

Feasibility was considered in terms of the retention of training-related improvements and compliance with individual CBAT. Although retention of post-training improvements was shown for a range of on-task and untrained measures at follow-up assessments up to 7 months post-training, the definition of retention varied across studies. The majority focused on the retention of improvements for trained tasks, not the retention of generalised improvements in untrained measures of speech intelligibility, cognition and communication. It is the latter that holds the most promise for individual CBAT to improve the everyday listening abilities of people with hearing loss.

Details of participant compliance with training were often underreported, appearing in less than half of the articles included in the review (6/13). Where reported, participant compliance rates were high. However, these reports of high compliance with training were not consistent with a large-scale study of more than 3000 clinical LACE trainees [80], where compliance (defined as completion of 10 or more training sessions) was around 30% [81]. This may suggest that rates of compliance with individual CBAT may be greater in smaller, controlled research-settings than may be typically expected in clinical environments.

Study Quality and Evidence of Bias

Study quality scores suggest that the articles included in this review offer very-low to moderate levels of evidence. None of the studies reported participant or tester blinding. Thus, where between-groups designs are employed and the control group received no intervention [38,39,41,44], we cannot be confident that any training improvements were not biased by placebo effects. The study by Sweetow and Henderson-Sabes [39] that obtained the highest quality score was the only study to report cognitive outcomes. Results showed significant generalisation of learning from trained stimuli (LACE) to untrained measures of speech intelligibility (QuickSIN), cognition (attention: Stroop Task, and working memory: listening span), and self-report of communication (HHIE, HHIA and CSOA).

The majority of studies failed to account for test-retest improvements in reported outcomes. When administering the outcomes across multiple test sessions, there is a possibility that improvement will occur as a result of procedural rather than perceptual learning [82,83]. It has been recommended for the HINT and QuickSIN sentences that practice with at least two sentence lists is needed to eliminate procedural learning effects at baseline sessions [83]. Only two of the articles repeated outcome measure assessments at baseline sessions. Studies by Fu and colleagues [36] administered outcomes for a minimum of two weeks prior to training, and Stacey and colleagues [43] repeated baseline measures for approximately three hours per participant, both until a performance asymptote was reached. The total number of occasions outcomes that administered was not reported in either study. Finally, two articles omitted findings from some outcome measures included in the studies [46,47]. Selective outcome reporting is likely to lead to inaccurate and misleading conclusions being reached [84].

Lack of High-quality Evidence as a Barrier to implementation

Results from this systematic review demonstrate robust on-task learning following individual CBAT. Generalisation of on-task learning to functional benefits for people with hearing loss is less robust. Evidence for the generalisation of on-task learning to improvements in speech intelligibility, cognition and self-report of hearing suggests that improvements are both small and inconsistent across studies and individual trainees. Inconsistencies in reported effects may in part be associated with inconsistencies in study designs, training protocols, participant samples, and outcome measures adopted. However, analysis of study quality has demonstrated some fundamental issues with scientific control, which may result in a range of biases in reported effects. Nevertheless, retention of learning from both trained and untrained stimuli was shown to persist where reported, up to seven months post-training. Furthermore, where participant compliance was reported, rates were high. This suggests that individual CBAT has the potential to be a feasible intervention, which may offer benefit to the auditory-perceptual abilities of people with hearing loss.

Nevertheless, some of the questions posed by Boothroyd [85] in a discussion of the potential role of formal training in adapting to changed hearing, remain unanswered in the current evidence-base. First, where benefits occur, what are the mechanisms of benefit of auditory training for people with hearing loss (i.e. where generalisation of learning is shown, what elements of on-task learning are these attributable to)? How do individual characteristics interact with training outcomes? And, do training-induced changes influence participation and quality of life for people with hearing loss? Although many of these questions are currently being explored in normally hearing listeners [86–88] there is a need for further research designed to specifically address these issues in people with hearing loss.

Recommendations for further research

Based on the reviewed evidence we propose key recommendations for future research:

1. High-level evidence. High quality studies that are randomised, blinded, with a sample size dictated by a power calculation, are crucial to adequately assess the efficacy of individual computer-based auditory training for people with hearing loss. Furthermore, the possible inclusion of an 'active' control group (that is a task comparable to the training group task, but for which no improvement in performance is expected), may help enable participant blinding to help ensure any training-related improvements are not influenced by placebo effects. Future research would ideally be reported in accordance with the CONSORT statement [89], which offers guidelines for the reporting of randomised controlled trials. This would result in sufficiently detailed reporting to allow for an adequate appraisal of the quality and applicability of published results. It is also important that future studies consider key factors pertinent to training intervention studies, including ecologically valid training environments, performance related feedback, and follow-up assessments to ascertain the long-term benefits of auditory training and adequate reporting of participant (non-) compliance as interventions can only ever be beneficial if individuals comply with them.

2. Outcome selection. Measures that are appropriate for and sensitive to CBAT effects should be adopted to allow accurate assessment of training efficacy. This includes a consideration of the magnitude of effect required for those outcomes to represent clinically significant improvements in listening abilities for people with hearing loss, for example, combining behavioural outcomes with questionnaires to assess self-reported benefits in everyday listening. In addition, the inclusion of cognitive outcomes in future studies assessing the efficacy of individual CBAT for people with hearing loss may be informative given that the only study to include such measures in this review reported significant post-training improvements in attention and auditory working memory [39]. Evidence from a study of LACE training with normally hearing adults suggested that training improves the neural representation of cues important for speech perception [86]. However, Tremblay and colleagues argue that at least that some of the physiological changes as a result of auditory training may not reflect sensory-specific fine-tuning, but other top-down modulatory influences that are activated during focused listening tasks, such as stimulus exposure, attention, memory, decision-making and task execution [88]. Thus, measurement of both auditory and cognitive outcomes may help to characterise the mechanisms of benefit for people with hearing loss following auditory training.

3. Standardisation of outcome measures. Standardisation of outcomes across auditory training studies would enable comparisons to be made between different training protocols. Furthermore, common outcome measures would enable meta-analyses of data from future training intervention studies.

4. Candidature. Published evidence suggests that post-training improvements in untrained outcomes are highly variable, and not everyone benefits from auditory training [39–41,44,45]. Thus, identification of those individuals most likely to benefit from auditory training would be of substantial clinical importance, enabling clinicians to individually target those for whom CBAT would be most effective, and consider alternative interventions for those who are least likely to benefit from training.

Summary and Conclusions

Individual computer-based auditory training (CBAT) is a time and cost efficient, flexible self-management intervention that has the potential to be delivered to people with hearing loss in their home environment. It is easily accessible to the target population via PCs and the internet [27], and can be tailored to individual needs. The present review identifies scientific, methodological and study quality issues in each of the 13 articles included in this systematic review. Our findings demonstrate that although individual CBAT is a feasible intervention for people with hearing loss, published evidence for the efficacy of individual CBAT to improve speech intelligibility, cognition and hearing abilities for adults with hearing loss is neither consistent nor robust. As such, the evidence cannot be used reliably to guide intervention at this time. Future high level evidence and the standardisation of outcome measures across different training studies will provide an evidence-base from which to adequately assess the efficacy of auditory training as an intervention for people with hearing loss.

Acknowledgments

We would like to thank Holly Thomas for her assistance with the systematic database search. We would also like to thank Dr Derek Hoare and Mark Edmondson-Jones and for their comments on earlier versions of this article. This paper presents independent research funded by the National Institute for Health Research (NIHR). The views expressed are those of the authors and not necessarily those of the NHS, the NIHR, or the Department of Health.

Author Contributions

Conceived and designed the experiments: HH MAF. Performed the experiments: HH MAF. Analyzed the data: HH MAF. Contributed reagents/materials/analysis tools: HH MAF. Wrote the paper: HH MAF.

References

1. World Health Organization (2004) The global burden of disease: 2004 update. Switzerland: WHO press.
2. Davis A, Smith P, Ferguson M, Stephens D, Gianopoulos I (2007) Acceptability, benefit and costs of early screening for hearing disability: a study of potential screening tests and models. Health Technology Assessment 11.
3. Scarinci N, Worrall L, Hickson L (2008) The effect of hearing impairment in older people on the spouse. International Journal of Audiology 47: 141–151.
4. Hétu R, Jones L, Getty L (1993) The impact of acquired hearing impairment on intimate relationships: Implications for rehabilitation. Audiology 32: 363–381.
5. Banh J, Singh G, Pichora-Fuller MK (2012) Age affects responses on the speech, spatial and qualities of hearing scale (SSQ) by adults with minimal audometric loss. Journal of the American Academy of Audiology 23: 81–91.
6. Action on Hearing Loss (2011) Statistics on deafness and hearing loss.
7. Davis A (1995) Hearing in Adults. London: Whurr Publishers Ltd.
8. Kochkin S (2008) MarkeTrak VIII: 25-year trends in the hearing health market. Hearing Review 16: 12–31.
9. Smeeth L, Fletcher AE, Ng ES, Stirling S, Nunes MB, et al. (2002) Reduced hearing, ownership and use of hearing aids in elderly people in the UK – the MRC trial of the assessment and management of older people in the community: a cross-sectional survey. Lancet 359: 1466–1070.
10. Kiessling J, Pichora-Fuller MK, Gatehouse S, Stephens D, Arlinger S, et al. (2003) Candidature for and delivery of audiological services: special needs of older people. International Journal of Audiology 42: S92–S101.
11. Pichora-Fuller MK, Schneider BA, Daneman M (1995) How young and old adults listen to and remember speech in noise. Journal of the Acoustical Society of America 97: 593–608.
12. Schneider BA, Daneman M, Murphy DR, Kwong-See S (2000) Listening to discourse in distracting settings: The effects of gaining. Psychology and Aging 15: 110–125.
13. Rönnberg J, Rudner M, Foo C, Lunner T (2008) Cognition counts: A working memory system for ease of language understanding (ELU). International Journal of Audiology 47: S99–S105.
14. Shinn-Cunningham BG, Best V (2008) Selective Attention in Normal and Impaired Hearing. Trends in Amplification 12: 283–299.
15. BSA (2012) Practice Guidance: common principles of rehabilitation for adults with hearing- and/or balance-related problems in routine audiologist services. Reading: British Society of Audiology.
16. Schow R, Nerbonne M (2007) Introduction to audiologic rehabilitation. Boston, MA: Pearson Education.
17. Wright BA, Zhang Y (2009) A review of the generalization of auditory learning. Philosophical Transactions of the Royal Society B: Biological Sciences 364: 301–311.
18. Sweetow RW, Palmer CV (2005) Efficacy of Individual Auditory Training in Adults: A Systematic Review of the Evidence. Journal of the American Academy of Audiology 16: 494–504.
19. Bode DL, Oyer JJ (1970) Auditory training and speech discrimination. Journal of Speech and Hearing Research 13: 839–255.
20. Kricos PB, Holmes AE (1996) Efficacy of audiologic rehabilitation for older adults. Journal of the American Academy of Audiology 7: 219–229.
21. Rubinstein A, Boothroyd A (1987) Effect of two approaches to auditory training on speech recognition by hearing-impaired adults. Journal of Speech, Language, and Hearing Research 30: 153–160.

22. Montgomery A, Walden B, Schwartz D, Prosek R (1984) Training auditory-visual speech recogntiion in adults with moderate sensorineural hearing loss. Ear & Hearing 5: 30–36.
23. Walden B, Erdman S, Montgomery A, Schwartz D, Prosek R (1981) Some effects of training on speech recognition by hearing-impaired adults. Journal of Speech and Hearing Research 24: 207–216.
24. Kricos P, Holmes A, Doyle D (1992) Efficacy of a communication training program for hearing impaired adults. Journal of the Academy of Rehabilitative Audiology 25: 69–80.
25. Ferguson MA, Henshaw H, Clark DA, Moore DR (2012) Auditory training improves listening and cognition in complex conditions. International Journal of Audiology 51: 220–227.
26. Chisolm T, Arnold M (2012) Evidence about the Effectiveness of Aural Rehabilitation Programs for Adults. In: L Wong, L Hickson (Eds.) Evidence-Based Practice in Audiology: Evaluating Interventions for Children and Adults with Hearing Impairment. Plural Publishing, San Diego. pp.237–266.
27. Henshaw H, Clark D, Kang S, Ferguson M (2012) Computer Skill and Internet Use in Adults Aged 50–74 years: Influence of Hearing Difficulties. Journal of Internet Medicine Research 14: e113.
28. Shipstead Z, Redick TS, Engle RW (2012) Is working memory training effective? Psychol Bull 138: 628–654.
29. Greenwald AG, Spangenberg ER, Pratkanis AR, Eskenazi J (1991) Double-blind tests of subliminal self-help audiotapes. Psychological Science 2: 119–122.
30. Cochrane (2012) The Cochrane Library. John Wiley & Sons Ltd.
31. Centre for Reviews and Dissemination (2008) Systematic Reviews: CRD's guidance for undertaking systematic reviews in health care. Centre for Research and Dissemination, University of York.
32. Moher D, Liberati A, Tetzlaff J, Altman DG (2009) Preferred Reporting Items for Systematic Reviews and Meta-Analyses: The PRISMA Statement. PloS Medicine 6: e1000097.
33. Amitay S, Halliday L, Taylor J, Sohoglu E, Moore DR (2010) Motivation and Intelligence Drive Auditory Perceptual Learning. PloS One 5: e9816.
34. Song JH, Skoe E, Banai K, Kraus N (2012) Training to improve hearing speech in noise: biological mechanisms. Cerebral Cortex 22: 1180–1190.
35. Group GW (2004) Grading quality of evidence and strength of recommendations. BMJ 328: 1490.
36. Fu QJ, Galvin J, Wang X, Nogaki G (2004) Effects of auditory training on adult cochlear implant patients: a preliminary report. Cochlear Implants International 5: 84–90.
37. Burk MH, Humes LE, Amos NE, Strauser LE (2006) Effect of Training on Word-Recognition Performance in Noise for Young Normal-Hearing and Older Hearing-Impaired Listeners. Ear & Hearing 27: 263–278.
38. Stecker GC, Bowman GA, Yund EW, Herron TJ, Roup CM, et al. (2006) Perceptual training improves syllable identification in new and experienced hearing aid users. Journal of Rehabilitation Research & Development 43: 537–551.
39. Sweetow RW, Henderson-Sabes J (2006) The Need for and Development of an Adaptive Listening and Communication Enhancement (LACETM) Program. Journal of the American Academy of Audiology 17: 538–558.
40. Burk MH, Humes LE (2008) Effects of Long-Term Training on Aided Speech-Recognition Performance in Noise in Older Adults. Journal of Speech, Language, and Hearing Research 51: 759–771.
41. Miller JD, Watson CS, Kistler DJ, Wightman FL, Preminger JE (2008) Preliminary evaluation of the speech perception assessment and training system (SPATS) with hearing-aid and cochlear-implant users. Proc Meet Acoust 2: 1–15.
42. Humes LE, Burk MH, Strauser LE, Kinney DL (2009) Development and efficacy of a frequent-word auditory training protocol for older adults with impaired hearing. Ear & Hearing 30: 613–627.
43. Stacey PC, Raine CH, O'Donoghue GM, Tapper L, Twomey T, et al. (2010) Effectiveness of computer-based auditory training for adult users of cochlear implants. International Journal of Audiology 49: 347–356.
44. Tyler RS, Witt SA, Dunn CC, Wang W (2010) Initial Development of a Spatially Separated Speech-in-Noise and Localization Training Program. Journal of the American Academy of Audiology 21: 390–403.
45. Oba SI, Fu Q, Galvin JJ (2011) Digit training in noise can improve cochlear implant users' speech understanding in noise. Ear & Hearing 32: 573–581.
46. Barcroft J, Sommers MS, Tye-Murray N, Mauze E, Schroy C, et al. (2011) Tailoring auditory training to patient needs with single and multiple talkers: Transfer-appropriate gains on a four-choice discrimination test. International Journal of Audiology 50: 802–808.
47. Ingvalson EM, Lee B, Fiebig P, Wong PC (2012) The Effects of Short-Term Computerized Speech-in-Noise Training on Post-Lingually Deafened Adult Cochlear Implant Recipients. Journal of Speech, Language and Hearing Research.
48. Zhang T, Dorman MF, Fu QJ, Spahr AJ (2012) Auditory training in patients with unilateral cochlear implant and contralateral acoustic stimulation. Ear and Hearing 33: e70–e79.
49. Studebaker GA (1985) A "Rationalized" Arcsine Transform. Journal of Speech and Hearing Research 28: 455–462.
50. Turner CW, Gantz BJ, Vidal C, Behrens A, Henry BA (2004) Speech recognition in noise for cochlear implant listeners: benefits of residual acoustic hearing. Journal of the Acoustical Society of America 115: 1729–1735.
51. Tyler RS, Noble W, Dunn C, Witt S (2006) Some benefits and limitations of binaural cochlear implants and our ability to measure them. International Journal of Audiology 45: S113–S119.
52. Spahr AJ, Dorman MF, Litvak LM, Van Wie S, Gifford RH, et al. (2012) Development and Validation of the AzBio Sentence Lists. Ear and Hearing 33: 112–117.
53. Bench J, Kowal A, Bamford J (1979) The BKB (Bamford-Kowal-Bench) sentence lists for partially-hearing children. British Journal of Audiology 13: 108–112.
54. Tye-Murray N, Sommers M, Spehar B, Myerson J, Hale S, et al. (2008) Auditory-visual discourse comprehension by older and young adults in favorable and unfavorable conditions. International Journal of Audiology 47 Supplement 2: S31–37.
55. Davis H, Silverman SR (1978) Hearing and Deafness. New York: Holt, Rinehart and Winston.
56. Hirsh IJ, Davis H, Silverman SR, Reynolds EG, Eldert E, et al. (1952) Development of Materials for Speech Audiometry. Journal of Speech and Hearing Disorders 17: 321–337.
57. Tillman TW, Carhart R (1966) An Expanded Test for Speech Discrimination Utilizing CNC Monosyllabic Words, Northwestern University Auditory Test No. 6. Texas: USAF School of Aerospace Medicine, Brooks Air Force Base. 1–12 p.
58. Peterson GE, Lehiste I (1962) Revised CNC lists for auditory tests. Journal of Speech and Hearing Disorders 27: 62–70.
59. Shannon RV, Jensvold A, Padilla M, Robert ME, Wang X (1999) Consonant recordings for speech testing. Journal of the Acoustical Society of America 106.
60. Kaplan H, Bally S, Brandt F, Busacco D, Pray J (1997) Communication Scale for Older Adults (CSOA). Journal of the American Academy of Audiology 8: 203–217.
61. Cox RM, Alexander GC, Gilmore C (1987) Development of the Connected Speech Test (CST). Ear & Hearing 8: 119S–126S.
62. Boothroyd A, Hanin L, Hnath T (1985) A sentence test of speech perception: Reliability, set equivalence, and short term learning. New York: City University of New York.
63. Dunn CC, Tyler RS, Witt SA (2005) Benefit of wearing a hearing aid on the unimplanted ear in adult users of a cochlear implant. Journal of Speech, Language, and Hearing Research 48: 668–680.
64. IEEE (1969) IEEE Recommended Practice for Speech Quality Measurements. IEEE Transactions on Audio and Electroacoustics 17: 225–246.
65. Robinson K, Gatehouse S, Browning GC (1996) Measuring patient benefit from otorhinolaryngological surgery and therapy. Annals of Otology, Rhinology and Laryngology 105: 415–422.
66. Newman CW, Weinstein BE, Jacobson GP, Hug GA (1990) The Hearing Handicap Inventory for Adults: psychometric adequacy and audiometric correlates. Ear & Hearing 11: 430–433.
67. Ventry IM, Weinstein BE (1982) The Hearing Handicap Inventory for the Elderly: A New Tool. Ear & Hearing 3: 128–134.
68. Nilsson M, Soli SD, Sullivan JA (1994) Development of the Hearing in Noise Test for the measurement of speech reception thresholds in quiet and in noise. The Journal of the Acoustical Society of America 95: 1085–1099.
69. Dubno JR, Levitt H (1981) Predicting consonant confusions from acoustic analysis. The Journal of the Acoustical Society of America 69: 249–261.
70. Killion MC, Niquette PA, Gudmundsen GI, Revit LJ, Banerjee S (2004) Development of a quick speech-in-noise test for measuring signal-to-noise ratio loss in normal-hearing and hearing-impaired listeners. Journal of the Acoustical Society of America 116: 2395–2405.
71. Wilson RH, McArdle R, Watts KL, Smith SL (2012) The Revised Speech Perception in Noise Test (R-SPIN) in a multiple signal-to-noise ratio paradigm. Journal of the American Academy of Audiology 23: 590–605.
72. Miller JD, Watson CS, Kewley-Port D, Sillings R, Mills W, et al. (2007) SPATS: Speech Perception Assessment and Training System. Journal of the Acoustical Society of America 122: 3063.
73. Kalikow DN, Stevens KN, Elliott LL (1977) Development of a test of speech intelligibility in noise using sentence materials with controlled word predictability. Journal of the Acoustical Society of America 61: 1337–1351.
74. Gatehouse S, Noble W (2004) The Speech, Spatial and Qualities of Hearing Scale (SSQ). International Journal of Audiology 43: 85–99.
75. Uttl B, Graf P (1997) Color-Word Stroop test performance across the adult life span. Journal of Clinical and Experimental Neuropsychology 19: 405–420.
76. Garofolo JS, Lamel LF, Fisher WM, Fiscus JG, Pallett DS, et al. (1993) DARPA TIMIT Acoustic-phonetic Continuous Speech Corpus. Philadelphia: Linguistic Data Consortium.
77. Bastiaanse R, Edwards S, Rispens J (2002) The verb and sentence test. Bury St Edmonds: Thames Valley Test Company.
78. Hillenbrand J, Getty LA, Clark MJ, Wheeler K (1995) Acoustic characteristics of American English vowels. Journal of the Acoustical Society of America 97: 3099–3111.
79. Tremblay K, Kraus N, McGee T (1998). The time course of auditory perceptual learning: neurophysiological changes during speech-sound training. Neuroreport 9: 3557–3560.
80. Sweetow R (2009) Integrating LACE into a busy clinical practice. American Academy of Audiology. Dallas, TX.

81. Sweetow RW, Sabes JH (2010) Auditory training and challenges associated with participation and compliance. Journal of the American Academy of Audiology 21: 586–593.
82. McArthur GM (2007) Test–Retest Effects in Treatment Studies of Reading Disability: The Devil is in the Detail. Dyslexia 13: 240–252.
83. Yund EW, Woods DL (2010) Content and Procedural Learning in Repeated Sentence Tests of Speech Perception. Ear & Hearing 31: 769–778.
84. Kirkham JJ, Dwan KM, Altman DG, Gamble C, Dodd S, et al. (2010) The impact of outcome reporting bias in randomised controlled trials on a cohort of systematic reviews. BMJ (Clinical research ed) 340: c365.
85. Boothroyd A (2010) Adapting to Changed Hearing: The Potential Role of Formal Training. Journal of the American Academy of Audiology 21: 601–611.
86. Song J, Skoe E, Banai K, Kraus N (2012) Training to improve speech in noise: Biological mechanisms. Cerebral Cortex 22: 1180–1190.
87. Wright BA, Wilson RM, Sabin AT (2010) Generalization lags behind learning on an auditory perceptual task. Journal of Speech, Language and Hearing Research 56: 31–43.
88. Tremblay K (2007) Training-related changes in the brain: Evidence from human auditory-evoked potentials. Seminars in Hearing 28: 120–132.
89. Schulz KF, Altman DG, Moher D (2010) CONSORT 2010 Statement: updated guidelines for reporting parallel group randomised trials. British Medical Journal 340: c869.

Permissions

All chapters in this book were first published in PLOS ONE, by The Public Library of Science; hereby published with permission under the Creative Commons Attribution License or equivalent. Every chapter published in this book has been scrutinized by our experts. Their significance has been extensively debated. The topics covered herein carry significant findings which will fuel the growth of the discipline. They may even be implemented as practical applications or may be referred to as a beginning point for another development.

The contributors of this book come from diverse backgrounds, making this book a truly international effort. This book will bring forth new frontiers with its revolutionizing research information and detailed analysis of the nascent developments around the world.

We would like to thank all the contributing authors for lending their expertise to make the book truly unique. They have played a crucial role in the development of this book. Without their invaluable contributions this book wouldn't have been possible. They have made vital efforts to compile up to date information on the varied aspects of this subject to make this book a valuable addition to the collection of many professionals and students.

This book was conceptualized with the vision of imparting up-to-date information and advanced data in this field. To ensure the same, a matchless editorial board was set up. Every individual on the board went through rigorous rounds of assessment to prove their worth. After which they invested a large part of their time researching and compiling the most relevant data for our readers.

The editorial board has been involved in producing this book since its inception. They have spent rigorous hours researching and exploring the diverse topics which have resulted in the successful publishing of this book. They have passed on their knowledge of decades through this book. To expedite this challenging task, the publisher supported the team at every step. A small team of assistant editors was also appointed to further simplify the editing procedure and attain best results for the readers.

Apart from the editorial board, the designing team has also invested a significant amount of their time in understanding the subject and creating the most relevant covers. They scrutinized every image to scout for the most suitable representation of the subject and create an appropriate cover for the book.

The publishing team has been an ardent support to the editorial, designing and production team. Their endless efforts to recruit the best for this project, has resulted in the accomplishment of this book. They are a veteran in the field of academics and their pool of knowledge is as vast as their experience in printing. Their expertise and guidance has proved useful at every step. Their uncompromising quality standards have made this book an exceptional effort. Their encouragement from time to time has been an inspiration for everyone.

The publisher and the editorial board hope that this book will prove to be a valuable piece of knowledge for researchers, students, practitioners and scholars across the globe.

List of Contributors

Liwei Chen, Ning Yu, Yan Lu, Daishi Chen, Weiwei Guo, Lidong Zhao, Mingbo Liu, Shiming Yang and Suoqiang Zhai
Department of Otolaryngology Head and Neck Surgery, Chinese PLA General Hospital, Beijing, China

Longjun Wu
Department of Otolaryngology Head and Neck Surgery, Wenzhou Medical College, Wenzhou, Zhejiang Province, China

Xuejun Sun
Department of Diving Medicine, Faculty of Naval Medicine, Second Military Medical University, Shanghai, China

Roland Schaette
Ear Institute, University College London, London, United Kingdom

Charlotte Turtle and Kevin J. Munro
School of Psychological Sciences, University of Manchester, Manchester, United Kingdom

Chuan-Jen Hsu
Department of Otolaryngology, National Taiwan University Hospital, Taipei, Taiwan

Chen-Chi Wu
Department of Otolaryngology, National Taiwan University Hospital, Taipei, Taiwan
Department of Medical Genetics, National Taiwan University Hospital, Taipei, Taiwan

Shin-Yu Lin
Department of Medical Genetics, National Taiwan University Hospital, Taipei, Taiwan

Chia-Cheng Hung and Yi-Ning Su
Department of Medical Genetics, National Taiwan University Hospital, Taipei, Taiwan
Graduate Institute of Clinical Genomics, National Taiwan University College of Medicine, Taipei, Taiwan

Wu-Shiun Hsieh and Po-Nien Tsao
Department of Pediatrics, National Taiwan University Hospital, Taipei, Taiwan

Chien-Nan Lee
Department of Obstetrics and Gynecology, National Taiwan University Hospital, Taipei, Taiwan

Ute Philipp, Bettina Lupp, Stefanie Mömke and Ottmar Distl
Institute for Animal Breeding and Genetics, University of Veterinary Medicine Hannover, Hannover, Germany

Veronika Stein and Andrea Tipold
Clinic for Small Animals, University of Veterinary Medicine Hannover, Hannover, Germany

Johanna Corinna Eule
Small Animal Clinic, Freie Universität Berlin, Berlin, Germany

Jürgen Rehage
Clinic for Cattle, University of Veterinary Medicine Hannover, Hannover, Germany

Shin-ichi Usami and Shin-ya Nishio
Department of Otorhinolaryngology, Shinshu University School of Medicine, Asahi, Matsumoto, Japan

Makoto Nagano, Satoko Abe and Toshikazu Yamaguchi
Department of Clinical Genomics, Biomedical Laboratories, Inc., Matoba, Kawagoe-shi, Saitama, Japan

Hyoung-Mi Kim and Philine Wangemann
Anatomy and Physiology Department, Kansas State University, Manhattan, Kansas, United States of America

Maiko Miyagawa, Shin-ya Nishio and Shin-ichi Usami
Department of Otorhinolaryngology, Shinshu University School of Medicine, Matsumoto, Japan

Shasha Huang, Yueshuai Song, Hongtian Wang, Deliang Huang and Dongyi Han
Department of Otolaryngology, PLA General Hospital, Beijing, People's Republic of China

Lujie Zuo and Guozheng Zhang
Department of Otolaryngology, PLA General Hospital, Beijing, People's Republic of China
Department of Otolaryngology, 3rd hospital of Hebei Medical University, Shijiazhuang, Hebei Province, People's Republic of China

Yongyi Yuan, Guojian Wang and Pu Dai
Department of Otolaryngology, PLA General Hospital, Beijing, People's Republic of China
Department of Otolaryngology, Hainan Branch of PLA General Hospital, Sanya, People's Republic of China

Xun Zhang
Department of Otolaryngology, 3rd hospital of Hebei Medical University, Shijiazhuang, Hebei Province, People's Republic of China

Oscar Diaz-Horta, Joseph Foster II, Aslı Sırmacı, Michael Gonzalez, Ibis Menendez, Rick H. Ulloa, Yvonne J. K. Edwards, Stephan Züchner, Susan Blanton and Mustafa Tekin
John P. Hussman Institute for Human Genomics and the Dr. John T. Macdonald Department of Human Genetics, University of Miami Miller School of Medicine, Miami, Florida, United States of America

Duygu Duman and Filiz Başak Cengiz
Division of Pediatric Genetics, Ankara University School of Medicine, Ankara, Turkey

Nikou Fotouhi and Mortaza Bonyadi
Faculty of Natural Sciences, Center of Excellence for Biodiversity, University of Tabriz, Tabriz, Iran

Mee Hyun Song
Department of Otorhinolaryngology, Kwandong University College of Medicine, Goyang, South Korea

Hyun-Ju Cho, Hee Keun Lee, Tae Jun Kwon and Un-Kyung Kim
Department of Biology, College of Natural Sciences, Kyungpook National University, Daegu, South Korea

Won-Sang Lee, Sanghee Oh and Jae Young Choi
Department of Otorhinolaryngology, Yonsei University College of Medicine, Seoul, South Korea

Jinwoong Bok
Department of Anatomy, BK 21 Project for Medical Science, Yonsei University College of Medicine, Seoul, South Korea

David Mann
College of Marine Science, University of South Florida, St. Petersburg, Florida, United States of America
Mote Marine Laboratory, Sarasota, Florida, United States of America

Charles Manire
Mote Marine Laboratory, Sarasota, Florida, United States of America

Mandy Hill-Cook
Department of Biology, Portland State University, Portland, Oregon, United States of America

Robert Lingenfelser
Marine Mammal Conservancy, Key Largo, Florida, United States of America

Abigale Stone
Clearwater Marine Aquarium, Clearwater, Florida, United States of America

Micah Brodsky
Dolphins Plus, Key Largo, Florida, United States of America

Kerry A. Miller and Louise H. Williams
Genetic Hearing Research, Murdoch Childrens Research Institute, Royal Children's Hospital, Melbourne, Victoria, Australia

Shehnaaz S. M. Manji
Genetic Hearing Research, Murdoch Childrens Research Institute, Royal Children's Hospital, Melbourne, Victoria, Australia
Department of Otolaryngology, University of Melbourne, Royal Victorian Eye and Ear Hospital, Melbourne, Victoria, Australia
The HEARing CRC, Audiology, Hearing and Speech Sciences, University of Melbourne, Melbourne, Victoria, Australia

Hans-Henrik M. Dahl
Genetic Hearing Research, Murdoch Childrens Research Institute, Royal Children's Hospital, Melbourne, Victoria, Australia
Department of Paediatrics, University of Melbourne, Melbourne, Victoria, Australia
The HEARing CRC, Audiology, Hearing and Speech Sciences, University of Melbourne, Melbourne, Victoria, Australia

Elizabeth Rose
Department of Otolaryngology, University of Melbourne, Royal Victorian Eye and Ear Hospital, Melbourne, Victoria, Australia

Michael Kuiper
Victorian Life Sciences Computation Initiative, University of Melbourne, Melbourne, Victoria, Australia

Davide Bottari and Francesco Pavani
Department of Cognitive Sciences and Education, University of Trento, Trento, Italy
Center for Mind/Brain Sciences, University of Trento, Trento, Italy

Anne Caclin and Marie-Hélène Giard
INSERM, U1028; CNRS, UMR5292; Lyon Neuroscience Research Center, Brain Dynamics and Cognition Team, Lyon, France
University Lyon 1, Lyon, France

Simone Jörs, Christian Grimm, Lars Becker and Stefan Heller
Departments of Otolaryngology - Head and Neck Surgery and Molecular and Cellular Physiology, Stanford University School of Medicine, Stanford, California, United States of America

Cherylea J. Browne, John W. Morley and Carl H. Parsons
Department of Anatomy and Cell Biology, School of Medicine, The University of Western Sydney, Sydney, New South Wales, Australia

Hyoung-Mi Kim and Philine Wangemann
Anatomy and Physiology Department, Kansas State University, Manhattan, Kansas, United States of America

Borum Sagong, Jeong-In Baek, Se-Kyung Oh, Jae Woong Bae and Un-Kyung Kim
Department of Biology, College of Natural Sciences, Kyungpook National University, Daegu, South Korea

Kyung Jin Na, Sang-Heun Lee and Kyu-Yup Lee
Department of Otorhinolaryngology-Head and Neck Surgery, College of Medicine, Kyungpook National University, Daegu, South Korea

Soo Young Choi
Department of Medicine, University of Pennsylvania, Philadelphia, Pennsylvania, United States of America

Ji Yun Jeong
Department of Endocrinology and Metabolism, Kyungpook National University Hospital, Kyungpook National University School of Medicine, Daegu, South Korea

Jae Young Choi
Department of Otorhinolaryngology, Yonsei University College of Medicine, Seoul, South Korea

Daniel Weiss, Alexis Bremer and Claudia Rudack
Department of Otorhinolaryngology, Head and Neck Surgery, University of Münster, Münster, Germany

Bruno Neuner
Department of Anaesthesiology and Intensive Care Medicine, Campus Virchow-Klinikum and Campus Charité-Mitte, Charité - University Medicine, Berlin, Germany

Kerstin Gorzelniak
Institute of Laboratory Medicine, Unfallkrankenhaus Berlin, Berlin, Germany

Michael Walter
Institute of Laboratory Medicine, Clinical Chemistry and Pathobiochemistry, Campus Virchow-Klinikum, Charité - University Medicine & Labor Berlin - Charite´ Vivantes Services GmbH, Berlin, Germany

Qian Zhang, Huizhan Liu, Garrett A. Soukup and David Z. Z. He
From the Department of Biomedical Sciences, Creighton University School of Medicine, Omaha, Nebraska, United States of America

JoAnn McGee and Edward J. Walsh
Boys Town National Research Hospital, Omaha, Nebraska, United States of America

Yu Su, Yong-Yi Yuan, Sha-Sha Huang, Yu Lu, Guo-Jian Wang and Fei Yu
Department of Otorhinolaryngology, Head and Neck Surgery, PLA General Hospital, Beijing, P. R. China

Ming-Yu Han, Yue-Shuai Song and Pu Dai
Department of Otorhinolaryngology, Head and Neck Surgery, PLA General Hospital, Beijing, P. R. China
Department of Otorhinolaryngology, Hainan Branch of PLA General Hospital, Sanya, P. R. China

Xue Gao
Department of Otorhinolaryngology, Head and Neck Surgery, PLA General Hospital, Beijing, P. R. China
Department of Otorhinolaryngology, Hainan Branch of PLA General Hospital, Sanya, P. R. China
Department of Otorhinolaryngology, the Second Artillery General Hospital, Beijing, P. R. China

Li-Ping Guan and Qing-Yan Zhu
BGI-Shenzhen, Beishan Industrial Zone, Yantian District, Shenzhen, P. R. China

Jing Wu
BGI-Tianjin, Tianjin, P. R. China

Aparna Ganapathy, Nishtha Pandey, Mohan Venkatappa, Arunima Chatterjee, Meenakshi Sharma, Rekha Santhanam and Anuranjan Anand
Molecular Biology and Genetics Unit, Jawaharlal Nehru Centre for Advanced Scientific Research, Bangalore, India

Arabandi Ramesh and C. R. Srikumari Srisailapathy
Department of Genetics, Dr. ALM Post Graduate Institute of Basic Medical Sciences, Chennai, India

Raghunath R. Rangasayee and Rajeev Jalvi
Department of Audiology, Ali Yavar Jung National Institute for the Hearing Handicapped, Mumbai, India

Shelly Chadha, Arun K. Agarwal and Vikas Malhotra
Department of ENT, Maulana Azad Medical College, New Delhi, India

A. Marceline van Furth
Department of Pediatric Infectious Diseases - Immunology, and Rheumatology, VU University Medical Center, Amsterdam, The Netherlands

Rogier C. J. de Jonge
Department of Pediatric Infectious Diseases - Immunology, and Rheumatology, VU University Medical Center, Amsterdam, The Netherlands
Department of Neonatology, Erasmus MC - Sophia Children's Hospital, Rotterdam, The Netherlands

Marieke S. Sanders
Department of Pediatric Infectious Diseases - Immunology, and Rheumatology, VU University Medical Center, Amsterdam, The Netherlands
Department of Medical Microbiology, Laboratory for Immunogenetics, VU University Medical Center, Amsterdam, The Netherlands
Department of General Medicine, Antonius Hospital, Nieuwegein, The Netherlands

Caroline B. Terwee and Martijn W. Heymans
Department of Epidemiology and Biostatistics and the EMGO Institute for Health and Care Research, VU University Medical Center, Amsterdam, The Netherlands

Reinoud J. B. J. Gemke
Department of Pediatrics, VU University Medical Center, Amsterdam, The Netherlands

Irene Koomen
Department of Pediatrics, Westfriesgasthuis, Hoorn, The Netherlands

Lodewijk Spanjaard
Department of Medical Microbiology, Netherlands Reference Laboratory for Bacterial Meningitis, Academic Medical Center, Amsterdam, The Netherlands

Hidekane Yoshimura, Yutaka Takumi, Shin-ya Nishio, Nobuyoshi Suzuki, Yoh-ichiro Iwasa and Shinichi Usami
Department of Otorhinolaryngology, Shinshu University School of Medicine, Matsumoto, Nagano, Japan

Robert J. Marano and Sharon L Redmond
Ear Science Institute Australia, Subiaco, Western Australia, Australia
Ear Sciences Centre, School of Surgery, The University of Western Australia, Nedlands, Western Australia, Australia

Jennifer Tickner
School of Pathology and Laboratory Medicine, QEII Medical Centre, The University of Western Australia, Nedlands, Western Australia, Australia

Sho Kanzaki and Kaoru Ogawa
Department of Otorhinolaryngology, Head and Neck Surgery, Keio University, School of Medicine, Shinjuku, Tokyo, Japan

Masafumi Sakagami
Department of Otorhinolaryngology, Hyogo College of Medicine, Nishinomiya, Hyogo, Japan

Hiroshi Hosoi
Department of Otorhinolaryngology, Nara Medical University, Kashihara, Nara, Japan

Shingo Murakami
Department of Otorhinolaryngology, Graduate School of Medical Sciences, Nagoya City University, Mizuho, Nagoya, Aichi, Japan

Helen Henshaw and Melanie A. Ferguson
NIHR Nottingham Hearing Biomedical Research Unit, Nottingham, United Kingdom

Index

www.ingramcontent.com/pod-product-compliance
Lightning Source LLC
LaVergne TN
LVHW060541210926
848485LV00005B/1237